4th edition

biochemistry

The National Medical Series for Independent Study

4th edition
biochemistry

EDITORS

Victor L. Davidson, Ph.D.

Professor
Department of Biochemistry
The University of Mississippi Medical Center
Jackson, Mississippi

Donald B. Sittman, Ph.D.

Professor
Department of Biochemistry
The University of Mississippi Medical Center
Jackson, Mississippi

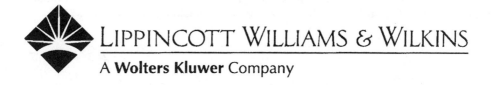

LIPPINCOTT WILLIAMS & WILKINS
A **Wolters Kluwer** Company

Editor: Elizabeth A. Nieginski
Editorial Director, Textbooks: Julie Scardiglia
Development Editors: Donna Siegfreid, Melanie Cann
Managing Editor: Darrin Kiessling
Marketing Manager: Jennifer Conrad

351 West Camden Street
Baltimore, Maryland 21201-2436 USA

227 East Washington Square
Philadelphia, PA 19106

Printed in the United States of America

Fourth Edition, 1999

Library of Congress Cataloging-in-Publication Data

Davidson, Victor L.,
    Biochemistry / Victor L. Davidson, Donald B. Sittman. — 4th ed.
        p.   cm — (The national medical series for independent study)
    Includes bibliographical references.
    ISBN 0–683–30503–4
    1. Biochemistry—Outlines, syllabi, etc.   2. Biochemistry—
Examinations, questions, etc.   I. Sittman, Donald B.   II. Title.
III. Series.
    QP518.3.D38 1999
    572—dc21   98–52792

To purchase additional copies of this book, call our customer service department at **(800) 638-3030** or fax orders to **(301) 824-7390.** International customers should call **(301) 714-2324.**

00 01 02 03
2 3 4 5 6 7 8 9 10

Contents

Section III   Metabolism

Preface

The fourth edition of NMS *Biochemistry* presents concise coverage of the fundamentals of biochemistry in a readily understandable outline format that emphasizes the relative importance of the facts presented. In this revised edition, an effort has been made to update material, infuse greater medical and clinical relevance, and increase the number of descriptive figures and tables with a concomitant reduction in text. Clinical case studies (more than in the third edition) are included in most of the chapters to emphasize the importance of the biochemical facts presented to the diagnosis, understanding, and treatment of medical problems.

This book will serve well as a supplement to either a formal medical biochemistry course or an integrated curriculum in which ready access to biochemical information is required. New and updated study questions should provide a solid base for preparing for the United States Medical Licensing Examination (USMLE) Step 1. We hope that senior medical students and physicians will also find this book to be a ready reference for biochemical information that is relevant to the study and practice of medicine.

Victor L. Davidson
Donald B. Sittman

Acknowledgments

We thank Donna Siegfried for the excellent editing of the manuscript, and Melanie Cann, Darrin Kiessling, and Elizabeth Nieginski for their assistance and guidance in the preparation of this text. We are also grateful to Susan Wellman, Ph.D., Associate Professor in the Department of Pharmacology at the University of Mississippi Medical Center, for helping to write several chapters.

STRUCTURE AND FUNCTION OF THE MAJOR CELL COMPONENTS

Chapter 1

Water, Acid–Base Equilibria, and Blood pH
Victor Davidson

Case 1-1

A patient has a history of emphysema, which has grown progressively worse over a period of years. The patient complains of chronic shortness of breath. Analysis of the patient's blood reveals the following: P_{CO_2} = 60 mm Hg; HCO_3^- = 34 mM; pH = 7.38.

- What is the most likely diagnosis?

- Are these symptoms normal for a patient with this history?

I. WATER

A. **Introduction.** In living cells, most chemical reactions occur in an aqueous environment. Approximately 75% of the mass of a living cell is water. Water is a reactant in many systems, and it is often a factor in determining the properties of macromolecules in cells.

B. **Dipole moment**

1. **Definition.** The water molecule is uncharged but the **distribution of electrons** within it is such that the portion of the molecule near the oxygen atom is slightly negative, and the portion near the hydrogen atoms is slightly positive. Such a molecule is called a **dipole** and has a **dipole moment.**

2. **Dipoles interact with charged ions.** In aqueous solutions, these ions are surrounded by shells of water. Thus, many inorganic ionic compounds dissolve in water and exist as separate ions surrounded by water (e.g., NaCl dissolves in water into Na^+ and Cl^-).

C. **Hydrogen bonds** are electrostatic interactions between hydrogen atoms and the unshared electron pairs of electronegative atoms, such as oxygen or nitrogen.

1. **Formation.** Hydrogen bonds may be formed between water molecules, or between two atoms without the involvement of water (Figure 1-1). Hydrogen bonds may be **intermolecular or intramolecular.**

2. **Bond strength.** Hydrogen bonds are weaker than covalent bonds. It requires **4.5 kcal/mol** of energy **to break a hydrogen bond** between molecules in water compared with **110 kcal/mol to break the covalent O—H bond** within the water molecule.

FIGURE 1-1. Examples of hydrogen bonds.

3. **Functions.** In biologic systems, hydrogen bonds play important roles in **stabilizing the three-dimensional structures of proteins and nucleic acids,** and in **enzyme catalysis.**

4. **Any molecule that is capable of forming hydrogen bonds can do so with water.** Thus, a variety of bio-organic molecules may dissolve in water.

D. **Dissociation of water**

1. Water molecules reversibly dissociate (i.e., ionize) into a hydrogen ion or proton (H^+) and a hydroxyl ion (OH^-).

$$H_2O \rightleftharpoons H^+ + OH^- \tag{1}$$

2. An alternative description of this dissociation is given by

$$2\ H_2O \rightleftharpoons H_3O^+ + OH^-$$

where H_3O^+ is referred to as a **hydronium ion.**

3. Undissociated water is present in great excess, and its concentration is virtually constant at 55.6 M (molar = mol/L).

4. The **ion product of water,** or K_w, is given by

$$K_w = [H^+][OH^-]$$

where the terms in brackets represent concentrations of H^+ and OH^-. At 25°C, $K_w = 1 \times 10^{-14}$ mol^2/L^2. This value is a constant for all aqueous solutions.
   a. If a large number of H^+ ions is added to water, the $[OH^-]$ must decrease so that the product $[H^+][OH^-]$ will remain 10^{-14} at 25°C.
   b. If a large number of OH^- ions is added, the $[H^+]$ must decrease.

II. **ACID–BASE EQUILIBRIUM**

A. **Dissociation of a weak acid**

1. **Strong and weak electrolytes**
   a. Strong electrolytes are fully dissociated in aqueous solution.
   b. Weak electrolytes are only partially dissociated (usually less than 5%) in aqueous solution.

2. **Brönsted-Lowry definitions. Acids** are **proton donors,** and **bases** are **proton acceptors.** An acid–base equilibrium system can be expressed as

$$HA \rightleftharpoons H^+ + A^-$$

TABLE 1-1. Physiologically Relevant Weak Acids and Their Conjugate Bases

Acid	Conjugate Base	pK$_a$
NH$_4^+$ Ammonium ion	NH$_3$ Ammonia	9.25
H$_2$CO$_3$ Carbonic acid	HCO$_3^-$ Bicarbonate ion	6.37
H$_2$PO$_4^-$ Dihydrogen phosphate ion	HPO$_3^{2-}$ Monophosphate hydrogen ion	6.86
CH$_3$CH(OH)COOH Lactic acid	CH$_3$CH(OH)COO$^-$ Lactate ion	3.86

where HA is the undissociated acid, and A$^-$ is its conjugate base (i.e., proton acceptor). If the acid form is ionized, this relation may be expressed as

$$BH^+ \rightleftharpoons H^+ + B$$

where BH$^+$ is the acid, and B is the conjugate base. Examples of physiologically relevant weak acids and their conjugate bases are given in Table 1-1.

3. The **dissociation of a weak acid** is described by

$$K_a = [A^-]\ [H^+]/HA \qquad (2)$$

where K$_a$ is the **dissociation constant** for a weak acid. The true (i.e., thermodynamic) dissociation constant requires the use of ion activities instead of molar concentrations. In biochemical and medical applications it is usual to designate the concentration in terms of moles per liter. In this case, the constant, K$_a$, is an **apparent dissociation constant, K$_a'$**.

B. The pH scale and pK$_a'$

1. **pH** is the negative logarithm of [H$^+$]; that is, pH = $-\log_{10}$[H$^+$].

2. **pK$_a'$** is the negative logarithm of the dissociation constant for a weak acid.

3. Equation (2) can be rearranged to give:

$$-\log H^+ = -\log K_a' - \log [HA]/[A^-] \qquad (3)$$

4. **Henderson-Hasselbalch equation.** Equation (3) becomes the following:

$$pH = pk_a' + \log [A^-]/[HA] \qquad (4)$$

This relation is the most useful formulation in acid–base equilibrium applications.

C. Behavior of weak acids in the presence of their salts

1. **Titration of a weak acid with a strong base**
   a. **Titration curve** (Figure 1-2). When a strong base is added in known increments to a weak acid (HA), and the pH is measured after each addition, a plot of pH against the amount of base added (or the degree of neutralization) can be prepared.
   b. As the strong base is added, several reactions occur.
      (1) Initially, the weak acid dissociates in the aqueous solution.

$$HA \rightleftharpoons H^+ + A^-$$

      (2) When OH$^-$ is added, it is neutralized by the H$^+$ to form H$_2$O.

$$H^+ + OH^- \rightleftharpoons H_2O$$

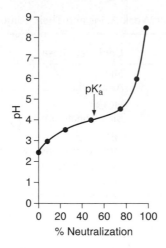

FIGURE 1-2. Titration curve for a weak acid (e.g., lactic acid, pK_a' = 3.86) titrated with increments of a strong base (e.g., sodium hydroxide).

    (3) In response to the removal of H^+, more HA ionizes to reestablish the equilibrium between HA and its ions. Thus, titration of a weak acid with a strong base is the sum of the prior two reactions.

$$HA + OH^- \rightleftharpoons H_2O + A^- \tag{5}$$

2. Determination of pH during the titration of a weak acid with a strong base
    a. Calculation of the initial pH depends solely on [HA] and the pK_a' value for that acid as given by:

$$pH = \frac{pK_a' - \log\ [HA]}{2} \tag{6}$$

    b. Calculation of intermediate values of pH
        (1) The pH at points on a titration curve between 10% and 90% of neutralization are calculated using equation (4). For example, after addition of 0.2 equivalents of strong base to a weak acid with a pK_a' of 3.9, pH can be calculated by using these values and equation (4).

$$pH = 3.9 + \log\ (0.2/0.8) = 3.3$$

        (2) At the midpoint of the titration curve (when the acid has been 50% neutralized), [HA] will equal [A⁻]. Because the ratio of acid to its conjugate base is 1, the log term in equation (4) becomes 0. Thus, at this point, pH = pK_a'.
    c. Final pH
        (1) The pH at the exact end (equivalence) point of the titration is not 7.0. This is because the reaction shown in equation (5) is an equilibrium reaction and is reversible.
        (2) In the absence of any remaining HA, A⁻ will react with H_2O to produce OH⁻ and HA and establish an equilibrium.
        (3) This increase in [OH⁻] explains why the pH of the solution at the end point of the titration is greater than 7.0.

3. Buffering is the resistance to change in pH, on the addition of H^+ or OH⁻.
    a. Near the 50% neutralization point, the pH changes very slowly with each increment of base added. The buffering effect is maximal at the midpoint of the titration when the pH is at the pK_a' of the acid–conjugate base pair.

    b. The extent to which a solution containing a weak acid and its salt can resist a change in pH on the addition of acid or base (i.e., how effective a buffer it is) depends on two factors.

        (1) The closer the buffer pH is to the pK_a' of the weak acid, the greater the **buffer capacity.**

        (2) The higher the buffer concentration is, the greater the buffer capacity.

D. **Other uses of the Henderson-Hasselbalch equation**

    1. The Henderson-Hasselbalch equation (4) may be used in the **preparation of buffer solutions of known pH,** which are prepared by mixing a weak acid with its corresponding salt.

        a. A weak acid is chosen, the pK_a' of which is close to the desired pH.

        b. The ratio of salt (A^-) to acid (HA) needed to give the desired pH is calculated using equation (4).

    2. The Henderson-Hasselbalch equation may be used to **calculate the degree of dissociation of weak acid–conjugate base pairs** at a particular pH. Given the pH of a solution and the pK_a' for the species in question, the degree of dissociation can be calculated. An example of this is given in III A 3.

III. **REGULATION OF BLOOD pH**

A. The relative levels of carbon dioxide (CO_2) and bicarbonate (HCO_3^-) in the blood are very important in maintaining proper blood pH.

    1. CO_2 dissolved in the blood is hydrated to yield H_2CO_3, which is unstable in aqueous solution and nearly completely dissociates to HCO_3^-.

    2. When CO_2 is dissolved in water, there is so little H_2CO_3 present that it can be ignored, and **CO_2 can be considered an acid with HCO_3^- as its conjugate base.**

$$CO_2 + H_2O \rightleftharpoons H^+ + HCO_3^-$$

    3. The pK_a' for this coupled system in blood under physiologic conditions is 6.1. The normal pH of blood is 7.4. Using equation (4), it is possible to calculate the relative levels of CO_2 and HCO_3^- that are necessary to maintain the physiologic pH.

$$pH = pK_a' + \log \frac{[base]}{[acid]}$$

$$7.4 = 6.1 + \log \frac{[HCO_3^-]}{[CO_2]}$$

$$1.3 = \log \frac{[HCO_3^-]}{[CO_2]}$$

$$antilog\ 1.3 = \frac{[HCO_3^-]}{[CO_2]} = 20$$

    4. **CO_2 levels are routinely expressed in terms of P_{CO_2},** where P stands for the partial pressure of the gas dissolved in the blood plasma. Under physiologic conditions, $[CO_2]$ and P_{CO_2} are related by the solubility constant for CO_2 in plasma at 38°C, which is 0.03 mM/mm Hg. **Normal values in blood are pH = 7.4, P_{CO_2} = 40 mm Hg,** and **$[HCO_3^-]$ = 24 mM.**

        a. CO_2 levels are regulated by the **lungs.**

        b. HCO_3^- levels are regulated by the **kidneys.**

TABLE 1-2. Acid–Base Abnormalities

Primary disorder	Effect on:			Compensation	Effect on:	
	Pco$_2$	HCO$_3^-$	pH		Pco$_2$	HCO$_3^-$
Respiratory acidosis	↑	—	↓	Metabolic alkalosis	—	↑
Respiratory alkalosis	↓	—	↑	Metabolic acidosis	—	↓
Metabolic acidosis	—	↓	↓	Respiratory alkalosis	↓	—
Metabolic alkalosis	—	↑	↑	Respiratory acidosis	↑	—

Note: ↑ = increased; ↓ = decreased.

B. **Clinical abnormalities of blood pH**

1. The pH of the blood may vary because of respiratory or metabolic disorders. If the pH falls below 7.4, the condition is called **acidosis.** If the pH of the blood rises above 7.4, the condition is called **alkalosis.**

2. A pH imbalance caused by a change in CO_2 levels is called **respiratory acidosis** or **respiratory alkalosis,** depending on whether the CO_2 levels increase or decrease.

3. A pH imbalance caused by a change in [HCO$_3^-$] is called **metabolic acidosis** or **metabolic alkalosis,** depending on whether [HCO$_3^-$] decreases or increases.

4. The body attempts to compensate for a pH imbalance by adjusting the activities of the lungs or kidneys. Respiratory acidosis or alkalosis may be counterbalanced by metabolic alkalosis or acidosis, and vice versa (Table 1-2).

Case 1-1 Revisited

Because of the patient's chronic lung disease (i.e., emphysema), the rate of respiration is depressed, and CO_2 is not being eliminated from the blood by the lungs as efficiently as it should. This causes the respiratory acidosis—elevated Pco$_2$. To compensate, his kidneys have increased secretion of H$^+$ and increased reabsorption of HCO$_3^-$. This has resulted in a compensatory metabolic alkalosis—high levels of serum HCO$_3^-$.

The patient's blood pH is slightly below normal, indicating that the body has not fully compensated for the respiratory acidosis. However, because this is a chronic condition, it can be assumed that the kidneys have had time to compensate as well as possible for this condition. Such values are common in individuals who suffer from chronic respiratory disorders.

STUDY QUESTIONS

DIRECTIONS: Each of the numbered items or incomplete statements in this section is followed by answers or by completions of the statement. Select the **one** lettered answer or completion that is **best** in each case.

1. A buffer solution contains a mixture of concentrations of 0.01 M of a weak acid and 0.001 M of its potassium salt. The pH of this solution is approximately

(A) pK_a'
(B) $pK_a' - 1$
(C) $pK_a' - 2$
(D) $pK_a' + 1$
(E) $pK_a' + 2$

2. A 0.1 M solution of lactic acid has a pH of 2.4. How much sodium hydroxide is required to titrate 100 ml of the solution to the end point?

(A) 100 Eq
(B) 100 mEq
(C) 100 ml of 0.1 M
(D) 2.4 mEq
(E) 0.1 mmol

3. If 0.1 M solutions of sodium dihydrogen phosphate (NaH_2PO_4) and disodium hydrogen phosphate (Na_2HPO_4) are mixed in equal proportions, what is the pH of the mixture? (The pK_a' values of orthophosphoric acid (H_3PO_4) are 2.0, 6.8, and 12.0.)

(A) 2.0
(B) 4.4
(C) 6.8
(D) 9.4
(E) 12.0

4. The pK_a' of acetic acid is 4.76. What is the pH of a 0.1 M solution of acetic acid?

(A) 5.76
(B) 2.88
(C) 2.43
(D) 1.88
(E) 4.76

Questions 5-6

A medical student becomes extremely anxious the night before a biochemistry examination and begins to hyperventilate uncontrollably.

5. What initial effects does hyperventilation have on the student's P_{CO_2} and blood pH?

(A) No effect
(B) P_{CO_2} increases and pH increases
(C) P_{CO_2} decreases and pH increases
(D) P_{CO_2} increases and pH decreases
(E) P_{CO_2} decreases and pH decreases

6. If the examination is postponed for 3 days and the student continues to hyperventilate, how may the body respond to this condition?

(A) The kidneys decrease secretion of H^+ and reabsorption of HCO_3^-
(B) Compensatory metabolic alkalosis occurs
(C) $[HCO_3^-]$ increases in the blood
(D) The kidneys increase secretion of H^+ and reabsorption of HCO_3^-
(E) Compensatory respiratory acidosis occurs

Questions 7-10

A man suffering from untreated diabetes mellitus is admitted to the hospital. Glucose and acetoacetate are present in his urine, and he exhibits shallow breathing. Analysis of his blood indicates $[HCO_3^-] = 16$ mM and $P_{CO_2} = 30$.

7. The most likely pH of his blood is

(A) 4.85
(B) 7.15
(C) 7.40
(D) 7.35
(E) 7.90

8. Which of the following actions best characterizes this man's condition?

(A) Respiratory acidosis that is partially compensated by metabolic alkalosis
(B) Respiratory alkalosis that is partially compensated by metabolic acidosis
(C) Metabolic alkalosis that is partially compensated by respiratory acidosis
(D) Metabolic acidosis that is partially compensated by respiratory alkalosis
(E) Uncompensated metabolic alkalosis

9. After insulin treatment, blood pH returns to normal and $[HCO_3^-]$ increases to 21 mM. The $[CO_2]$ in the blood plasma is

(A) 35.0 mM
(B) 12.5 mM
(C) 0.95 mM
(D) 0.03 mM
(E) 1.05 mM

10. A sample of this man's urine contains 30 mmol of total acetoacetic acid–acetoacetate ($pK_a' = 4.8$). The pH of the urine is 4.8. Assuming that Na^+ is excreted as a counter-ion with equivalent amounts of the conjugate base, how much Na^+ is excreted with this keto acid?

(A) 5 mmol
(B) 10 mmol
(C) 15 mmol
(D) 20 mmol
(E) 25 mmol

ANSWERS AND EXPLANATIONS

1. The answer is B [II B, D 2]. The pH of a buffer solution of a weak acid and its salt depends on the ratio of dissociated conjugate to undissociated weak acid. The relation between this ratio, the pK_a' of the weak acid, and the pH of the solution is given by the Henderson-Hasselbalch equation. If the ratio is 0.1, the pH is approximately equal to the pK_a - 1, which is determined by substituting the log of 0.1 into the following equation: $pH = pK_a' + \log [A^-]/[HA]$.

2. The answer is C [II C 1]. The complete neutralization of the dissociable hydrogen of a lactic acid solution with sodium hydroxide requires an amount of hydroxyl ions equivalent to the hydrogen ions potentially available from the lactic acid. Lactic acid is a weak acid with one dissociable proton, and 100 ml of a 0.1 M solution contains 10 mEq of potential hydrogen ions. Therefore, 10 mEq of sodium hydroxide are required, which is the amount contained in 100 ml of 0.1 M sodium hydroxide.

3. The answer is C [II C 2, D 1]. Orthophosphoric acid (H_3PO_4) has three dissociable protons with pK_a' values of 2.0, 6.8, and 12.0. The dissociation relevant to this question of $H_2PO_4^-$ to the HPO_4^{2-} species has a pK_a' of 6.8. When sodium dihydrogen phosphate (NaH_2PO_4) and disodium hydrogen phosphate (Na_2HPO_4) are mixed in equal proportions, $H_2PO_4^{2-}$ and HPO_4^{2-} are present in equal concentrations. The pH is, therefore, at the pK_a' value of 6.8.

4. The answer is B [II C 2 a]. Because only the weak acid and no added base is present, the initial pH will depend solely on the concentration of acetic acid and its pK_a' value. The answer is obtained by substituting these values into the following equation: $pH = (4.76 - \log[0.1])/2 = 2.88$.

5-6. The answers are: 5-C, 6-A [III]. The increased rate of respiration causes the lungs to remove more CO_2 from the blood than normal, which decreases P_{CO_2}. In the initial stages of hyperventilation, the kidneys have not yet had enough time to compensate by adjusting HCO_3^- levels. The decrease in CO_2 (an acid in plasma) relative to HCO_3^- (its conjugate base) causes an increase in pH. This is an example of respiratory alkalosis. With time, the kidneys decrease HCO_3^- levels, decreasing secretion of H^+ and reabsorption of HCO_3^-. This is a compensatory metabolic acidosis that should decrease the blood pH to normal or near-normal levels.

7-10. The answers are: 7-D, 8-D, 9-E, 10-C [II B; III]. The pH of the blood is calculated using the following equation—$pH = pK_a' + \log [A^-]/[HA]$—with P_{CO_2} converted to $[CO_2]$, CO_2 considered an acid, and HCO_3^- its conjugate base. Therefore, $pH = 6.1 + \log 16/(30 \times 0.03) = 7.35$.

The primary cause of this condition is metabolic acidosis, which results from the ketoacidosis caused by the diabetes. The lungs respond by increasing the rate of respiration to lower CO_2 levels to compensate for the decrease in pH. This is a compensatory respiratory alkalosis. The pH did not return to normal because the lungs were able to only partially compensate. Without compensation, the pH would be significantly lower.

After treatment, HCO_3^- levels begin to increase toward normal. The $[CO_2]$ can also be determined by $pH = pK_a' + \log [A^-]/[HA]$; that is, $7.4 = 6.1 + \log (24/[CO_2])$.

The pH of the urine is the same as the pK_a' of the acetoacetic acid conjugate acid–base pair. At this pH, 50% of the acetoacetic acid is present as acetoacetate ion, which carries a single negative charge. Sodium will be excreted as the positively charged counter-ion in equivalent amount; that is, 50% of 30 mmol, or 15 mmol.

Chapter 2

Amino Acid and Protein Structure
Donald Sittman

Case 2-1

A black 2-year-old boy is brought to the emergency room having very painful swelling of his hands and feet. A detailed family history reveals that both parents have relatives with sickle cell disease. This disease is caused by a change of one amino acid (glutamine is replaced by valine) in the sixth position of the β chain of hemoglobin [see Chapter 3 II B 4 b (1)].

■ What clinical tests can be run to definitively diagnose this child as having sickle cell disease?

I. NATURE OF PROTEINS

A. **Structure**

1. Proteins are linear, unbranched polymers constructed from 20 different α-amino acids that are encoded in the DNA of the genome.

2. All living organisms use the same 20 amino acids and, with few exceptions, the same genetic code (see Chapter 10 I B).

B. **Size.** Proteins are diverse in size. The mass of single-chain proteins is typically 10–50 kilodaltons (kdal), although proteins as small as 350 dal and greater than 1000 kdal are known to exist. Multichain protein complexes of greater than 200 kdal are frequently encountered.

C. **Function.** Proteins serve a wide range of functions in living organisms. A few of their functions include:

1. **Enzymatic catalysis**—Most enzymes are proteins.

2. **Transport and storage** of small molecules and ions

3. **Structural elements of the cytoskeleton.** Proteins make up the cytoskeleton, which:
   a. Provides **strength and structure** to cells
   b. Forms the **fundamental mechanistic components** for **intracellular and extracellular movement**

4. **Structure of skin and bone.** Proteins such as **collagen** (see Chapter 3 V), the most abundant protein in the body, give these structures high tensile strength.

5. **Immunity.** The **immune defense system** is composed of proteins such as **antibodies,** which mediate a protective response to pathogens.

6. **Hormonal regulation.** Hormones coordinate the metabolic actions within the body (see Chapter 15).
   a. Some **hormones** are proteins [e.g., somatotropin (pituitary growth hormone) and insulin].
   b. The **cellular receptors** that recognize hormones and neurotransmitters are proteins.

7. **Control of genetic expression.** Activators, repressors, and many other regulators of gene expression in prokaryotes and eukaryotes are proteins (see Chapter 12).

D. **Unique conformation**

1. **Specificity.** Proteins show an exquisite specificity of biologic function—a consequence of the uniqueness of the three-dimensional structural shape, or **conformation,** of each protein.

2. In humans, **disease states** are often related to the altered function of a protein, which is often attributed to an anomaly in the protein's structure. Examples of diseases caused by abnormal protein structure and function include:
   a. **Hemoglobinopathies,** in particular **sickle cell anemia** (see Chapter 3 II B 4 b)
   b. **Marfan syndrome,** which appears to be caused by single amino acid changes in an elastic connective tissue protein called **fibrillin**
   c. **Cystic fibrosis,** the major form of which arises because of a single amino acid deletion in the adenosine triphosphate (ATP)-binding domain of a transmembrane conductance regulatory protein

II. **AMINO ACIDS** are the fundamental units of proteins.

A. **Composition**

1. Amino acids are composed of an **amino group** ($-NH_2$), a **carboxyl group** ($-COOH$), a hydrogen atom, and a distinctive **side chain,** all bonded to a carbon atom (the **α-carbon**). Table 2-1 lists the 20 fundamental amino acids according to their side chains.

2. One of the 20 amino acids, **proline,** is an **imino acid** ($-NH-$), not an **α-amino acid** as are the other 19.

3. **Post-translational modification.** Other amino acids are found in a number of proteins but are not coded for in DNA (see Chapter 10); they are derived from some of the 20 fundamental amino acids after these have been incorporated into the protein chain (i.e., post-translational modification). More than 100 different kinds of amino acids that arise from post-translational modifications have been identified. Examples of a few of the major post-translational modifications of amino acids are:
   a. Addition of **hydroxyl** ($-OH$) groups to some prolines and lysines in collagen and gelatin
   b. Addition of **methyl** ($-CH_3$) groups to some lysines and histidines in muscle myosin
   c. Addition of **carboxyl** ($-COOH$) groups to glutamates in blood clotting and bone proteins
   d. Addition of **phosphate** ($-PO_3$) groups to some serine, threonine, and tyrosine molecules. **Reversible phosphorylation** is a common method of regulating the activity of many enzymes, cell-surface receptors, and other regulatory molecules.

4. There are many **nonprotein amino acids** found throughout nature. In some cases, these amino acids serve as antibiotics or toxins.

B. **Optical activity**

1. With the exception of glycine, all amino acids contain at least one **asymmetric carbon** atom and are, therefore, optically active.

2. **Enantiomers.** Amino acids exist as stereoisomeric pairs called enantiomers. These amino acid isomers are typically called L (levorotatory) or D (dextrorotatory) depending on the direction they rotate plane-polarized light.
   a. L-**Amino acids** are the only optically active amino acids that are incorporated into proteins.

TABLE 2-1. The 20 Amino Acids Used for Building Protein Chains

Name	Symbol	Structural Formula
Aliphatic nonpolar side chains		
Glycine	Gly (G)	$H-CH-COO^-$ \ NH_3^+
Alanine	Ala (A)	$H_3C-CH-COO^-$ \ NH_3^+
Valine	Val (V)	$\begin{matrix} H_3C \\ H_3C \end{matrix}CH-CH-COO^-$ \ NH_3^+
Leucine	Leu (L)	$\begin{matrix} H_3C \\ H_3C \end{matrix}CH-CH_2-CH-COO^-$ \ NH_3^+
Isoleucine	Ile (I)	$\begin{matrix} CH_3 \\ CH_2 \\ CH \\ CH_3 \end{matrix}-CH-COO^-$ \ NH_3^+
Aromatic side chains		
Phenylalanine	Phe (F)	$\bigcirc-CH_2-CH-COO^-$ \ NH_3^+
Tyrosine	Tyr (Y)	$HO-\bigcirc-CH_2-CH-COO^-$ \ NH_3^+
Tryptophan	Trp (W)	indole$-C-CH_2-CH-COO^-$ \ NH_3^+
Hydroxyl-containing side chains		
Serine	Ser (S)	$HO-CH_2-CH-COO^-$ \ NH_3^+
Threonine	Thr (T)	$CH_3-CH-CH-COO^-$ \ $OH \quad NH_3^+$
Acidic side chains		
Aspartate	Asp (D)	$^-OOC-CH_2-CH-COO^-$ \ NH_3^+

TABLE 2-1. Continued

Name	Symbol	Structural Formula
Glutamate	Glu (E)	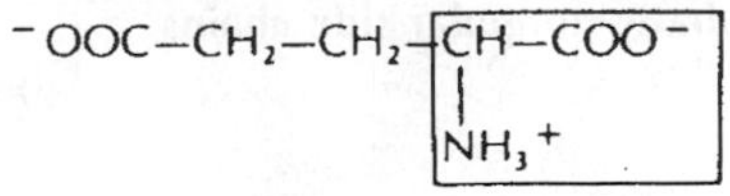 $^-OOC-CH_2-CH_2-\boxed{CH-COO^-}$ with NH_3^+

Amidic amino acids

Asparagine	Asn (N)	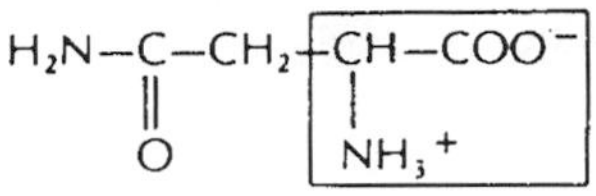 $H_2N-\underset{O}{\overset{\parallel}{C}}-CH_2-\boxed{CH-COO^-}$ with NH_3^+
Glutamine	Gln (Q)	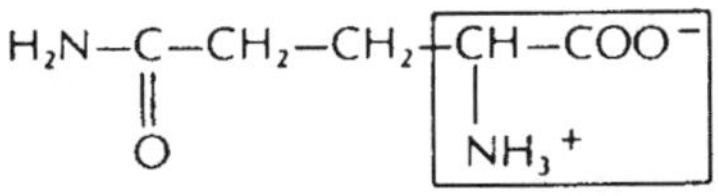 $H_2N-\underset{O}{\overset{\parallel}{C}}-CH_2-CH_2-\boxed{CH-COO^-}$ with NH_3^+

Basic side chains

Lysine	Lys (K)	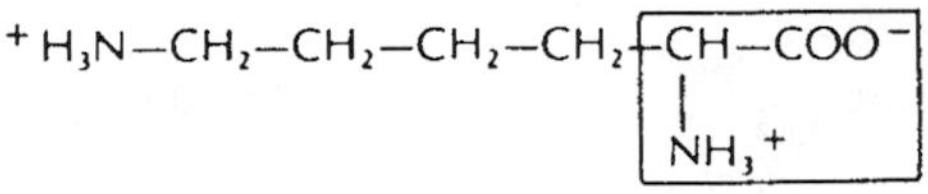 $^+H_3N-CH_2-CH_2-CH_2-CH_2-\boxed{CH-COO^-}$ with NH_3^+
Arginine	Arg (R)	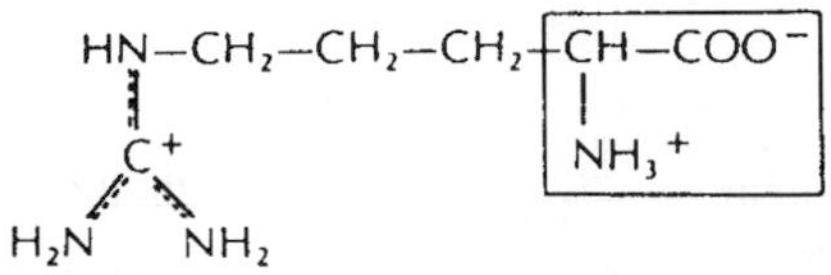 $HN-CH_2-CH_2-CH_2-\boxed{CH-COO^-}$ with NH_3^+; $\underset{H_2N \quad NH_2}{C^+}$
Histidine	His (H)	$\boxed{\underset{CH_2}{\overset{NH_3^+}{|}}-\overset{}{CH-COO^-}}$ ... $C=CH$ ... $^+HN \quad NH$ ... $\underset{H}{C}$

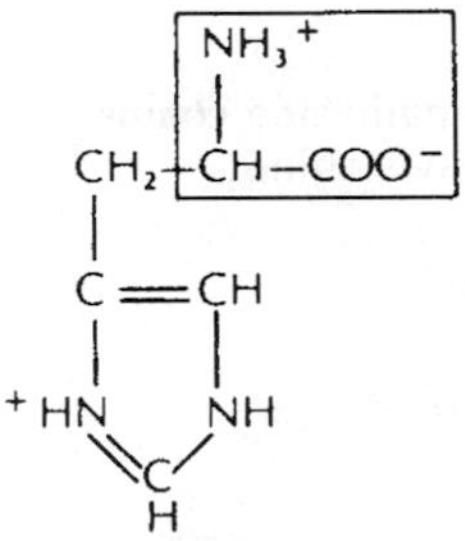

Sulfur-containing side chains

Cysteine	Cys (C)	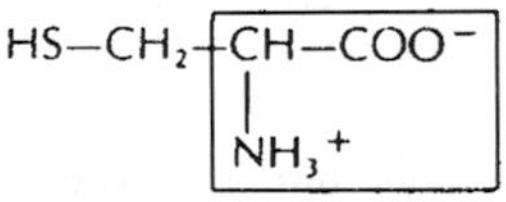 $HS-CH_2-\boxed{CH-COO^-}$ with NH_3^+
Methionine	Met (M)	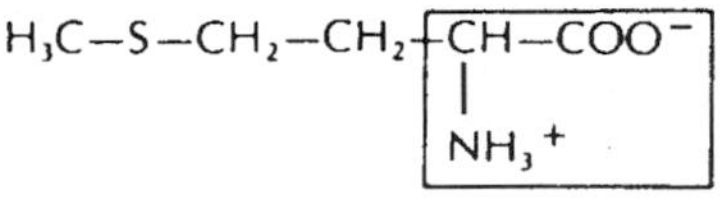 $H_3C-S-CH_2-CH_2-\boxed{CH-COO^-}$ with NH_3^+

Imino acid

Proline	Pro (P)	$\boxed{\overset{COO^-}{\underset{^+H_2N-CH}{|}}}$ ... $H_2C \quad CH_2$ ... CH_2

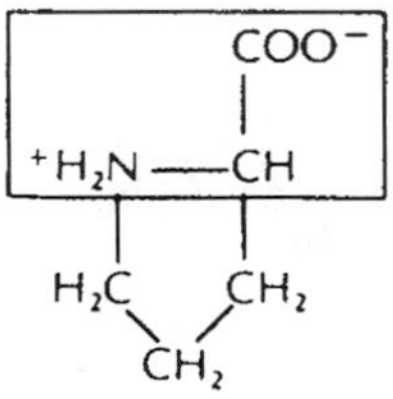

    b. D-Amino acids are found in bacterial products (e.g., in cell walls) and in many peptide antibiotics, but they are not incorporated into proteins via the ribosomal protein synthesizing system.

C. Amphoteric properties

1. Amino acids are **amphoteric molecules;** that is, they have both basic and acidic groups.

2. Monoamino–monocarboxylic acids exist in aqueous solution as **dipolar molecules (zwitterions),** which means that they have both positive and negative charges.
    a. The **α-carboxyl group** is dissociated and negatively charged.
    b. The **α-amino group** is protonated and positively charged.
    c. Thus, the overall molecule is **electrically neutral.**

3. At **low pH** (i.e., high concentrations of hydrogen ion), the carboxyl group accepts a proton and becomes uncharged, so that the overall charge on the molecule is positive.

4. At **high pH** (i.e., low concentrations of hydrogen ion), the amino group loses its proton and becomes uncharged; thus, the overall charge on the molecule is negative.

Low pH   High pH

$$H_3N^+ - CH - COOH \rightleftharpoons H_3N^+ - CH - COO^- \rightleftharpoons H_2N - CH - COO^-$$

$$\qquad\qquad | \qquad\qquad\qquad\qquad\qquad | \qquad\qquad\qquad\qquad | $$
$$\qquad\qquad R \qquad\qquad\qquad\qquad\qquad R \qquad\qquad\qquad\qquad R$$

Overall charge 1+   0   1–

5. Some amino acids have **side chains** that contain **dissociating groups.**
    a. Side chains
        (1) Those of aspartate and glutamate are acidic; those of histidine, lysine, and arginine are basic.
        (2) Two others, cysteine and tyrosine, have a negative charge on the side chain when dissociated.
    b. Dissociating groups
        (1) Whether these groups are dissociated depends on the prevailing pH and the apparent dissociation constant (pK_a') of the dissociating groups.
        (2) These dissociating amino acids also exist in solution as zwitterions. For example, glutamate has three dissociable protons with pK_a' values of 2.19, 4.25, and 9.67. As the pH increases above each of these pK_a' values, protons dissociate and the charge changes as shown:

$$H_3N^+ - CH - COOH \quad\quad H_3N^+ - CH - COO^- \quad\quad H_3N^+ - CH - COO^- \quad\quad H_2N+ - CH - COO^-$$

$$\qquad | \qquad\qquad\qquad\qquad\qquad\qquad | \qquad\qquad\qquad\qquad\qquad\qquad | \qquad\qquad\qquad\qquad\qquad\qquad | $$
$$CH_2 \quad\quad pK_{a_1}' = 2.19 \quad\quad CH_2 \quad\quad pK_{a_2}' = 4.25 \quad\quad CH_2 \quad\quad pK_{a_3}' = 9.67 \quad\quad CH_2$$
$$\qquad | \qquad\qquad\quad\rightleftharpoons\qquad\qquad\quad | \qquad\qquad\quad\rightleftharpoons\qquad\qquad\quad | \qquad\qquad\quad\rightleftharpoons\qquad\qquad\quad |$$
$$CH_2 \qquad\qquad\qquad\qquad\quad CH_2 \qquad\qquad\qquad\qquad\quad CH_2 \qquad\qquad\qquad\qquad\quad CH_2$$
$$\qquad | \qquad\qquad\qquad\qquad\qquad\qquad | \qquad\qquad\qquad\qquad\qquad\qquad | \qquad\qquad\qquad\qquad\qquad\qquad | $$
$$COOH \qquad\qquad\qquad\qquad\quad COOH \qquad\qquad\qquad\qquad\quad COO^- \qquad\qquad\qquad\qquad\quad COO^-$$

Overall charge 1+   0   1–   2–

III. PEPTIDES AND POLYPEPTIDES

A. Formation. The linking together of amino acids produces **peptide** chains, also called **polypeptides** if many amino acids are linked.

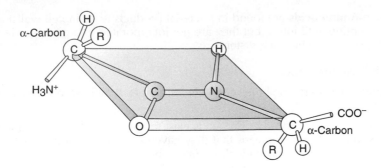

FIGURE 2-1. The planar nature of the peptide bond. H = hydrogen; R = side group; C = carbon; N = nitrogen; O = oxygen.

1. The **peptide bond** is the bond formed between the α-carboxyl group of one amino acid and the α-amino group of another. In the process, water is removed.

$$H_3N^+ \!\!-\!\! CH \!\!-\!\! COO^- + H_3N^+ \!\!-\!\! CH \!\!-\!\! COO^- \rightarrow H_3N^+ \!\!-\!\! CH \overset{\text{Peptide bond}}{\fbox{$-CO-NH-$}} CH \!\!-\!\! COO^- + H_2O$$

$$\qquad\qquad R_1 \qquad\qquad\qquad R_2 \qquad\qquad\qquad\quad R_1 \qquad\qquad\qquad R_2$$

2. Peptide bond formation is highly **endergonic** (i.e., energy-requiring) and requires the concomitant hydrolysis of high-energy phosphate bonds.

3. The peptide bond is a **planar** structure with the two adjacent α-carbons, a carbonyl oxygen, an α-amino nitrogen and its associated hydrogen atom, and the carbonyl carbon all lying in the same plane (Figure 2-1). The —CN— bond has a partial double-bond character that prevents rotation around the bond axis.

4. Amino acids, when in polypeptide chains, are customarily referred to as **residues.**

B. **Amphoteric properties**

1. The **formation of the peptide bond** removes two dissociating groups, one from the α-amino and one from the α-carboxyl, per residue.

2. Although the N-terminal and C-terminal α-amino and α-carboxyl groups can play important roles in the formation of protein structures, and thus in protein function, the amphoteric properties of a polypeptide are mainly governed by the **dissociable groups** on the amino acid **side chains.**

3. **Laboratory use.** These properties of proteins are not only important in terms of protein structure and function but are also useful in a number of analytic procedures, such as ion exchange or high-performance liquid chromatography (see V B 3), for the purification and identification of proteins.

IV. **CONFORMATION OF PROTEINS.** Every protein in its **native state** has a unique **three-dimensional structure,** which is referred to as its **conformation.** The function of a protein arises from its conformation. Protein structures can be classified into four levels of organization: primary, secondary, tertiary, and quaternary.

A. The **primary structure** is the covalent "backbone" of the polypeptide formed by the **specific amino acid sequence.**

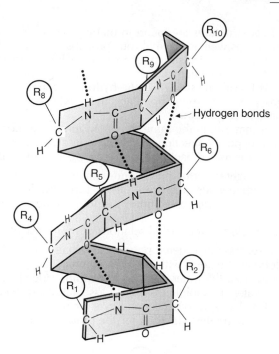

FIGURE 2-2. The right-handed α-helix shows planar peptide bonds and hydrogen bonds between every fourth bond. The numbered circles represent the varied side chains (R) of the different amino acids.

1. This sequence is coded for by DNA and determines the final three-dimensional form adopted by the protein in its native state.

2. By convention, peptide sequences are written from left to right, starting with the amino acid residue that has a free α-amino group (the so-called **N-terminal amino acid**) and ending with the residue that has a free α-carboxyl group (the **C-terminal amino acid**). Either the three-letter abbreviations (e.g., Ala-Glu-Lys) or, for long peptides, the single-letter abbreviations given in Table 2-1 are used.

B. The **secondary structure** is the spatial relation of neighboring amino acid residues.

1. **Secondary structure is dictated by the primary structure.** The secondary structure arises from interactions of neighboring amino acids. Because the DNA-coded primary sequence dictates which amino acids are near each other, secondary structure often forms as the peptide chain comes off the ribosome (see Chapter 10 V B; VI).

2. **Hydrogen bonds.** An important characteristic of secondary structure is the formation of hydrogen bonds (H bonds) between the —CO group of one peptide bond and the —NH group of another nearby peptide bond.
   a. If the H bonds form between peptide bonds in the same chain, either **helical** structures, such as the **α-helix,** develop or turns, such as **β-turns,** are formed.
   b. If H bonds form between peptide bonds in different chains, **extended** structures form, such as the **β-pleated sheet.**

3. **The α-helix** is a rod-like structure with the peptide bonds coiled tightly inside and the side chains of the residues protruding outward (Figure 2-2).
   a. Each —CO is hydrogen bonded to the —NH of a peptide bond that is **four residues away** from it along the **same chain.**
   b. There are 3.6 amino acid residues per turn of the helix, and the helix is **right-handed** (i.e., the coils turn in a clockwise fashion around the axis).

4. β-Pleated sheet structures are found in many proteins, including some globular, soluble proteins, as well as some fibrous proteins (e.g., silk fibroin).
    a. They are more extended structures than the α-helix and are "pleated" because the C—C bonds are tetrahedral and cannot exist in straight lines (Figure 2-3).
    b. The chains lie side by side, with the **hydrogen bonds** forming between the —CO group of one peptide bond and the —NH group of another peptide bond in the **neighboring chain.**
    c. The chains may run in the same direction, forming a **parallel β-sheet,** or they may run in opposite directions, as they do in a globular protein in which an extended chain is folded back on itself, forming an **antiparallel β-structure.**

5. A **β-turn** is the tightest turn a polypeptide chain can make, although there are many ways a polypeptide chain can turn. β-Turns result in a complete reversal in the direction of a polypeptide chain in just four amino acid residues.

C. **Tertiary structure** refers to the spatial relations of more distant residues.

    1. Folding. The secondarily ordered polypeptide chains of soluble proteins tend to fold into globular structures with the hydrophobic side chains[1] in the interior of the structure away from the water and the hydrophilic side chains on the outside in contact with water. This folding is due to associations between segments of α-helix, extended β-chains, or other secondary structures and represents a state of lowest energy (i.e., of **greatest stability**) for the protein in question.

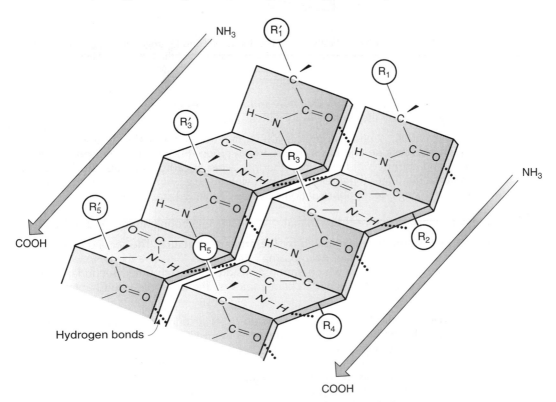

FIGURE 2-3. Parallel β-pleated sheet. Planar peptide bonds are shown with hydrogen bonds between parallel adjacent peptide chains. The numbered circles represent the varied side chains (R and R') of the different amino acids on each peptide chain. The adjacent arrows indicate the directionality of the peptide chains from their amino to carboxyl ends.

---

[1] Amino acids with long, nonpolar side chains (e.g., valine, leucine, isoleucine, phenylalanine, tryptophan, and methionine) are hydrophobic in nature.

2. The conformation results from:
  a. Hydrogen-bonding within a chain or between chains
  b. The **flexibility** of the chain at **points of instability,** allowing water to obtain maximum entropy and thus govern the structure to some extent
  c. The formation of **other noncovalent bonds** between side-chain groups, such as salt linkages, or π-electron interactions of aromatic rings
  d. The sites and numbers of **disulfide bridges** between Cys residues within the chain (Cys residues linked by disulfide bonds are termed **cystine** residues)

3. A peptide chain free in solution will not achieve its biologically active tertiary structure as rapidly or properly as within the cell. Within the cell, some of the proteins that facilitate proper folding are:
  a. Protein disulfide isomerase. This protein catalyzes the formation of proper disulfide bond formation between cysteine residues.
  b. Chaperones. This family of proteins catalyzes the proper folding of proteins in part by inhibiting improper folding and interactions with other peptides.

D. **Quarternary structure** refers to the spatial relations between individual polypeptide chains in a multichain protein; that is, the characteristic noncovalent interactions between the chains that form the native conformation of the protein as well as occasional disulfide bonds between the chains.

1. Many proteins larger than 50 kdal have more than one chain and are said to contain **multiple subunits,** with individual chains known as **protomers.**

2. Many multisubunit proteins are composed of different kinds of **functional subunits** [e.g., the regulatory and catalytic subunits of regulatory proteins (see Chapter 4)].

V. PURIFICATION OF PROTEINS

A. **General considerations.** A protein in biologic fluids may require some degree of purification before it can be specifically measured, studied, or used.

1. Separation of a protein from other proteins and molecules is achieved by applying a combination of several methods based on properties such as solubility, molecular size, molecular charge, and specific binding of the protein to a specific substance.

2. Diagnostic and therapeutic purposes. Clinical laboratories routinely separate proteins for diagnostic purposes. Plasma proteins, for example, are routinely examined by gel electrophoresis. Similar techniques are used to purify proteins for therapeutic purposes.

B. **Separation procedures**

1. Protein solubility is influenced by the **salt concentration** of the solution.
  a. Salting out. Adding salts, such as ammonium sulfate, to a solution of a protein mixture precipitates some proteins at a given salt concentration but not others. This type of separation is performed to increase the amount of a given protein in a fraction of a highly complex mixture, such as a tissue homogenate or a sample of blood plasma.
  b. Salting in. Some proteins require inorganic ions for water solubility. Extensive **dialysis** (see V B 2 a) against a solution with a low salt concentration may, therefore, cause certain proteins from a mixture to precipitate out of solution.

2. Separation on the basis of molecular size
  a. Dialysis. A mixture of proteins and small solutes can be separated by dialysis through a **semipermeable membrane.** The point at which molecules are excluded or prevented from passing through the membrane depends on the **pore size** of the dialysis membrane.

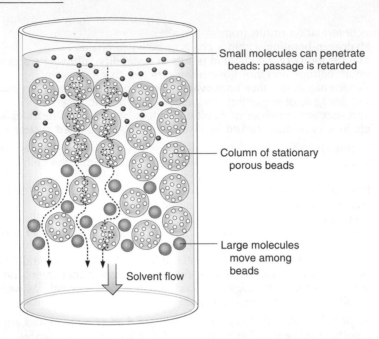

Small molecules can penetrate beads: passage is retarded

Column of stationary porous beads

Large molecules move among beads

Solvent flow

FIGURE 2-4. Gel filtration chromatography. Columns of porous insoluble gel beads can separate molecules according to size. When a mixture of large and small molecules flows through the column, the large molecules do not enter the pores in the beads but the small molecules do. The large molecules, therefore, flow through faster than do the small molecules, which take a longer, more tortuous path through the beads. Intermediate-size molecules flow through the gel at an intermediate rate.

    b. Gel filtration (molecular exclusion chromatography, molecular sieving) uses a column of insoluble carbohydrate polymer in the form of porous beads (Figure 2-4). Small molecules can enter the pores, but large molecules cannot. Therefore, the volume of the solvent available for the small molecules is greater than that for the large molecules, so the small molecules flow through the column more slowly. Accordingly, the rate at which a molecule flows through the column depends on its size and shape. Gel filtration is used to estimate the molecular weight of a protein as well as to separate proteins.

    c. Ultracentrifugation. High-speed centrifugation can separate a protein solution into multiple components.

      (1) The rate at which a protein sediments in a centrifugal field depends on its size and shape. For proteins of similar shape, the larger the molecular weight, the faster it sediments.

      (2) The data from an ultracentrifugation study are often expressed in terms of **Svedburg units (S),** which are related to the rate of sedimentation of the protein in the centrifugal field.

    d. Sodium dodecyl sulfate (SDS) polyacrylamide gel electrophoresis, done on a cross-linked polyacrylamide gel in the presence of SDS and a reducing agent, such as β-mercaptoethanol, separates proteins on the basis of their molecular weight (Figure 2-5).

      (1) SDS, a 12-carbon–chain anionic detergent, denatures the protein, while the reducing agent breaks the disulfide bonds (see IV C 2 d), thereby minimizing the effects of the protein's shape on the molecular weight determination. The SDS dissociates quaternary structures (see IV D) into protomers.

      (2) Because the SDS forms negatively charged micelles with the protein, the effect of the protein charge is lost, and the **shape** of all molecules becomes **rod-like.**

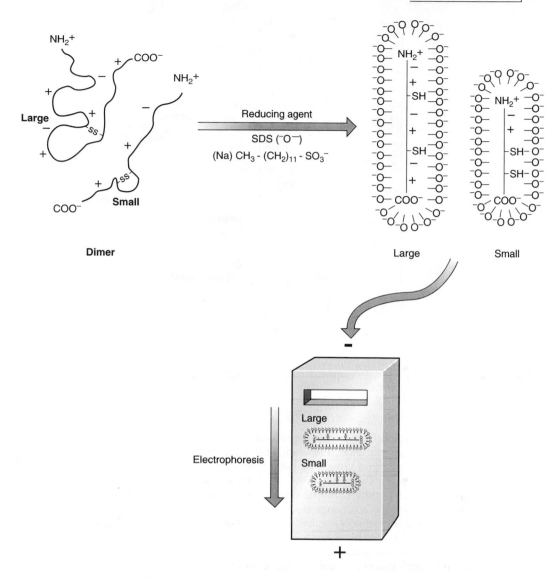

FIGURE 2-5. Proteins can be separated on the basis of their size by sodium dodecyl sulfate (SDS) polyacrylamide gel electrophoresis. Proteins are heated with SDS and a reducing agent, which breaks the disulfide bonds. The SDS forms negatively charged micelles around the protein. When these proteins are run through a cross-linked polyacrylamide gel in an electric field, all micelle-protein molecules move toward the positive pole. The small molecules migrate through the gel faster than the large molecules.

    (3) The SDS–protein micelles are separated according to size by gel electrophoresis (see V B 3 c). The SDS–protein micelles migrate to the positive pole with the cross-linked polyacrylamide acting as a molecular sieve. Smaller molecules migrate through the gel faster than larger molecules.

3. Separation on the basis of molecular charge
    a. Ion-exchange chromatography (Figure 2-6)
        (1) Proteins are bound to the ion-exchange resin in the column. The tightness of binding of particular proteins depends on how many residues are available to interact with the ion-exchange resin.

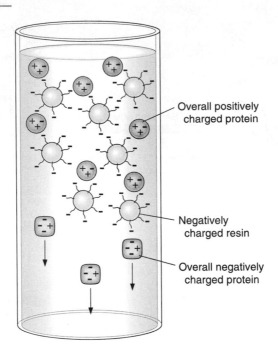

Overall positively
charged protein

Negatively
charged resin

Overall negatively
charged protein

FIGURE 2-6. Ion-exchange chromatography. A column of insoluble ion-exchange resin retains oppositely charged molecules by ionic interactions.

(2) A column of insoluble ion-exchange material carrying either polyanionic or polycationic groups is used. At the appropriate pH, these groups bind oppositely charged groups by ionic interactions.

(a) Proteins may be eluted from the exchanger by washing with a solution containing salts that disrupt the electrostatic interactions of the proteins and ion-exchange resin.

(b) If a gradually increasing salt concentration (i.e., a salt gradient) is applied to the column, weakly bound proteins are eluted before tightly bound proteins.

b. **High-performance liquid chromatography (HPLC)**

(1) HPLC is similar to ion-exchange chromatography and other chromatographic methods in that solutions of proteins are passed through special resins that have attached side groups, which can interact either ionically or hydrophobically with proteins, depending on the type of resin.

(2) HPLC differs from conventional chromatography in that it is done under high pressure (typically 5000–10,000 pounds per square inch). This high-pressure chromatography is faster and results in better resolution than conventional low-pressure chromatography.

c. **Electrophoresis.** Methods that use an electric field to drive the movement of any molecule with a net charge are termed electrophoresis. Charged molecules move in an electric field at a rate determined by their charge-to-mass ratio and their shape.

(1) In an electric field, proteins migrate in a direction determined by the net charge on the molecule. The **net charge on a protein** is determined by the nature of the ionizing groups on the protein and the prevailing pH (see II C 5).

(2) For each protein, there is a pH, called the **isoelectric point (pI),** at which the molecule has no net charge and does not move in an electric field.

(3) At pH values **more acidic** than the pI, the protein bears a **net positive charge,** behaves as a **cation,** and moves toward the negatively charged pole.

(4) At **pH values higher than the pI,** the protein has a **net negative charge** and behaves as an **anion,** moving toward the positively charged pole.

(5) The migration of a protein in an electric field is defined by its **electrophoretic mobility (μ),** which is a ratio of the velocity of migration (V) to the electric field strength (E), or $\mu = V/E$, measured in cm^2 per volt-second. Proteins migrate much more slowly than simple ions because they have a much smaller **ratio of charge-to-mass.**

(6) Electrophoretic procedures

　(a) Gel electrophoresis is often used to separate plasma proteins for diagnostic purposes. The sample is layered on a matrix as a thin zone and is then electrophoresed through the matrix, which is usually made of polyacrylamide or agarose gels. After electrophoresis, the proteins are stained. Different proteins appear in different zones (bands) depending on their overall charge, size, and shape.

　　(i) The matrix tends to stabilize the sample against convection during electrophoresis.

　　(ii) The matrix also provides a sieving component that plays a role in separating proteins according to their size and shape.

　(b) In **isoelectric focusing,** polyamino–polycarboxylic acids (i.e., amphoteric molecules called **ampholines**) with known pI values are used to set up a pH gradient in an electric field. A protein migrates to the part of the gradient that has the same pI as the protein.

　(c) SDS polyacrylamide gel electrophoresis separates proteins on the basis of size (see V B 2 d; Figure 2-5).

　(d) Free zone capillary electrophoresis is a technique in which electrophoretic separation of charged molecules is achieved free in solution in very small-bore (0.05–0.3 mm) capillary tubes. A matrix is not needed to stabilize against convection forces because the heat of electrophoresis is rapidly dissipated in these capillary tubes.

　　(i) Because of the efficient dissipation of heat, very high voltages (10 kV) can be used to quickly separate charged biomolecules.

　　(ii) This relatively new technology is being increasingly used for diagnostic purposes because of its speed and the need for very small amounts (i.e., typically nanoliters) of starting material.

4. Separation by specific affinity binding

a. Affinity (absorption) chromatography

　(1) This technique is based on a property that some proteins possess, that of binding strongly to another molecule (called the **ligand**) by specific, noncovalent bonding.

　(2) The ligand is covalently attached to the surface of large, hydrated particles of porous material to make a chromatographic column. If a solution containing a mixture of proteins is passed through the column, the protein to be selectively absorbed binds tightly to the ligand molecules, whereas the other proteins flow through the column unhindered. After traces of the other proteins are washed out, the absorbed protein can be eluted by a solution with a high concentration of pure ligand, which competes for the protein with the bound ligand.

b. Precipitation by antibodies

　(1) Antibodies to specific proteins can be prepared and used to react with the desired protein in a mixture of proteins (e.g., a tissue extract or body fluid). The interaction of protein and antibody may produce an antigen–antibody complex large enough to be centrifuged out of solution, allowing recovery of the protein.

(2) It is often necessary to create a larger complex than the antigen–antibody complex by adding rabbit anti-gamma globulin (anti-IgG) to the antibody–protein mixture and then recovering the triple complex by centrifugation.

(3) Like ligands (see V B 4 a), antibodies can be attached to hydrated matrices and made into affinity chromatography columns.

Case 2-1 Revisited

If the patient has sickle cell disease, a microscopic analysis of his blood might reveal red blood cell (RBC) lysis and some sickle-shaped RBCs. Although characteristic of sickle cell disease, such a blood profile is not diagnostic of sickle cell disease because other hemoglobinopathies may have the same characteristics. The single Glu to Val mutation that causes sickle cell disease alters the tertiary structure of the β chain of hemoglobin. This change affects the solubility properties of the mutated β chain [i.e., hemoglobin S (Hb S)].

A simple solubility test can be run in which, under the appropriate conditions, RBCs are lysed, Hb S becomes insoluble, and normal hemoglobin A remains soluble. The presence of insoluble Hb S results in a measurably turbid solution. Again, this test is not definitively diagnostic because other hemoglobinopathies and conditions can result in false positives of sickle cell disease with this assay.

Because different types of hemoglobins are made of subunits with different charges and structures due to their primary sequence differences, they can be differentially separated by several specialized electrophoretic techniques. Electrophoresis of hemoglobin on cellulose acetate membranes at an alkaline pH separates most types of hemoglobin subunits. A few rare, abnormal hemoglobin subunits cannot be separated by cellulose acetate electrophoresis. Fortunately, these subunits can be separated by electrophoresis through a citrate agar gel at an acidic pH. Other electrophoretic techniques can be used to identify even rarer forms of hemoglobin subunits.

More recently, HPLC has begun to be used to identify mutated forms of hemoglobin subunits. Recombinant DNA techniques, such as the polymerase chain reaction (see Chapter 11 IV F), can also be used to diagnose sickle cell disease. Such techniques may not, however, identify other hemoglobin defects if they happen to coexist with the sickle cell mutation.

■ STUDY QUESTIONS

DIRECTIONS: Each of the numbered items or incomplete statements in this section is followed by answers or by completions of the statement. Select the **one** lettered answer or completion that is **best** in each case.

1. Which of the following amino acids is an imino acid?

(A) Leucine
(B) Lysine
(C) γ-Carboxyglutamate
(D) Glycine
(E) Proline

2. With the exception of glycine, all amino acids found in proteins are

(A) dextrorotatory
(B) of the D configuration
(C) optically inactive
(D) of the L configuration
(E) either L or D

3. For the partial structure shown below, which letter indicates the group that is not in a plane with the other lettered groups?

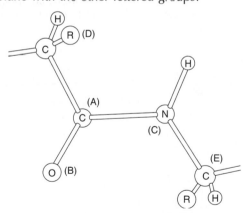

4. Which one of the following electrophoretic analytic procedures depends least on the charge of the protein?

(A) Free zone capillary electrophoresis
(B) Gel electrophoresis
(C) Polyacrylamide gel electrophoresis in sodium dodecyl sulfate (SDS)
(D) Isoelectric focusing

5. Which one of the following statements about protein structure is correct?

(A) The extended β-configuration is not found in globular proteins
(B) The stability of the α-helix is mainly due to hydrophobic interactions
(C) Globular proteins tend to fold into configurations that keep hydrophobic side chains in the interior of the molecule
(D) The protomers of polymeric proteins are linked by covalent bonds
(E) The primary structure of a peptide does not influence the formation of the native three-dimensional configuration

6. Compositional analyses from a large diversity of proteins from humans reveals

(A) that they are all made of only 20 amino acids
(B) the presence of a few D-amino acids
(C) that none of the amino acids contains phosphate
(D) that some of the glutamates from blood proteins have an additional carboxyl group

7. Which one of the following ionic species of glutamate would be prevalent at pH 10?

(A) $HOOC-CH-(CH_2)_2-COOH$
       $|$
       $^+NH_3$

(B) $^-OOC-CH-(CH_2)_2-COOH$
       $|$
       $^+NH_3$

(C) $HOOC-CH-(CH_2)_2-COO^-$
       $|$
       $^+NH_2$

(D) $^-OOC-CH-(CH_2)_2-COO^-$
       $|$
       $^+NH_3$

(E) $^-OOC-CH-(CH_2)_2-COO^-$
       $|$
       NH_2

8. Which interaction may play a role in the formation of quarternary structure by covalently linking different polypeptide chains?

(A) Hydrogen bonds
(B) Electrostatic interactions
(C) Disulfide bridges
(D) Peptide bonds
(E) Hydrophobic interactions

Each set of matching questions in this section consists of a list of lettered options followed by several numbered items. For each numbered item, select the appropriate lettered option(s). Each lettered option may be selected once, more than once, or not at all.

Questions 9-10

(A) Leucine
(B) Aspartate
(C) Isoleucine
(D) Cysteine
(E) Proline
(F) Arginine
(G) Glutamate
(H) Lysine
(I) Valine

For each property, select the amino acids that exhibit it.

9. These three amino acids are hydrophobic and have a tendency to be located away from the surface of proteins.

10. These two amino acids are basic and have a tendency to be found on the surface of proteins.

ANSWERS AND EXPLANATIONS

1. The answer is E [II A 2]. Of the 20 fundamental amino acids found in proteins, 19 are α-amino acids. That is, they have an amino group ($-NH_2$), a carboxyl group ($-COOH$), a hydrogen group, and a distinctive side group bonded to a central carbon atom named the α-carbon. Therefore, it is named an α-amino acid because the amino group is linked to the α-carbon. In proline, the nitrogen is not in the form of an amino group but instead is present as an imino ($-NH-$) group. The side group ($CH_2)_3$ off of the α-carbon cyclizes through the nitrogen.

2. The answer is D [II B]. A given amino acid may be either levorotatory (L) or dextrorotatory (D). With the exception of the optically inactive glycine, all amino acids derived from proteins by hydrolysis are of the L configuration. Glycine is not optically active because it does not have an asymmetric carbon atom.

3. The answer is D [III A 3]. The peptide bond is a planar structure with the two adjacent α-carbons, a carbonyl oxygen, an α-amino nitrogen and its associated hydrogen atom, and the carbonyl carbon all lying in the same plane. The distinct side chains (R groups) for each amino acid lie outside the planar structure of the peptide bond.

4. The answer is C [V B 2 d, 3 c (6)]. Electrophoresis carried out on a crosslinked polyacrylamide gel in the presence of the detergent sodium dodecyl sulfate (SDS), separates reduced proteins primarily on the basis of their molecular weight rather than their charge. The SDS forms negatively charged micelles with the protein so that the effect of the protein charge is lost. The SDS-protein micelles migrate to the positive pole with the crosslinked polyacrylamide gel acting as a molecular sieve; the smaller the protein, the faster its migration rate. Free zone capillary electrophoresis does not require a matrix. Although it can be done in the presence of a reducing agent and SDS, and it can separate proteins according to size, free zone capillary electrophoresis is often performed under nondenaturing conditions in which the migration

of the protein depends on the charge. Both gel electrophoresis and isoelectric focusing depend on the charge of the protein.

5. The answer is C [IV A, B 2 b, 3 a, C 1, D 1]. The primary structure of a protein (i.e., its amino acid sequence) dictates the final three-dimensional form adopted by the protein. Globular proteins may contain peptide chains, which in part may be extended β-configurations. Some of these might fold back on themselves, forming antiparallel β-sheet conformations in part of the protein. The α-helix is stabilized by intrachain hydrogen bonds that form between peptide bonds that are four residues apart. Globular proteins fold so that the hydrophobic side chains are kept away from water in the interior of the molecule, and the polar side chains are on the outside in contact with water. The individual chains, or protomers, of multisubunit proteins associate by noncovalent bonding, which is frequently largely hydrophobic in nature.

6. The answer is D [II A 3].
There are only 20 fundamental amino acids. However, more than 100 different kinds of amino acids have been identified in proteins that arise by post-transitional modification. The major modifications of amino acids found are hydroxylation, methylation, carboxylation, and phosphorylation of particular amino acids. All proteins are not post-transitionally modified to the same extent. For instance, carboxylation of glutamates is rare on most proteins but commonly found on many of the blood clotting proteins. None of the basic amino acids contains phosphates yet post-transitional phosphorylation of serines, threonines, and tyrosines is a common method of regulating the activity of many amino acids. D-Amino acids are found in bacterial cell walls and in peptide antibiotics but are not incorporated into proteins via the ribosomal protein synthesizing system (see II B 2 b).

7. The answer is E [II C 5 b (2)]. Glutamate has three dissociable protons, two with pK_a' values well below pH 7, and one with a pK_a' value well above pH 7. At pH 10, both the α-carboxyl ($pK_a' = 2.19$) and the γ-carboxyl (pK$_a$′ = 4.25) will have lost a proton and will, therefore, carry a negative charge. The α-amino group (pK$_a$′ = 9.67) will also have lost a proton and will be uncharged.

8. The answer is C [III A, IV D]. Quarternary structure is the interaction of the many polypeptide chains in a multichain protein. These interactions are usually noncovalent (e.g., hydrogen bonds), electrostatic, or hydrophobic, but covalent interactions (e.g., disulfide bridges) may occur occasionally. Peptide bonds form the backbone of polypeptides. They do not link polypeptides to each other.

9. The answers are A, C, and I [IV C 1; Table 2-1]. Of the 20 amino acids, 3 have sufficiently long carbon chains to be significantly hydrophobic: valine, leucine, and isoleucine. Phenylalanine and methionine are also not polar and are very hydrophobic. Other amino acids exhibit different degrees of hydrophobicity, but these five amino acids have the strongest aversion to combining with water and are, therefore, often found in the interior portion of globular proteins.

10. The answers are F and H [II C 5 a (1); Table 2-1]. The three basic amino acids are lysine, arginine, and histidine. Charged amino acids, both basic and acidic, are very hydrophilic in nature and, accordingly, have a tendency to be found on the surface of proteins.

Chapter 3

Protein Structure–Function Relationships
Donald Sittman

Case 3-1

A thin, 50-year-old indigent white male (a "street person") comes to the emergency department with a knife cut on his right forearm. A routine physical examination reveals that previous wounds have either not healed or are regressing, and some are also bleeding. The patient has many missing teeth, and his gums are red, swollen, bleeding, and showing signs of infection. The skin at the base of many of his hair follicles appears red and inflamed. He also has an enlarged and tender liver.

- What is the possible diagnosis of the patient's skin and oral symptoms?
- What blood test would confirm this diagnosis?
- What treatment would correct these problems?

I. **INTRODUCTION.** Structure, and changes in structure, are crucial to the function of most proteins. To demonstrate this point, five classic, well-described, medically relevant protein families are presented in this chapter. Understanding their structure and the structural changes that they undergo leads to an understanding of how they function.

A. The **first three** descriptions are of two globular protein families: the **oxygen transport proteins** of the body (i.e., myoglobin and hemoglobin), **albumin,** which is the most abundant serum transport protein, and **immunoglobulins.** Cellular immunity cannot be understood without knowledge of the structure and function of antibodies.

B. The **fourth** classic model described is of **collagen,** the major fibrous structural protein of the body.

C. The **fifth** model describes the mechanism by which an enzymatic activity drives a structural change in a very precisely organized complex of both globular and fibrous proteins that leads to muscle contraction.

II. **OXYGEN TRANSPORT PROTEINS.** Oxygen enters cells by diffusion, and the availability of oxygen is limited by the distance over which diffusion must occur. As the size of cells and organisms has increased, circulatory systems with oxygen-binding molecules have evolved to carry oxygen to cells and subcellular areas that cannot get oxygen by direct diffusion. In higher animals, oxygen transport is mediated by two oxygen-binding globular proteins: myoglobin and hemoglobin (Figure 3-1).

A. **Myoglobin**

   1. Function. Myoglobin is found in muscle cells, where it stores oxygen and transports oxygen to the mitochondria. To perform its function, myoglobin must be able to bind oxygen well at the relatively low oxygen tension in the tissues where hemoglobin releases oxygen. This ability to bind oxygen at low oxygen tension is seen by looking at its oxygen-binding curve.

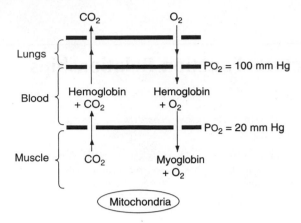

FIGURE 3-1. Diagram of oxygen (O_2) transport. Oxygen is picked up by hemoglobin in the lungs, where the partial pressure of oxygen (PO_2) is 100 mm Hg. Hemoglobin releases the oxygen at the tissues, where the PO_2 is approximately 20 mm Hg. The oxygen then diffuses into the cell and is used. In muscles, the oxygen can be bound and stored in myoglobin until needed. Carbon dioxide (CO_2) diffuses out of the cell and is carried by hemoglobin back to the lungs, where it is released and exhaled.

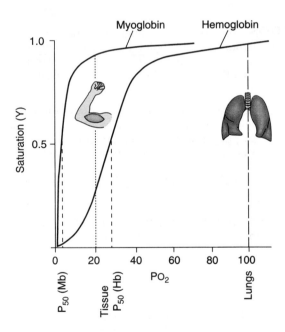

FIGURE 3-2. Oxygen-binding curves for myoglobin (Mb) and hemoglobin (Hb). P_{50}(Hb) = 50% saturation of hemoglobin; P_{50}(Mb) = 50% saturation of myoglobin; PO_2 = partial pressure of oxygen.

  a. The **oxygen-binding curve** (also called an oxygen-dissociation curve) for myoglobin is a rectangular hyperbola (Figure 3-2) with the binding sites 90% saturated at 20 mm Hg (torr), which is the partial pressure of oxygen (PO_2) in muscle.
  b. This relationship can be expressed as

$$Y = \frac{[MbO_2]}{[Mb] + [MbO_2]}$$

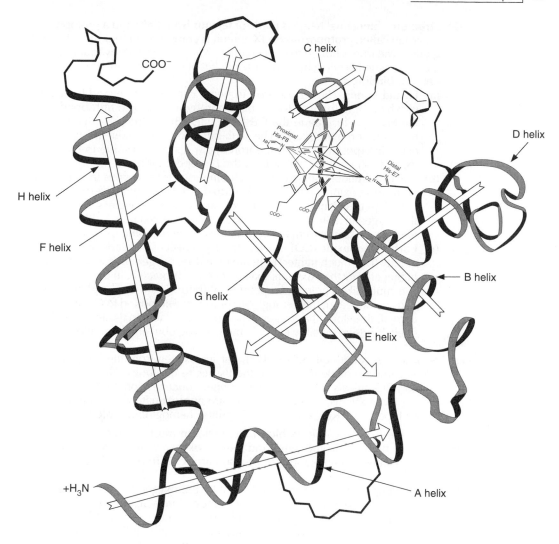

FIGURE 3-3. Model of myoglobin. The heme molecule shows bound oxygen between the seventh amino acid (histidine) in the E-helix and the eighth amino acid (histidine) in the F-helix.

where Y is the fraction of myoglobin saturated with oxygen, [MbO_2] is the concentration of oxygenated myoglobin, and [Mb] is the concentration of deoxygenated myoglobin.

2. Structure

    a. Myoglobin is a compactly folded, single peptide chain that is 153 residues in length (Figure 3-3).

    b. Approximately 75% of the structure of myoglobin consists of eight α-helical segments (lettered A through H in Figure 3-3). The polar (hydrophilic) residues tend to be on the outside of the molecule, whereas almost all of the nonpolar (hydrophobic) residues are on the inside of the molecule.

    c. Heme

        (1) Function. Heme is **a prosthetic group** that **enables the binding of oxygen to myoglobin and hemoglobin** (see II B 2). Without the heme group (**apoprotein** form), myoglobin will not bind oxygen.

      (2) **Structure.** Functional heme is made of **ferrous iron (Fe^{2+})** and a protoporphyrin group called **protoporphyrin IX,** which is composed of four linked pyrrole groups. The iron is bound to the center of protoporphyrin IX by four nitrogen groups. Heme fits into a hydrophobic pocket of the myoglobin molecule.

      (3) **Oxygen-binding site**

          (a) **Ligand bonds.** The ferrous iron in heme can form six ligand bonds, four of which bind the iron to the protoporphyrin ring. The fifth bond is to the histidine residue in the F α-helix (His-F8), on the proximal side of the protoporphyrin plane. The sixth bond forms between an oxygen molecule interposed between the iron and a histidine residue in the E α-helix (His-E7) on the distal side of the protoporphyrin ring.

          (b) The **hydrophobic pocket** of myoglobin protects the ferrous iron group in heme from oxidizing to the ferric form (Fe^{3+}). Heme with a ferric iron is called **metmyoglobin,** and it cannot carry oxygen. A water group replaces the oxygen in metmyoglobin. Ferric iron is oxidized iron. With the extra electron, it cannot form the coordinates needed to bind oxygen.

          (c) **Carbon monoxide (CO)** is a very toxic gas because it binds with a higher affinity (i.e., much tighter) to heme than does oxygen. Because CO has a higher affinity than oxygen, oxygen cannot displace it. In this way, CO acts much like a potent competitive inhibitor. There can be plenty of oxygen available, but the hemoglobin or myoglobin bound to CO will not carry it; therefore, the oxygen is not made available to tissues. CO effectively binds irreversibly to the heme in myoglobin and hemoglobin.

B.   **Hemoglobin,** found in **red blood cells (RBCs),** carries oxygen from the lungs to the tissues and carries carbon dioxide (CO_2) from the tissues to the lungs. The packaging of hemoglobin into RBCs allows it to be present at high concentrations without osmotic pressure or viscosity problems. In humans, there are approximately five billion RBCs per milliliter of blood. Each RBC contains 280 million hemoglobin molecules.

    1. Function. As the oxygen carrier in blood, hemoglobin must be able to bind oxygen at the relatively high P_{O_2} in the lungs and release oxygen at the relatively low P_{O_2} in the tissues. Likewise, hemoglobin must also carry CO_2 from the tissues and release it in the lungs.

      a. Oxygen-binding curve (see Figure 3-2). Unlike the oxygen-binding curve for myoglobin, the oxygen-binding curve for hemoglobin is **sigmoidal.**

        (1) A comparison of the myoglobin and hemoglobin oxygen-binding curves shows that hemoglobin very efficiently binds oxygen at the P_{O_2} levels found in lungs, and it releases the oxygen at the P_{O_2} levels found in tissues (e.g., muscle).

        (2) In contrast, myoglobin binds oxygen very efficiently at the low P_{O_2} levels at which hemoglobin releases oxygen.

      b. Cooperative oxygen binding. The shape of the oxygen-binding curve of hemoglobin is sigmoidal because oxygen binding is cooperative. That is, as oxygen binds to some sites on hemoglobin, the binding of more oxygen to hemoglobin becomes easier (see II B 3 a).

      c. Hill coefficient (n). The degree of cooperativity in the binding reaction is expressed by the Hill coefficient, *n,* in the following expression, where *Y* is the fraction of myoglobin or hemoglobin saturated with oxygen and P_{50} is the partial pressure of oxygen at which myoglobin is 50% saturated with oxygen.

$$Y = \frac{(P_{O_2})^n}{(P_{O_2})^n + P_{50}}$$

As *n* increases, the cooperativity of binding increases. For hemoglobin, the value of *n* is 2.8, whereas for myoglobin it is 1.

    2. Structure. Hemoglobin is a tetramer of four noncovalently linked subunits, each of which is structurally and evolutionarily similar to myoglobin. Like myoglobin, each hemoglobin subunit has a hydrophobic pocket that contains heme and serves as

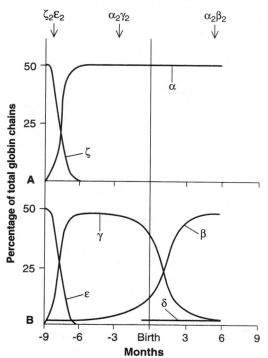

Predominant hemoglobin

FIGURE 3-4. Expressions of genes for different globin chains during early development. *(A)* Alpha (α) and zeta (ζ) genes. *(B)* Beta (β), gamma (γ), delta (δ), and epsilon (ε) genes. At conception the $\zeta_2\epsilon_2$ hemoglobin is predominant; during the last trimester, the $\alpha_2\gamma_2$ hemoglobin is predominant; and shortly after birth the $\alpha_2\beta_2$ hemoglobin becomes predominant. (Reprinted with permission from Stryer L: *Biochemistry,* 3rd ed. New York, W.H. Freeman, 1988, p 151.)

the site of oxygen binding. The heme prosthetic groups of myoglobin and hemoglobin are identical.

a. Structural diversity of hemoglobin. Several different forms of hemoglobin can be found in adult humans and during early human development. The early developmental forms are particularly suited for the oxygen transport needs at the stage of development in which they are expressed (see II B 3 d). The various hemoglobin forms differ in the primary structure of the subunits that form the hemoglobin tetramer.

b. Genetic variation. The different subunits of various hemoglobins are products of different globin genes. Figure 3-4 shows when during early development the genes for different hemoglobin subunits are expressed.

(1) **Hemoglobin A₁** is the major (98%) form found in human adults. It is a tetramer of two identical α subunits and two identical β subunits (abbreviated $\alpha_2\beta_2$). The α and β chains are composed of 141 and 146 residues, respectively.

(2) **Hemoglobin A₂** is a minor (2%) form found in human adults. It is a tetramer of two α subunits and two delta (δ) subunits ($\alpha_2\delta_2$).

(3) **Fetal hemoglobins.** The first hemoglobin formed during embryogenesis is a tetramer of two zeta (ζ) subunits, which are evolutionarily similar to α subunits, and two epsilon (ε) subunits ($\zeta_2\epsilon_2$). Through the first 6 months of development, the ζ subunits are replaced by α subunits, and the ε subunits are replaced by the γ subunits forming hemoglobin F ($\alpha_2\gamma_2$). Through later embryonic development and just after birth, the γ subunits are replaced by β subunits.

3. **Structure–function relationships.** The mechanism of cooperative binding of oxygen to hemoglobin and the fact that protons (H^+), carbon dioxide, and 2,3-bisphospho-glycerate (2,3-BPG; see II B 3 c) are allosteric effectors of hemoglobin emphasizes the role that structure plays in the function of hemoglobin. The importance of structure's effect on function is also seen in fetal hemoglobin, in which a subunit that differs from adult hemoglobin changes its oxygen affinity because it does not bind 2,3-BPG well.

a. **Cooperative oxygen binding**

(1) In **deoxyhemoglobin** (i.e., hemoglobin with **no bound oxygen**), the iron is slightly (0.4 Å) out of the heme plane. This is due in part to steric repulsion between the proximal histidine [see II A 2 c (3) (a)] and the nitrogen atoms of the porphyrin ring. On oxygenation, the iron atom moves into the plane of the porphyrin ring so that it can form a strong bond with oxygen.

(2) **Structural change** increases the oxygen-binding affinity constants.

(a) The movement of the iron into the plane of the porphyrin ring results in the pulling of the His-F8 residue toward the heme. This in turn significantly changes the interaction of the F-helix with the C-helix of the adjacent subunit.

(b) This change in structure, which is transmitted to the adjacent subunit, increases the affinity constant for the binding of oxygen of the adjacent subunit. Therefore, the binding of the first oxygen cooperatively enhances the binding of subsequent oxygens to the other heme groups in hemoglobin.

(3) **Two forms of hemoglobin that bind oxygen with different affinities**

(a) In the deoxyhemoglobin state, the quarternary conformation of hemoglobin is said to be in the **tight** or **T form.**

(b) Because of the change in structure induced by the initial binding of oxygen (which changes hemoglobin to oxyhemoglobin), the quarternary conformation is said to be in the **relaxed** or **R form.**

b. **Protons (H^+) and carbon dioxide.** The **Bohr effect** describes the relationship of hemoglobin's oxygen affinity to P_{CO_2} levels and pH.

(1) The **oxygen-binding affinity of hemoglobin is decreased by an increase in hydrogen ion concentration.** The binding affinity of hemoglobin for oxygen is also decreased by an **increase in P_{CO_2}.** These changes in binding affinity are reflected in a rightward shift in the oxygen-binding curve of hemoglobin with increases in proton or carbon dioxide concentrations (Figure 3-5).

(2) Because an increase in P_{CO_2} and a decrease in pH are both characteristic of actively metabolizing cells, these cells promote the release of oxygen from hemoglobin.

(3) **Protons bind to specific sites on hemoglobin.** Binding of protons causes hemoglobin to shift from the R form to the T form. In the lungs, at pH 7.4 and high P_{O_2}, hemoglobin shifts to the R form, with a lower affinity for protons. The protons are subsequently released.

(4) Carbon dioxide binds to the terminal amino group of the hemoglobin subunits as a **carbamate:**

$$-NH_3 + CO_2 \leftrightarrow -\overset{\overset{\textstyle H}{\textstyle |}}{N}-COO^- + 2H^+$$

The binding of carbon dioxide is also higher in the T conformation, so, like the binding of protons, it favors a shift of hemoglobin from the R form to the T form. This effect is increased because the formation of carbamate also increases the proton concentration, and likewise the Bohr effect. In the lungs, at high P_{O_2}, a shift to the R form and subsequent release of carbon dioxide is promoted by the binding of oxygen.

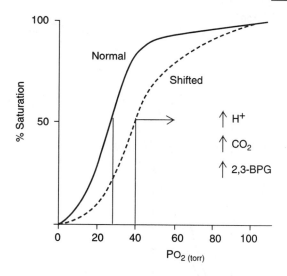

FIGURE 3-5. Rightward shift of the hemoglobin oxygen-binding curve in the presence of an increased concentration of protons (H+; decreased pH), carbon dioxide (CO_2), or 2,3-bisphosphoglycerate (2,3-BPG).

(5) The effect of a decrease in tissue concentration of carbon dioxide levels is seen in patients with **hyperventilation.** Rapid breathing promotes the loss of carbon dioxide and a lowering of the tissue P_{CO_2}. This decrease in tissue carbon dioxide levels means less oxygen is delivered to the tissues. The decrease in oxygen delivery can lead to numbness, dizziness, muscle cramps, and other symptoms.

c. Role of 2,3-BPG

(1) 2,3-BPG is found in RBCs at nearly the same concentration as hemoglobin. It is responsible for significantly lowering the oxygen affinity of hemoglobin and allowing the hemoglobin to more efficiently release oxygen at the typical P_{O_2} of tissues.

(2) Only one molecule of 2,3-BPG interacts with each hemoglobin tetramer. The 2,3-BPG molecule specifically binds to hemoglobin by interacting with three positively charged groups on each β chain, effectively cross-linking these subunits.

(3) **A rise of 2,3-BPG in RBCs promotes the shift of hemoglobin to the T form** and the subsequent release of oxygen. In RBCs, 2,3-BPG levels rise as they adapt to conditions of tissue hypoxia (e.g., from anemia, high altitudes, or pulmonary dysfunction).

(4) During storage of blood to be used for transfusions, RBCs fail to maintain high levels of 2,3-BPG. This increases the stored blood's affinity for oxygen and, therefore, decreases its ability to release oxygen in tissues.

d. Fetal hemoglobin differs from adult hemoglobin by having a **much higher affinity for oxygen.**

(1) **Function.** The fetus must pick up oxygen at the lower P_{O_2} of the placenta, so its hemoglobin must be different from the maternal hemoglobin that releases it in the placenta.

(2) **Structure. Hemoglobin F (Hb F),** the predominant hemoglobin through much of fetal life, has two γ subunits instead of two β subunits (therefore $\alpha_2\gamma_2$). The higher oxygen affinity of Hb F arises because the γ subunits do not bind 2,3-BPG well. This means that the oxygen affinity-binding curve of Hb F is shifted to the left as compared with hemoglobin A_1 (Hb A_1; Figure 3-6). In the absence of 2,3-BPG, Hb F has a slightly lower oxygen affinity than Hb A_1.

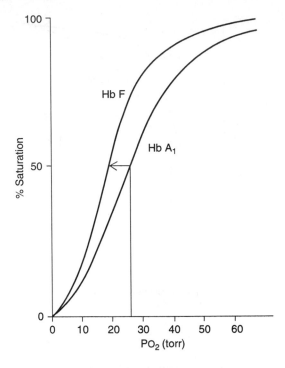

FIGURE 3-6. Comparison of hemoglobin F (Hb F) and hemoglobin A_1 (Hb A_1) oxygen-binding curves. Po_2 = partial pressure of oxygen.

4. **Clinical aspects of hemoglobin**
   a. **Glycosylation of Hb A_1 and diabetes mellitus**
      (1) Hb A_1 reacts spontaneously with glucose to form a derivative known as **hemoglobin A_{1c} (Hb A_{1c}).**
      (2) Normally the concentration of Hb A_{1c} in blood is very low, but in patients with diabetes mellitus, in whom blood sugar levels may be high, the concentration of Hb A_{1c} may reach 12% or more of the total hemoglobin.
      (3) Because the average life of an RBC is 120 days, the amount of Hb A_{1c} becomes a good indicator of blood glucose levels over a 2- to 4-month period. For example, determination of the amount of Hb A_{1c} can tell a physician if patients have maintained their blood glucose levels over the preceding months or have lowered their glucose levels just before their clinical examination.
   b. **Hemoglobinopathies** are genetic diseases in which the globin subunits of hemoglobin are mutated. Hundreds of hemoglobinopathies have been described. In some there are no symptoms or impairment, whereas in others there may be severe impairment. Table 3-1 presents a few examples of hemoglobinopathies with different mutations that cause different effects. Major hemoglobinopathies include the following.
      (1) **Sickle cell anemia, or hemoglobin S (Hb S)** was one of the first hemoglobinopathies to be described. It occurs when valine (Val) replaces glutamic acid (Glu) in the sixth position of the β chains. The α chains are normal.
         (a) Hb S is the **most common hemoglobinopathy** in the United States; 0.3% of the black population is homozygous for Hb S (**sickle cell disease**) and 8%–13% are heterozygous (**sickle cell trait**).
         (b) On deoxygenation, Hb S polymerizes within the RBC. This polymerization leads to the characteristic **sickle-shaped cell.** In other respects, Hb S appears to be normal, exhibiting good cooperative oxygen binding.

TABLE 3-1. Examples of Hemoglobinopathies and Their Properties

Hemoglobin	Mutation		Properties
Hb S	β6	Glu → Val	Red blood cell sickling, hemolytic anemia
Hb C	β6	Glu → Lys	Mild anemia, Hb C crystals in red blood cells
Hb E	β26	Glu → Lys	Mild anemia
Hb M-Boston	β58	His → Tyr	Methemoglobin, cyanosis
Hb M-Saskatoon	β63	His → Tyr	Methemoglobin, cyanosis
Hb Rainier	β145	Tyr → Cys	Increased oxygen affinity, polycythemia
Hb Chesapeake	α92	Arg → Leu	Increased oxygen affinity, polycythemia
Hb Kansas	β102	Asn → Thr	Decreased oxygen affinity, mild cyanosis
Hb Köln	β98	Val → Met	Unstable β subunit, hemolysis

Note. Hemoglobinopathies were originally identified by different electrophoretic mobilities of the globin subunits and were named with a capital letter. After realization that all mutant proteins did not have different electrophoretic mobilities and that many more existed than could be named with letters, the convention was established that called for naming the hemoglobins after the location of the patient in which they were discovered. The mutation position is listed by the chain, α or β, followed by the amino acid position. *Arg* = arginine; *Asn* = asparagine; *Cys* = cysteine; *Glu* = glutamate; *Hb S* = hemoglobin S; *Hb C* = hemoglobin C; *Hb E* = hemoglobin E; *Hb M* = hemoglobin M; *His* = histidine; *Leu* = leucine; *Lys* = lysine; *Met* = methionine; *Thr* = threonine; *Tyr* = tyrosine; *Val* = valine.

    (c) The **symptoms** of sickle cell disease can be severe. The patients are anemic, and their RBCs have an average life span of 10–15 days instead of the normal 120 days. A **sickle cell crisis** can be extremely painful and can lead to cumulative organ damage. Death often occurs in early adulthood.

    (d) People with sickle cell trait are usually symptom free except under conditions of low P_{O_2}. Persons with sickle cell trait show an **increased resistance to malaria,** and the world distribution of sickle cell anemia closely parallels the distribution of malaria.

  (2) **Hemoglobin C (Hb C)** is the second most common hemoglobinopathy in the United States. As in Hb S, the glutamic acid (Glu) at position 6 in the β chain is mutated to a lysine (Lys). The RBCs of people with Hb C do not sickle; however, crystals of Hb C may form within them.

    (a) **Homozygotes.** Individuals homozygous for Hb C are found in the black population at a frequency of 0.01%–0.02%.

    (b) **Heterozygotes** are present in the black population at a frequency of 2.0%–2.5%. Clinically, Hb C heterozygotes are asymptomatic.

  (3) **Hemoglobin M (Hb M).** A number of rare hemoglobinopathies lead to a high percentage of methemoglobins in red blood cells. These usually arise due to mutations in either the proximal or distal histidines of either the α or β chains, which bond with the iron in the heme group. These mutations stabilize the iron in the ferric form (Fe^{3+}), which cannot bind oxygen. Only patients who are heterozygous for these mutations have been found. Presumably, homozygosity is lethal.

 c. **Thalassemias** are **hemolytic anemias** that arise from insufficient production of either the α or β subunits of hemoglobin. α-Thalassemia is due to insufficient production of α globin, and β-thalassemia is due to insufficient production of β globin.

  (1) **Insufficient production of globin subunits** has been shown to arise from any of a number of causes:

    (a) Deletion of one or more of the globin genes

        (b) Mutations in the promoter or gene regulatory regions of any of the globin genes

        (c) Mutations that destabilize the globin messenger RNAs (mRNAs) or that result in defective processing of the globin mRNA

        (d) Nonsense or frameshift mutations that cause premature termination of translation or the translation of an aberrant globin that is either unstable or nonfunctional

    (2) Classes of thalassemias. Thalassemias are classified according to the number of copies of mutated genes that the patient carries. Individuals with thalassemias may have either one (heterozygous) or two (homozygous) mutated genes. Because the α-globin genes are duplicated, from one to four α-globin genes may be mutated.

        (a) Thalassemia minor. Heterozygotes carrying one mutated β-globin gene have thalassemia minor. This is the **most common** thalassemia in the United States. The loss of expression of a β-globin gene is partially compensated for by increased formation of Hb A_2 and Hb F. These patients have only mild anemia and few associated problems. Most will have a normal life span.

        (b) Thalassemia major. Homozygotes carrying two mutated β-globin genes have thalassemia major. These patients have severe hemolytic anemia with many complications. They rarely live to adulthood.

        (c) α-Thalassemias

            (i) Patients deficient in the expression of a single α-globin gene are completely normal and are only carriers of α-thalassemia.

            (ii) Patients deficient in the expression of two α-globin genes are said to have **α-thalassemia trait.** They suffer from only mild anemia with few complications.

            (iii) Patients with deficient expression of three α-globin genes have hemoglobin H (Hb H) disease. They have somewhat more severe anemia than patients with α-thalassemia trait.

            (iv) Homozygous α-thalassemia is the deletion of four α-globin genes, which is always a lethal condition. Affected individuals are either stillborn, or they die soon after birth.

III. ALBUMIN

ALBUMIN is produced by the liver, and, at 55%–60% of the total plasma protein, it is the most abundant protein in the blood plasma.

A.

Function. Albumin is a multifunctional protein.

1. Transport. Because of albumin's ability to bind to many diverse molecules, it serves as a low-specificity transport protein. Some of the types of molecules that it binds and transports in the bloodstream are:

    a. Metal ions such as calcium and copper. Half of the blood calcium ions are bound to albumin.

    b. Free fatty acids. Albumin binds to the free fatty acids (see Chapter 22) released by adipocytes and facilitates their transfer to other tissues.

    c. Bilirubin is bound very tightly by albumin. This protects from the toxic side effects of unconjugated bilirubin (see Chapter 25 VII C).

    d. Bile acids. Albumin carries the bile acids that are recycled from the intestines to the liver in the hepatic portal vein (see Chapter 23 IV C).

    e. Hormones such as thyroid hormones and the steroid hormones

2. Maintenance of osmotic pressure in the capillaries and movement of interstitial fluid back into the bloodstream also involves the transport of molecules by albumin.

B. **Structure**

1. **Shape.** Albumin's ellipsoid shape does not significantly increase the blood viscosity. This means that it is easily transported through the bloodstream.

2. **Charge.** Albumin is a very acidic protein with a large negative charge at the blood pH. This helps it bind cationic molecules and enhances its ability to draw water from the interstitial fluid back into the bloodstream.

3. **Domains.** Albumin has at least three major domains, each of which has two subdomains. The diversity of its domains may account for why it binds to different classes of molecules.

C. **Clinical aspects**

1. Albumin binds to a wide array of different drugs and strongly affects the turnover or pharmacokinetics of these drugs.

2. The antimicrobial sulfonamides, by competitive binding, cause the release of unconjugated bilirubin from albumin. If given to infants, sulfonamides may lead to kernicterus (see Chapter 25).

3. In cases of liver disease or starvation, albumin synthesis decreases. This leads to edema or the retention of water in tissues, because albumin is no longer available to maintain the proper tissue osmotic pressure.

IV. **HUMORAL IMMUNITY.** The humoral immune system is responsible for secreting soluble immunoglobulins, or antibodies, into the bloodstream. Typically, foreign substances, which are antigenic, elicit an immune response, which comprises the processes that lead to the removal of antigens from the body.

A. **Definitions**

1. **Antigen.** An antigen is any substance that binds to antibodies and induces the production of antibody or immune cell function.
   a. **Epitope.** An epitope, or determinant, is the specific site on an antigen to which an antibody binds. An antigen may have one or more epitopes. Antibodies are capable of binding epitopes through hydrophobic, ionic, or Van der Waals forces, but not through covalent bonding.
   b. **Haptens** can bind to antibodies but cannot elicit an immune response on their own. Haptens are usually small molecules such as drugs. If they are linked to a larger molecule, or **carrier,** then haptens can elicit an immune response. Drugs such as penicillin are haptens that link to serum proteins and may elicit an immune response.

2. **Antibodies,** or **immunoglobulins,** are secreted from **plasma cells,** which develop from bone-marrow–derived lymphocytes (i.e., **B cells**). Antibodies bind to antigens and elicit or effect an immune response. The body can produce greater than 10^8 different antibodies, each of which is capable of recognizing and binding a different antigen. Chapter 12 VIII C describes how antibody diversity is achieved.

B. **Basic antibody structure.** The five major classes of antibodies (see IV C) share a common structural form, which is shown in Figure 3-7.

1. **Functional domains.** Functionally, antibodies can be divided into two domains:
   a. **Binding domain.** This is the region of the antibody responsible for binding the antigen.

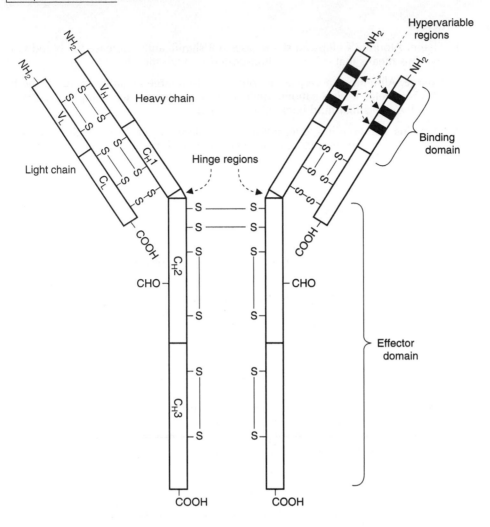

FIGURE 3-7. Diagrammatic structure of an antibody monomer. There are two light (L) chains and two heavy (H) chains linked by disulfide bonds (S–S). The L chains are made of two regions: one a region of variable amino acid sequence (V_L) and one of constant amino acid sequence (C_L). The H chains also have a variable region (V_H) and a constant region that is divided into multiple domains (e.g., C_H1, C_H2, and C_H3 for IgG). The binding and effector domains are indicated. CHO = carbohydrate; COOH = carboxy-terminal end; NH_2 = amino-terminal end.

    b. Effector domain. This region of the antibody is responsible for the following actions:
        (1) Initiating the processes that rid the body of antibody-bound antigens
        (2) Designating the class of the antibody, and likewise its distribution in the body

  2. Basic structural unit. The basic structural unit of an antibody is referred to as a **monomer,** although it is made of two pairs of polypeptide chains. An antibody monomer is made of two identical **light (L) chains** and two identical **heavy (H) chains.** Each H chain is paired in the same orientation—amino to carboxyl—with an L chain.

  3. Disulfide bonds. The H and L chains are held together by disulfide bonds, which occur between H chains, between H and L chains, and, in some antibodies, between L chains. Intrachain disulfide bonds play a role in dividing antibodies into structural domains (e.g., C_H1, C_H2, C_H3; see Figure 3-7).

4. **Variable and constant regions**
   a. **Variable region.** The NH_2-terminal portion of both the L and H chains has a variable structure that differs in sequence considerably between different antibodies. The variable regions of paired L and H chains are adjacent to each other and form the **antibody-binding site,** which binds antigen. The amino acid sequence of the variable region is the sole determinant of the specificity of binding of an antibody with an antigen.
   b. **Hypervariable region.** There are subregions within the variable region that exhibit highly variable amino acid sequence. These sequences are primarily responsible for antigen binding and are called hypervariable regions, or **complementarity-determining regions (CDRs).**
   c. **Constant region.** The COOH-terminal domains of the H and L chains have a constant structure that is similar between different antibodies of the same class. The amino acid sequence in this region shows very little difference between different antibodies. The effector domain lies within the constant region.

5. **Hinge.** The H chains contain a hinge region between the first two structural domains (C_H1 and C_H2; see Figure 3-7) of the constant region. As the name implies, this region is flexible and allows movement between the two antibody-binding sites. The hinge region is digested by proteases such as papain, and it allows the antibody to be split into three fragments.
   a. Two **identical antigen-binding fragments (Fab fragments)** contain the antigen-binding site.
   b. The **crystallizable fragment (Fc fragment)** contains the effector domain.

C. **Classes of antibodies.** There are five basic classes, or **isotypes,** of antibodies. The constant region of the H chains determines the class of an antibody.

1. **Immunoglobulin M (IgM)**
   a. **Function.** IgM is the first antibody produced by a B cell upon induction of an immune response and is present on the surface of most B cells. IgM is also present in the serum at 8%–10% of the total antibody level. It is the most abundant antibody produced by the fetus. IgMs avidly bind viruses and bacteria and provide the first line of defense against infections.
   b. **Structure.** IgM exists either as a **monomeric or pentameric** structure. The monomer form is found on B cells. The pentameric form is found in the serum. The pentameric form of IgM is made of five monomeric antibodies that are linked together by disulfide bonds. The disulfide linkages occur at the C-terminal ends of the H chains as well as at an additional polypeptide called the **joining (J) chain.**

2. **Immunoglobulin D (IgD)**
   a. **Function.** IgD is expressed with IgM on the surface of B cells before their activation (see Chapter 12 VIII C 4). It is a low-abundance antibody in serum, present at less than 1% of the total antibody in serum. Because of its low abundance, the function of IgD is controversial.
   b. **Structure.** IgD is a monomer.

3. **Immunoglobulin G (IgG)**
   a. **Function.** IgG is the main serum antibody, accounting for approximately 75% of the total antibody in serum. As the most abundant serum antibody, IgG plays a major role in eliciting an immune response to antigens. It is also the only maternal antibody that can pass through the placenta to protect the fetus.
   b. **Structure.** There are four subtypes of IgG (IgG1–IgG4), all of which are monomers.

4. **Immunoglobulin E (IgE)**
   a. **Function.** IgE is found in trace amounts (0.004%) in the serum. It is primarily found in tissues of the spleen, tonsils, and adenoids and in mucosal membranes of the lungs and gastrointestinal tract. Bound to antigens, it elicits many allergic responses by inducing mast cells to release histamines. It is involved in providing immunity in mucosal membranes and to intestinal parasites.

    b. Structure. IgE is a monomer.

5. Immunoglobulin A (IgA)
    a. Function. IgA is abundant in secretions such as saliva and tears, as well as in secretions of the respiratory and intestinal tract. It provides an early defense against infection by binding pathogens and preventing them from adhering to tissues and colonizing. It also makes them susceptible to removal by phagocytosis.
    b. Structure. There are two subtypes of IgA (IgA1 and IgA2). IgAs can exist as a monomer, dimer, or trimer. The monomeric subunits are joined by disulfide bonds at the COOH-terminal ends of the H chains as well as by disulfide bonds to a J chain. The dimers are the predominant secreted form. A polypeptide in the secretion of IgA, called **secretory component,** is bound to the dimer by disulfide bonds.

D. **Antibody-deficiency disorders.** The human immune system has far more complex functions than the simple production of antibodies described in this section. Numerous medical problems such as allergic reactions, overproduction of antibodies, and autoimmune diseases can arise from a malfunctioning immune system. Several disorders also lead to a deficiency in antibody production, such as:

1. Infantile X-linked (Bruton's) agammaglobulinemia
    a. Symptoms. Patients present after 5-6 months of age with severe, recurrent bacterial infections.
    b. Molecular basis of the disorder. Bruton's agammaglobulinemia is a recessive trait linked to the X chromosome. The maturation of pre–B-cells in the bone marrow to circulating B cells, which can produce IgM, is blocked in patients with this disorder. These patients have low levels of all five classes of antibodies. This disorder presents at 5–6 months of age, which is approximately the time when the infant's supply of maternal IgG is depleted.
    c. Treatment includes regular injection of either antibodies (called gamma globulin because it contains mainly IgG) or fresh frozen plasma. Prophylactic antibiotic treatment is also often necessary.

2. Transient hypogammaglobulinemia of infancy
    a. Symptoms. At 5–6 months of age, patients present with recurrent bacterial infections.
    b. Molecular basis of the disorder. The cause of the disorder is unknown, but the infants show a delayed production of IgG between 5–6 months of age, when a decrease of maternal IgG levels occurs.
    c. Treatment includes injections of gamma globulin and antibiotics.

3. Selective IgA deficiency
    a. Symptoms. Selective IgA deficiency is the most common immunodeficiency disorder. Patients can be symptom free or can suffer recurrent sinopulmonary infections and gastrointestinal problems, such as diarrhea and malabsorption.
    b. Molecular basis of the disorder. Selective IgA deficiency is a genetic disorder that occurs in 0.1%–0.2% of Caucasians. The B cells of patients with this disorder are unable to mature to plasma cells, which produce IgA. Serum levels of all other classes of antibodies are normal in these patients.
    c. Treatment includes antibiotics as necessary. Gamma globulin, which may contain IgA, should not be given to these patients. The patient could develop antibodies to IgA because they do not normally have it in their circulation and potentially go into anaphylactic shock.

V. **COLLAGEN.** Many **structural proteins** such as elastin, which forms ligaments, the keratins, which form hair, fibrin, which forms blood clots (see Chapter 4 VII), and collagen, which is the body's major framework protein, are rod-shaped, fibrous proteins that are insoluble in water. Of the fibrous structural proteins, collagen is the most abundant. In fact, collagen is the most abundant of all the human proteins: A 150-pound human contains 25–30 pounds of protein, of which 13–15 pounds is collagen.

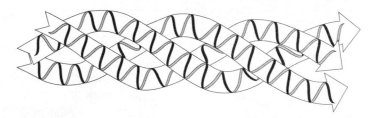

FIGURE 3-8. Right-handed collagen triple helix formed from three left-handed alpha (α)-chain helices.

A. **Function.** Collagen is found in all tissues and organs, where it serves as the major extracellular structural protein. Collagen is not a single protein of one structural form; rather, it is a class of proteins of which there are at least 12 types. These diverse types provide the variability in physical properties that is required of different tissues.

B. **Basic structure of type I collagen.** Type I collagen was the first collagen type to be structurally described. Its basic triple-helix structure is the prototype for most collagen types. The other types of collagen differ from type I collagen in the length of their triple helix and the presence or absence of globular domains at their amino- or carboxyl-terminal ends.

1. **Amino acid composition and sequence**
    a. **Amino acids.** Collagen has a unique amino acid composition with 33% of the total residues being glycine (Gly), 10% proline (Pro), 10% hydroxyproline (Hyp), and 1% hydroxylysine (Hyl).
    b. **Composition.** The basic structural unit of collagen is **tropocollagen,** which is crosslinked to form large fibers of collagenous tissues. Tropocollagen is made of three polypeptide chains called α chains, each of which is made of 1050 amino acids.
    c. **Sequence.** Every third amino acid in the α chain is a glycine. Sixty percent of the α chains are made of either the sequence Gly-Pro-X or the sequence Gly-X-Hyp, where X may be any amino acid. The remaining forty percent of the α chains are various sequences of amino acids, with every third amino acid being a glycine.

2. **Structure of tropocollagen**
    a. **Each α chain forms a left-handed helix,** where every third amino acid repeat makes one turn of the helix. This helix is unlike the typical α helix (see Chapter 2 IV B 3; Figure 2-2) in that there is no intrachain peptide hydrogen bonding.
        (1) Synthetic peptides made only of proline form a similar structure.
        (2) These polyproline helices and the α chains that form tropocollagen may be stabilized by steric repulsion of the pyrrolidine rings of the proline residues.
    b. The three α chains wind around each other to form a tight, right-handed triple helix (Figure 3-8).
    c. The triple-helical structure of collagen is such that only a Gly, with its small hydrogen side chain, can fit into the central region of the helix. This is why every third amino acid must be glycine.
    d. Interchain hydrogen bonding between glycine's NH group in the peptide bond and the carbonyl (C=O) groups of amino acids in adjacent peptides stabilizes the triple-helical structure.

C. **Biosynthesis.** An overview of the multistep process leading to the formation of mature collagen is shown in Figure 3-9.

1. **Synthesis on the endoplasmic reticulum (ER).** Like all proteins that are destined to be secreted, the translation of the collagen α-chain mRNAs takes place on the rough ER (see Chapter 10 VII B).

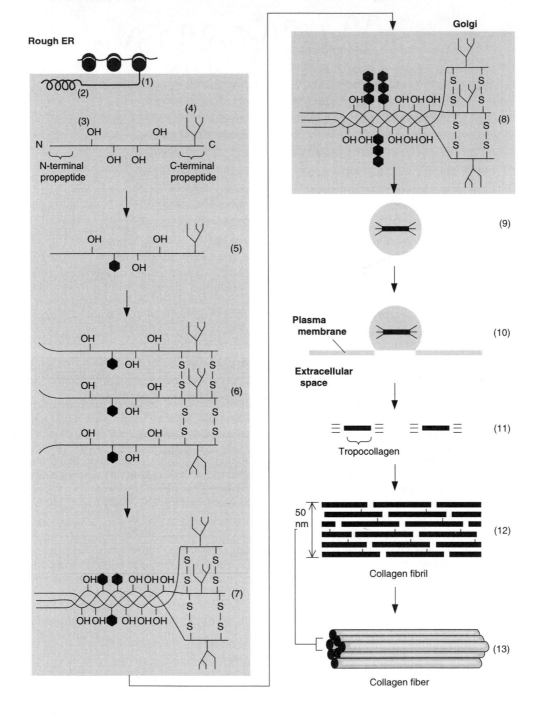

FIGURE 3-9. Synthesis and formation of mature collagen. *(1)* Synthesis and entry of preprocollagen into lumen of rough endoplasmic reticulum (ER). *(2)* Cleavage of signal peptide to form procollagen. *(3)* Hydroxylation of selected proline and lysine residues. *(4)* Addition of N-linked oligosaccharides. *(5)* Initial glycosylation of hydroxylysine residues. *(6)* Chain alignment and formation of disulfide bonds. *(7)* Formation of triple-helical procollagen. *(8)* Completion of O-linked oligosaccharide chains. *(9)* Transport vesicle. *(10)* Exocytosis. *(11)* Removal of N- and C-terminal propeptides. *(12)* Lateral association of collagen molecules followed by covalent cross-linking. *(13)* Aggregation of fibrils. (Reprinted with permission from Darnell J, Lodish H, Baltimore D: *Molecular Cell Biology,* 2nd ed. New York, Scientific American Books, 1990, p 911.)

    a. The earliest α chains formed are in the preprocollagen form. The "pre" prefix in this nomenclature refers to the signal peptide sequences, which direct the translation of the α-chain mRNAs to the ER.

    b. Propeptides. In addition to the signal peptide sequences, there are 150 residues at the N-terminus and 250 amino acids at the C-terminus that are required for proper collagen assembly, but they are removed on conversion of procollagen to collagen. These sequences are called propeptides.

2. Post-translational processing in the lumen of the ER. Post-translational processing of the α-chain preprocollagen polypeptides must take place within the lumen of the ER before they can properly associate and assemble into a triple helical form.

    a. Removal of the signal peptide. One of the first events after the newly translated preprocollagen α chains enter the lumen of the ER is the removal of their signal peptide sequences by **signal peptidase.** This converts the preprocollagen form of the α chains to the procollagen form.

    b. Hydroxylation of proline and lysine residues. A subset of particular proline and lysine residues in the region where triple-helix formation occurs is hydroxylated before assembly can take place.

        (1) Three enzymes are required for proper hydroxylation of procollagen.

            (a) Lysyl hydroxylase converts lysines in the sequence X-Lys-Gly to 5-hydroxylysine.

            (b) Prolyl-4-hydroxylase converts prolines in the sequence X-Pro-Gly to 4-hydroxyproline.

            (c) Prolyl-3-hydroxylase converts prolines in the sequence Hyp-Pro-Gly to 3-hydroxyproline.

        (2) These hydroxylation reactions require **Fe^{2+}, ascorbic acid (vitamin C), oxygen, and α-ketoglutarate** in the reaction:

$$\text{AA residue} + \text{Ascorbic acid} + O_2 + \alpha\text{-Ketoglutarate}$$
$$\textit{Hydroxylase} \rightarrow \text{Hydroxy-AA} + \text{Succinate}$$

    c. Glycosylation. In addition to hydroxylation reactions, the formation of stable triple helices requires glycosylation.

        (1) Galactose residues are removed from uridine diphosphate (UDP)-galactose and added to specific hydroxylysyl residues by galactosyl transferase.

        (2) Glucose residues are removed from UDP-glucose and added to some of these modified hydroxylysyl residues by glucosyl transferase.

        (3) N-linked glycosylation takes place on certain asparagines in the C-terminal propeptide.

    d. Formation of disulfide bonds. Oxidation of cysteine residues to form intrachain and interchain disulfide bonds in the propeptides takes place before triple helix formation. The correct interchain disulfide bonds in the C-terminal propeptides must be formed for correct alignment of the α chains before triple helix formation.

    e. Formation of triple helix. A triple helix forms between α chains on the completion of disulfide bond formation, glycosylation, and hydroxylation. After completion of triple helix formation, the procollagen is transported to the Golgi body.

    f. Post-translational processing in the Golgi complex and export from the cell. In the Golgi complex, O-linked glycosylation is completed, and the procollagen molecules are packaged into transport vesicles for export from the cell.

3. Extracellular processing

    a. Formation of tropocollagen. On secretion of procollagen, the N- and C-terminal propeptides are removed by procollagen peptidases to form tropocollagen. For each form of collagen there is a set of peptidases—one for each end—to remove the propeptides.

    b. Collagen fibril and fiber formation. The newly formed tropocollagen molecules self assemble into collagen fibrils. Each tropocollagen associates in a parallel,

staggered array with four other tropocollagens to form a **collagen fibril.** These fibrils are then packed together to form **collagen fibers.**
  c. **Collagen maturation.** Intra- and intermolecular cross-links of tropocollagen form with time, resulting in a slow maturation of collagen.
    (1) **Cross-links** can occur between aldehydes of lysine or hydroxylysine. Aldehydes of lysine and hydroxylysine are formed by the enzyme **lysyl oxidase.**

$$
\begin{array}{ccc}
\overset{|}{NH} & & \overset{|}{NH} \\
\overset{|}{HC}-(CH_2)_3-CH_2-NH_3^+ & \xrightarrow[\substack{O_2}]{\substack{Lysyl \\ oxidase \\ +Cu^{++}}} & \overset{|}{HC}-(CH_2)_3-C\overset{\diagup O}{\diagdown H} \\
\overset{|}{CO} & & \overset{|}{CO}
\end{array}
$$

    (2) **Covalent aldol cross-links,** which give mature collagen some of its tensile strength, can then form between these aldehydes. These cross-links are made slowly but continuously throughout life. As the number of cross-links increase, collagen begins to lose some of its elasticity, an unfortunate side effect of aging.

$$
\begin{array}{ccc}
\overset{|}{NH} & & \overset{|}{NH} \\
\overset{|}{HC}-(CH_2)_3-\overset{H}{C}=C-(CH_2)_2-\overset{|}{CH} & & \\
\overset{|}{CO} & & \overset{|}{CO}
\end{array}
$$

D. **Disorders related to collagen metabolism**

  1. **Scurvy** is a nutritional disorder caused by a deficiency in ascorbic acid (vitamin C). It arises in bottle-fed babies whose milk is not supplemented with vitamin C and in people who are on fad diets that are deficient in vitamin C.
    a. **Symptoms** include:
      (1) Abnormal bone development in infants and children
      (2) Easy bruising and bleeding due to fragile capillaries
      (3) Loosening of teeth and swollen gums
      (4) Poor wound healing
      (5) Osteoporosis
    b. **Molecular basis of the disorder.** Because vitamin C plays an important role in metabolic processes other than collagen metabolism, its effects are not strictly confined to deficiencies in proper collagen formation.
      (1) Vitamin C plays a role in collagen metabolism by acting as a cofactor in the enzymatic reactions involved in the hydroxylation of proline and lysine (see V C 2 b).
      (2) Without the hydroxylation of lysine and proline, proper aligned stable helices of the α chains are not formed, so the procollagen that is formed is unstable and degraded.
      (3) A deficiency in collagen arises, which results in many of the symptoms of scurvy.
    c. **Prevention and treatment.** Daily ingestion of vitamin C from fresh fruits and vegetables should prevent scurvy. If a person's diet is such that scurvy develops, vitamin C supplementation serves as the treatment.

TABLE 3-2. Identified Defects of Some Types of Ehlers-Danlos Syndrome

Type	Defect	Major Symptom
IV	Autosomal dominant defect resulting in a deficiency or structural alteration in type III procollagen	Easily ruptured arteries and internal viscera; thin skin but no hyperelasticity of skin or joints
VI	Autosomal recessive lysyl hydroxylase deficiency	Scoliosis; hyperextensible, soft, velvety skin; hypermobile joints; prone to ocular injury
VII	Autosomal dominant mutation that leads to deficient removal of the N-terminal propeptide, resulting in tissue accumulation of propeptide	Hypermobile joints, prone to joint dislocations; soft skin
IX	X-linked recessive deficiency in lysyl oxidase, resulting in decreased cross-linking of collagen	Soft, hyperextensible skin; bladder diverticulae; skeletal deformities

2. **Osteogenesis imperfecta** is a genetic disorder resulting in structurally weak bones and skeletal deformities. There are many different types of osteogenesis imperfecta, each of which is caused by a different genetic defect.
   a. **Symptoms.** Depending on the specific defect, the symptoms of osteogenesis imperfecta can vary in their severity. In all cases there is a weakening of the bones, which in milder cases leads to crippling deformities and in the most severe cases results in death in utero or shortly after birth.
   b. **Molecular basis of the disorder.** Osteogenesis imperfecta arises from mutations in either the $\alpha1(I)$ or $\alpha2(I)$ genes, which produce the α chains of type I collagen. Known mutations range from shortened α chains to single glycine mutations. These mutations can lead to improperly formed, unstable procollagen helices, which become degraded or cannot be exported from the ER. The importance of a glycine in every third position of type I collagen is demonstrated by the fact that glycine substitutions often lead to the most severe forms of this disorder. Because there are two $\alpha1(I)$ chains in type I collagen, mutations in this gene are usually more severe than in the $\alpha2(I)$ gene.
   c. **Treatment.** There is currently no treatment for osteogenesis imperfecta beyond bracing and other orthopedic repair.

3. **Ehlers-Danlos syndrome** is a group of connective tissue disorders of which there are at least 10 known types (Table 3-2). Most are genetic disorders.
   a. **Symptoms.** In Ehlers-Danlos syndrome, an inherited weakness of connective tissue leads to symptoms such as hyperextensibility of skin and joints; deformities; laxity in the musculoskeletal system; and thin, fragile skin.
   b. **Molecular basis of the disorders.** Each of the different types of Ehlers-Danlos syndrome results in different mutations that affect some component essential for proper collagen formation. The known defects are listed in Table 3-2.
   c. **Treatment.** Most of the different types of Ehlers-Danlos syndrome are genetic disorders for which there are currently no treatments.
      (1) However, in **type VI,** some patients have a mutant form of lysyl hydroxylase, which has an increased Michaelis constant (K_m) for ascorbic acid, and these patients respond to therapy with ascorbic acid.
      (2) It is also possible to mimic type V through reduced levels of copper, which is required for lysyl hydroxylase activity. The drug D-penicillamine binds copper and can generate the side effect of hyperextensible skin.

VI. **MUSCLE CONTRACTION** is made possible by both globular and fibrous proteins.

A. **Muscle morphology.** Striated muscles are made of bundles of highly specialized cells that are capable of contraction (Figure 3-10). The striated appearance arises because of the near-perfect alignment of the contractile units within muscle cells, which are called **muscle fibers.**

1. **Muscle fibers.** Each muscle fiber is a single, large, multinucleate (i.e., syncytial) cell.
   a. **Myoblasts.** Developmentally, muscle fibers arise from the fusion of many single-nucleate cells called myoblasts.
   b. **Myofibrils.** Muscle fibers are made of many separate myofibrils, each of which is 1–2 μm in diameter.
   c. **Sarcolemma. The plasma membrane of a muscle fiber** is an electrically excitable organelle called the sarcolemma.
   d. **Sarcoplasm.** The **cytoplasm of a muscle** fiber is called the sarcoplasm.
   e. **Sarcoplasmic reticulum.** The ER of muscle cells, the sarcoplasmic reticulum, has evolved into a specialized organelle that plays a key role in the regulation of contraction (see VI C 3). The sarcoplasmic reticulum is connected to the sarcolemma by way of the **transverse (T) tubule.**

2. **Sarcomeres.** Myofibrils consist of repeating units called sarcomeres. The parallel alignment of myofibrils with their sarcomeres in register give muscle fibers a periodic pattern of alternating light and dark bands (i.e., striations) as observed with a light microscope. The molecular structure of sarcomeres and the reasons for striations are described here.
   a. The **A band** refers to the band that appears **dark** through the light microscope.
      (1) Within the A band is a lighter, less dense **H zone.**
      (2) In the middle of this H zone is a darker **M line.**
      (3) The M line is made of **M protein** and joins the fibers that make the A band.
   b. The **I band** refers to the band that appears **light** through the light microscope.
      (1) The I band separates adjacent sarcomeres along a very dark, dense, narrow **Z line,** which demarcates the ends of sarcomeres (i.e., a sarcomere is a Z line-to-Z line repeat).
      (2) The Z line is made of the proteins α-actinin and desmin.
   c. The dark A band is made of **thick filaments** that extend the length of the A band. Thick filaments do not change length (1.6 μm) or width (15 μm) during muscle contraction. The primary component of thick filaments is **myosin.**
   d. **Thin filaments** extend from the Z line, across the I band and through the A band up to the H zone. The thin filaments do not change length (1 μm) or width (7 nm) during contraction. The primary components of thin filaments are **actin, tropomyosin,** and **troponin.**
   e. **Thick and thin filaments overlap** and interact in the A band.
      (1) The region in which thick and thin filaments overlap is the **darkest portion of the A band** as seen with a light microscope.
      (2) The **H zone** is the portion of the A band where there is **no overlap** between the thin filaments and the thick filaments. The H zone gets shorter on contraction.
      (3) A cross-sectional view of the A band, where the thick and thin filaments overlap, shows a **precisely ordered array of filaments** (see Figure 3-10). Each thick filament is surrounded by six thin filaments, and each thin filament is likewise surrounded by three thick filaments.
      (4) **Cross-bridges** can occasionally be seen through an electron microscope connecting thick and thin filaments in the overlap region.

B. **Molecular components of the contractile unit**

1. **Thick filaments.** The primary component of thick filaments is **myosin,** of which

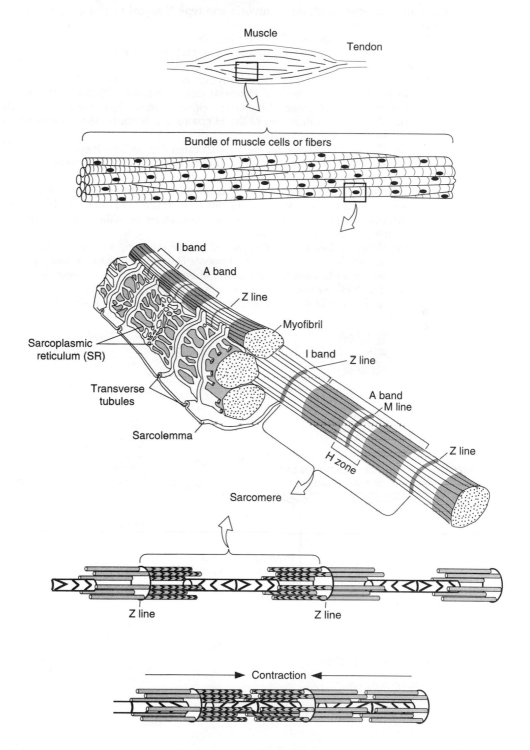

FIGURE 3-10. Muscle structure and organization showing the sliding filament model of contraction. (Adapted from Alberts B et al: *Molecular Biology of the Cell,* 2nd ed. New York, Garland Publishing, 1989, p 615; and Darnell J, Lodish H, Baltimore D: *Molecular Cell Biology,* 2nd ed. New York, Scientific American Books, 1990, pp 866, 871.)

there are two types: Both **type I myosin** and **type II myosin** participate in cellular movement processes.

a. Type I myosin is not found in muscle cells.

b. Type II myosin is required for muscle contraction, but it can also be found in nonmuscle cells.

    (1) Structure (Figure 3-11). Type II myosin is a large protein (470,000 MW) that contains two identical H chains (approximately 230,000 MW each) and two pairs of different L chains (approximately 18,000 and 20,000 MW).

        (a) The NH_2-terminal end of the H chains is a globular structure to which the L chains are bound.

        (b) The two H chains are attached through the coiling of each of their α-helical tails around each other to form what is called a **coiled-coil structure.**

    (2) Function. Type II myosin can be digested with different proteases (e.g., trypsin, papain) to yield separate regions (see Figure 3-11) that exhibit different activities. Type II myosin exhibits three separate activities that are important structurally and functionally.

        (a) When isolated myosin is placed at a physiologic salt concentration, it aggregates to form a thick filament. This **self-assembly activity lies solely within the COOH-terminal end region** of the myosin molecule.

        (b) The **NH_2-terminal, globular ends of myosin can bind to filamentous (F) actin** (see VI B 2 a). The cross bridges between thick and thin filaments,

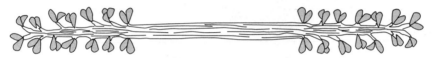

Thick filament

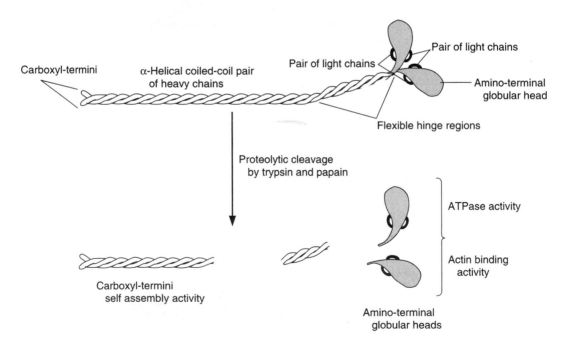

Carboxyl-termini

α-Helical coiled-coil pair of heavy chains

Pair of light chains

Pair of light chains

Amino-terminal globular head

Flexible hinge regions

Proteolytic cleavage by trypsin and papain

Carboxyl-termini self assembly activity

ATPase activity

Actin binding activity

Amino-terminal globular heads

FIGURE 3-11. Structure and regions of type II myosin. The thick filament is made of hundreds of myosin molecules. ATPase = adenosine triphosphatase. (Adapted with permission from Warrick HM, Spudich J: *Ann Rev Cell Bio* 3:379, 1987; and Pollard T: *The Journal of Cell Biology,* 1981, Vol 91, p 156 by copyright permission of The Rockefeller University Press.)

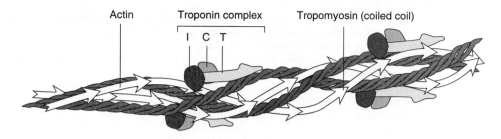

Actin   Troponin complex   Tropomyosin (coiled coil)

I   C   T

Thin filament

FIGURE 3-12. Organization of thin filaments.

seen in the A band, result from the binding of the myosin amino-terminal head groups to the actin of thin filaments.
- (c) The **amino-terminal, globular ends of myosin exhibit adenosine triphosphatase (ATPase) activity,** which is enhanced 200-fold by actin. Actin specifically enhances the rate at which myosin head groups release the products of adenosine triphosphate (ATP) hydrolysis, adenosine diphosphate (ADP), and inorganic phosphate (P_i). The products of this catalysis must be released before more substrate ATP can be bound.

$$ATP + H_2O \rightarrow ADP + P_i + H^+$$

2. **Thin filaments.** The primary components of thin filaments are actin, tropomyosin, and the troponins (Figure 3-12).
   a. **Actin**
      (1) **Structure**
         (a) Actin is a polymer of globular-shaped subunits (called **G actin**), which are 43,000 MW in size. One molecule of ATP is bound to each G actin.
         (b) At physiologic salt concentrations, G actin polymerizes to form filaments of actin called F actin, which is a helical structure of linked G-actin molecules.
         (c) The hydrolysis of **ATP** on conversion of G actin to F actin is not essential for polymerization. It serves to increase the rate of formation of F actin. The ADP that is formed remains bound to, and stabilizes, F actin.
         (d) **Polarity.** If globular head groups of myosin bound to F actin [see VI B 1 b (2) (b)] are viewed with an electron microscope, a structure is seen resembling linked arrowheads that are aligned in the same direction. This observation indicates there is a polarity to F actin. Polarity is important to the directionality of contraction.
      (2) **Function.** Actin is one of the most abundant proteins in the cell. It is the major structural component of microfilaments, which are part of the cytoskeleton. In association with other proteins (e.g., myosin), actin plays a major role in many types of cellular movement processes, including muscle contraction.
         (a) There are at least six forms of actin, called **isoforms,** which have small sequence differences.
         (b) Actin isoforms are involved in **different contractile functions.** For instance, in striated muscles there is a type of actin that differs from the type found in heart muscle, which differs from several types found in smooth muscles and several other types found in nonmuscle cells.
   b. **Tropomyosin**
      (1) **Structure**

  (a) Tropomyosin is made of two subunit polypeptides, α and β, which are twisted around each other to form a rod-shaped coiled-coil structure with a molecular weight of 66,000.
  (b) Tropomyosin molecules lie end-to-end in a helical groove of the actin filament (see Figure 3-12).
  (c) There is one tropomyosin molecule for every seven actin monomers.
 (2) Function. Tropomyosin plays an integral role in contraction by regulating the interaction of actin and myosin.
 c. Troponin
  (1) Structure. Troponin is a 73,000 MW complex of three polypeptides: **troponin T, troponin I,** and **troponin C.** There is one troponin complex for every tropomyosin.
  (2) Function. The troponin complex in conjunction with tropomyosin mediates the regulation of contraction by calcium (see VI C 3). Each polypeptide of the troponin complex exhibits a different activity that is essential to the overall function of the complex.
  (a) Troponin T binds to tropomyosin.
  (b) Troponin I binds to actin.
  (c) Troponin C binds to calcium.

C. **Mechanism of contraction**

 1. The **sliding filament model** describes mechanistically the contraction of muscles (see Figure 3-10).
  a. Each sarcomere of a myofibril shortens when the thin filaments "slide" across the thick filaments.
  b. Both thin and thick filaments exhibit polarity. The thick filaments are bipolar. The oppositely oriented thin filaments, which surround each end of the thick filaments, move across the thick filaments pulling the Z discs of each sarcomere closer together.
  c. Shortening all the sarcomeres can result in a significant reduction in the length of myofibrils.

 2. Basic contraction reaction (Figure 3-13). Contraction can be described as a cycle of four basic steps.
  a. Myosin, with the bound products of ATP hydrolysis, ADP, and P_i, diffuses and makes contact with actin. The P_i is lost upon initial binding, and **myosin** then **binds tightly to actin.**
  b. The tight binding of myosin to actin induces a **conformational change in myosin,** which with actin bound to myosin results in a pulling of actin across the thick filament. ADP is released, accompanying the change in conformation of myosin.
  c. If ATP is present, it binds to myosin, which causes the **release of myosin from actin.**
  d. Myosin then hydrolyzes ATP to ADP and P_i and resumes a conformation in which it is free to bind actin. The cycle then continues as long as regulatory calcium (see VI C 3) and ATP are present. (ATP is required for the release of myosin and actin binding. If ATP is depleted, as it is upon death, myosin remains bound to actin, and **rigor mortis** takes place.)

 3. Regulation of contraction. The key regulatory molecule of contraction in striated muscles is **calcium.**
  a. In the **absence of calcium,** tropomyosin lies in the groove of the actin helix in such a way that the myosin-ADP-P_i complex cannot bind.
  b. When calcium is present, it binds to troponin C, which causes a conformational change in the whole troponin–tropomyosin complex. This results in the tropomyosin moving away from the myosin binding site on actin, which allows myosin to bind and contraction to proceed.
  c. In **resting muscle,** calcium is sequestered in the **sarcoplasmic reticulum.**

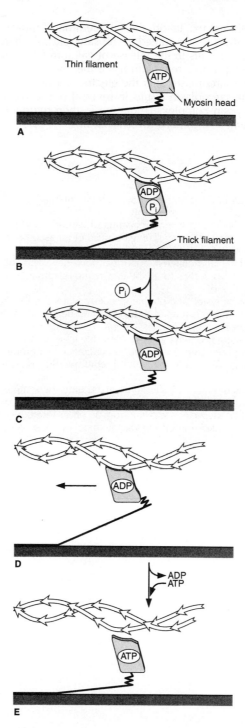

FIGURE 3-13. Basic steps of muscle contraction. In *A,* the bound adenosine triphosphate (ATP) hydro-lyzes to adenosine diphosphate (ADP) and inorganic phosphate (Pᵢ), which in *B* remain associated with the myosin head. The myosin head releases Pᵢ and binds tightly to the actin filament *(C).* The myosin head undergoes a large conformational change, which creates the "powerstroke" *(D).* ADP is then released, and ATP binds to the myosin head, which causes it to reduce its affinity for actin *(E).* The cycle can then begin again.

(1) On electrical excitation, the sarcolemma of muscles is depolarized. This **depolarization** is transmitted to the sarcoplasmic reticulum by way of the T tubules and results in the release of calcium from the sarcoplasmic reticulum.

(2) The sarcoplasmic reticulum has a **membrane enzyme** that removes calcium from the sarcoplasm after the electric impulse is fired. Removal of calcium from the sarcoplasm results in reversal of the conformation of the troponin–tropomyosin complex. Tropomyosin then returns to the groove of the actin helix, where it inhibits myosin binding.

Case 3-1 Revisited

The fact that this patient is an indigent street person with an enlarged liver indicates that he is likely a chronic alcoholic. (It is not uncommon for chronic alcoholics to have enlarged, fatty livers, possibly with cirrhosis and alcoholic hepatitis.) The poor healing of wounds, oral problems, and other skin lesions are consistent with the patient having scurvy because of an ascorbic acid (vitamin C) deficiency. Other symptoms of vitamin C deficiency include easy bruising and bleeding because of fragile capillaries, osteoporosis, and, in infants and children, abnormal bone development. Vitamin C plays a role in collagen metabolism by acting as a cofactor in the enzymatic reactions involved in the hydroxylation of proline and lysine (see V C 2 b).

Without the hydroxylation of lysine and proline, properly aligned stable helices of the α chains are not formed, so the procollagen that is formed is unstable and degraded. A deficiency in collagen arises after long-term deprivation of vitamin C (i.e., 4–7 months), which results in many of the symptoms of scurvy. However, because vitamin C plays an important role in other metabolic processes besides collagen metabolism, its effects are not strictly confined to deficiencies in proper collagen formation.

If scurvy is the correct diagnosis, a follow-up blood report would reveal little-to-undetectable vitamin C in the plasma.

Large, multiple daily doses of vitamin C should be given until the symptoms of scurvy disappear. Daily ingestion of vitamin C from fresh fruits and vegetables prevents scurvy. Chronic alcoholics often have a poor diet, and many of their calories come from alcohol. Vitamin deficiencies are not uncommon. A recurrence of scurvy is likely unless the chronic alcohol abuse is stopped.

STUDY QUESTIONS

DIRECTIONS: Each of the numbered items or incomplete statements in this section is followed by answers or by completions of the statement. Select the **one** lettered answer or completion that is **best** in each case.

1. Which one of the following statements about oxygen binding and release by hemoglobin is correct?

(A) On binding oxygen, the iron of the heme prosthetic group is oxidized to the ferric state

(B) Lowering the pH accelerates the release of oxygen from oxyhemoglobin

(C) A high concentration of 2,3-bisphosphoglycerate in the erythrocyte enhances the binding of oxygen by hemoglobin

(D) Oxygen binding by any one of the four heme groups occurs independently of the other three

(E) The formation of carbamate decreases the proton concentration

2. What effect does hyperventilation have on the oxygen binding affinity of hemoglobin?

(A) P_{50} and oxygen affinity decrease

(B) P_{50} and oxygen affinity increase

(C) P_{50} decreases and the oxygen affinity increases

(D) P_{50} increases and the oxygen affinity decreases

(E) P_{50} and oxygen affinity remain the same

3. Sulfonamides may lead to kernicterus in infants by displacing a molecule that is normally bound to albumin; that is,

(A) copper

(B) testosterone

(C) fatty acids

(D) bilirubin

(E) bile acid

4. Which one of the following substances is involved in the formation of hydroxyproline and hydroxylysine during collagen synthesis?

(A) Pyridoxal phosphate (vitamin B_6)

(B) Biotin

(C) Thiamine pyrophosphate (vitamin B_1)

(D) Ascorbic acid (vitamin C)

(E) Methylcobalamin (vitamin B_{12})

5. A deficiency of copper affects the formation of normal collagen by reducing the activity of

(A) glucosyl transferase

(B) galactosyl transferase

(C) prolyl hydroxylase

(D) lysyl hydroxylase

(E) lysyl oxidase

6. The antibody class that can pass through the placenta to protect the fetus is

(A) immunoglobulin A (IgA)

(B) immunoglobulin G (IgG)

(C) immunoglobulin M (IgM)

(D) immunoglobulin D (IgD)

(E) immunoglobulin E (IgE)

7. The primary component(s) of thin filaments include which one of the following?

(A) Actin

(B) Myosin

(C) Tropomyosin and myosin

(D) Actin, tropomyosin, and troponin

(E) Myosin and M protein

8. Which one of the following does not change length during muscle contraction?

(A) The A band

(B) The I band

(C) The H zone

(D) The sarcomere

(E) The myofibril

DIRECTIONS: The group of items in this section consists of lettered options followed by a set of numbered items. For each item, select the **one** lettered option that is most closely associated with it. Each lettered option may be selected once, more than once, or not at all.

Questions 9-12

Match the following disorders with the correct molecular basis of the disorder.

(A) Absence of a subunit
(B) Single amino acid mutation leading to a structural change
(C) Short halflife of protein
(D) Deficiency in processing enzyme
(E) Absence of specialized cells

9. Infantile X-linked (Bruton's) agammaglobulinemia

10. Ehlers-Danlos syndrome type V

11. Hemoglobin C (Hb C)

12. Hemoglobin H (Hb H) disease

ANSWERS AND EXPLANATIONS

1. The answer is B [II B 3 b (2)]. The iron in heme must be in the ferrous state to bind oxygen reversibly. On binding oxygen, the iron does not change its valence. A reduction in pH, such as occurs at the tissues relative to the lung, enhances the release of oxygen from oxyhemoglobin. This is the Bohr effect. The formation of carbamate increases the proton concentration. The binding of 2,3-bisphosphoglycerate to hemoglobin increases the stability of the deoxy form, thus promoting the unloading of oxygen. Oxygen binding by hemoglobin exhibits cooperativity with the binding of oxygen to the first heme iron, facilitating the binding of oxygen by the other three heme iron molecules.

2. The answer is C [II B 3 b]. The Bohr effect describes the relationship of hemoglobin's oxygen affinity to P_{CO_2} levels and pH. As proton or CO_2 levels increase, there is a rightward shift in the oxygen-binding curve of hemoglobin. A rightward shift means there is an increase in the P_{50} and likewise a decrease in the oxygen-binding affinity of hemoglobin. The reverse is true as proton levels or CO_2 levels decline, which happens during hyperventilation. This means hemoglobin binds oxygen more tightly and releases less oxygen in the tissues.

3. The answer is D [III C]. Albumin binds to a wide variety of drugs including the sulfonamides. The binding site on albumin of the sulfonamides is the same as the binding site of bilirubin. This means that in high doses the sulfonamides can cause the release of bound bilirubin. If too much free unconjugated bilirubin is present in the bloodstream of infants, they may develop kernicterus.

4. The answer is D [V C 2 b]. The enzymes prolyl-3-hydroxylase, prolyl-4-hydroxylase, and lysyl hydroxylase form 3-hydroxyproline, 4-hydroxyproline, and 5-hydroxylysine, respectively, from proline and lysine residues in procollagen molecules as they pass through the lumen of the endoplasmic reticulum during synthesis. Ascorbic acid (vitamin C) is required by these hydroxylases, possibly to

keep the essential iron component of the system in the reduced state. The reaction also requires molecular oxygen and α-ketoglutarate, but none of the other vitamin-derived cofactors listed (vitamins B_1, B_6, B_{12}, and biotin) are involved.

5. The answer is E [V C 3 c (1), D 3 c (2)]. After tropocollagen is secreted from the cell, and the nonhelical NH_2 and COOH-terminal regions are proteolytically removed, a number of intermolecular cross-links are gradually formed to produce mature collagen. Only one enzymatic reaction is involved, the oxidative deamination of lysyl and hydroxylysyl residues to yield aldehydes. The enzyme involved is lysyl oxidase, which requires copper and molecular oxygen. A deficit of lysyl oxidase activity can result from poisoning with β-aminopropionitrile (found in sweet pea seeds), from a copper-deficient diet, or from therapy with D-penicillamine, a chelator of copper. Copper deficiencies do not influence the activity of the glucosyl or galactosyl transferases or the prolyl or lysyl hydroxylases, all of which act on tropocollagen while it is still intracellular (i.e., in the lumen of the endoplasmic reticulum), whereas lysyl oxidase activity is extracellular.

6. The answer is B [IV C 3 a]. Immunoglobulin G (IgG) is the major serum antibody of adults, and it is the only maternal antibody that can pass through the placenta to protect the fetus. Immunoglobulin A (IgA) is abundant in saliva, tears, and secretions of the respiratory and intestinal tract. Immunoglobulin M (IgM) is the first antibody produced by B cells when an immune response is elicited. It is accordingly the first and most abundantly produced antibody of the fetus. The function of immunoglobulin D (IgD) is controversial. Immunoglobulin E (IgE) is responsible for eliciting allergic responses, and it is involved in providing immunity in mucosal membranes and against intestinal parasites.

7. The answer is D [VI A 2 d, B 2]. The primary components of thin filaments are actin, tropomyosin, and troponin. Actin forms the primary structure of thin filaments. Tropomyosin lies in a helical groove in the actin filament. Troponin is a complex of three polypeptides: troponin T, which binds to tropomyosin; troponin I, which binds to actin; and troponin C, which binds to the contraction regulatory molecule, calcium. The primary component of thick filaments is myosin. M protein joins thick filaments at the middle of a sarcomere.

8. The answer is A [VI A 2 a, e]. The A band is made of thick filaments, and it does not shorten on contraction. The I band is the portion of the thin filaments that does not overlap with the thick filaments. Although the thin filaments themselves do not change length on contraction, they slide across the thick filaments. This movement increases the degree of overlap and decreases the length of the region that did not overlap before contraction. The H zone is the central area of the A band in which there is no overlap of thin and thick filaments. The length of the H zone must decrease as the thin filaments slide over the thick filaments during contraction. The sarcomere is the repeating structural unit of myofibrils that shortens on contraction.

9-12. The answers are: 9E [IV D 1], **10D** [V D 3; Table 3-2], **11B** [II B 4 b (2)], **12A** [II B 4 c (2)(c)]. Infantile X-linked (Bruton's) agammaglobulinemia appears in infants older than 5 months of age. Infants with Bruton's agammaglobulinemia are deficient in all classes of antibodies because the pre-B-cells in their bone marrow fail to mature to circulating B cells, which are specialized antibody-producing cells.

Ehlers-Danlos syndrome is a group of connective tissue disorders. Individuals affected with type V have a deficiency in lysyl oxidase, which is a collagen-processing enzyme that cross-links collagen. These cross-links provide mature collagen with much of its tensile strength.

Hemoglobin C (Hb C) is the second most common hemoglobinopathy in the United States. It results from a glutamate to lysine change at position 6 of β-globin, which structurally changes the Hb C subunits so that they crystallize in the red blood cells.

Hemoglobin H (Hb H) disease is an α-thalassemia in which the patients have a deficient expression of three α-globin genes. This leads to a significant absence of α globins and therefore low levels of Hb A_1.

Many diseases lead to a short halflife of particular proteins, which may often be a secondary result of the defect. For instance, Hb S has a short halflife only because the altered structure of sickle-cell-shaped red blood cells leads to their rapid turnover. Also, in osteogenesis imperfecta, mutations in different α chains lead to improperly formed collagen that is unstable in the body.

Chapter 4

Enzymes
Victor Davidson and Donald Sittman

Case 4-1

A 60-year-old man is admitted to the hospital with complaints of severe chest pain and difficulty breathing. A blood sample is taken, and his serum levels of certain enzymes and isozyme patterns are determined. Analysis reveals high levels of the MB isozyme of creatine kinase (CK-MB) relative to other CK isozymes. Analysis of lactate dehydrogenase (LDH) isozymes indicates that serum levels of the H-containing isozymes, particularly H_4, are elevated such that the H_4: H_3M ratio was greater than 1.

- What is the diagnosis for this patient?
- Are there alternative explanations for these isozyme patterns?

I. GENERAL CHARACTERISTICS OF ENZYMES

A. Biologic catalysts

1. **Shared properties with chemical catalysts**
   a. Enzymes are neither consumed nor produced during the course of a reaction.
   b. Enzymes do not cause reactions to take place, but they greatly enhance the rate of reactions that would proceed much slower in their absence. They alter the rate but not the equilibrium constants of reactions that they catalyze.

2. **Differences between enzymes and chemical catalysts**
   a. Enzymes are proteins.
   b. Enzymes are highly specific and produce only the expected products from the given reactants, or **substrates** (i.e., there are no side reactions).
   c. Enzymes may show a high specificity toward one substrate or exhibit a broad specificity, using more than one substrate.
   d. Enzymes usually function within a moderate pH and temperature range.

B. Measures of enzyme activity

1. **Specific activity** is usually expressed as μmol of substrate transformed to product per minute per milligram of enzyme under optimal conditions of measurement.

2. **Turnover number,** or k_{cat}, is the number of substrate molecules metabolized per enzyme molecule per unit time with units of min^{-1} or s^{-1}.

C. Enzyme nomenclature

1. Enzymes are divided into **six major classes** with several subclasses (Table 4-1).
   a. **Oxidoreductases** are involved in oxidation and reduction.
   b. **Transferases** transfer functional groups (e.g., amino or phosphate groups).
   c. **Hydrolases** transfer water; that is, they catalyze the hydrolysis of a substrate.
   d. **Lyases** add (or remove) the elements of water, ammonia, or carbon dioxide (CO_2) to (or from) double bonds.
   e. **Isomerases** catalyze rearrangements of atoms within a molecule.
   f. **Ligases** join two molecules.

TABLE 4-1. Six Major Classes of Enzymes and Examples of Their Subclasses

Classification	Distinguishing Feature
Oxidoreductases	
Oxidases	Use oxygen as an electron acceptor but do not incorporate it into the substrate
Dehydrogenases	Use molecules other than oxygen (e.g., NAD^+) as an electron acceptor
Oxygenases	Directly incorporate oxygen into the substrate
Peroxidases	Use H_2O_2 as an electron acceptor
Transferases	
Methyltransferases	Transfer one-carbon units between substrates
Aminotransferases	Transfer NH_2 from amino acids to keto acids
Kinases	Transfer PO_3^- from ATP to a substrate
Phosphorylases	Transfer PO_3^- from inorganic phosphate (P_i) to a substrate
Hydrolases	
Phosphatases	Remove PO_3^- from a substrate
Phosphodiesterases	Cleave phosphodiester bonds such as those in nucleic acids
Proteases	Cleave amide bonds such as those in proteins
Lyases	
Decarboxylases	Produce CO_2 via elimination reactions
Aldolases	Produce aldehydes via elimination reactions
Synthases	Link two molecules without involvement of ATP
Isomerases	
Racemases	Interconvert L and D stereoisomers
Mutases	Transfer groups between atoms within a molecule
Ligases	
Carboxylases	Use CO_2 as a substrate
Synthetases	Link two molecules via an ATP-dependent reaction

ATP = adenosine triphosphate; CO_2 = carbon dioxide; H_2O_2 = hydrogen peroxide; NAD^+ = oxidized nicotinamide adenine dinucleotide; NH_2 = amino group; O_2 = molecular oxygen; PO_3^- = phosphate.

    2. Trivial names (e.g., trypsin, pepsin), which give no indication of the function of the enzyme, are commonly used. In some cases, the trivial names are the names of substrates with the suffix -*ase* added (e.g., carboxypeptidase, ribonuclease).

II. MECHANISM OF ENZYME CATALYSIS

A. Chemical reactions

    1. Free-energy changes that occur during a chemical reaction when the reaction is catalyzed (lower curve) and uncatalyzed (upper curve) are illustrated in Figure 4-1.

    2. Energy of activation is required to sufficiently energize a substrate molecule to reach a **transition state** in which there is a high probability that a chemical bond will be made or broken to form the product. Enzymes increase the rate of reaction by decreasing the energy of activation.

B. Specificity

    1. The specificity of an enzyme is determined by the functional groups of the substrate, the functional groups of the enzyme, and the physical proximity of these functional groups.

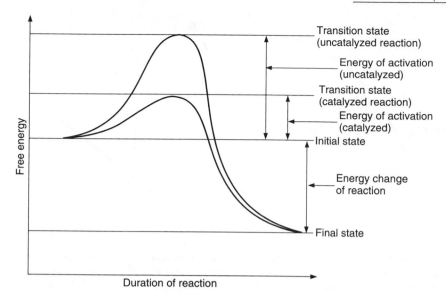

FIGURE 4-1. Diagrammatic representation of the free energy of activation of a chemical reaction.

   2. Two theories have been proposed to explain the specificity of enzyme action.
      a. Lock and key theory. The enzyme active site is complementary in conformation to the substrate, so that enzyme and substrate recognize one another.
      b. Induced-fit theory. The enzyme changes shape on binding substrate, so that the conformation of substrate and enzyme is only complementary after binding.

 III.   **ENZYME KINETICS**

A.   **Michaelis-Menten kinetic theory of enzyme action**

   1. Effect of enzyme concentration on reaction velocity. If the substrate concentration is held constant, the velocity of the reaction is proportional to the enzyme concentration.

   2. Effect of substrate concentration on reaction velocity (Figure 4-2A)
      a. When the substrate concentration ([S])is low, the reaction velocity (v) is **first-order** with respect to substrate (i.e., v is directly proportional to [S]).
      b. At high substrate concentration, the reaction is **zero-order** (i.e., v is independent of [S]).
      c. At mid-[S], the reaction is mixed-order (i.e., the proportionality is changing).

   3. Michaelis-Menten kinetic model. An enzyme-catalyzed reaction involves the reversible formation of an enzyme–substrate complex [ES], which breaks down to form free enzyme [E] and product [P].

$$E + S \underset{k_1}{\overset{k_2}{\rightleftharpoons}} ES \xrightarrow{k_3} E + P \qquad (1)$$

In equation (1), k_1 is the rate constant for ES formation, k_2 is the rate constant for the dissociation of ES back to E + S, and k_3 is the rate constant for the dissociation of ES to E + P.

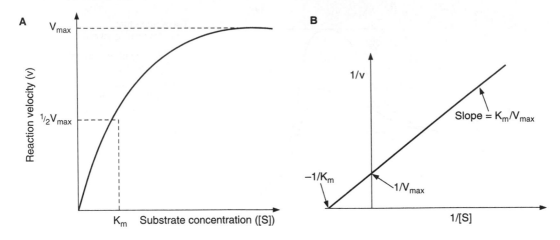

FIGURE 4-2. *(A)* The hyperbolic dependence of velocity (v) on substrate concentration ([S]) for a typical enzyme-catalyzed reaction. K_m is the substrate concentration at $\frac{1}{2}V_{max}$. V_{max} is the maximum rate at which the enzyme can catalyze the reaction. *(B)* A Lineweaver-Burk plot of 1/v against 1/[S] for an enzyme-catalyzed reaction.

4. **The Michaelis-Menten equation**
   a. **The relationship of substrate concentration to velocity** for many enzymes may be described by equation (2), where v is the initial velocity of the reaction, $V_{max} = k_3[E]_T$, and $K_m = (k_2 + k_3)/k_1$. E_T is the total [E] present. [It should be noted that capital V is used only with the abbreviation for the maximum reaction velocity (V_{max}).]

$$v = V_{max} \ [S]/([S] + K_m) \tag{2}$$

   b. **The Michaelis-Menten equation is based on three key assumptions.**
      (1) [S] is very large compared with [E], so that when all E is bound in the form ES, there is still an excess of S.
      (2) Only initial velocity conditions are considered. Thus, there is very little accumulation of P, and the formation of ES from E + P is negligible.
      (3) **Steady-state assumption.** The rate of breakdown of ES equals the rate of formation of ES.

B. **Using the Michaelis-Menten equation**

1. **Significance of the Michaelis constant (K_m)**
   a. If K_m is set equal to [S] and substituted into equation (2), then $v = \frac{1}{2}V_{max}$. Therefore, K_m is equal to the substrate concentration at which the velocity is half-maximal.
   b. K_m is not a true dissociation constant, but it does provide a measure of the affinity of an enzyme for its substrate. The lower the value of K_m, the greater the affinity of the enzyme for enzyme–substrate complex formation.

2. **Lineweaver-Burk linear transform.** Because it is difficult to estimate V_{max} from the position of an asymptote, as in the plot of a rectangular hyperbola (see Figure 4-2A), this linear transform of the Michaelis-Menten equation is often used.

$$1/v = 1/V_{max} + K_m/V_{max} \cdot 1/[S] \tag{3}$$

3. **Graphical analysis.** Figure 4-2B shows the straight-line graph obtained by plotting 1/v against 1/[S], where the y-intercept = $1/V_{max}$, the x-intercept = $-1/K_m$, and the slope = K_m/V_{max}.

IV. ENGZYME INHIBITION

A. **Reversible inhibition**. Different types of reversible enzyme inhibition are easily distinguished by analysis of Lineweaver-Burk plots (Figure 4-3 and Table 4-2).

1. **Competitive inhibition**
   a. Inhibitors compete directly with substrate for binding to the active site (i.e., the catalytic site).
   b. For a competitive inhibitor, the inhibition constant [K_i] is defined as the dissociation constant for the enzyme–inhibitor complex.

2. **Uncompetitive inhibition**
   a. Inhibitors bind only to the ES complex at a site distinct from the active site (i.e., the allosteric site).
   b. For an uncompetitive inhibitor, K_i is defined as the dissociation constant for the ES–inhibitor complex.

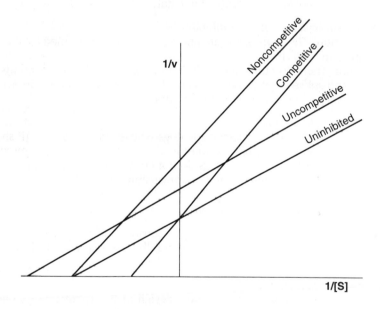

FIGURE 4-3. Lineweaver-Burk plots showing the effects of uncompetitive, competitive, and noncompetitive inhibitors on the kinetics of enzyme-catalyzed reactions.

TABLE 4-2. Types of Reversible Enzyme Inhibition

Type of Inhibition	Enzyme–Inhibitor Interactions	Effect On		
		K_m	V_{max}	Lineweaver-Burk Plot
Competitive	$E + I \rightleftharpoons EI$	Increases	None	Slope varies Intercept constant
Uncompetitive	$ES + I \rightleftharpoons ESI$	Decreases	Decreases	Slope constant Intercept varies
Noncompetitive	$E + I \rightleftharpoons EI$ $ES + I \rightleftharpoons ESI$	None	Decreases	Slope varies Intercept varies

E = enzyme; *I* = inhibitor; *S* = substrate.

3. Noncompetitive inhibition
   a. Inhibitors bind both to the free enzyme and to the ES at the allosteric site, which is distinct from the active site.
   b. For a **"pure" noncompetitive inhibitor,** the dissociation constants for the binding of the inhibitor to the enzyme and ES are identical.
   c. For a **"mixed" noncompetitive inhibitor,** the dissociation constants for the binding of the inhibitor to the enzyme and ES are not equal.

B. **Irreversible competitive inhibitors** bind covalently or so tightly to the active site that the enzyme is inactivated irreversibly. Irreversible inhibition does not obey Michaelis-Menten kinetics.

1. Affinity labels
   a. **Definition.** These are substrate analogs that possess a highly reactive group that is not present on the natural substrate.
   b. **Action.** The active site is permanently blocked from the substrate because the group reacts covalently with an amino acid residue. The residue that is modified is not necessarily involved in catalysis.

2. Mechanism-based or suicide inhibitors
   a. **Definition.** These are substrate analogs that are transformed by the catalytic action of the enzyme.
   b. **Action.** Their structures are such that the product of this reaction is highly reactive and subsequently combines covalently with an amino acid residue in the active site, thus inactivating the enzyme.

3. Transition-state analogs
   a. **Definition.** These are substrate analogs whose structures closely resemble the transition state of the natural substrate.
   b. **Action.** Transition-state analogs do not covalently modify the enzyme but bind the active site so tightly that they irreversibly inactivate it.

C. **Medical relevance of enzyme inhibitors**

1. Toxicity. Many highly toxic, naturally occurring, and man-made compounds are irreversible enzyme inhibitors. For example, the nerve gas, sarin, is an acetylcholinesterase inhibitor.

2. Therapeutic applications (Table 4-3)
   a. **Synthetic compounds. The rational design of therapeutic drugs** often involves the synthesis of inhibitors of certain enzymes (e.g., fluorouracil).
   b. **Natural compounds** used as drugs can also inhibit enzymes (e.g., penicillin).

TABLE 4-3. Examples of Enzyme Inhibitors with Therapeutic Applications

Inhibitor	Target Enzyme	Effect or Application
Allopurinol	Xanthine oxidase	Treatment of gout
Aspirin	Cyclooxygenase	Anti-inflammatory agent
5-Fluorouracil	Thymidylate synthetase	Antineoplastic agent
Lovastatin	HMG-CoA reductase	Cholesterol-lowering agent
Pargyline	Monoamine oxidase	Antihypertensive agent
Penicillin	Transpeptidase	Antibacterial agent

HMG-CoA = 3-hydroxy-3-methylglutaryl coenzyme A.

V. REGULATION OF ENZYMES

 A. **pH.** A change in pH can alter the rates of enzyme-catalyzed reactions, with many enzymes exhibiting a bell-shaped curve when enzyme activity is plotted against pH (Figure 4-4A). Changes in pH can alter the following:

1. The **ionization state** of the substrate or the enzyme-binding site for substrate

2. The ionization state at the catalytic site on the enzyme

3. **Protein molecules** so that their conformation and catalytic activity change

B. **Temperature.** The rate of an enzyme-catalyzed reaction usually increases with increasing temperature up to an **optimum point** (see Figure 4-4B), then it decreases because enzymes are **thermolabile.**

C. **Product inhibition.** If the product accumulates, it can inhibit some enzymes. This form of control limits the rate of formation of the product when the product is underused.

D. Covalent modification

1. **Phosphorylation**
   a. **Effect on enzyme activity.** In certain enzymes, the addition of a phosphate group to a specific amino acid residue [usually serine (Ser), tyrosine (Tyr), or threonine (Thr)] by specific protein kinases dramatically enhances or depresses activity.
   b. **This modification is reversible.** The phosphorylated enzyme may be dephosphorylated by specific phosphatases.

2. **Nucleotidylation**
   a. **Effect on enzyme activity.** The activities of certain enzymes are regulated by the reversible addition of a nucleotide (e.g., adenosine) to a specific amino acid.
   b. **This modification is reversible.** For example, an adenylated enzyme may be deadenylated by a specific enzyme.

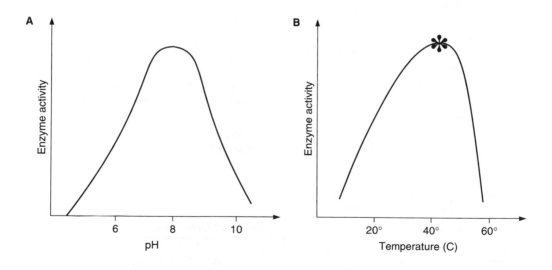

FIGURE 4-4. *(A)* A typical pH-activity plot of an enzyme-catalyzed reaction. *(B)* Effect of temperature on the activity of an enzyme. The apparent optimum point (*) shown here is the result of an initial increase in reaction rate due to a rise in temperature, followed by a decrease in enzymatic activity as the temperature continues upward with increasing thermal denaturation of the enzyme molecule.

3. **Proteolytic cleavage.** Certain enzymes are synthesized as **proenzymes,** or **zymogens,** which are inactive forms of enzymes that become active only after being cleaved at a specific site in their polypeptide chain by specific **proteases.**
   a. Many **digestive enzymes that hydrolyze proteins** (e.g., trypsin, pepsin) are synthesized as zymogens in the stomach and pancreas.
   b. **Blood clotting** is mediated by a series of proteolytic zymogen activities of several serum enzymes (see VII).

E. **Allosteric regulation of metabolic pathways.** The activity of enzymes that catalyze key regulatory reactions (**committed steps**) of metabolic pathways are often subject to allosteric regulation. Their activity can be **modulated by the binding of allosteric effectors** to a site on the enzyme that is distinct from the active site (i.e., allosteric site).

1. **Effectors** are positive if they enhance the rate of a reaction (i.e., activators) and negative if they decrease the rate of reaction (i.e., inhibitors).

2. **Feedback inhibition** is negative modulation of the committed step of a metabolic pathway by its end product. This prevents unnecessary production of an excess of end product by shutting down the pathway until more is needed.

VI. **ENZYMES IN CLINICAL DIAGNOSIS** (Table 4-4)

A. **Isozymes**

1. **Definition.** Isozymes are different molecular forms of enzymes that may be isolated from the same or different tissues.

2. **Clinical use.** Analysis of the distribution of isozymes of particular enzymes is sometimes a useful tool in clinical diagnosis.

B. **Serum enzyme levels**

1. **Description.** Many enzymes are present in serum, and their activity can be easily assayed without purification.

2. **Clinical use.** Elevation or depression of the levels of activity of specific enzymes may indicate either the presence of a disease or damage to a specific tissue.

C. **Enzymes as diagnostic reagents**

1. **Description.** Many purified enzymes are now commercially available for use in the determination of components in blood and tissues. Such enzymatic assays are usually more specific, more sensitive, and faster than chemical determinations.

2. **Clinical use.** Examples of clinically relevant compounds that can be determined enzymatically include glucose, urea, ethanol, and triglycerides.

TABLE 4-4. Enzyme Activities Useful in Clinical Diagnosis

Assayed Enzyme	Diagnostic Uses
Acid phosphatase	Prostate cancer
Alanine aminotransferase	Viral hepatitis, liver damage
Alkaline phosphatase	Liver disease, bone disorders
Amylase	Acute pancreatitis
Creatine kinase	Muscle disorders, heart attack
Lactate dehydrogenase	Heart attack

VII. **BLOOD CLOTTING** is an excellent example of a medically relevant process that is controlled by a sequence of critically regulated enzymatic reactions.

A. **Proper clot formation,** and the necessary regression of clots, is a tightly regulated process involving many activating and inhibiting factors. In a healthy individual, all of the precursors needed for the formation of a clot—except for the initiators of clot formation—are present throughout the bloodstream.

1. **Cascade mechanism of activation.** The coagulation phase of the response to blood vessel damage involves **a cascade of zymogen activations** (see V D 3), which leads to the formation of a blood clot.

2. **Clotting pathways.** In normal clotting, two pathways, the **intrinsic** and the **extrinsic,** which are initiated by different activators, converge to activate a final **common pathway,** which leads to the final clot formation. Figure 4-5 presents an overview of the major components of the clot formation pathways.

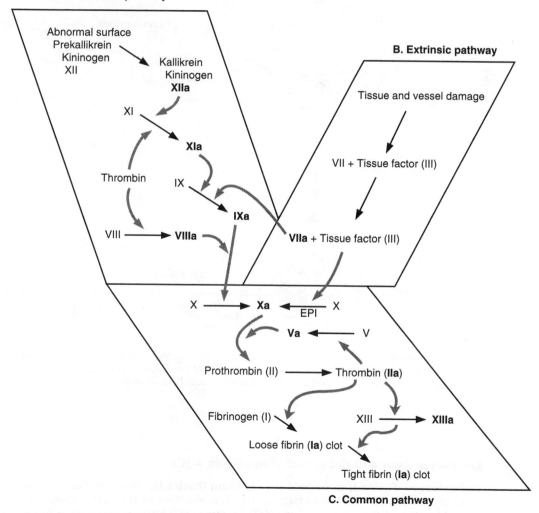

FIGURE 4-5. Blood clotting pathways. Blood clot formation arises from a series of zymogen activation cascades. Two cascade pathways, the intrinsic and extrinsic, each activate a common cascade pathway, which leads to clot formation. The active forms in the cascades are bold. *EPI* = extrinsic pathway inhibitor.

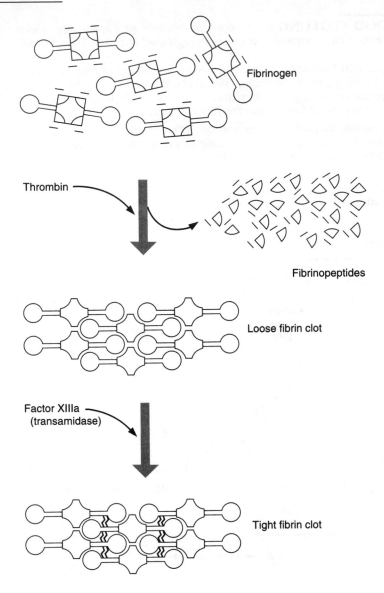

FIGURE 4-6. The conversion of fibrinogen to a tight clot. The large negative charge of the fibrinopeptide domains keeps the fibrinogen monomers in solution. The removal of the fibrinopeptides by thrombin allows fibrin to aggregate to a loose clot. Factor XIIIa covalently cross-links aggregated fibrin to form a tight clot.

B. **Common pathway and clot formation** (see Figure 4-5C)

1. **Fibrinogen (Factor I)** is the precursor to **fibrin (Factor Ia,** the lower case "a" refers to the active form of clotting factors), which forms the clot structure (Figure 4-6).
   a. **Structure.** Fibrinogen is a long (460 Å), large (340 kdal), water-soluble molecule made of three pairs of polypeptides (two α's, two β's, and two γ's).
   b. **Function.** Fibrinogen is converted to insoluble fibrin by the action of **thrombin** (see VII B 2 c). Fibrinogen cleavage by thrombin causes the release of two pairs of peptides, the **A and B fibrinopeptides,** from the α and β polypeptides.

(1) Fibrinopeptides have a large negative charge that, while the fibrinopeptides were still part of the fibrinogen molecule, was responsible for keeping fibrinogen in solution and keeping it from aggregating.

(2) The release of the fibrinopeptides facilitates the aggregation of fibrin molecules into a fragile, **loose clot.**

c. **Fibrin-stabilizing factor (Factor XIIIa)** is a **transamidase,** which covalently links fibrin monomers between specific glutamine (Gln) and lysine (Lys) residues. It converts loose clots to **tight clots.**

2. **Prothrombin (Factor II)** is the precursor to **thrombin (Factor IIa).**
   a. **Structure.** The amino end of prothrombin contains many **carboxylated glutamate (Gla) residues.**

$$\begin{array}{c} \text{COOH} \\ \diagdown \\ \text{CH}-\text{CH}_2-\text{CH} \\ \diagup \hspace{2.5cm} \diagdown \text{COOH} \\ \text{NH}_2 \hspace{3.5cm} \text{COOH} \end{array}$$

γ-carboxyglutamate

   (1) The Gla residues **enable prothrombin to bind calcium** and have a subsequent affinity for activated platelets.

   (2) The Gla residues are carboxylated by a **vitamin K-dependent enzyme,** which is inhibited by several vitamin K antagonists that are commonly used as anticoagulant drugs (see IX B). These anticoagulant drugs effectively slow the association with platelets of prothrombin and other vitamin K-dependent, Gla-containing clotting factors, such as Factors VII, IX, and X.

   b. **Functions**
   (1) **Prothrombin binds calcium,** which facilitates its binding to negatively charged phospholipids that are on the surface of activated platelets. Activated platelets form the platelet plug at the site of bleeding early in the response to injury.
      (a) **Colocalization event.** The binding of prothrombin to activated platelets puts it in close proximity to **Factors Xa and Va,** which, in the presence of calcium, also bind to platelet phospholipids.
      (b) **Accelerated conversion to thrombin.** A 10,000-fold acceleration of conversion of prothrombin to thrombin occurs because of this colocalization event.
   (2) **Prothrombin is converted to thrombin** by the action of Factor Xa in conjunction with Factor Va.
      (a) **Factor Va** is a modifier protein that serves to accelerate the conversion of prothrombin to thrombin by Factor Xa.
      (b) **Factor V** is converted to Factor Va by thrombin.

   c. **Thrombin** is a very specific protease that is responsible for activating a number of factors in the clotting cascade:
   (1) **Fibrinogen (Factor I)**
   (2) **Fibrin-stabilizing factor (Factor XIII)**
   (3) **Factor V**
   (4) **Factor VIII**
   (5) **Factor XI**

C. The extrinsic pathway (see Figure 4-5B) is short-lived and is primarily responsible for the initiation of clotting. This clotting activation pathway is triggered by **tissue factor,** or **thromboplastin (Factor III),** which is not normally found in circulating blood. The extrinsic pathway can be inhibited by a circulating blood lipoprotein.

1. **Tissue factor (thromboplastin, Factor III)** is a membrane-bound glycoprotein located in the tissue adventitia. When exposed upon vessel injury, tissue factor tightly binds Factor VII.

2. **Factor VII.** While bound to tissue factor, Factor VII is converted to Factor VIIa by trace amounts of circulating, active proteases.

    3. Tissue factor–Factor VIIa complex
      a. Common pathway. The complex of tissue factor and Factor VIIa catalyzes the conversion of Factor X of the common pathway to Factor Xa.
      b. Intrinsic pathway. The tissue factor–Factor VIIa complex also converts Factor IX of the intrinsic pathway to Factor IXa.

    4. Extrinsic pathway inhibitor (EPI), or **lipoprotein-associated coagulation inhibitor (LACI),** is a circulating blood lipoprotein that inhibits the conversion of Factor X to Xa by the tissue factor–Factor VIIa complex. This is one reason why people affected with hemophilia (see VII E) who have normal extrinsic pathways do not form effective clots.

D. **The intrinsic pathway** (see Figure 4-5A) is responsible for most of the growth and maintenance of clots.

    1. Initiation of the intrinsic pathway. All of the factors needed for this activation pathway are in the bloodstream before initiation of clotting. The pathway is initiated by the interaction of the appropriate factors in blood with abnormal surfaces.
      a. When a **complex of Factor XII, prekallikrein, and high molecular weight kininogen** makes contact with an abnormal surface, such as collagen in an open wound, the prekallikrein is converted to kallikrein, which converts Factor XII to Factor XIIa.
      b. Factor XIIa then initiates the activation cascade shown in Figure 4-5A.
      c. Factor VIII is a crucial modifier protein that, at the end of the intrinsic pathway, accelerates 200,000-fold the conversion of Factor X to Xa by Factor IXa.

    2. Feedback activation. The intrinsic pathway is enhanced by the feedback activation of Factors VIII and XI by thrombin, as is Factor V of the common pathway.

    3. Clinical correlation. The activation of the intrinsic pathway by abnormal surfaces presents instances when anticoagulation therapy is necessary.
      a. Anticoagulation therapy is needed to prevent clots from forming on prosthetic heart valves (see IX B 3).
      b. An anticoagulant is needed to keep blood from coagulating in test tubes that hold blood samples (see IX B 1).

E. **Hemophilias** are inherited clotting disorders in which there are deficiencies or abnormalities in various clotting factors. Many of the clotting factors were identified through the study of patients with bleeding disorders. The two most prevalent forms of hemophilia in the United States are:

    1. Classic hemophilia (hemophilia A) is an X-linked recessive trait that is the predominant form of hemophilia in the United States (80%). It arises from a deficiency in the modifier protein **Factor VIII,** which in its active form (Factor VIIIa) interacts with Factor IXa and significantly accelerates the conversion of Factor X to Factor Xa.

    2. Hemophilia B is an X-linked recessive trait that accounts for 10% of the cases of hemophilia in the United States. It arises from a deficiency in Factor IX of the intrinsic pathway.

VIII. **REGULATION OF CLOTTING** is necessary so that clots do not expand beyond the site of injury or exist longer than necessary. Regulation is controlled by inhibiting clot formation and degrading clots at the proper time.

A. **Natural inhibition of clot formation.** The large volume and flow of blood assures that factors such as thrombin, which are released from platelets on activation, are quickly removed from the clotting site and carried to the liver where they are degraded.

1. **EPI** (see VII C 4) shifts clot formation from the extrinsic to the intrinsic pathway, although it is not a general inhibitor of clotting.

2. **Antithrombin III** is a slow inhibitor (i.e., it allows clots to form before it acts) of the following factors:
   a. Thrombin
   b. Factor IXa
   c. Factor Xa
   d. Factor XIa

3. **Activated protein C** is a vitamin K-dependent, Gla-containing protease that inactivates the modifying proteins, Factors Va and VIIIa. This activity is stimulated by another vitamin K-dependent protein, **protein S.**

4. **Thrombomodulin** converts thrombin from an enzyme that is crucial to clot formation to one that inhibits clot formation.
   a. Thrombomodulin is bound to the plasma membrane of endothelial cells and prevents clot formation from extending to normal, healthy vascular tissue.
   b. Thrombomodulin binds and changes the substrate specificity of thrombin. Thrombin bound to thrombomodulin no longer carries out its normal functions; instead, it activates circulating protein C.

B. **Clot degradation (fibrinolysis).** A clot is a transient component of wound healing that begins to be degraded soon after formation.

1. **Plasmin,** the active form of the zymogen plasminogen, is the protease that specifically degrades clots.

2. **Tissue plasminogen activator (t-PA)** is the protease that converts plasminogen to plasmin.
   a. Both plasminogen and t-PA become localized to clots because they bind to clots with a high affinity.
   b. **Plasminogen activator inhibitors** regulate the activity of t-PA.

IX. DRUGS THAT AFFECT CLOTTING

A. **Procoagulants** promote the formation of clots. Although there are numerous hemostatic agents that are used at the site of a wound to reduce bleeding and promote healing, few directly affect the clotting cascade.

1. **Thrombin** can be used therapeutically to promote clot formation if it is added topically to wounds.

2. Hemophiliacs often require blood **plasma** or **purified clotting factors** to inhibit a bleeding event. Unfortunately, this has left hemophiliacs susceptible to numerous blood-borne diseases. However, clotting factors produced by recombinant DNA technology (see Chapter 11) are becoming available.

B. **Anticoagulants** inhibit the formation of clots.

1. **Heparin** is an anticoagulant that binds to and increases the inhibitory activity of antithrombin III (see VIII A 2).
   a. It is commonly used postsurgically to prevent clots from forming on prosthetic implants.
   b. Heparin is also used in test tubes to keep blood drawn for clinical laboratory analysis from clotting.

2. **Hirudin,** which is synthesized by the European medicinal leech, is the most potent natural inhibitor of thrombin.

3. **Coumarins** act by inhibiting the vitamin K-dependent γ-carboxylation of Gla resi-

dues in several of the clotting factors [see VII B 2 a (2)].

    a. Because coumarins can be taken orally, they are prophylactically used in patients with prosthetic implants that are in direct contact with blood.

    b. Coumarins reduce the chance of clot formation on the abnormal surfaces of the prosthesis.

 C.   **Fibrinolytics** are agents that use enzymatic reactions to dissolve clots. Two fibrinolytics commonly used to dissolve clots that cause heart attacks include streptokinase and t-PA.

    1. Streptokinase is an enzyme from β-hemolytic streptococci that facilitates the breakdown of clots by binding to and activating plasminogen. This activation does not occur through proteolysis of plasminogen. Streptokinase induces a conformational change in plasminogen, which makes plasminogen active without cleavage. This "active" plasminogen can convert "inactive" plasminogen to plasmin, which is proteolytically active.

    2. t-PA (see VIII B 2) binds to fibrin clots and becomes a potent activator of plasminogen. It is now produced by recombinant DNA technology (see Chapter 11).

Case 4-1 Revisited

CK occurs as a dimer of two subunits that can be present as two distinct molecular forms: brain type (B) and muscle type (M). Thus, three isozymes are possible: CK-MM, CK-BB, and CK-MB. These isozymes can be readily distinguished and quantitated by electrophoresis. CK-MB is normally present in trace amounts only in the myocardium. Elevation of CK-MB levels to greater than 6% of the total CK is diagnostic of a myocardial infarction. LDH is a tetramer of four subunits that can be present as two distinct molecular forms. Type H is found primarily in the heart, and type M is found primarily in muscle or liver. Five isozymes of LDH composed of different combinations of these subunits are possible: M_4, HM_3, H_2M_2, H_3M, and H_4. In normal serum, the H_3M isozyme is present in the highest concentration. In an individual who has suffered a myocardial infarction, the serum levels of the H-containing isozymes, particularly H_4, are elevated. A ratio of H_4:H_3M greater than 1 confirms the diagnosis that the patient suffered a myocardial infarction.

    Conditions other than myocardial infarction can cause similar changes in the isozyme patterns of either CK or LDH, but it is unlikely that both patterns would be affected in this manner. Therefore, clinical results such as these can be reliably used to distinguish between the occurrence of myocardial infarction and other conditions that may have caused the reported symptoms.

STUDY QUESTIONS

DIRECTIONS: Each of the numbered items or incomplete statements in this section is followed by answers or by completions of the statement. Select the **one** lettered answer or completion that is **best** in each case.

1. A Lineweaver-Burk plot exhibits a slope of 5×10^{-4} M $\cdot$ min/mol and a y-intercept of 0.1 min/mol. Which one of the following conclusions is correct?

(A) $K_m/V_{max} = 200$
(B) The turnover number for the enzyme is 100 min^{-1}
(C) The equilibrium constant for the dissociation of the enzyme-substrate complex to enzyme and product is 0.005 M
(D) When the concentration of substrate = 0.005 M, v = 5 mol/min
(E) The rate of reaction increases linearly with substrate concentration

2. Which one of the following characteristics best applies to an allosteric effector? It

(A) competes with substrate for the catalytic site
(B) binds to a site on the enzyme molecule distinct from the catalytic site
(C) changes the nature of the product formed
(D) changes the substrate specificity of the enzyme
(E) covalently modifies the enzyme

Questions 3-5

An alcoholic has consumed antifreeze as a substitute for ethanol. Ethylene glycol, an ingredient in antifreeze, is also a substrate for the enzyme alcohol dehydrogenase (ADH), which normally converts ethanol to acetaldehyde. Ethylene glycol, however, is converted by ADH to a highly toxic product. Ethanol is administered as a treatment in this case of poisoning.

3. Why is ethanol an effective treatment for ethylene glycol poisoning?

(A) ADH exhibits a much higher affinity (K_m) for ethanol than for ethylene glycol
(B) Ethanol is an allosteric effector of ADH
(C) Ethanol combines with the toxic product formed by the reaction of ADH with ethylene glycol and renders it harmless
(D) Acetaldehyde is of therapeutic value
(E) Ethanol induces another enzyme that is capable of metabolizing ethylene glycol

4. If one compares Lineweaver-Burk plots for the reactions of ADH with ethanol and ethylene glycol, which of the following would be observed?

(A) They exhibit identical slopes
(B) They exhibit identical y-intercepts
(C) They exhibit identical x-intercepts
(D) Only the plot for the reaction of ethanol is linear
(E) Only the plot for the reaction of ethylene glycol is linear

5. Blood was taken from this patient and analyzed for the serum levels of certain enzymes. Which one of the following enzymes will most likely be present at elevated levels?

(A) Amylase
(B) Creatine kinase
(C) Alanine aminotransferase
(D) Acid phosphatase
(E) Lactate dehydrogenase

6. Which one of the following drugs would be best for a patient who has just had a heart attack?

(A) Heparin
(B) Tissue plasminogen activator
(C) Dicoumarol
(D) Desmopressin
(E) Thrombin

DIRECTIONS: The group of items in this section consists of lettered options followed by a set of numbered items. For each item, select the **one** lettered option that is most closely associated with it. Each lettered option may be selected once, more than once, or not at all.

Questions 7-9

For each statement, select the blood clotting factor to which it is most closely associated.

(A) Factor VIII
(B) Factor IX
(C) Factor V
(D) Factor XIII
(E) Factor VII

7. The zymogen form of a transamidase

8. Deficient in patients with hemophilia B

9. Its active form is inhibited by antithrombin III

Each set of matching questions in this section consists of a list of lettered options followed by several numbered items. For each numbered item, select the appropriate lettered option(s). Each lettered option may be selected once, more than once, or not at all.

Questions 10-12

(A) Factor I
(B) Factor II
(C) Factor III
(D) Factor V
(E) Factor VII
(F) Factor VIII
(G) Factor IX
(H) Factor X
(I) Factor XI

For each blood clotting pathway, select the factors that are part of that pathway.

10. Intrinsic pathway (select 3 factors)

11. Extrinsic pathway (select 2 factors)

12. Common pathway (select 4 factors)

ANSWERS AND EXPLANATIONS

1. The answer is D [III B]. The Lineweaver-Burk plot is a graph of a linear transform of the Michaelis-Menten equation given by:

$$1/v = 1/V_{max} + K_m/V_{max} \times 1/[S]$$

where v is reaction velocity, V_{max} is the maximum reaction velocity, K_m is the Michaelis constant, and [S] is the substrate concentration. K_m/V_{max} is equal to the slope, not 200. The intercept on the y-axis is equal to $1/V_{max}$. Therefore, V_{max} = 10 mol/min, and K_m = 0.005 M. The turnover number cannot be determined from this data. K_m is not a true dissociation constant. It is the value of [S] at which $v = V_{max}/2$ (choice D). Choice E is incorrect because the direct plot of v versus [S] would be hyperbolic.

2. The answer is B [IV A; V E]. Allosteric means "other site," indicating that the effector binds reversibly to a site distinct from the catalytic active site. The substrate specificity is not changed, and the product formed is not different in the presence of the effector.

3-5. The answers are: 3-A [III B; IV A], **4-B** [III B; IV A], **5-C** [VI A, B]. Aldehyde dehydrogenase (ADH), which exhibits a broad substrate specificity for alcohols, has a much higher affinity for ethanol [i.e., a lower K_m] than for ethylene glycol. Saturating ADH with ethanol by administration of therapeutic levels prevents it from converting ethylene glycol to the toxic aldehyde, and allows ethylene glycol to eventually be excreted unmetabolized.

If ADH obeys Michaelis-Menten kinetics, then the Lineweaver-Burk plot, which is a linear transform of the Michaelis-Menten equation, will be linear for both substrates. ADH exhibits different K_m values for ethanol and ethylene glycol. Therefore, the x-intercept (1/K_m) and the slope (K_m/V_{max}) are different. If only the affinity for the alternative substrate is different, then the V_{max} will be the same as will the y-intercept (1/V_{max}).

Chronic alcoholics are likely to exhibit signs of liver damage. Alanine aminotransferase is present in the cytosol of liver cells, and its release into the serum is diagnostic of hepatocellular damage. Lactate dehydrogenase and creatine kinase isozymes are analyzed to diagnose heart attacks. Amylase levels are elevated in patients with acute pancreatitis, and elevated acid phosphatase levels may be diagnostic of prostate cancer.

6. The answer is B [IX A-B]. Heart attacks, or myocardial infarctions, may occur because a clot, or thrombosis, blocks the blood flow in a coronary artery. The amount of heart muscle damage caused by the subsequent reduced blood flow can be lessened by treatment with tissue plasminogen activator (t-PA), which binds to fibrin clots and activates the conversion of plasminogen to plasmin, which specifically degrades clots. Both heparin and dicoumarol are anticoagulants and, as such, can do nothing to remove a clot once it has formed. Desmopressin and thrombin are procoagulants; therefore, they increase clot formation.

7-9. The answers are: 7-D [VII B 1 c], **8-B** [VII E 2], **9-B** [VIII A 2]. Proteolytic cleavage by thrombin converts inactive Factor XIII to active Factor XIIIa. Factor XIIIa is a transamidase that converts loose clots to tight clots by covalently linking fibrin monomers between specific glutamine and lysine residues.

Hemophilias are inherited disorders in which patients are deficient in particular clotting factors. Patients deficient in Factor VIII have hemophilia A. Patients with hemophilia B are deficient in Factor IX.

Antithrombin III is important in the regulation of clot formation; it inhibits thrombin as well as Factors IXa, Xa, and XIa. Factors V and VIII are modifier proteins, which enhance the conversion of prothrombin to thrombin by Factor Xa and the conversion of Factor X to Xa by Factor IXa, respectively. Factor VII is the zymogen form of Factor VIIa that, with tissue factor, converts Factor X to Xa.

10-12. The answers are: 10-F,G,I [VII D], **11-C,E** [VII C], **12-A,B,D,H** [VII B]. These are all of the inactive forms of factors in the three pathways of clotting. Factor VII and tissue factor (Factor III) are part of the extrinsic pathway. Along with prekallikrein and kininogen, Factors XII, XI, IX, and VIII make up the intrinsic pathway. Either of these two pathways may activate the common pathway, which is made up of Factors X, V, II (prothrombin), I (fibrinogen), and XIII (fibrin-stabilizing factor).

Chapter 5

Carbohydrate Function and Structure

Victor Davidson

Case 5-1

A young adult complains of intestinal problems. The symptoms, which present shortly after drinking milk or consuming certain dairy products, include bloating, gas, cramps, and diarrhea.

- What is the most likely diagnosis?
- How can the diagnosis be confirmed?
- What is the treatment for this disorder?

I. CARBOHYDRATE FUNCTIONS

A. Carbohydrates **provide the majority of energy** in most organisms (simple carbohydrates are sugars; complex carbohydrates can be broken down into simple sugars).

B. Carbohydrates are **structural components** of cell walls and cell membranes.

C. Carbohydrates **serve as metabolic intermediates** (e.g., glucose-6-phosphate).

D. Carbohydrates (e.g., ribose, deoxyribose) are **components of the nucleotides that form DNA and RNA.**

E. Carbohydrates **play roles in lubrication, cellular intercommunication, and immunity.**

II. CARBOHYDRATE CLASSIFICATION AND NOMENCLATURE

A. **Classification**

1. **Monosaccharides (e.g., glucose)** are simple sugars. They may be connected by **glycosidic linkages** (see IV) to form the following **glycosides.**
   a. **Disaccharides (e.g., sucrose)** are composed of two monosaccharides.
   b. **Oligosaccharides (e.g., blood group antigens)** are composed of two to ten monosaccharides.
   c. **Polysaccharides (e.g., glycogen)** are composed of more than 10 monosaccharides.

2. **Aldoses and ketoses.** The reactive group (i.e., aldehyde or ketone) on a carbohydrate determines whether it is an aldose or a ketose.
   a. **Aldoses (e.g., glucose)** possess a reactive aldehyde (CHO) group.
   b. **Ketoses (e.g., fructose)** possess a reactive ketone (C=O) group.

Open-chain forms

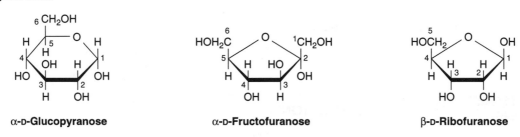

Cyclic forms

FIGURE 5-1. Representations of monosaccharide molecules. The numbering system for identifying carbons in the *open-chain* and *cyclic* structural representations is indicated, as is the system for designating the anomeric carbon as α or β.

B. **Nomenclature**

1. **Carbon numbering system.** In the general formula for monosaccharides—$C_nH_{2n}O_n$—n is the number of carbons. Carbons are numbered sequentially with the carbon possessing the aldehyde or ketone group assigned the lowest possible number (Figure 5-1).

2. The total number of carbons determines whether a monosaccharide is a **triose** (3 carbons), a **tetrose** (4 carbons), a **pentose** (5 carbons), or a **hexose** (6 carbons).

3. Monosaccharide and reactive-group names can be combined to designate compounds. For example, **glucose** is an **aldohexose** (i.e., a hexose possessing an aldehyde group).

III. **STRUCTURES**

A. **Open-chain forms**

1. **Asymmetric carbons.** All monosaccharides are optically active because they contain at least one asymmetric carbon (i.e., a carbon bonded to four different atoms or groups of atoms). For the purposes of nomenclature, monosaccharides are designated L or D by comparison with the structure of glyceraldehyde.

$$\text{L-Glyceraldehyde} \qquad \text{D-Glyceraldehyde}$$

A D-sugar is one that matches the configuration of D-glyceraldehyde around the asymmetric carbon that is farthest from the aldehyde or ketone group. An L-sugar matches L-glyceraldehyde.

2. **Isomers** are compounds with the same chemical formula. **Optical isomers** are alike with respect to what atoms are bonded to each other but different in how the atoms are oriented in space.

3. **Epimers** are isomers with conformations that differ only at one carbon atom.

4. **Enantiomers** are isomers that are mirror images. They rotate the same plane of polarized light to exactly the same extent, but in opposite directions. Their physical properties are otherwise identical.
   a. If light is rotated to the **right** (i.e., clockwise), the compound is **dextrorotatory.**
   b. If light is rotated to the **left** (i.e., counterclockwise), the compound is **levorotatory.**

B. **Cyclic hemiacetals and hemiketals.** Hemiacetals are formed when an alcohol reacts with an aldehyde, and can occur in linear or cyclic forms. In glucose, the hydroxyl group on the C-5 carbon can react intramolecularly with the carbonyl group on C-1 to form a stable cyclic hemiacetal (see Figure 5-1). The analogous reaction between a ketone and an alcohol forms a hemiketal. Cyclic hemiketals are formed by ketoses such as fructose (see Figure 5-1).

1. Cyclic forms of sugar occur much more frequently than do open-chain sugar structures.

2. **Ring structures** of sugars can have a five-membered ring called a **furanose** or a six-membered ring called a **pyranose** (see Figure 5-1).

3. **Anomeric carbons** are new asymmetric carbons (e.g., C-1 in glucose) that are created by cyclization during hemiacetal and hemiketal formation.
   a. If the −OH on the anomeric carbon is **below** the plane of the ring, the sugar is α (see Figure 5-1).
   b. If the −OH on the anomeric carbon is **above** the plane of the ring, the sugar is β.

4. **Mutarotation** is the process by which α and β sugars, in solution, slowly change into an equilibrated mixture of both.

IV. GLYCOSIDIC LINKAGES

A. **Glycosides.** A sugar can react with an alcohol to form a glycoside. If the sugar residue is glucose, the derivative is a **glucoside.** If the residue is galactose, the derivative is a **galactoside,** and so forth.

B. **Disaccharides** are glycosides formed by the reaction of a sugar with an -OH of another sugar. Much of the sugar in our diet is in the form of disaccharides (Table 5-1). If a disaccharide reacts with another sugar, the glycoside is a **trisaccharide,** and so forth.

TABLE 5-1. Physiologically Important Disaccharides

Disaccharide	Components	Sources
Lactose	Galactose + glucose	Milk, dairy products
Maltose	Glucose + glucose	Hydrolysis of starch
Sucrose	Glucose + fructose	Cane and beet sugar

 C. **Nomenclature.** By convention, glycosidic linkages are named by reading from left to right. Therefore, sucrose has an α-1,2-glycosidic linkage.

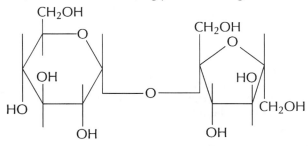

Sucrose (α-D-glucopyranosyl-β-D-fructofuranoside)

1. **A reducing sugar** possesses a free anomeric carbon atom that is not involved in a glycosidic linkage. The free aldehyde or ketone group reduces an alkaline copper reagent such as Fehling's solution.

2. In contrast to the linkages in most simple carbohydrates, the oxygen bridge between glucose and fructose in sucrose is between the anomeric carbons. Therefore, **sucrose is not a reducing sugar.**

 D. **Polysaccharides** (Table 5-2)

1. **Starch** is a mixture of amylose and amylopectin. It is the storage form of glucose in plants (i.e., fruits and vegetables).

2. **Glycogen** is the major storage form of carbohydrate in animals, found mostly in liver and muscle. It is a more highly branched form of amylopectin.

3. **Cellulose** is a structural component of plant cells. It is not hydrolyzed or digested by human enzymes, but it is an important source of bulk fiber in the diet.

TABLE 5-2. Physiologically Important Polysaccharides Composed of Glucose

Polysaccharide	Linkages	Importance
Amylose	α-1,4 linear	Component of dietary starch
Amylopectin	α-1,4-linear + α-1,6 branching*	Component of dietary starch
Cellulose	β-1,4 linear	Nondigestible component of plants
Glycogen	α-1,4 linear + α-1,6 branching*	Major storage form of carbohydrate in animals

*In amylopectin, branching points occur every 25–30 glucose residues. In glycogen, they occur every 8–10 residues.

V. CARBOHYDRATE DERIVATIVES

A. **Phosphoric acid esters of monosaccharides** (phosphorylated sugars), such as D-glucose-1-phosphate (Figure 5-2), are **metabolic intermediates. Phosphorylation** is the initial step in the metabolism of sugars.

B. **Amino sugars** have a hydroxyl group replaced by an **amino** or an **acetylamino** group.

1. **Glucosamine** (see Figure 5-2) is the product of the hydrolysis of chitin, the major polysaccharide of the shells of insects and crustaceans.

2. **Galactosamine** is found in the polysaccharide of cartilage, chondroitin sulfate.

C. **Sugar acids** are produced by oxidation of the aldehydic carbon, the terminal hydroxyl carbon, or both.

1. **Ascorbic acid** (vitamin C) is a sugar acid.

2. **Glucuronic acid** (see Figure 5-2) is a component of proteoglycans (see VI C) and is involved in the metabolism of bilirubin (see Chapter 25).

D. **Deoxy sugars** possess a hydrogen atom in place of one of their hydroxyl groups. These include 2-deoxyribose, which is found in DNA.

E. **Sugar alcohols**

1. **Structure.** Aldoses and ketoses may be reduced at the carbonyl carbon to the corresponding polyhydroxy alcohols (sugar alcohols).
   a. **Aldoses** yield the corresponding alcohols.
      (1) D-**Glucose** yields D-**sorbitol.**
      (2) D-**Mannose** yields D-**mannitol.**
   b. **Ketoses** form two alcohols because a new asymmetric carbon is formed in the process. For example, D-fructose, a ketose, yields D-mannitol and D-sorbitol.

2. **Function.** The sugar alcohols function mainly as intermediates in minor pathways. However, overproduction of sorbitol is clinically important in patients with uncontrolled diabetes (see Chapter 27).

VI. GLYCOPROTEINS are proteins that possess a covalently attached polysaccharide chain.

A. **Physiologic functions of glycoproteins**

1. Structural molecules (e.g., components of cell walls and membranes)

2. Lubricants (e.g., components of mucus)

3. Cell attachment and recognition sites

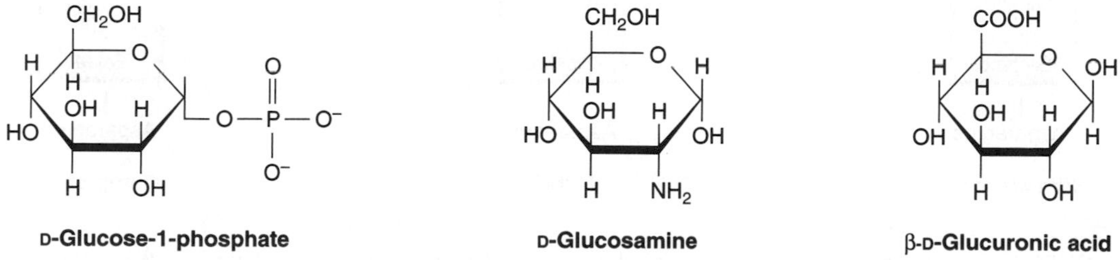

D-**Glucose-1-phosphate**   D-**Glucosamine**   β-D-**Glucuronic acid**

FIGURE 5-2. Examples of carbohydrate derivatives.

4. Certain hormones [e.g., human chorionic gonadotropin (hCG), thyrotropin]

5. Immunologic components (e.g., immunoglobulins, complement, interferon)

B. **Protein–carbohydrate linkages**

1. **O-linked glycoproteins.** Sugars are attached via the hydroxyl group of a serine (Ser) or threonine (Thr) residue.

2. **N-linked glycoproteins.** Sugars are attached via the amide NH_2 group of an asparagine residue. There are three major classes of N-linked glycoproteins (Figure 5-3).
   a. Each class contains a common **pentasaccharide core (core oligosaccharide),** which is linked to asparagine via N-acetylglucosamine.
   b. Depending on which other sugars are attached to this core, it is termed high mannose, complex, or hybrid.

C. **Proteoglycans (mucopolysaccharides)** are distinguished from other glycoproteins by the nature of the attached polysaccharide.

1. **Glycosaminoglycans** are the polysaccharide portions of proteoglycans.
   a. **Structure.** Glycosaminoglycans consist of repeating disaccharide units in which D-glucosamine or D-galactosamine, or a derivative, is always present.
   b. **Heparin,** a free glycosaminoglycan and an anticoagulant, is an **intracellular component** of mast cells, found near the walls of blood vessels and on the surface of endothelial cells.

2. **Function.** Proteoglycans are present in several tissues and fluids (Table 5-3). In many cases they form the **ground substance** (i.e., extracellular medium) of connective tissues.

3. **Mucopolysaccharidoses** are genetic disorders of proteoglycan metabolism. They are characterized by the excessive accumulation and excretion of glycosaminoglycans.
   a. **Cause.** Deficiencies of lysosomal enzymes that are responsible for the degradation of mucopolysaccharides cause these disorders (Table 5-4).
   b. **Clinical manifestations** include skeletal deformities, mental retardation, and early death in severe cases.

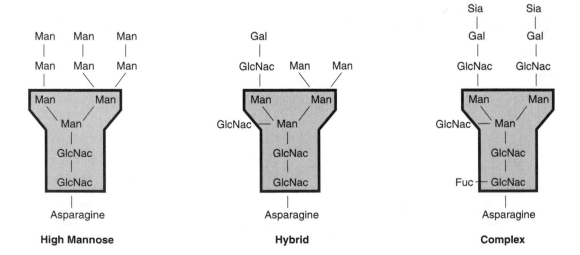

FIGURE 5-3. Structures of the major types of oligosaccharides present in N-linked glycoproteins. The abbreviations are as follows: *Fuc* = fucose; *Gal* = galactose; *GlcNac* = N-acetylglucosamine; *Man* = mannose; *Sia* = sialic acid. The *shaded areas* indicate the common pentasaccharide core.

TABLE 5-3. Structure and Occurrence of Glycosaminoglycans

Glycosaminoglycan	Repeating Unit	Tissue Distribution
Hyaluronic acid	Glucuronic acid–N-acetylglucosamine	Joint fluid, eye fluid
Chondroitin sulfate	Glucuronic acid–N-acetylgalactosamine*	Cartilage, bone
Keratan sulfate	Galactose–N-acetylgalactosamine*	Cartilage
Heparan sulfate	Glucuronic acid*–glucosamine*	Lung, muscle, liver
Dermatan sulfate	Iduronic acid*–N-acetylgalactosamine*	Skin, lung

*Indicates that the sugar residue is sulfated.

TABLE 5-4. Mucopolysaccharidoses

Type	Syndrome	Enzymatic Defect	Accumulated Metabolite
I	Hurler or Scheie	α-L-Iduronidase	Dermatan sulfate
			Heparan sulfate
II	Hunter	Iduronate sulfatase	Dermatan sulfate
			Heparan sulfate
IIIA	Sanfilippo A	Heparan N-sulfatase	Heparan sulfate
IIIB	Sanfilippo B	N-Acetylglucosaminidase	Heparan sulfate
IV	Morquio	N-Acetylgalactosamine-6-sulfatase	Keratan sulfate
VI	Maroteaux-Lamy	N-Acetylgalactosamine-4-sulfatase	Dermatan sulfate
VII	Sly	β-Glucuronidase	Dermatan sulfate
			Heparan sulfate

VII. **BLOOD GROUP ANTIGENS** are **specific classes of oligosaccharides** that may be bound to proteins, lipids, or membranes. More than 20 different blood groups and more than 150 different antigens have been described.

A. **Clinical relevance.** Before a patient can be given a blood transfusion or a tissue transplant, the blood or tissue types must be matched with the donor. Use of mismatched blood or tissue could be fatal to the patient. The specific blood type corresponds to the presence of a specific blood group antigen.

B. **Antigen–antibody response.** A **like antigen** is normally present in the host, and the host will not produce antibodies against it. A **foreign antigen** is not normally present in the host, and the host will produce antibodies against it.

C. **ABO blood group.** This blood group is comprised of the ABO antigens, which are distinguished by a different single-sugar moiety on an otherwise common oligosaccharide core (Figure 5-4).

1. **Blood type O.** People with type O blood make antibodies against type A and type B antigens. They can only receive blood from another type O individual but may donate blood to an individual with any other blood type (i.e., **type O individuals are universal donors**).

2. **Blood type A.** People with type A blood make antibodies only to type B antigens. They can receive blood from type O or type A donors, but may donate blood to either type A or type AB recipients.

3. **Blood type B.** People with type B blood make antibodies only to type A antigens. They can receive blood from type O or type B donors, but may donate blood to either type B or type AB recipients.

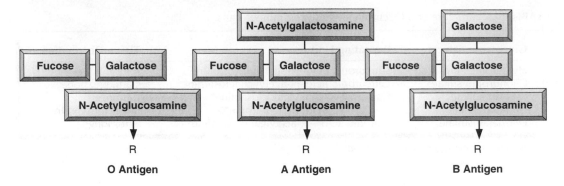

FIGURE 5-4. Representation of the oligosaccharide structures of the ABO blood group antigens. *R* represents either a protein or lipid molecule to which the oligosaccharide is bound, sometimes via other sugar residues.

4. Blood type AB. People with type AB blood make no antibodies to type A or B antigens. They may receive blood from any donor (i.e., **type AB individuals are universal recipients),** but may donate blood only to other type AB individuals.

Case 5-1 Revisited

The patient has a lactase deficiency. To be absorbed from the intestine, disaccharides must first be hydrolyzed to monosaccharides by enzymes (i.e., disaccharidases) of the intestinal microvilli. The enzyme required to hydrolyze lactose (the major carbohydrate in milk) is lactase. In lactase deficiency, the lactose is not hydrolyzed or absorbed and will pass into the colon. An osmotic imbalance results, which causes fluid to enter the intestinal tract and leads to diarrhea. Bacteria present in the colon use the lactose as a substrate for fermentation, producing gas that causes cramps and bloating. Lactase activity in humans typically declines during childhood and adolescence to 5%–10% of the levels present at birth. For this reason, a deficiency may not present until after childhood.

The diagnosis may be confirmed by a lactose tolerance test. This involves oral administration of lactose followed by determinations of blood glucose. In patients with a lactase deficiency, no increase in glucose levels is observed.

The treatment is avoidance of lactose in the diet, primarily avoidance of dairy products. Yogurt can be consumed because the microorganism that converts milk to yogurt also metabolizes much of the lactose. This provides a good source of dietary calcium. Over-the-counter products that contain the enzyme that hydrolyzes lactose may be added to dairy products so that they can be consumed by lactose-intolerant individuals.

STUDY QUESTIONS

DIRECTIONS: Each of the numbered items or incomplete statements in this section is followed by answers or by completions of the statement. Select the **one** lettered answer or completion that is **best** in each case.

1. The monosaccharide glucose is best described by which one of the following statements?

(A) It usually exists in the furanose form
(B) It is a ketose
(C) It possesses an anomeric C-2 carbon atom
(D) It forms part of the disaccharide sucrose
(E) It is reduced to form mannitol

2. The oligosaccharide portions of all N-linked glycoproteins are best described by which one of the following statements?

(A) They are attached to the protein via linkage to a serine or threonine residue
(B) They possess a common linear pentasaccharide core
(C) They are attached to the protein via linkage of mannose to asparagine
(D) They contain both mannose and N-acetylglucosamine
(E) They are comprised of at least 50% mannose residues

3. The sugar residues of amylose are best described as

(A) β-1,4 linkages
(B) α-1,4 linkages
(C) galactose units only
(D) fructose units only
(E) both galactose and fructose units

4. Certain amino sugars may be components of

(A) DNA
(B) glycogen
(C) the ABO blood group antigens
(D) vitamin C
(E) cellulose

DIRECTIONS: The group of items in this section consists of lettered options followed by a set of numbered items. For each item, select the **one** lettered option that is most closely associated with it.

Questions 5-8

Match the following characteristics of sugars to the correct lettered structure.

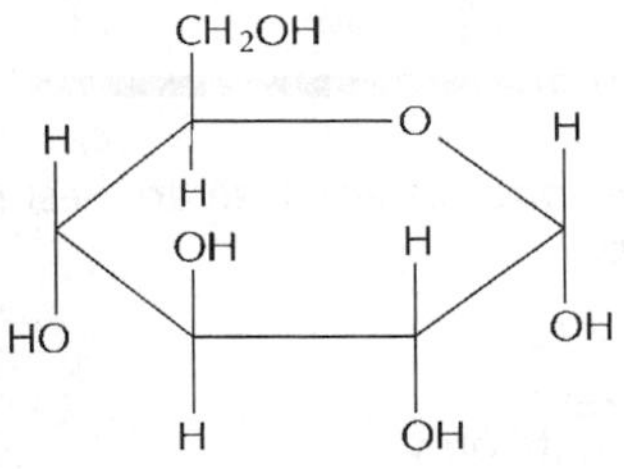

(A)

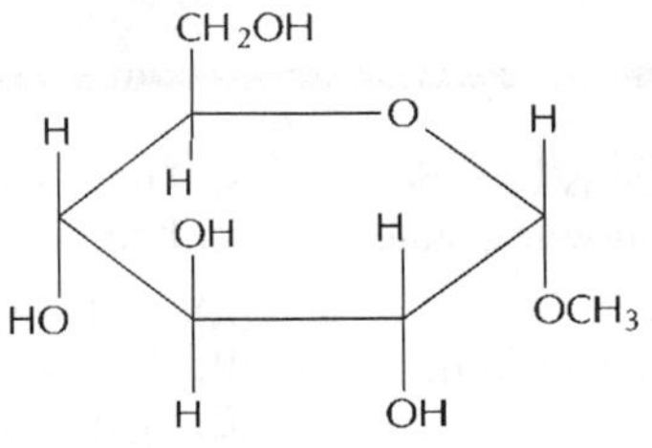

(B)

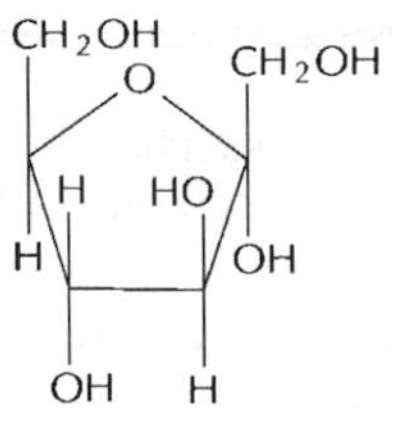

(C)

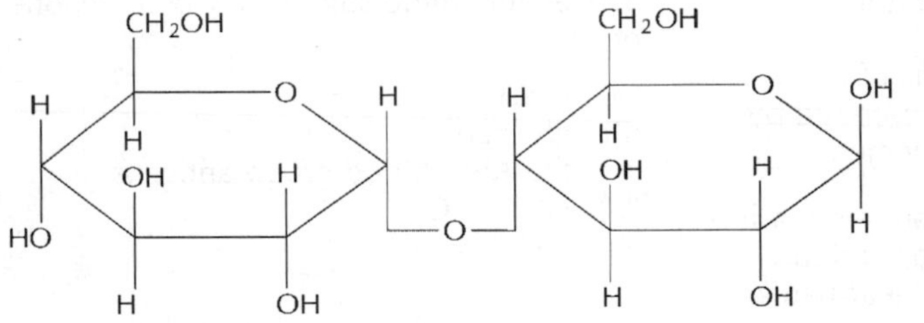

(D)

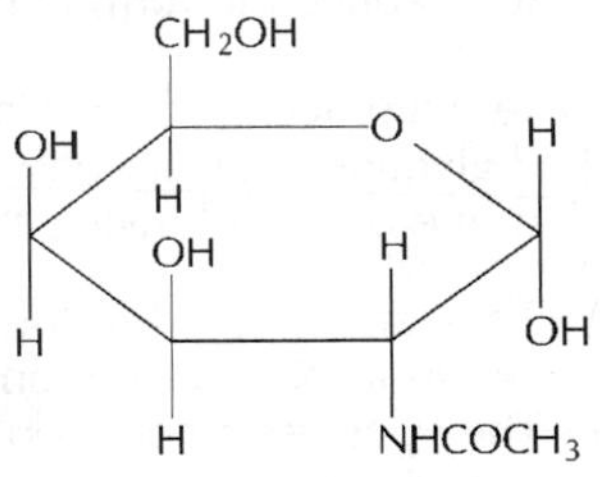

(E)

5. Possesses a β-anomeric carbon

6. Is not a reducing sugar

7. Is most likely to be present in proteoglycans

8. Is a ketose

ANSWERS AND EXPLANATIONS

1. The answer is D [II B 2; IV C; V E]. Glucose is an aldose sugar and forms a six-membered pyranose ring. The C-1 carbon is the anomeric carbon. Sucrose is α-D-glucopyranosyl-β-D-fructofuranoside, a disaccharide of glucose and fructose. Glucose may be reduced to form the sugar alcohol sorbitol.

2. The answer is D [VI B 2; Figure 5-3]. The oligosaccharide portions of N-linked glycoproteins share a common branched pentasaccharide core comprised of three mannose and two N-acetylglucosamine residues. This portion is attached to the protein via a linkage between N-acetylglucosamine and asparagine. O-linked glycoproteins are attached to the protein by a glycosidic linkage to the hydroxyl group of a serine or threonine residue. High-mannose and hybrid N-linked glycoproteins contain primarily mannose, but those of complex N-linked glycoproteins possess less than 50% mannose.

3. The answer is B [IV D; Table 5-2]. Amylose is a linear unbranched polymer of α-D-glucose units in a repeating sequence of α-1,4-glycosidic linkages. β-1,4-glycosidic linkages join chains of D-glucose units to form cellulose.

4. The answer is C [IV D 3; V C; VII]. Glycogen and cellulose are polymers of D-glucose found in animals and plants, respectively. Vitamin C is a sugar acid. The sugar components of DNA are deoxy sugars. N-Acetylglucosamine, an amino sugar, is a component of the core oligosaccharide structure of the ABO blood group antigens.

5-8. The answers are: 5-D [III B 3], **6-B** [IV C 2], **7-E** [IV B; VI C 1], **8-C** [II A 2]. The anomeric carbon is created by cyclization at the carbon bound to oxygen in hemiacetal formation. The carbon is in the beta position when the hydroxyl group on that carbon is above the plane of the ring. This is true regardless of whether the sugar is a monomer or a disaccharide such as maltose.

A reducing sugar must possess a free aldehyde or ketone group. In other words, the hydroxyl group on the anomeric carbon must have nothing attached to it. Option (B) has a glycosidic linkage at its anomeric carbon and, therefore, is not a reducing sugar.

The polysaccharide portion of the proteoglycan, is made up of a repeating disaccharide unit that contains glucosamine or galactosamine, or one of their derivatives. N-Acetylgalactosamine, (E), and its sulfated derivatives are present in several glycosaminoglycans.

In fructose, (C), cyclization has occurred between carbons 2 and 5. Therefore, the carbonyl function on that sugar must have been present on carbon 2, which defines it as a ketone group. The other sugars each possess the carbonyl function on carbon 1, which defines it as an aldehyde.

Chapter 6

Nucleic Acids
Donald Sittman

I. **NUCLEIC ACIDS ARE POLYMERS OF NUCLEOTIDES.** Nucleic acids are responsible for the storage and passage of the information needed for the production of proteins.

A. **Types of nucleic acids.** Nucleic acids are found in two basic structural forms: **deoxyribonucleic acid (DNA)** and **ribonucleic acid (RNA).** Each plays a different role in the storage and passage of cellular information.

1. **Role of DNA.** In most organisms DNA serves as the genetic material.

2. **Role of RNA.** RNA plays multiple roles.
   a. RNA serves as the **genetic material** for some viruses (e.g., tobacco mosaic virus, poliovirus, and influenza virus).
   b. RNA serves as the **carrier of genetic information** to the site of protein synthesis (see messenger RNA, Chapter 9).
   c. RNA forms the crucial **link between messenger RNA and amino acids** being coupled in protein synthesis (see transfer RNA, Chapter 10 II).
   d. RNA is an essential component of **ribosomes** (see Chapter 10 IV) and some enzymes [see small nuclear ribonucleoprotein particles (SNRPS), Chapter 9]. In fact, RNA can have catalytic activity without interacting with proteins.

B. **Nucleotide structure** (Figure 6-1). Nucleic acids, both DNA and RNA, are polymers of **nucleotides (nucleoside monophosphates).** Each nucleotide consists of a pentose sugar, a nitrogenous base, and a phosphate group.

1. A **pentose sugar** is a five-carbon sugar in a pentose ring form. DNA and RNA have different sugar moieties.
   a. **Ribose sugar.** RNA nucleotides, or **ribonucleotides,** contain ribose sugars, which have a hydroxyl group in both the 2′ and 3′ position of the sugar ring.
   b. **Deoxyribose sugar.** DNA nucleotides, or **deoxyribonucleotides,** have 2′-deoxyribose sugars. These sugars have only a single hydroxyl group, in the 3′ position of the sugar ring.

2. **Base.** A nitrogenous base is attached by a glycosidic bond to the 1′ carbon atom of the nucleotide's sugar. The bases of nucleic acids are of two structural types (see Figure 6-1).
   a. **Purines** consist of linked five-membered and six-membered rings. There are two purines commonly found in nucleic acids: **adenine (A)** and **guanine (G).** Each can be found in DNA or RNA.
   b. **Pyrimidines** consist of six-membered rings. There are three pyrimidines commonly found in nucleic acids: **cytosine (C), thymine (T),** and **uracil (U).** Cytosines can be found in DNA or RNA. Thymines are found in DNA. Uracils are found in RNA.

3. **Phosphate.** A nucleotide contains a single phosphate group, which is a strong acid. The phosphate can be attached through the oxygen of a hydroxyl at either the 5′ or 3′ position of the sugar. It is more commonly attached to the 5′ position.

4. The **nomenclature of nucleotides and nucleosides** is presented in Table 6-1. A nucleoside is the term for a sugar and a base (see Figure 6-1). From one to three phosphates can be attached to nucleosides to form nucleoside mono-, di-, or triphosphates (see Figure 6-1). A nucleoside monophosphate can also be called a nucleotide.

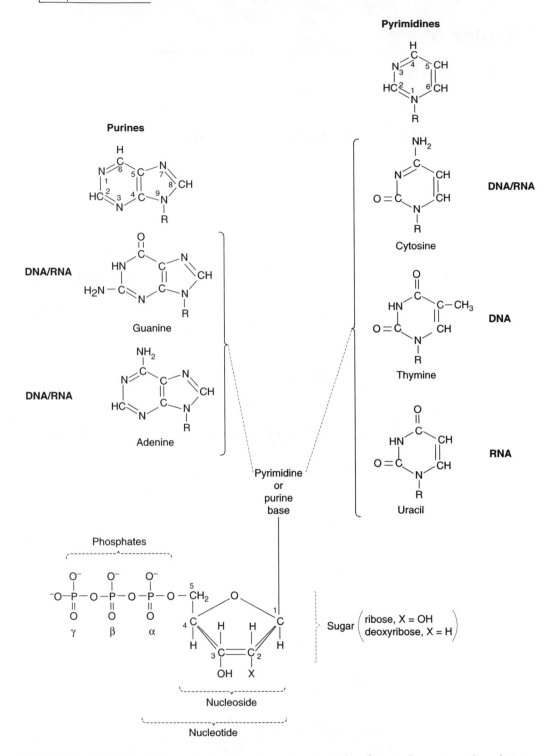

FIGURE 6-1. Nucleotide structure. A drawing of a nucleoside triphosphate is shown. A nucleoside is a base and sugar. A nucleotide is a base, sugar, and phosphate. Up to three phosphates (α, β, and γ) can be added to the sugar. In RNA, nucleotides have a hydroxyl (OH) group in the 2′ position of the sugar. In DNA, the nucleotides have a hydrogen (H) in the 2′ position of the sugar. The five common pyrimidine and purine bases in nucleic acids can be attached to the 1′ carbon of the sugar. R = the attachment site to the sugar.

TABLE 6-1. Nomenclature of Nucleotides and Nucleosides

Bases		Purines		Pyrimidines	
		Adenine (A)	Guanine (G)	Cytosine (C)	Uracil (U) (Thymine [T])
Nucleosides	In RNA	Adenosine	Guanosine	Cytidine	Uridine
	in DNA	Deoxyadenosine	Deoxyguanosine	Deoxycytidine	Deoxythymidine
Nucleotides	In RNA	Adenylate (AMP)	Guanylate (GMP)	Cytidylate (CMP)	Uridylate (UMP)
	in DNA	Deoxyadenylate (dAMP)	Deoxyguanylate (dGMP)	Deoxycytidylate (dCMP)	Thymidylate (dTMP)

C. **Primary polymeric structure** (Figure 6-2)

1. **Linkage of nucleotides.** Nucleotides are linked together by **phosphodiester bonds** between the 3′ hydroxyl on the sugar of one nucleotide through a phosphate molecule to the 5′ hydroxyl on the sugar of another nucleotide. The sugar–phosphate linkages form a symmetrical "backbone," with the 5′ end of one sugar always linked through a phosphate molecule to the 3′ end of the adjacent sugar. The bases are variable and stick out from the backbone. The order of bases determines the coding or structural capacity of the nucleic acid.

2. **Polarity.** The symmetry of the sugar–phosphate backbone imparts a polarity to nucleic acid polymers. The terminal nucleotide of one end usually has a free 3′-hydroxyl group on its sugar moiety, and the other end usually has a free phosphate group attached to the 5′ position of the sugar.

3. **Notation.** It is standard to use the one-letter abbreviation for the bases (see Table 6-1) when writing the order of a nucleic acid polymer. By convention, DNA sequences are written in the 5′ to 3′ direction. The sequence of the nucleic acid presented in Figure 6-2 is written as GCA.

II. DNA SECONDARY STRUCTURE

A. **Double-helical (B-form) DNA** (Figure 6-3). In 1953, Watson and Crick, using x-ray diffraction data of Franklin and Wilkins, proposed a structure for DNA that became known as the **double helix.** It is now known that DNA can adopt different conformations; however, Watson and Crick's double helix is the predominant conformation and is now referred to as **B-form DNA.**

1. **Two antiparallel strands form a right-handed helix.** B-form DNA consists of two polymers, or strands, of DNA paired to each other and coiled around a common axis in a right-handed manner. Each strand has an opposite polarity to the other. That is, where one sugar–phosphate backbone has a 5′ to 3′ symmetry, the adjacent, paired strand is oriented oppositely in a 3′-to-5′ direction. The two strands are said to be **antiparallel.**

2. **Complementary base pairing.** The two DNA strands of the double helix are held together by complementary base pairing. Specific hydrogen bonds can only form between complementary bases in a double helix (see Figure 6-3). The purine adenine pairs with the pyrimidine thymine through two hydrogen bonds (AT), and the purine guanine pairs with the pyrimidine cytosine through three hydrogen bonds (GC). Therefore, in double-helical DNA, there are always the same number of adenine bases as thymine bases, and always the same number of guanosine bases as there are cytosine bases.

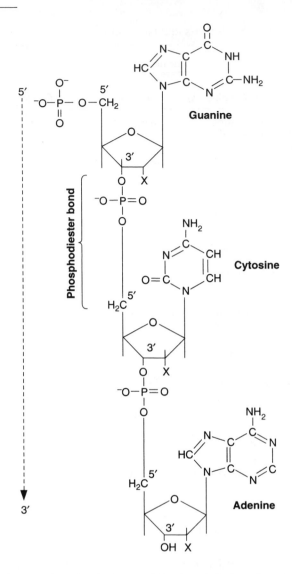

FIGURE 6-2. Structure of a trinucleotide. The bases of the three linked nucleotides are guanine, cytosine, and adenine. If X is OH, then the sugar is ribose, and the structure is RNA. If X is H, then the sugar is deoxyribose, and the structure is DNA.

3. **Base stacking.** The complementary base pairs lie inside the helix, perpendicular to the sugar–phosphate backbone, which lies outside the helix. The base pairs inside the helix are stacked one above the other. The hydrogen bonding of the base pairs and the van der Waals interactions of the stacked base pairs provide the thermodynamic stability of the double helix.

4. **Spiral staircase.** Each base pair is offset approximately 36° from its neighboring base pairs. The helix therefore appears much like a spiral staircase in which **there are 10 steps or base pairs for each complete turn of the helix.**

5. **Dimensions.** The B-form double helix is 20 Å wide. There are 3.4 Å between each stacked base pair. A turn of the helix (10 base pairs) is therefore 34 Å long. From outside the helix, two grooves are apparent: a **major groove** (22 Å wide) and a **minor groove** (12 Å wide). It is through these grooves that many drugs and proteins can make contact with the bases without requiring the helix to open.

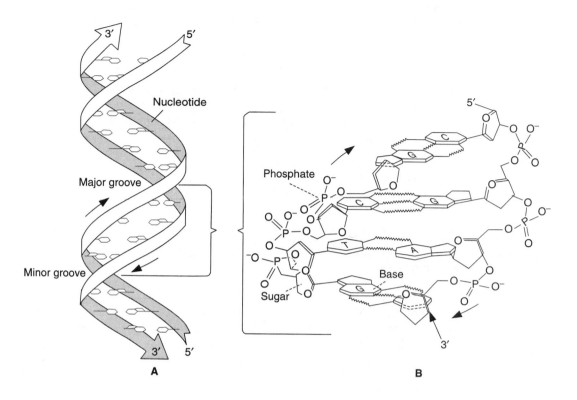

FIGURE 6-3. Structure of B-form DNA. *(A)* Two complementary strands of DNA base pair to form a double helix. The antiparallel sugar–phosphate backbones are presented as ribbons. *(B)* An expanded view of a subregion of the helix showing the paired bases (〜 = hydrogen bonds between bases) and their position in relation to the sugar groups of the sugar–phosphate backbone. (Adapted from Lewin B: *Genes IV,* Cambridge, Massachusetts, Cell Press, 1990, p 66.)

B. **Alternate structural forms of DNA.** In the aqueous environment of the cell, DNA is a dynamic structure that can bend and adopt many alternate structures. B-form DNA remains the predominant form of duplex DNA in the cell, although in the cell it is believed to be a slightly more tightly compacted molecule. Other structures of DNA have been described and are believed to be present in the cell, at least for short distances. Two well-described structures are A-form DNA and Z-form DNA.

1. **A-form DNA** is more compact than B-form DNA, with 11 base pairs per turn. This structure is probably the structure that double-stranded RNA adopts (see IV B 1).

2. **Z-form DNA** is dramatically different from B-form or A-form DNA. It is a left-handed helix and is more elongated than B-form DNA. There are 12 base pairs per turn. Z-form DNA only occurs in sequences of alternating purines and pyrimidines. In particular, if the cytosine residues in a stretch of alternating guanines and cytosines are methylated (see II C), then Z-form DNA can exist under physiologic conditions.

C. **Modification of DNA.** Just as amino acids in proteins can be modified after translation, so can the bases in DNA be modified after DNA synthesis. The most common base modification in eukaryotic DNA is the **methylation of cytosines** that precede guanosines (i.e., in CG doublets that are adjacent on the same strand) to produce methylcytosine.

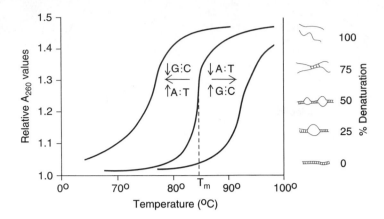

FIGURE 6-4. Melting curve of DNA. As the percentage of guanine–cytosine (G:C) base pairs increases, the melting temperature (T_m) increases. As the percentage of adenine–thymine (A:T) base pairs increases, the T_m decreases. As the temperature increases, the DNA becomes more denatured, and the absorbance value at 260 nm (A_{260}) increases.

1. **Frequency of methylation.** This modification occurs in less than 10% of all cytosines. The cytosines that are methylated vary among different tissue types.

2. **Function of methylation.** The presence of methylcytosines in genes is strongly correlated with transcriptionally inactive genes (see Chapter 12 V). Also, methylcytosine in sequences of alternating CG doublets favors the transition of DNA from the B-form to the Z-form.

D. **Dissociation (denaturation) and reassociation (renaturation) of DNA.** Double-helical strands of DNA have a remarkable ability to dissociate from one another and to reassociate again. This behavior is essential to the process of **replication** (see Chapter 8) and **transcription** (see Chapter 9).

1. **Denaturation.** The hydrogen bonds that hold the two strands of a double helix together can be broken with an **increase in temperature (melting)** or by **treatment with alkali.** When all the hydrogen bonds holding the two strands together are broken, the strands separate, or denature.

   a. **Hyperchromic effect.** DNA absorbs ultraviolet light maximally at the wavelength of 260 nm. The absorption of light at 260 nm by DNA increases upon denaturation. This is called the hyperchromic effect.

   b. **Melting curve.** The denaturation of DNA can be studied by measuring the increase in its absorption of ultraviolet light as temperature is increased (Figure 6-4). The **melting temperature (T_m)** is the temperature at which half of the DNA is unwound or denatured.

   c. **Base composition affects the T_m.** It takes more heat energy to disrupt the three hydrogen bonds of a GC base pair than to disrupt the two hydrogen bonds of an AT base pair. Therefore, the higher the percentage of GC base pairs in DNA, the higher is its T_m (see Figure 6-4). The GC content of the DNA from various organisms differs, as determined by melting curves. Mammalian DNA has approximately 40% GC base pairs and, under standard solution conditions, has a T_m of 87°C.

2. **Renaturation.** Denaturation is reversible. The process whereby denatured, complementary strands of DNA can reform a duplex DNA structure is called renaturation or **annealing.**

   a. **Hypochromic effect.** As single-stranded, complementary DNA reforms a duplex structure, its absorbance at 260 nm decreases. This is called the hypochromic effect.

b. Reassociation kinetics. To reassociate, the denatured, complementary strands of DNA must make contact in such a manner that initial base pairing occurs. After base pairing occurs over a short range of properly realigned, complementary bases, the rest of the molecule renatures quickly, much like a "zipper." Reassociation of denatured, complementary DNA molecules **depends on several factors.**

    (1) Temperature. For reassociation to take place, the temperature of the solution of complementary strands of DNA must be **below the T_m** of their duplex form. However, the temperature should not be so low that intrastrand base pairing (see IV B 2) prevents interstrand complementary sequences from pairing.

    (2) Concentration. Before initial base pairing occurs, complementary strands randomly diffuse in solution until they make contact. Therefore, the rate at which renaturation takes place depends strongly on the concentration of the complementary strands.

    (3) Cot analysis. Reassociation kinetic studies, often called Cot analyses [because they measure the dependence of DNA renaturation on the initial concentration (Co) of denatured DNA with time (t)], have been used to predict the overall organization of the human genome (see II E).

c. Hybridization originally defined the process whereby hybrid duplexes of complementary DNA and RNA combined. This terminology now extends to the analysis of the duplex formation ability of any DNA or RNA molecules, even if they are not perfectly complementary. Although there are many ways to do hybridization analysis, all methods fundamentally measure the degree to which different nucleic acids can form duplex structures. Hybridization technology is a powerful tool; one of its many uses has led to the cloning of many different genes and other DNA sequences from different organisms (see Chapter 11 III).

E. **Organization of eukaryotic genomic DNA.** Humans have 3.3×10^9 base pairs of DNA per haploid genome. It has been estimated that less than 10% of this DNA codes for a product. Cot analysis and later recombinant DNA studies elucidated the nature and location of much of this "extra" DNA in the genome, although the function, if any, of much of it is still unknown.

1. Three major classes of DNA have been indicated by Cot analysis of the human genome.

    a. Nonrepetitive sequences. Approximately 60% of the DNA of many eukaryotes consists of sequences that are found in only one or a few copies in the genome.

        (1) Most protein-coding sequences are in this class of DNA.

        (2) Genes that code for proteins are interspersed with middle repetitive sequences, which are typically not transcribed (see II E 1 b).

        (3) The genes for most proteins are divided into expressed regions (**exons**) that are split up by intervening regions (**introns**), which are transcribed with the exons but are then removed by a process called **splicing** (see Chapter 9 III).

    b. Middle repetitive sequences. Approximately 30% of the DNA of many eukaryotes consists of sequences that are repeated anywhere from ten to hundreds of times. These sequences are used in DNA fingerprinting (see Chapter 11 IV D).

    c. Highly repetitive sequences. Approximately 10% of the DNA of many eukaryotes consists of sequences that are repeated from hundreds to hundreds of thousands of times.

2. Further classification of repetitive DNAs. The characteristics of the DNAs that are known to be in the middle and highly repetitive DNA classes are not clearly distinguishable based solely on their repetitiveness. Based on what has been learned about repetitive DNA from recombinant DNA studies, most can be assigned to one of several classes.

    a. Tandemly repeated genes. A number of genes, such as the ribosomal RNA (rRNA) genes and the transfer RNA (tRNA) genes exist in **tandem repeats** of hundreds to thousands of copies. Usually these genes are identical copies of each other separated by some noncoding DNA called **spacer sequences.** The number of copies of these genes depends on the gene and the organism.

   (1) Humans have approximately 250 copies of the genes for 45S pre-rRNA, 2000 5S rRNA genes, and 1300 tRNA genes.

   (2) Tandemly repeated genes share the trait of producing products that are needed abundantly in most cell types, although not all genes that can be abundantly expressed exist in multiple copies.

  b. Noncoding repetitive DNA

   (1) Simple sequence repeats. Some regions of genomic DNA are made of **short, tandemly repeated sequences.** Their basic repeating unit can be from 5–200 base pairs, and their overall length can reach 10^5 base pairs.

    (a) Structure. Although the function of these sequences is unknown, it is believed that they may play a structural role in the chromosome because they are located at the centromeres and telomeres (see Chapter 8 III D).

    (b) Function. Some simple sequence repeats have a lower repeat number than those in centromeres and telomeres. They are interspersed throughout the chromosome, and their function is unknown. These sequences are called **hypervariable regions** because the number of repeats, but not the sequence of the repeating units, varies considerably between individuals. Because of this variation, these sequences are the basis of a very specific identification test called **DNA fingerprinting** (see Chapter 11 IV D).

   (2) Interspersed repeats. Much of the middle repetitive DNA is made of interspersed sequences that exist throughout the genome in apparently random locations. Their length can vary between 150 and 300 base pairs, called **short interspersed repeats (SINES),** and between 1000 and 6000 base pairs called **long interspersed repeats (LINES).** There can be up to 500,000 copies of any one of these repeats. Many of these sequences are **mobile elements,** which can move to different positions in the genomic DNA.

III. **HIGHER ORDER (TERTIARY) STRUCTURE OF DNA.** The DNA in a single human cell, if stretched to its full length, is 1.74 meters. Clearly, to get DNA into a cell's nucleus, it must be packaged into a more tightly compacted form. The structural flexibility of DNA allows it to adopt more compacted structures than simple linear B-form DNA.

A. **Supercoils**

  1. Description. Studies of circular DNA have shown that it can be twisted into a compact supercoiled or superhelical form. DNA supercoils can be either **right-handed (positive)** or **left-handed (negative).**

   a. Positive supercoils are twisted in the same direction as the right-handed helix of B-form DNA about its axis, whereas **negative supercoils** are twisted in the opposite direction.

   b. Supercoils have a **higher free energy** than nonsupercoiled, "relaxed" DNA.

  2. Supercoils exist naturally. Bacterial genomic DNA and plasmid DNA (see Chapter 11 III B 2 a) are supercoiled. Eukaryotic DNA also becomes supercoiled as it becomes packaged into higher order chromatin structures (see III B). Most of these naturally occurring supercoils are negative.

  3. Topoisomerases. Enzymes responsible for altering the superhelicity of cellular DNA are called topoisomerases because they affect the topology of DNA. These enzymes are very important to the process of replication (see Chapter 8).

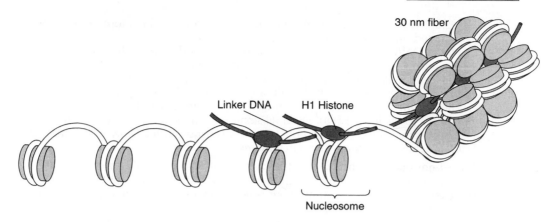

FIGURE 6-5. Illustration of nucleosomes showing the core particle and where the histone H1 binds, if present. *Linker DNA* joins the core particles. A *nucleosome* is the repeating unit of core particle, H1, and linker DNA. The core particle consists of two histones H2a, two histones H2b, two histones H3, and two histones H4; wrapped around these core histones are 146 base pairs of DNA. In the presence of the *H1 histone,* nucleosomes condense into a 30-nm fiber, which is shown here in the *solenoid* model.

B. **Chromatin.** In humans, DNA is divided and packaged into 46 separate structures known as chromosomes, which during mitosis are visible with a light microscope. The packing of DNA in a mitotic chromosome represents a 10,000-fold shortening of its length from primary B-form DNA. During interphase, when DNA needs to be accessible to the transcription and replication enzymes, it is packaged less densely than in mitotic chromosomes, in a structure known as **chromatin.** Chromatin was originally detected by its ability to be stained with a variety of microscopy stains. The DNA of chromatin is packaged with approximately double its mass of protein.

1. **Histones.** The major class of proteins associated with chromatin is the histones, which exist in a mass approximately equal to DNA in the chromatin.
   a. Histones are **small (11,000–21,000 MW), basic proteins** that bind to the acidic DNA by noncovalent interactions to form nucleosomes (see III B 2).
   b. There are **five types of histones:**
      (1) The **four core histones: H2a, H2b, H3,** and **H4**
      (2) The **one linker histone: H1**
   c. **Evolution.** Evolutionarily, the histones are **highly conserved.** For example, the histone H4 of the pea plant and the cow only differ by 2 out of 102 amino acids. This degree of evolutionary conservation implies that histones play a very important functional role in the chromatin of all eukaryotes.
   d. In many eukaryotes there are **amino acid sequence variants of all of the histones except H4.** These variants likely have slightly different functional roles in chromatin.
   e. All of the **histones are post-translationally modified** (e.g., phosphorylated, methylated, acetylated) at various stages of the cell cycle. These modifications are expected to play a functional role in changing the structure of chromatin. However, the specific role of each type of modification is not yet known.

2. **Nucleosomes.** If chromatin is placed in a low salt buffer and viewed with an electron microscope, it resembles a "string of beads." The repeating beads-on-a-string structure is also called the **10-nm fiber,** based on measurements of its width, and represents a sevenfold shortening of linear, B-form DNA. The repeating, bead-like structures are the **basic packaging unit of chromatin** called nucleosomes, and they occur an average of once for every 200 base pairs of DNA.
   a. **Core particles** (Figure 6-5). The fundamental **structural feature of nucleosomes** is the core particle, the structure of which has been determined by x-ray crystal-

lography. It consists of two each of the core histones, which form a disc that is wrapped, in two turns, by 146 base pairs of DNA.

b. **Linker DNA.** The amount of DNA wrapped around core particles is constant. However, the **DNA that connects core particles,** called linker DNA, is variable in length. Linker DNA averages 60 base pairs in length; however, depending on the organism and tissue, its length ranges from 8–120 base pairs.

c. **The histone H1** binds to core particles at the point where DNA enters and exits the core particle (see Figure 6-5). Histone H1 may sometimes be present in nucleosomes. Its presence in nucleosomes is **required for DNA to be packaged in a higher order form than nucleosomes.**

3. **The 30-nm fiber.** The next level of packaging leads to a 40-fold shortening of B-form DNA. The formation of 30-nm fibers requires the presence of the histone H1. The exact structure of the 30-nm fiber is not known but it is believed to look much like a **solenoid** (see Figure 6-5).

4. **Higher-order chromatin structure.** Few details are known of how DNA is condensed and packaged beyond the 30-nm fiber to its ultimate packaged form in mitotic chromosomes. It is, however, known that all DNA is not packaged equally. There are at least three forms of packaged DNA in most cells.

a. **Heterochromatin.** Portions of chromatin stain darkly and represent **densely packaged DNA.** These DNA regions, called heterochromatin, are thought to be **transcriptionally inactive** and do not appear to be unpackaged from their mitotic chromosome form.

b. **Euchromatin.** Portions of the chromatin stain poorly and are not tightly packaged like heterochromatin. These portions of the chromatin are thought to be **transcriptionally active** and are called euchromatin.

c. **Loop domains.** There is some evidence that DNA is attached to a proteinaceous matrix, called a **scaffold** in mitotic chromosomes, or a **nuclear matrix** in interphase nuclei. The DNA projects out as **loops** from these matrices, which are believed to contain active genes.

5. **Nonhistone chromatin proteins.** In addition to the histones and the enzymes and factors needed for transcription (see Chapter 9 II) and replication (see Chapter 8), other proteins are associated with chromatin.

a. **High-mobility group (HMG) proteins** are abundant chromatin-associated proteins that share the property of showing fast mobility upon electrophoresis. The specific function of HMG proteins is unknown beyond the fact that they affect chromatin structure and folding.

b. **Scaffold proteins.** Several scaffold proteins have been found. One is the enzyme called **topoisomerase II.** Presumably it is needed to relieve torsional stress in the loops of DNA projecting from the scaffold or nuclear matrix upon replication or during mitosis. Another is the filamentous **lamins** that are also part of the lamina that lines the inner membrane of the nucleus. Presumably they link the chromatin scaffold structure to the nuclear membrane.

IV. **RNA STRUCTURE.** RNA plays multiple roles in the cell that mostly are clearly distinct from the role of DNA. The fundamental structural units of RNA differ little from DNA (see I B), yet RNA has greater structural versatility than DNA, which to a large extent confers the functional versatility of RNA.

A. **Primary structure.** RNA is initially synthesized as a single-stranded polymer by the process of transcription. Ribonucleotides are linked into a polar molecule by **phosphodiester bonds** between the 3′ hydroxyl on the sugar of one ribonucleotide through a phosphate to the 5′ hydroxyl on the sugar of another ribonucleotide, like those in DNA (see I C). The sugar–phosphate linkages form a symmetrical **"backbone,"** with the 5′ end of one sugar always linked through a phosphate to the 3′ end of the adjacent sugar. The bases are variable and stick out from the backbone.

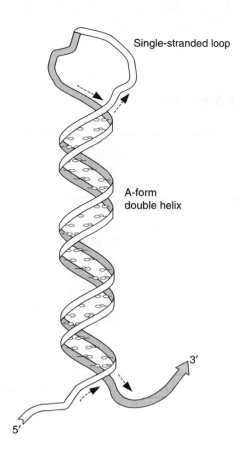

Single-stranded loop

**A-form
double helix**

3′

5′

FIGURE 6-6. An RNA stem-loop structure. A *single-stranded* RNA molecule may fold back on itself to form an *A-form double helix* by base pairing between complementary sequences.

B. **Secondary structure.** Complementary RNA sequences can base pair (see II A 2). In RNA helices, **adenine pairs with uridine** through two hydrogen bonds, and **guanine pairs with cytosine** through three hydrogen bonds. The nature of the RNA double helix is similar to DNA in that the strands must be antiparallel.

1. **Double-stranded RNA is an A-form helix** (see II B 1). B-form RNA cannot form because the 2′ hydroxyl on the ribose sugar sterically hinders its formation.

2. **Stem-loop structures.** If two regions within a single-stranded piece of RNA are complementary, they can base pair and form a stem-loop structure (Figure 6-6).

C. **Tertiary structure.** Some RNAs serve structural roles, some interact extensively with specific proteins, and a few have catalytic functions requiring that they be able to form very complex structures (see Chapter 9).

1. **Modification of RNA.** The bases in RNA can be modified after RNA is synthesized. **Methylations** at numerous positions of the different bases are the most common of these modifications, which allow for unusual base pairings that enhance the structural diversity of RNA.

2. **Transfer RNA (tRNA).** The most heavily modified RNA is tRNA (see Chapter 10 II). Modifications are required to achieve the unique structural features of tRNA, which are crucial to its highly specialized function.

STUDY QUESTIONS

DIRECTIONS: Each of the numbered items or incomplete statements in this section is followed by answers or by completions of the statement. Select the **one** lettered answer or completion that is **best** in each case.

1. If the base sequence of a segment of DNA is CAGTTAGC, which of the following sequences is complementary?

(A) GCTAACTG
(B) CGATTGAC
(C) TAGCCAGT
(D) GCUAACUG

2. The structure shown below is which one of the following compounds?

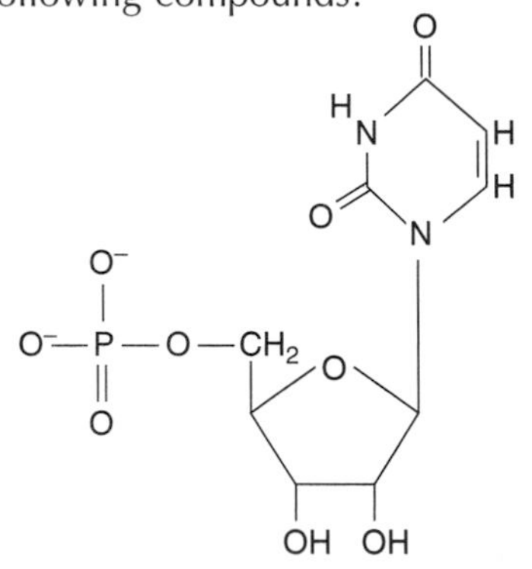

(A) Adenosine
(B) Deoxyguanylate
(C) Thymidylate
(D) Cytidine
(E) Uridylate

3. Which one of the following statements is true of double-helical DNA?

(A) The planes of the bases lie parallel to the helix axis
(B) The chains have a backbone of linked glycosides
(C) Unless the DNA is circular, the 3'-hydroxyl groups of each chain are at opposite ends of the molecule
(D) The duplex structure is stabilized only by hydrogen bonding between bases
(E) Although they are associated in antiparallel fashion, the two chains have an identical base sequence

4. Most protein-coding sequences are found in which class of DNA?

(A) Long interspersed repeats
(B) Highly repetitive sequences
(C) Middle repetitive sequences
(D) Nonrepetitive sequences
(E) Tandem repeats

5. If a sample of DNA is found to have the base composition (mole ratios) of adenine = 40; thymine = 22; guanine = 19; and cytosine = 19, what conclusion can be drawn?

(A) The DNA is a circular duplex
(B) The DNA is a linear duplex
(C) The DNA is single-stranded
(D) The DNA has highly repetitive sequences
(E) The DNA has a high melting point

6. If the cytosine content of double-helical DNA is 20% of the total bases, the adenine content would be

(A) 10%
(B) 20%
(C) 30%
(D) 40%
(E) 50%

7. The hyperchromic effect is best described by which one of the following statements?

(A) The increase in the melting temperature (T_m) of DNA with increasing guanine-cytosine content
(B) A maximum rate of denaturation versus temperature for double-helical DNA
(C) An increase in the absorbance of light at 260 nm upon denaturation of DNA
(D) An increase in the absorbance of light at 260 nm when DNA-RNA hybrids are annealed

8. The melting temperature (T_m) of DNA is best defined as being

(A)   proportional to the length of DNA
(B)   proportional to the guanine-cytosine (GC) content of DNA
(C)   the temperature at which all of the DNA is denatured
(D)   proportional to the purine content of DNA
(E)   the same in all animals

9. Nucleosomes are best described by which one of the following statements?

(A)   They are the basic packaging unit of chromatin
(B)   They are found only in euchromatin
(C)   They are comprised of histones, high-mobility-group (HMG) proteins, and DNA
(D)   They condense DNA by wrapping two each of the core histones around 146 base pairs of DNA
(E)   They package DNA into a 10-nm solenoid-shaped fiber

10. The histone H1 is best described by which one of the following statements?

(A)   It is one of the four histones that make up the nucleosome core particle
(B)   It is an abundant, acidic protein found in the nucleus
(C)   It is required to package DNA beyond the 10-nm fiber
(D)   It links chromatin to the nuclear matrix
(E)   It has no post-translationally modified amino acids

11. Which one of the following statements concerning RNA is correct?

(A)   The mole fraction of adenine (A) equals the mole fraction of uracil (U)
(B)   In RNA helices, A can base pair with U through three hydrogen bonds
(C)   Double-stranded RNA is an A-form helix
(D)   The sugar group of ribonucleotides has two hydrogens at the 2′ position
(E)   Ribonucleotides are linked into a polar molecule by phosphodiester bonds between the 2′ position on the sugar of one ribonucleotide through a phosphate to the 5′ hydroxyl on the sugar of another ribonucleotide

ANSWERS AND EXPLANATIONS

1. The answer is B [I C 3; II A 2]. Adenine (A) pairs with thymine (T) [or with uridine (U), if base pairing with RNA], and guanine (G) pairs with cytosine (C). By convention, DNA and RNA sequences are written in the 5′ to 3′ direction. Because DNA strands are antiparallel, the complementary sequence must be written in the reverse, or 5′ to 3′ direction.

2. The answer is E [I B 1-4; Figure 6-1; Table 6-1]. The structure is uridylate, which is a nucleotide with a pyrimidine base and a ribose sugar. Adenosine is a purine ribonucleoside. Deoxyguanylate is a purine deoxyribonucleotide. Thymidylate is a pyrimidine deoxyribonucleotide. Cytidine is a pyrimidine ribonucleoside.

3. The answer is C [II A]. Double-helical DNA molecules are formed from two antiparallel, complementary, polydeoxyribonucleotide chains wound around one another with the purine and pyrimidine bases on the inside of the helix and the deoxyribose and phosphates on the outside. Because linear DNA molecules are antiparallel, the 3′-hydroxyl groups lie at opposite ends of each molecule. The base sequences complement one another in terms of Watson-Crick base pairing (i.e., adenine with thymine and guanine with cytosine); therefore, they are not identical in sequence. Double-helical formation is made possible by hydrogen bonding between base pairs, but the stability of the double helix owes much to the van der Waals interactions of the stacked bases that lie perpendicular to the helix axis, which is composed of deoxyribose-phosphate chains. The bases are attached to the deoxyribose by glycosidic bonds.

4. The answer is D [II E 1 a]. Most protein-coding sequences are found in the nonrepetitive fraction of the genome. Some protein-coding sequences can also be found in repetitive-sequence DNAs, except for some of the most highly repeated sequences. The tandem repeats contain some genes, such as for the histones and ribosomal RNAs, which are expressed abundantly.

5. The answer is C [II A 2, D 1 b]. The mole fraction of any one of the four standard bases—adenine (A), guanine (G), thymine (T), and cytosine (C)—in double-helical DNA establishes the content of each of the other three. Because A = T and G = C in all double-helical DNAs, the sample cannot be a double-helical molecule. The DNA could have highly repetitive sequences, but this conclusion cannot be drawn from the data given. Melting of DNA refers to the dissociation of double-helical DNA and does not apply to single-stranded DNA.

6. The answer is C [II A 2]. Because the mole fraction of cytosine (C) equals the mole fraction of guanine (G) in double-helical DNA, G + C = 40%. The remaining 60% must be divided equally between adenine (A) and thymine (T) because the mole fraction of A equals the mole fraction of T in double-helical DNA. Thus, the adenine content must be 30% of the total bases.

7. The answer is C [II D 1 a]. The bases in double-helical DNA are sequestered inside the double helix away from water. Interaction between the stacked, planar ring structures reduces their absorbance of ultraviolet light at 260 nm. Upon denaturation, the bases lose interaction with one another, and the absorbance of light at 260 nm increases, which is the hyperchromic effect of denaturation. The base composition does affect the melting temperature (T_m) of DNA but it does not affect the magnitude of the increase in absorbance upon denaturation.

8. The answer is B [II D 1 b-c]. Dissociation of the two chains of double-helical DNA occurs when temperature is increased beyond a certain point and is referred to as melting. The melting temperature (T_m) of DNA is the temperature at which one half of the DNA is denatured. The T_m of a particular piece of DNA, measured under standard conditions of pH and salt concentration, increases with an increase in guanine-cytosine (GC) content of the DNA. The T_m of DNA is not directly proportional to the length of DNA, nor is it the same for all animals. The percentage of purines is the same for all DNAs so the T_m cannot be proportional to the number of purines in DNA.

9. The answer is A [III B]. Nucleosomes are the basic repeating unit of chromatin. They consist of two each of the core histones (H2a, H2b, H3, and H4), which form a disc that is wrapped in two turns by 146 base pairs of DNA. Nucleosomes are the basic packaging unit of DNA in both euchromatin and heterochromatin. The solenoid structure of chromatin occurs when nucleosomes package beyond their normal 10-nm fiber size to a 30-nm fiber size in the presence of the H1 histones. The high-mobility group (HMG) proteins are abundant chromatin-associated proteins; however, they are not part of the basic nucleosome structure.

10. The answer is C [III B 2 c]. The histone H1 is the linker histone that is required in the packaging of DNA beyond the 10-nm fiber. Although it is abundant and basic like the other (core) histones, it is not part of the nucleosomal core particle. Another class of proteins, the lamins, play a role in forming the nuclear scaffold and linking it to the nuclear membrane. All of the histones are post-translationally modified.

11. The answer is C [I B 1 a; IV]. RNA differs from DNA by having a hydroxyl group attached to the 2' carbon of the sugar moiety. As in DNA, the nucleotides are linked into a polar molecule by phosphodiester bonds between the 3' hydroxyl on the sugar of one nucleotide through a phosphate to the 5' hydroxyl on the sugar of another nucleotide. Complementary RNA sequences can base pair to generate an A-form helix. In RNA helices, adenine-uracil (AU) base pairs can be formed with two hydrogen bonds, and guanine-cytosine (GC) base pairs can be formed with three hydrogen bonds. Only complementary stretches of RNA can base pair to form a double-stranded helix; therefore, the mole fraction of complementary bases is not likely to be equal.

Chapter 7

Lipids and Related Compounds

Victor Davidson

Case 7-1

A 15-year-old girl is admitted to the hospital because of easy bruising and bleeding and an apparent mass in her abdomen. Physical examination reveals that the mass is due to a greatly enlarged spleen. Enlargement of the liver is also observed. Blood analysis indicates a decrease of all blood cells including platelets. Bone marrow analysis reveals the presence of enlarged cells.

- What is the diagnosis, and how may it be confirmed?
- What is the basis for the patient's symptoms?
- Is this condition treatable?

I. **NATURE OF LIPIDS.** Lipids have a hydrophobic nature because of the predominance of hydrocarbon chains ($-CH_2-CH_2-CH_2-$) in their structure. They are insoluble or only poorly soluble in water, but readily soluble in nonpolar solvents such as ether and benzene. Some common classifications of lipids and their general biologic functions are listed in Table 7-1.

II. **FATTY ACIDS**

A. **Nature and nomenclature.** Fatty acids are water-insoluble, saturated or unsaturated, long-chain hydrocarbons with a carboxyl group at the end of the chain (Table 7-2).

1. **Saturated fatty acids** do not have double bonds in the chain.
   a. **Nomenclature.** The **systematic name** gives the number of carbons, with the suffix *-anoic* appended. Palmitic acid, for example, has 16 carbons and has the systematic name hexadecanoic acid.
   b. **Structure.** The **general formula** of saturated fatty acids is $CH_3-(CH_2)_n-COOH$, where *n* is the number of methylene groups between the methyl and carboxyl carbons.

TABLE 7-1. Classifications and Functions of Lipids

Lipid	Primary Functions
Fatty acids	Energy sources, biosynthetic precursors
Triacylglycerols	Storage, transport
Phosphoglycerides	Membrane components
Ketone bodies	Energy sources
Sphingolipids	Membrane components
Eicosanoids	Modulators of physiologic activity
Cholesterol	Membrane component
Steroid hormones	Modulators of physiologic activity

TABLE 7-2. Predominant Fatty Acids Found in Mammalian Tissues

Common Name	Systematic Name	No. Carbon Atoms	No. Double Bonds	Melting Point (°C)
Lauric	Dodecanoic	12	0	43.5
Myristic	Tetradecanoic	14	0	54.4
Palmitic	Hexadecanoic	16	0	62.8
Stearic	Octadecanoic	18	0	69.6
Pamitoleic	cis-Δ^9-Hexadecenoic	16	1	1.0
Oleic	cis-Δ^9-Octadecenoic	18	1	13.0
Linoleic	all cis-Δ^9,Δ^{12}-Octadecadienoic	18	2	−11.0
Linolenic	all cis-Δ^9,Δ^{12},Δ^{15}-Octadecatrienoic	18	3	−11.2
Arachidonic	all cis-Δ^5,Δ^8,Δ^{11},Δ^{14}-Eicosatetraenoic	20	4	−49.5

  2. **Unsaturated fatty acids** have one or more double bonds. In naturally occurring fatty acids, these bonds are always in a *cis* as opposed to a *trans* configuration (i.e., the single hydrogens bonded to each carbon are oriented in the same direction). The most commonly used system for designating the position of double bonds in an unsaturated fatty acid is the delta (Δ) numbering system.
     a. **Numbering system.** The terminal carboxyl carbon is designated C-1, and the double bond is given the number of the carbon on the carboxyl side of the double bond. For example, palmitoleic acid, which has 16 carbons and a double bond between C-9 and C-10, is designated 16:1:Δ^9, or 16:1:9.
     b. The **systematic name** gives the number of carbon atoms, number of double bonds (unless it has only one), and bears the suffix -*enoic* (see Table 7-2). Thus, linoleic acid, with 18 carbons and two *cis* double bonds, is *cis*-Δ^9,Δ^{12}-octadecadienoic acid.

B. Source

  1. **Nonessential fatty acids.** Nonessential fatty acids can be synthesized from products of glucose oxidation (see Chapter 22 I) and do not, therefore, have to be included in the diet.
  2. **Essential fatty acids.** Fatty acids of the linoleic ($18:2:\Delta^{9,12}$) and linolenic ($18:3:\Delta^{9,12,15}$) families must be obtained from the diet.

C. Physical properties

  1. Fatty acids are detergent-like because of their **amphipathic nature.** They have nonpolar (CH_3) and polar (−COOH) ends. In biphasic systems, they orient with the polar end associated with water and the nonpolar end associated with the hydrophobic phase.
  2. The melting point of fatty acids is related to chain length and degree of unsaturation. The longer the chain length, the higher the melting point; the greater the number of double bonds, the lower the melting point (see Table 7-2).

D. Triacylglycerols (triglycerides)

  1. **Structure.** Triacylglycerols are triesters of glycerol and three fatty acids (Figure 7-1).
  2. **Function.** Fatty acids are converted to triacylglycerols for transport between tissues and for storage of metabolic fuel.
     a. The main stores of metabolic fuel in humans are the fat deposits in fat cells (**adipocytes**). These serve long-term needs for metabolic fuel.
     b. Triacylglycerols have two major advantages over other forms of metabolic fuel.
        (1) Triacylglycerols provide a concentrated form of fuel because their complete combustion to carbon dioxide (CO_2) and water releases 9 kcal/g as opposed to 4 kcal/g for carbohydrate.

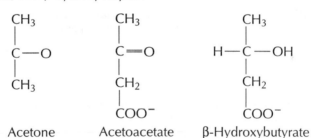

FIGURE 7-1. Structures of lipids derived from glycerol. R = a fatty acid; X = a hydroxy-containing compound.

    (2) Because they are water insoluble, triacylglycerols present no osmotic problems to the cell when stored in large amounts.

  c. **Lipolysis** involves the **hydrolysis of triacylglycerols to free glycerol and free fatty acids** (also known as **nonesterified fatty acids**) with both products leaving the adipocyte. The appearance of fatty acids in the blood during fasting is due to the mobilization of fat stores by this process.

    (1) **Utilization of fatty acids.** Fatty acids are used by most tissues, except the brain, as a metabolic fuel.

    (2) **Utilization of glycerol.** Glycerol is used by the liver as a substrate for gluconeogenesis (see Chapter 20 II).

E. **Ketone bodies,** which are formed from fatty acids and carbohydrates, include acetone, acetoacetate, and β-hydroxybutyrate.

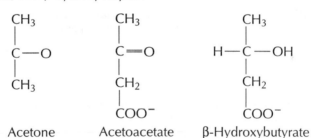

Acetone   Acetoacetate   β-Hydroxybutyrate

1. Synthesis of ketone bodies (see Chapter 22 IV)

  a. Ketone bodies are synthesized in liver mitochondria and released into the blood for use as metabolic fuel by other tissues. **The liver does not use ketone bodies.**

  b. Levels of synthesis are high when the rate of fatty acid oxidation is high and carbohydrate utilization is low. This occurs during fasting, starvation, untreated diabetes, and prolonged alcohol abuse.

2. **Ketoacidosis** is an imbalance of blood pH (see Chapter 1 III B) caused by the excessive accumulation of acetoacetate or β-hydroxybutyrate, which are weak acids.

  a. **Ketosis** refers to **ketonuria** (high urine levels of ketone bodies) and **ketonemia** (high blood levels of ketone bodies).

  b. During starvation, ketone bodies are the only source of fuel, so they are consumed by the body, and there is no excess to accumulate. In contrast, in untreated diabetes, blood levels of ketone bodies may become high enough to produce life-threatening ketoacidosis.

III. **PHOSPHOLIPIDS** are the major lipid constituents of cellular membranes. They comprise approximately 40% of the lipids in the erythrocyte membrane and more than 95% of the lipids in the inner mitochondrial membrane.

A. **Phosphoglycerides** are triesters of glycerol-3-phosphate in which two esters have been formed between the two hydroxyl groups and fatty acid side chains (R_1 and R_2), and a third ester has been formed between the phosphate group and a hydroxyl-containing compound, X (see Figure 7-1).

B. **Classification of phosphoglycerides.** Phosphoglycerides include the following compounds:

1. **Phosphatidylcholine** (lecithin)

2. **Phosphatidylethanolamine** (a cephalin)

3. **Phosphatidylserine** (a cephalin)

4. **Phosphatidylinositol**

5. **Cardiolipin,** which comprises approximately 20% of the lipids of the inner mitochondrial membrane

C. **Characteristics of phosphoglycerides**

1. Phosphoglycerides are the most polar lipids and are **amphipathic,** possessing **both hydrophilic and hydrophobic groups.** They inhabit transition regions between aqueous and nonaqueous phases.

2. Phosphoglycerides are **amphoteric,** bearing **both negatively and positively charged groups.**

IV. **SPHINGOLIPIDS** are present in nearly all human tissues. The greatest concentration of sphingolipids is found in the central nervous system (CNS), particularly in white matter.

A. **Sphingomyelin**

1. **Function.** Sphingomyelin is the major phospholipid component of membranes in neural tissues.

2. **Structure.** Sphingomyelin, which is derived from the amino alcohol, sphingosine, is the only sphingolipid that contains phosphate and has no sugar moiety. It is formed from **ceramide,** which is the **core structure** of naturally occurring sphingolipids, including the glycosphingolipids.

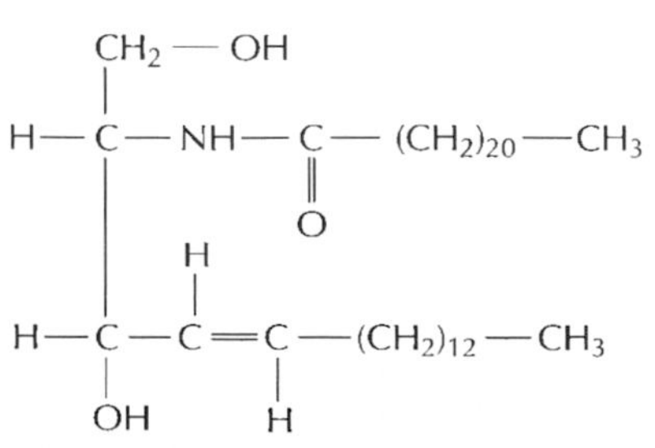

Ceramide 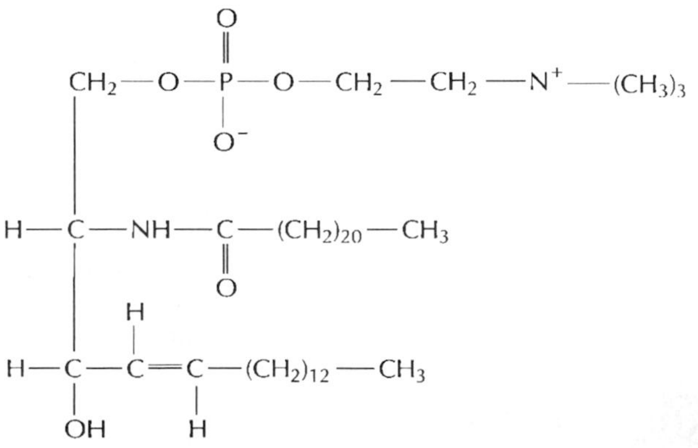   Sphingomyelin

B. **Glycosphingolipids** are sphingolipids that contain carbohydrate moieties.

1. **Cerebrosides** are ceramide monohexosides, the most important being **galactocerebroside** and **glucocerebroside.** Cerebrosides are found in neural tissue membranes, particularly the myelin sheath.

Glucocerebroside

2. **Sulfatides** are cerebrosides that contain sulfated sugars. **β-Sulfogalactocerebroside** accounts for approximately 15% of the lipids in white matter of the brain.

3. **Globosides** are ceramide oligosaccharides that contain two or more sugar molecules, most often galactose, glucose, or N-acetylgalactosamine, attached to ceramide. They are found in serum, the spleen, the liver, and erythrocytes. For example, **lactosylceramide** is found in erythrocyte membranes.

4. **Gangliosides**
   a. **Nature.** Gangliosides are glycosphingolipids that contain one or more neuraminic acid residues, usually as the N-acetyl derivative [i.e., **N-acetylneuraminic acid (NANA)**], which is **sialic acid.** They are found in high concentration in ganglion cells of the CNS and in lower concentration in the membranes of most cells.
   b. **Nomenclature**
      (1) The letter G is used to denote a ganglioside, with M, D, T, or Q to indicate, respectively, mono-, di-, tri-, or quatrosialic acid contents. Numerical subscripts are based on their chromatographic migration. For example:

$$GM_1 = Gal\text{-}(N\text{-}AcGal)\text{-}Gal\text{-}Glc\text{-}Cer$$
$$GM_2 = (N\text{-}AcGal)\text{-}Gal\text{-}Glc\text{-}Cer$$
$$GM_3 = Gal\text{-}Glc\text{-}Cer$$

where *Cer* = ceramide, *Glc* = glucose, *Gal* = galactose, and *N-AcGal* = N-acetylgalactosamine.
      (2) For example, the GM_2 ganglioside is:

$$(N\text{-}AcGal)\text{-}Gal\text{-}Glc\text{-}Cer$$
$$|$$
$$NANA$$

C. **Sphingolipidoses** are inherited genetic disorders referred to as **lipid storage diseases,** in which there is a deficiency of an enzyme that is involved in the normal catabolism of a particular sphingolipid. This results in the intracellular accumulation of that lipid to harmful levels (Table 7-3).

V. EICOSANOIDS are products of arachidonic acid (see Table 7-2).

A. **Prostaglandins**
1. **Structure.** Prostaglandins are analogs of **prostanoic acid.**

TABLE 7-3. Sphingolipidoses

Disease	Lipid Accumulated	Enzyme Deficiency	Primary Organ Affected
Niemann-Pick	Sphingomyelin	Sphingomyelinase	Brain, liver, spleen
Gaucher's	Glucocerebroside	β-Glucosidase	Brain, liver, spleen
Krabbe's	Galactocerebroside	β-Galactosidase	Brain
Metachromatic leukodystrophy	β-Sulfogalacto- cerebroside	Sulfatide sulfatase	Brain
Fabry's	Ceramide trihexoside	α-Galactosidase	Kidneys
Tay-Sachs	Ganglioside GM_2	Hexosaminidase A	Brain

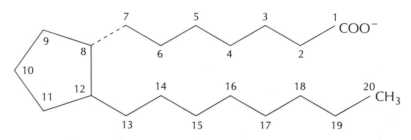

Prostanoic acid

2. **Nomenclature. Prostaglandins** are abbreviated **PG,** with an additional capital letter that denotes the ring type and a numeral (or, in one case, a Greek letter) as a subscript.

    a. **Substitutions on the ring.** Seven kinds of rings are found in naturally occurring prostaglandins (Figure 7-2).

    b. **Hydrocarbon structure.** The **subscript number** (e.g., PGE_1, PGE_2, and PGE_3) denotes the **number of unsaturated bonds** that a prostaglandin contains in the **hydrocarbon** chains. In the 1 series, the double bond is $\Delta^{13,14}$; in the 2 series, they are $\Delta^{5,6}$ and $\Delta^{13,14}$; and in the 3 series, they are $\Delta^{5,6}$, $\Delta^{13,14}$, and $\Delta^{17,18}$.

3. **Function.** Prostaglandins are widely distributed in tissues, but their role is not fully understood. At low concentrations, prostaglandins have been shown to modulate a wide range of biologic activities, including:

    a. Smooth muscle contraction and relaxation
    b. Gastric secretion
    c. Platelet aggregation
    d. Inflammatory response
    e. Response to trophic hormones
    f. Sodium and water retention by kidney tubules

B. **Thromboxanes**

1. **Structure and nomenclature.** Thromboxanes are analogs of prostanoic acid that possess a six-membered, oxygen-containing ring (see Figure 7-2). Thromboxanes are abbreviated **TX,** with different capital letters used to designate different ring substituents. A subscript, if present, denotes the number of unsaturated bonds.

2. **Function**

    a. Thromboxane A_2 (TXA_2) is produced by platelets. It causes contraction of arteries and triggers platelet aggregation.

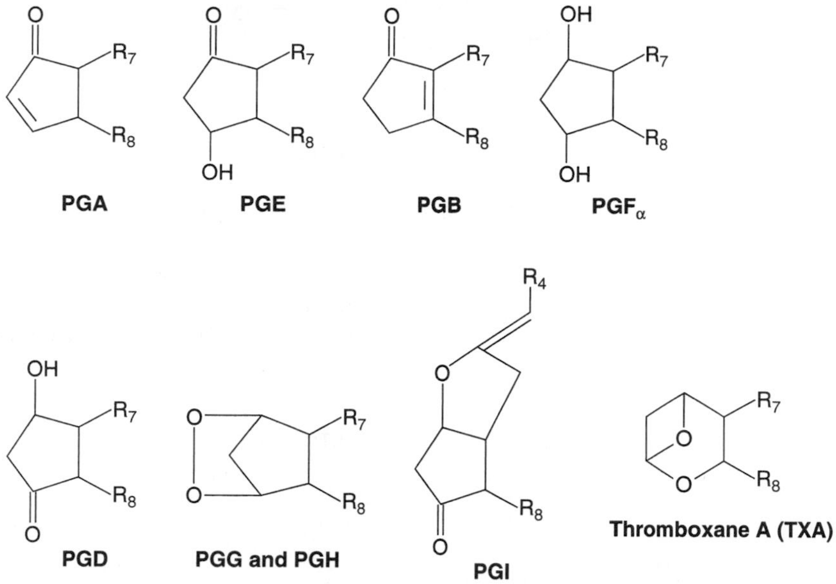

FIGURE 7-2. Structures of the seven prostaglandin (*PG*) families and thromboxane (*TX*). Each has a different characteristic type of ring substitution. The subscript *4, 7,* or *8* on the side group (*R*) refers to the number of carbons present on the attached carbon chain.

    b. These effects are exactly the opposite of those caused by prostacyclin (PGI_2), which is produced by the endothelial cells of the vascular system.

    c. TXA_2 and PGI_2 are antagonistic and have a balanced working relationship.

C. **Hydroperoxyeicosatetraenoic acids (HPETEs)**

    1. Structure. HPETEs are hydroxy fatty acid derivatives of arachidonic acid that do not contain a ring structure (Figure 7-3).

    2. Nomenclature. Hydroperoxy substitution may occur at positions 5, 8, 9, 11, or 15, and the HPETE is named accordingly.

    3. Function. It is not clear whether HPETEs are biologically active; however, **they can be converted to active compounds such as leukotrienes.**

D. **Leukotrienes**

    1. Structure and nomenclature

        a. Leukotrienes are formed from HPETEs by lipoxygenase and have a common feature of **three conjugated double bonds.**

        b. All leukotrienes are abbreviated **LT.** Those derived from **arachidonic acid** have a subscript numeral four to denote that they contain a total of **four double bonds.** An additional letter is included to indicate modifications to the carbon chain of the parent compound (see Figure 7-3).

        c. Some leukotrienes (e.g., LTC_4, LTD_4, and LTE_4) have one or more amino acids covalently attached.

    2. Functions

        a. Leukotrienes are involved in chemotaxis, inflammation, and allergic reactions.

        b. Leukotriene D_4 (LTD_4) has been identified as the **slow-reacting substance of anaphylaxis (SRS-A),** which causes smooth muscle contraction and is approximately 1000 times more potent than histamine in constricting the pulmonary airways. SRS-A also increases fluid leakage from small blood vessels and constricts coronary arteries.

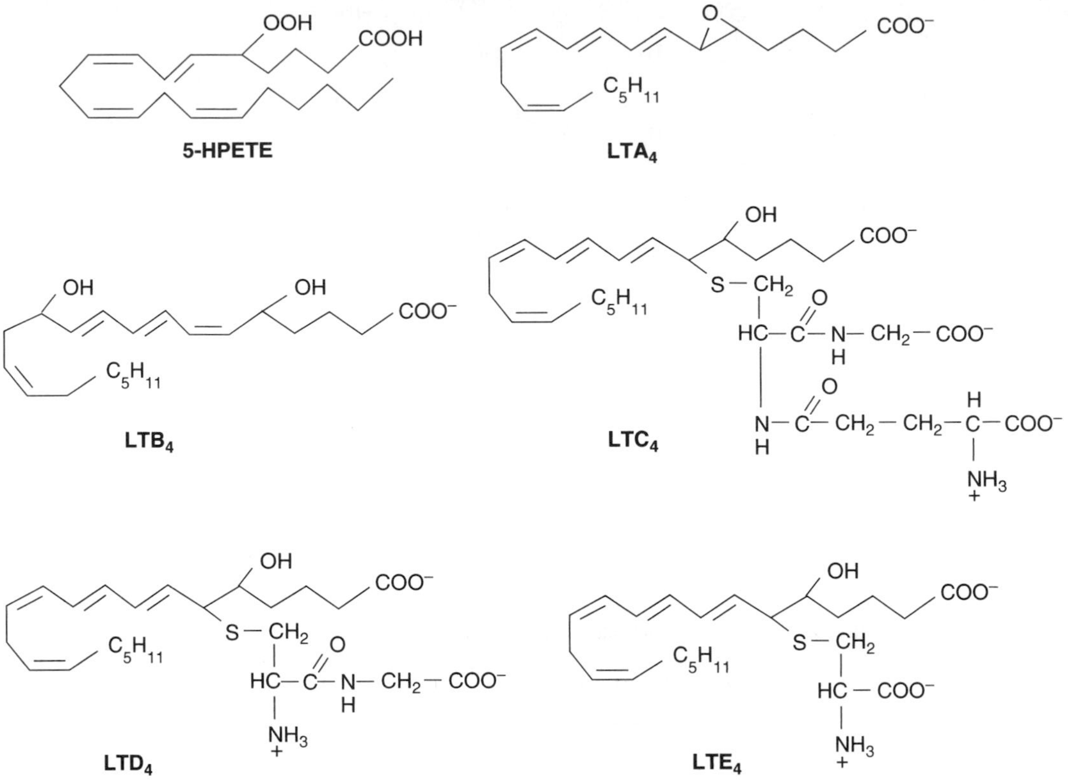

FIGURE 7-3. Hydroperoxyeicosatetraenoic acid (*HPETE*) and leukotriene (*LT*) structures. Letters *A–E* appended to the LT abbreviation indicate modifications. The subscript *4* indicates four double bonds.

    c. Leukotriene B$_4$ (LTB$_4$) attracts neutrophils and eosinophils, which are found in large numbers at sites of inflammation.

VI. **STEROIDS** are lipids that contain four fused carbon rings that form the cyclopentanoperhydrophenanthrene steroid nucleus.

A. **Cholesterol** (Figure 7-4) is the major **sterol** in the human body. Sterols are a class of steroids characterized by a hydroxyl group at carbon 3, and an aliphatic chain of at least eight carbons at C-17.

    1. Cholesterol is a **structural component** of cell membranes and plasma lipoproteins.

    2. It is the **precursor** from which steroid hormones and bile acids are synthesized.

B. **Steroid hormones** produced in humans are formed and secreted by the **adrenal cortex,** the **testis,** the **ovary,** and the **placenta.**

    1. The **adrenal cortex** produces hormones with two kinds of physiologic activities.
        a. The zona fasciculata of the adrenal cortex primarily produces **cortisol** (see Figure 7-4) in humans. Cortisol regulates a number of key metabolic steps and also inhibits the inflammatory response. It is called a **glucocorticoid,** and its 11-keto derivative **cortisone** is a clinically equivalent steroid.

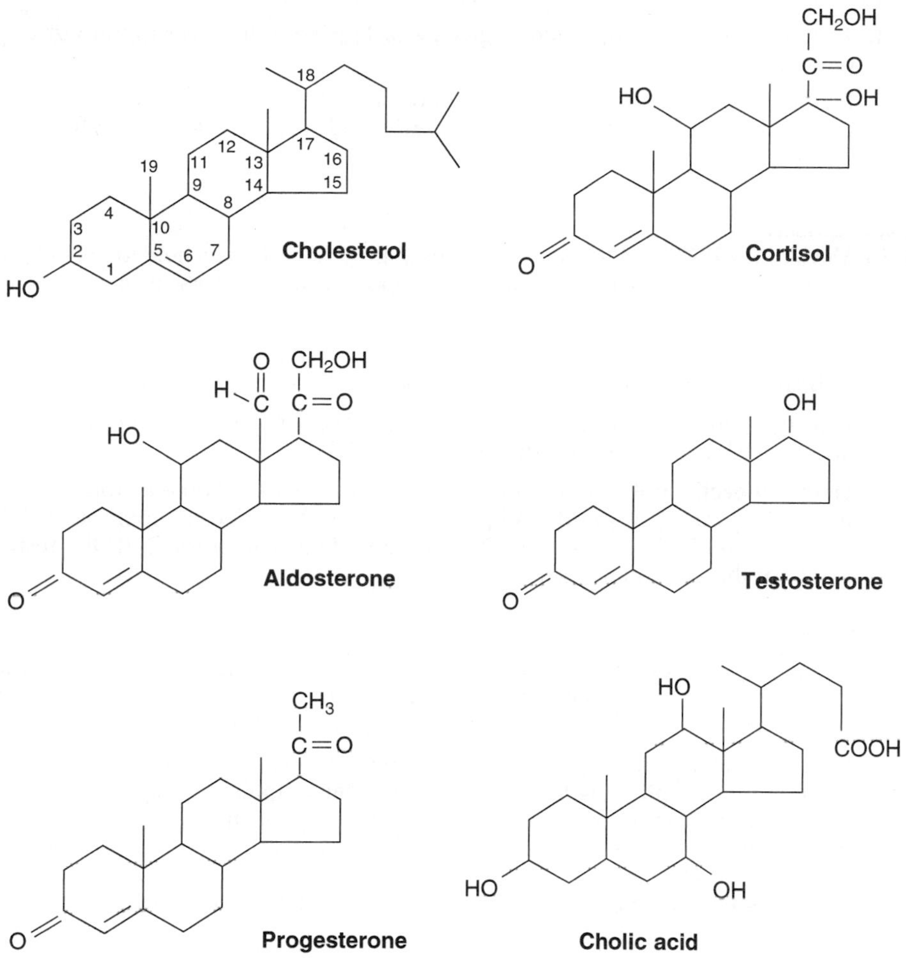

FIGURE 7-4. Structures of cholesterol and important cholesterol derivatives. The *numbering system* for the cyclopentanoperhydrophenanthrene steroid nucleus is indicated on the structure of cholesterol.

    b. The adrenal zona glomerulosa produces **aldosterone** (see Figure 7-4), which controls the reabsorption of Na⁺ in the kidney. Aldosterone is called a **mineralocorticoid.**

  2. Gonadal steroids
    a. The Leydig cells of the **testis** produce **testosterone** (see Figure 7-4), the hormone responsible for the development of the male secondary sexual characteristics.
    b. The **ovary** produces **estradiol** in the thecal cells of the graafian follicle and **progesterone** (see Figure 7-4) in the corpus luteum; progesterone is also formed by the **placenta** in pregnancy.

C.   **Bile acids are derived from cholesterol.** The predominant bile acids in humans are cholic (see Figure 7-4), **chenodeoxycholic, deoxycholic,** and **lithocholic acids.**

  1. Primary bile acids. Cholic and chenodeoxycholic acids are formed in the liver from cholesterol.

  2. Secondary bile acids. Deoxycholic acid and lithocholic acid are formed from the primary bile acids in the intestine through the action of intestinal bacterial enzymes.

3. The bile acids are conjugated to **glycine** or **taurine** in the liver to form glyco- or taurocholate.

4. **Function.** Continuous conversion of cholesterol to bile acids prevents the excessive accumulation of cholesterol in tissues. **Bile acids are excreted in the feces.**

VII. PLASMA LIPOPROTEINS are complexes of protein and lipids held together by noncovalent bonds. They function as clinically important transporters of lipids (see Chapter 23 V).

A. **Classification.** Two systems for classifying plasma lipoproteins are in use.

1. **Density.** This system is the most commonly used. Five fractions are distinguished, and their characteristics are shown in Table 7-4.

2. **Electrophoretic mobility.** The other classification is based on electrophoretic mobility. In this system, α, pre-β, and β correspond to high-density lipoprotein (HDL), very low-density lipoprotein (VLDL), and low-density lipoprotein (LDL), respectively, in the commonly used system.

B. **Structure**

1. Lipoprotein components do not have an exact stoichiometric relationship, but the different classes have characteristic **lipid:protein ratios,** and characteristic lipid classes are associated with different apoproteins (see Table 7-4).

2. Volume calculations suggest that the lipoprotein complex (Figure 7-5) can be thought of as a **sphere with the protein plus the amphipathic lipid** (phosphatidylcholine and unesterified cholesterol) forming an outer shell.
   a. The **apolar** segments of the shell are directed inward, and the polar segments face the water outside.
   b. The **nonpolar** lipids (triacylglycerols and esterified cholesterol) form the inside of the sphere.

TABLE 7-4. Properties of Major Plasma Lipoproteins

	HDL	LDL	IDL	VLDL	Chylomicron
Density (g/ml)	1.06–1.2	1.02–1.06	1.01–1.02	0.95–1.01	<0.95
Diameter (nm)	5–20	20–25	25–30	30–90	90–1000
% Lipid	50–55	75–80	80–85	90–95	98
% Total lipid as:					
Cholesterol (free)	3–4	7–10	8	5–10	1–3
Cholesterol ester	12	35–40	22	10–12	3–5
Phospholipid	20–25	15–20	22	15–20	7–9
Triacylglycerol	3	7–10	30	50–65	84–89
% Protein content	45–50	20–25	15–20	5–10	2
% Total protein as apoprotein (Apo):					
ApoA-1,A-2,A-4	90–95	0	0	0–3	0–3
ApoB-48,B-100	0–2	95–100	50–60	40–50	20–22
ApoC-1,C-2,C-3	4–6	0–5	20	35–40	60–65
ApoD	0–2	0	0	0	1
ApoE	0–5	0	15–20	5–10	5

HDL = high-density lipoprotein; *IDL* = intermediate-density lipoprotein; *LDL* = low-density lipoprotein; *VLDL* = very low-density lipoprotein; *nm* = nanometer.

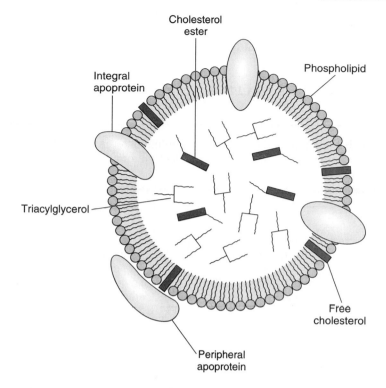

Cholesterol
ester

Integral
apoprotein

Phospholipid

Triacylglycerol

Free
cholesterol

Peripheral
apoprotein

FIGURE 7-5. Schematic representation of the structure of a plasma lipoprotein.

3. When the lipids are extracted from a lipoprotein by organic solvents, the **apoproteins** remain. At least 10 major apoproteins have been identified (see Table 7-4).

4. Because it is spherical, an increase in the nonpolar lipid:protein ratio occurs as the size of the lipoprotein particle increases. Because polar lipids and proteins are found only on the surface, any increase in size results primarily from an increase in the amount of nonpolar lipid that comprises the bulk of the particle.

Case 7-1 Revisited

The diagnosis for this 15-year-old girl is Gaucher's disease, the most commonly observed sphingolipidosis. Patients are deficient in β-glucosidase, which is needed to degrade glucocerebroside. To confirm the diagnosis, extracts of leukocytes that were isolated from her blood were assayed for β-glucosidase activity.

Glucocerebroside is stored mostly in the liver, spleen, and bone marrow. It is derived primarily from the membranes of red and white blood cells, the turnover of which generates significant amounts of glucocerebroside. When glucocerebroside is not degraded, it cannot be readily excreted because it is not very soluble in water or body fluids. Therefore, it accumulates in cells of the spleen and liver, which accounts for the enlargement of these organs. It also accumulates in bone marrow cells. These enlarged cells, termed Gaucher's cells, are readily observable during microscopic examination of bone marrow aspirates. The enlarged spleen and liver further complicate this disorder by prematurely destroying red and white blood cells and platelets. A loss of red blood cells can lead to anemia, and a loss of platelets, which are important for coagulation, contributes to bruising and bleeding.

Until recently, treatment had been essentially symptomatic (e.g., splenectomy). Some success has been achieved with treatment by enzyme replacement therapy, in which the patient receives an intravenous infusion of a functional enzyme. The replacement must be repeated on a regular basis because the infused enzyme is eventually degraded. Methods of treatment involving gene replacement therapy are currently being studied and offer promise for the future.

STUDY QUESTIONS

DIRECTIONS: Each of the numbered items or incomplete statements in this section is followed by answers or by completions of the statement. Select the **one** lettered answer or completion that is **best** in each case.

Questions 1-2

A patient is suspected of having a lipid storage disease. Extracts of cells from the patient were incubated with appropriate substrates and assayed for enzyme activities. The cells were deficient in hexosaminidase A activity.

1. This patient suffers from which one of the following diseases?

(A) Gaucher's disease
(B) Niemann-Pick disease
(C) Krabbe's disease
(D) Fabry's disease
(E) Tay-Sachs disease

2. Which of the following lipids accumulates in this disease?

(A) Sphingomyelin
(B) Glucocerebroside
(C) Ganglioside GM_2
(D) Ceramide trihexoside
(E) Galactocerebroside

3. Which one of the following pairs of lipids and related compounds exhibits opposite biologic activities?

(A) 5-Hydroperoxyeicosatetraenoic acid (5-HPETE) and leukotriene D_4
(B) Cholic acid and lithocholic acid
(C) Thromboxane A_2 and prostacyclin (PGI_2)
(D) Lactosylceramide and galactocerebroside
(E) Acetone and β-hydroxybutyrate

DIRECTIONS: The group of items in this section consists of lettered options followed by a set of numbered items. For each item, select the **one** lettered option that is most closely associated with it.

Questions 4-9

Match the following descriptions of function with the correct lipids.

(A) Prostaglandins
(B) Leukotrienes
(C) Sphingomyelin
(D) Steroids
(E) Ketone bodies
(F) Triacylglycerols
(G) Gangliosides
(H) Phosphoglycerides
(I) Bile acids

4. Primarily used as a source of metabolic energy

5. May contain a carbohydrate moiety and is present in most cell membranes

6. Are the primary lipids present in very low-density lipoproteins

7. Are derived from 5-hydroperoxyeicosatetraenoic acid (5-HPETE) and modulate a variety of biologic functions

8. Are found in cell membranes and contain two fatty acid moieties esterified to a glycerol backbone

9. Are derived from arachidonic acid, contain four double bonds, and may contain amino acids

ANSWERS AND EXPLANATIONS

1-2. The answers are: 1-E, 2-C [IV B 4, C; Table 7-3]. Accumulation of specific sphingolipids is characteristic of each different sphingolipidosis. Glucocerebroside accumulates in Gaucher's disease because of β-glucosidase deficiency. Galactocerebroside accumulates in Krabbe's disease because of β-galactosidase deficiency. Ceramide trihexoside accumulates in Fabry's disease due to α-galactosidase deficiency. Sphingomyelin accumulates in Niemann-Pick disease due to sphingomyelinase deficiency. Ganglioside GM_2 accumulates in Tay-Sachs disease because of hexaminidase A deficiency.

3. The answer is C [V B 2]. Thromboxane A_2 (TXA_2) is produced by platelets, causes contraction of arteries, and triggers platelet aggregation, exactly the opposite of effects caused by prostacyclin (PGI_2). 5-Hydroperoxyeicosatetraenoic acid (5-HPETE) is a precursor of leukotrienes. Cholic and lithocholic acid are bile acids. Lactosylceramide and galactocerebroside are glycosphingolipids, which perform structural roles. Acetone and β-hydroxybutyrate are ketone bodies, which are used as a source of energy.

4-9. The answers are: 4-E [II E], **5-G** [IV B 4], **6-F** [VII B 2 b, 4; Table 7-4], **7-B** [V D], **8-H** [III A], **9-B** [V D; Figure 7-3]. Ketone bodies and triacylglycerols are involved in energy metabolism; triacylglycerols are the primary storage form of energy that must be hydrolyzed to free fatty acids and glycerol to be used for energy. Ketone bodies are used directly. Steroids, primarily cholesterol, sphingomyelin, phospholipids, and gangliosides, may be found in cell membranes. Gangliosides, which are found in most cells, are the only one of these lipids that also contains carbohydrate.

The lipid fractions of the different classes of lipoproteins contain variable amounts of cholesterol, cholesterol esters, phospholipids, and triacylglycerols. For very low-density lipoproteins, triacylglycerols comprise more than 50% of the total lipid present.

Prostaglandins, leukotrienes, and certain steroids modulate biologic functions. Only leukotrienes are derived from 5-hydroperoxyeicosatetraenoic acid (5-HPETE).

Steroids, primarily cholesterol, sphingomyelin, phosphoglycerides, and gangliosides, may be found in cell membranes. Only phosphoglycerides contain fatty acids esterified to the glycerol backbone. Triacylglycerols also contain fatty acids esterified to the glycerol backbone; however, they are a storage lipid, not a membrane component.

The leukotrienes are formed from arachidonic acid by the action of lipoxygenase, which first forms 5-HPETE. They contain four double bonds, three of which are conjugated. Leukotriene C_4 (LTC_4), LTD_4, and LTE_4 each contain one or more amino acids bound to the core structure of the leukotrienes.

STORAGE AND EXPRESSION OF GENETIC INFORMATION

Chapter 8

DNA Replication and Repair
Donald Sittman

Case 8-1

A 65-year-old white man is diagnosed, by liver biopsy, with hepatocellular carcinoma present in both lobes of his liver. The patient, a retired worker from a plastics factory, is negative for hepatitis B and C. Because the biopsy report indicates that the cancer spread throughout the liver, surgical resection of the tumor is ruled out as a treatment. The patient is entered into a combination chemotherapeutic treatment program using doxorubicin, fluorouracil, and intrahepatic-arterial cisplatin.

- What is the mechanism of action of doxorubicin, fluorouracil, and cisplatin?
- Do these drugs affect only cancer cells?

Hepatocellular carcinoma is strongly associated with hepatitis B and C infections. Because this patient is negative for these viral infections, the physician suspects that exposure to a chemical, such as vinyl chloride, which is a solvent used in plastics manufacturing, may have caused this patient's cancer.

- Prior to animal testing, how is the carcinogenic potential of chemicals tested?

I. **THE STRUCTURE OF DNA REVEALS A MECHANISM FOR ITS REPLICATION.** Genetic material must be able to be accurately replicated and passed on from one generation to the next. Although elegant experiments indicated that DNA could carry genetic information from one generation to the next, not until Watson and Crick discovered the structure of DNA was it understood how DNA might be replicated. The **double-helical model** of DNA suggested that the **strands can separate and act as templates for the formation of a new, complementary strand.** However, the structure of DNA did not reveal whether the DNA was replicated conservatively or semiconservatively.

A. **Conservative replication** would occur if, after replication and cell division, the parental DNA strands remained together in one of the daughter cells, and the newly synthesized DNA strands went to the other daughter cell (Figure 8-1).

B. **Semiconservative replication** was shown in experiments by Meselson and Stahl to be the mechanism by which replication takes place. After replication and cell division, each daughter cell receives one parental DNA strand and one newly synthesized complementary strand for which the parental strand was the template (see Figure 8-1).

II. **PROKARYOTIC REPLICATION.** The mechanism of replication in prokaryotes is much better understood than in eukaryotes. The basic requirements and components of replication are the same for prokaryotes as for eukaryotes. Therefore, an understanding of how prokaryotes replicate provides much insight into the understanding of how eukaryotes replicate.

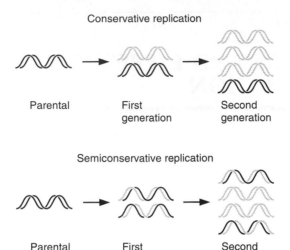

Conservative replication

Parental · First generation · Second generation

Semiconservative replication

Parental · First generation · Second generation

FIGURE 8-1. Conservative versus semiconservative replication. If the DNA of parental cells is labeled with the heavy isotope of nitrogen (^{15}N) or with a radioisotope, and the cells are then allowed to divide in medium without isotope, a detailed analysis of the DNA from subsequent daughter cells reveals that replication takes place semiconservatively. Isotopically labeled parental DNA is indicated with *heavy lines.* Newly synthesized DNA, which forms upon replication in the absence of isotope, is indicated with a *light line.*

 Basic requirements for DNA synthesis (Figure 8-2)

1. **Substrates.** The four deoxynucleoside triphosphates (dNTPs)—deoxyadenosine triphosphate (dATP), deoxyguanosine triphosphate (dGTP), deoxycytidine triphosphate (dCTP), and deoxythymidine triphosphate (dTTP)—are needed as substrates for DNA synthesis. Cleavage of the high-energy phosphate bond between the α and β phosphates provides the energy for the addition of the nucleotide.

2. **Template.** DNA replication cannot occur without a template. A template is required to direct the addition of the appropriate complementary deoxynucleotide to the newly synthesized DNA strand. In semiconservative replication, each strand of parental DNA serves as a template. Then, each template strand and its newly synthesized complementary strand serve as the DNA in daughter cells.

3. **Primer.** DNA synthesis cannot start without a primer, which prepares the template strand for the addition of nucleotides. Because new nucleotides are added to the 3′ end of a primer that is properly base paired to the template strand of DNA, **new synthesis is said to occur in a 5′ to 3′ direction.**

4. **Enzyme.** The DNA synthesis that occurs during the process of replication is catalyzed by enzymes called **DNA-dependent DNA polymerases.** These enzymes depend on DNA to the extent that they require a DNA template. They are more commonly called DNA polymerases.

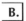 **Multiple DNA polymerases with multiple enzymatic activities.** The bacteria *Escherichia coli* contains three separate DNA polymerases. These enzymes are capable of catalyzing other reactions in addition to DNA synthesis. The other reactions catalyzed by these three DNA polymerases play an important role in replication and DNA repair. Table 8-1 summarizes some of the properties of these enzymes.

1. **DNA polymerase I (pol I)** was the first DNA polymerase discovered.
   a. **Function.** Pol I functions in the **replication of DNA** (see II D 2 d) and in the **repair of damaged DNA** [see VI A 1 a (2), 2, 3 c].

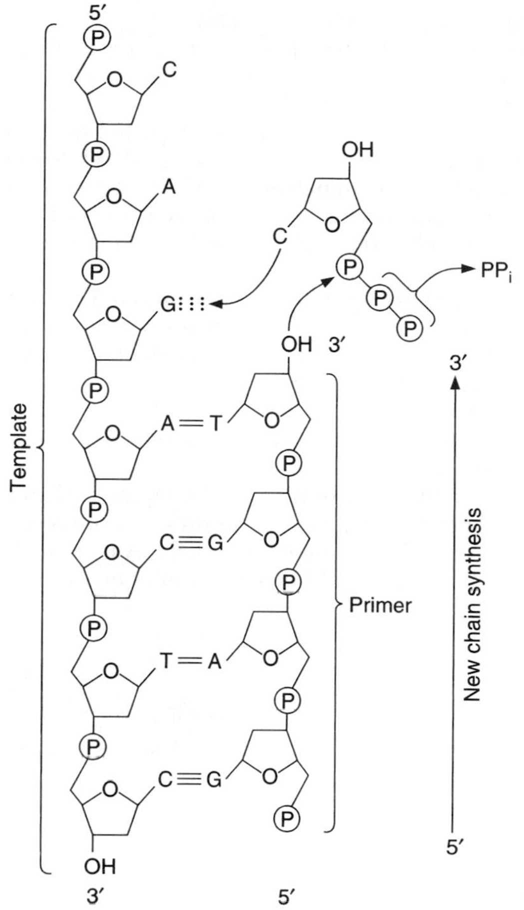

FIGURE 8-2. Addition of a deoxynucleotide to a strand of DNA during replication. The template directs the addition of the newly added complementary deoxynucleotide. Further synthesis requires the 3′ deoxynucleotide of the primer to be properly base paired with the template. New chain synthesis is in a 5′ to 3′ direction. A = adenine; C = cytosine; G = guanine; OH = hydroxyl; P = phosphate; PP$_i$ = inorganic pyrophosphate; T = thymine.

TABLE 8-1. Properties of Prokaryotic DNA Polymerases

Feature	DNA Polymerase		
	I	II	III
5′ → 3′ exonuclease activity	+	−	−
3′ → 5′ exonuclease activity	+	+	+
Synthesis rate (nucleotides/minute)	600	30	30,000
Molecules/cell	400	?	10
Replication	+	−	+
Repair	+	+	−

b. **Structure.** Pol I is a single polypeptide.
c. **Other enzymatic activities.** Pol I has two enzymatic activities—besides DNA polymerase activity—that are important to its cellular function.
  (1) **Proofreading** (Figure 8-3A). Pol I does not typically add a nucleotide to the growing DNA chain that cannot properly base pair with the template strand. If a mismatched nucleotide is added, the enzyme halts polymerization. **A 3'- to 5'-exonuclease** activity removes the mismatched nucleotide, and polymerization resumes. This activity is called proofreading, and it assures the high-level fidelity of replication that is a desirable trait of genetic material.
  (2) **Excision–repair** (Figure 8-3B). **Pol I has a 5' to 3' exonuclease activity,** called excision–repair activity, that can hydrolytically remove a segment of DNA from the 5' end of a strand of duplex DNA.
    (a) From 1–10 nucleotide segments of DNA can be removed simultaneously.
    (b) This activity is essential for the removal of primers in DNA replication (see II D 2 d).
    (c) This activity is essential for the repair of damaged DNA (see VI A).
  (3) **Nick-translation** (Figure 8-4). A **nick** is a break in a phosphodiester bond of one strand of DNA in a double helix. A nick leaves a free 3'-hydroxyl and a free 5'-phosphate. Pol I can function at nicks as an exonuclease and a poly-

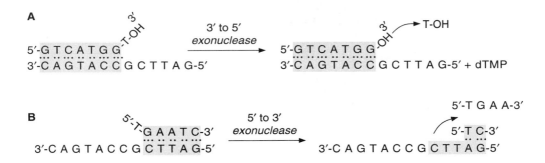

FIGURE 8-3. *(A)* 3' to 5' exonuclease (proofreading) activity. *(B)* 5' to 3' exonuclease (excision–repair) activity. dTMP = deoxythymidine monophosphate.

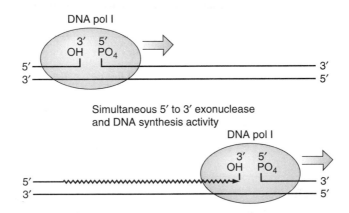

FIGURE 8-4. Nick-translation by DNA polymerase I (pol I). During nick-translation, the 5' to 3' exonuclease-containing domain is believed to precede the DNA polymerase domain with its associated proofreading domain. In this way, it can remove and replace DNA simultaneously at a nick, causing the nick to be moved or translated in a 5' to 3' direction. New DNA synthesis is represented with a *squiggly line*.

merase at the same time. As the 5′-phosphate nucleotide is removed or displaced by pol I, it is replaced with the polymerase activity of pol I. Pol I cannot reseal the nick; therefore, the nick is moved, or **translated,** along the DNA in the direction of synthesis.

2. **DNA polymerase II (pol II)** is a minor DNA polymerase in *E. coli.*
    a. **Function.** Pol II may be involved in some DNA repair processes, but *E. coli* mutants lacking this enzyme show no replication or growth deficiencies.
    b. **Structure.** Pol II is a single polypeptide.
    c. **Other enzymatic activities.** Pol II has proofreading (3′ to 5′ exonuclease) activity but lacks excision–repair (5′ to 3′ exonuclease) activity.

3. **DNA polymerase III (pol III) is the primary DNA polymerase involved in cellular replication.**
    a. **Function.** Pol III catalyzes leading and lagging strand synthesis (see II D 1–2).
    b. **Structure.** Pol III is structurally complex. The **pol III core enzyme,** made of three different polypeptides, was first isolated. Gentle purification schemes and careful reconstitution showed that the active cellular form of pol III, called **pol III holoenzyme,** is made of 10 subunit polypeptides. The subunits are organized into an asymmetric dimeric structure with two catalytic centers. This is important in understanding how it catalyzes both leading and lagging strand syntheses at the replication fork (see II C 3, D).
    c. **Other enzymatic activities.** Pol III holoenzyme has proofreading (3′ to 5′ exonuclease) activity but no excision–repair (5′ to 3′ exonuclease) activity. The two α subunits both contain the DNA polymerase activity, and the two ε subunits both contain the 3′ to 5′ exonuclease activity. The two β subunits form a dimer that circles around the DNA. This β_2 "DNA clamp" enables the pol III holoenzyme to stay bound to the DNA and facilitates its high rate of replication.

C. **Origin of replication.** In prokaryotes, replication starts at particular DNA sequences called **origins** (an origin is often called by its genetic abbreviation, **ori**).

1. **OriC** is the single origin in *E. coli.* OriC is a sequence of approximately 240 base pairs, which is required to direct the initiation of replication that takes place within the oriC region.

2. **dnaA protein** is specific protein in *E. coli* that is required for proper initiation of replication at the origin. It binds to specific sequences within oriC, and in the presence of ATP and the other components of replication (see II D, E), dnaA protein facilitates initiation of replication.

3. **Replication forks.** After initiation, replication has been observed (using radiographic electron microscopic techniques) proceeding away from the origin. In most organisms, replication proceeds **bidirectionally** from the origins as **replication forks** (Figure 8-5). Replication forks represent unwound parental template DNA strands to which newly synthesized complementary DNA is paired.

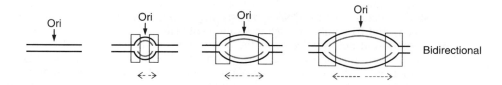

FIGURE 8-5. Bidirectional replication from a single origin of replication *(Ori).* Active DNA synthesis takes place at the replication forks, which are indicated within the *boxes.*

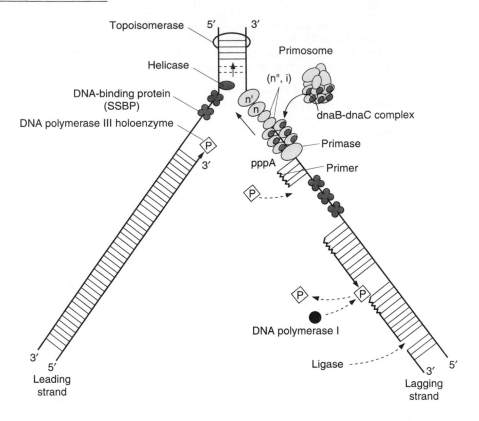

FIGURE 8-6. Schematic diagram of the basic molecular events at the replication fork of *Escherichia coli.* The primosome is a complex of proteins that comprises primase, a hexamer of the helicase *dnaB* protein, *dnaC* protein, and several other proteins: *n, n', n"*, and *i. pppA* = 5' terminal adenosine with three 5' phosphates; *SSBP* = single-strand binding protein.
(Reprinted with permission from Kornberg A, Baker TA: *DNA Replication,* 2nd ed. New York, WH Freeman, 1992, plate 15.)

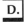 **D.** **Basic molecular events at replication forks** (Figure 8-6). Because the molecular events that occur at replication forks in *E. coli* are well described, there is a good understanding of how new DNA synthesis takes place on both of the parental DNA strands at replication forks.

1. **Leading strand synthesis** is the continuous synthesis of one of the daughter strands in a 5' to 3' direction. **Pol III catalyzes leading strand synthesis.**

2. **Lagging strand synthesis**
   a. **Okazaki fragments.** One of the newly synthesized daughter strands is made **discontinuously.** The resulting short fragments are called Okazaki fragments. These fragments are later joined by DNA ligase to make a continuous piece of DNA. This is called lagging strand synthesis. Discontinuous synthesis of the lagging strand occurs because DNA synthesis always occurs in a 5' to 3' direction (see II A 3). **Pol III catalyzes lagging strand synthesis.**
   b. **Direction of new synthesis.** As the replication fork moves forward, leading strand synthesis follows. A gap forms on the opposite strand because it is in the wrong orientation to direct continuous synthesis of a new strand. After a lag period, the gap that forms is filled in by 5' to 3' synthesis. This means that new DNA synthesis on the lagging strand is actually moving away from the replication fork.
   c. **Priming of Okazaki fragment synthesis**

(1) Enzyme. An enzyme called **primase** is the catalytic portion of a **primosome** that makes the RNA primer needed to initiate synthesis of Okazaki fragments (see II E 4). It also makes the primer that initiates leading strand synthesis at the origin.

(2) Primers provide a 3'-hydroxyl group that is needed to initiate DNA synthesis (see II A 3). The primers made by primase are small pieces of RNA (4–12 nucleotides) complementary to the template strand.

d. **The role of pol I in replication.** On completion of lagging strand synthesis by pol III, **the RNA primer is then removed by pol I and replaced with DNA.** Synthesis of each new Okazaki fragment takes place until it reaches the RNA primer of the preceding Okazaki fragment. This effectively leaves a nick between the newly synthesized Okazaki fragment and the RNA primer. DNA pol I uses its nick-translation properties to hydrolyze the RNA (5' to 3' exonuclease activity) and replace it with DNA.

e. **Joining of Okazaki fragments.** After pol I has removed the RNA primer and replaced it with DNA, an enzyme called **DNA ligase** catalyzes the formation of phosphodiester bonds between the adjoining fragments by the following reaction:

$$\text{—DNA—}^{3'}\text{OH} + {}^-\text{O—}\overset{\overset{\displaystyle O}{\|}}{\underset{\underset{\displaystyle O^-}{|}}{P}}\text{—O—DNA—} \xrightarrow[\substack{+\text{ATP} \\ \text{or} \\ \text{NAD}^+}]{\substack{\text{DNA} \\ \text{Ligase}}} \text{—DNA—O—}\overset{\overset{\displaystyle O}{\|}}{\underset{\underset{\displaystyle O^-}{|}}{P}}\text{—O—DNA—}$$

E. **Other factors needed for propagation of replication forks**

1. **Helicases** are enzymes that catalyze the unwinding of the DNA helix. A helicase derives energy from cleavage of high-energy phosphate bonds of nucleoside triphosphates, usually ATP, to unwind the DNA helix. **Helicase activity provides single-strand templates for replication.**
   a. **Proteins with helicase activity.** A number of proteins have been isolated that have helicase activity. Most of these proteins play a role in DNA repair, recombination, or bacteriophage replication.
   b. The **dnaB protein** is the principal helicase of *E. coli* replication and is a component of the primosome (see II E 4).

2. **Gyrase.** Positive supercoils would build up in advance of a moving replication fork without the action of gyrase, which is a topoisomerase (see Chapter 6 III A 3).

3. **Single-strand binding protein** (SSBP) is an important component of replication. As its name implies, it binds to single-stranded DNA.
   a. **Function**
      (1) SSBP **enhances the activity of helicase and binds to single-strand template DNA** until it can serve as a template.
      (2) SSBP may serve to protect single-strand DNA from degradation by nucleases, and it may block formation of intrastrand duplexes of hairpins that can slow replication.
   b. **Release.** SSBP is displaced from single-strand DNA when the DNA undergoes replication.

4. **Primosome**
   a. **Definition.** The primosome is a complex of proteins that comprises primase (see II D 2 c), a hexamer of the helicase dnaB protein, dnaC protein, and several other proteins: n, n', n", and i.
   b. **Function.** The primosome complex primes DNA synthesis at the origin. Driven by ATP hydrolysis, the primosome moves with the replication fork, making RNA primers for Okazaki fragment synthesis.

F. **The replisome** (Figure 8-7). It is believed that all the replication enzymes and factors are part of a large macromolecular complex called a replisome. It has been suggested

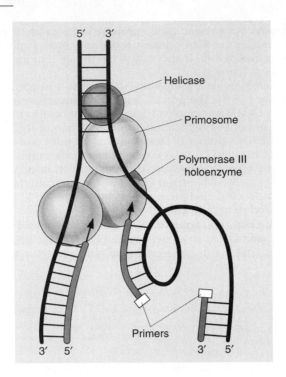

FIGURE 8-7. Replisome model of replication. Looping of the lagging strand template effectively allows the lagging strand synthesis to take place in the same direction as leading strand synthesis. This allows the replisome to concurrently synthesize both leading and lagging strands. (Reprinted with permission from Kornberg A: DNA replication. *J Biol Chem.* 1988, 263:1–4.)

that the replisome may be attached to the membrane and that instead of the replisome moving along the DNA during replication, DNA is passed through the stationary replisome.

G. **Termination of replication.** Termination sequences (e.g., ter) direct termination of replication. A specific protein—the termination utilization substance **(Tus) protein**—binds to these sequences and prevents the helicase dnaB protein from further unwinding DNA. This facilitates the termination of replication.

III. **EUKARYOTIC REPLICATION.** Eukaryotes represent a diversity of organisms that may utilize slightly different mechanisms of replication. However, most of these mechanisms are very similar to those in prokaryotic replication. This section reviews replication only in mammalian cells. As with prokaryotic replication, mammalian replication is semiconservative and proceeds **bidirectionally from many origins.**

A. **Replicons** are basic units of replication.

1. **Function.** A replicon encompasses the entire DNA replicated from the growing replication forks that share a single origin.

2. **Size.** Replicons may vary in size from 50–120 μm. The *E. coli* genome, with its single origin, is essentially one large replicon. There are estimated to be anywhere from 10,000–100,000 replicons per cell in mammals. The large number of replicons is needed to replicate the large mammalian genomes in a reasonable period

TABLE 8-2. Properties of Eukaryotic DNA Polymerases

Feature	DNA Polymerase*				
	α	β	δ	γ	ε
Location	Nucleus	Nucleus	Nucleus	Mitochondria	Nucleus
5′ → 3′ exonuclease activity	−	−	−	−	−
3′ → 5′ exonuclease activity	−	−	+	+	+
Primase activity	+	−	−	−	−
Replication	+	−	+	+	+
Repair	−	+	−	−	−

*The nomenclature of the DNA polymerases is for the mammalian enzymes. Analogous, but differently named, DNA polymerases are present in all eukaryotes.

of time. It takes approximately 8 hours to replicate the human genome.

3. **Replication rate**
    a. **Prokaryotes.** An *E. coli* replication fork progresses at approximately 1000 base pairs per second.
    b. **Eukaryotes.** The eukaryotic replication rate is about 10 times slower than the prokaryotic replication rate. Eukaryotic replication forks progress at approximately 100 base pairs per second. Each replicon completes synthesis in approximately 1 hour. Therefore, during the total period of eukaryotic replication, not every replicon is active. The slow rate of eukaryotic replication is likely due to interference of nucleosomes and chromosomal proteins. Heterochromatin is known to replicate slower than euchromatin (see Chapter 6 III B 4).

B. **Multiple eukaryotic DNA polymerases.** Eukaryotes contain at least four different nuclear DNA polymerases (i.e., α, β, δ, and ε) and one mitochondrial DNA polymerase (γ). Table 8-2 summarizes the cellular role and properties of these DNA polymerases.

1. **DNA polymerase α is essential for replication.**
    a. DNA polymerase α has three associated subunit polypeptides. Two of these have primase activity, and the function of the third is unknown.
    b. DNA polymerase α is responsible for initiation at origins and of Okazaki fragments. It is therefore required for both leading and lagging strand synthesis.

2. **DNA polymerase δ also is essential for replication.** It is required for both leading and lagging strand synthesis.
    a. Pol δ is associated with another protein called **proliferating cell nuclear antigen (PCNA).** PCNA is analogous to the dimeric β subunits of *E. coli* pol III (see II B 3 c). It also forms a DNA clamp that enables pol δ to stay bound to DNA and sustain a high rate of replication.
    b. After pol α has initiated replication, a protein called **replication factor C (RF-C)** facilitates the inhibition and replacement of pol α with both PCNA and pol δ in an ATP-dependent manner.

3. **DNA polymerase β plays no role in replication and acts only in DNA repair synthesis.**

4. **DNA polymerase ε also is essential for replication,** although its exact role is not clearly defined. It behaves similarly to pol δ and may support some component of lagging strand synthesis.

5. **DNA polymerase γ resides in and replicates mitochondrial DNA.**

C. **Other factors involved in eukaryotic replication.** Eukaryotic DNA has all of the topologic constraints to replication that prokaryotic replication has. To deal with these constraints, eukaryotes have all of the DNA polymerase-associated factors and enzymes found in prokaryotes that are known to be needed for proper replication.

1. **5′ to 3′ exonucleases** [see II B 1 c (2)] have been isolated from eukaryotes. One is known to be associated with DNA polymerase β.

2. **3′ to 5′ exonuclease activity.** DNA polymerases δ, ε, and γ have proofreading capability [see II B 1 c (1)]. Other enzymes exhibiting only 3′ to 5′ exonuclease activity have also been isolated.

3. **Ligase.** Four ligases have been isolated from eukaryotes: One is involved in replication and repair, and one is involved in DNA repair synthesis only. The function of the other two is not clear. Unlike prokaryotic ligases that use nicotinamide adenine dinucleotide (NAD) as an energy source, eukaryotic ligases use ATP.

4. **Helicases.** Although not well characterized as to which ones play a role in replication, a number of helicases have been isolated from eukaryotes.

5. An SSBP called **replication protein A (RP-A)** has been isolated from mammalian cells.

6. **Topoisomerases.** Eukaryotes have several well-characterized topoisomerases that relieve positive supercoils that build up in advance of replication forks. There are two basic types of eukaryotic topoisomerases.
   a. **Topoisomerase I** is the major topoisomerase used to relieve supercoils. It resolves or "unknots" DNA by breaking one strand of DNA, passing the other strand though the break, and then re-ligating the broken strand.
   b. **Topoisomerase II** also is required during replication. It is needed to resolve the final knots that form when adjacent replication forks meet. It also is required before mitosis can proceed to separate the two daughter strands formed by replication. Topoisomerase II separates double helical strands of DNA by cutting both strands of one of the helices and passing the other strand though the break before re-ligating the cut helix.

D. **Telomeres.** Unlike prokaryotes, eukaryotic DNA is linear and not circular. Because all DNA synthesis requires a primer, DNA would be lost at the lagging strand ends unless replication of ends proceeds by a different mechanism than all other DNA. Eukaryotic chromosomes have unique sequences at their ends called telomeres. A specialized DNA polymerase called **DNA telomerase** replicates telomeric ends.

1. **Structure of telomeres.** Mammalian telomeres are short, tandem repeats of the sequence TTAGGG. The 3′ end of these repeats is single stranded.

2. The **mechanism of telomere replication** is shown in Figure 8-8. The essence of this mechanism is that the telomerase provides an RNA template complementary to the telomeric repeat, and the free 3′ end of the telomere is the primer for new DNA synthesis. After elongation of the telomere by telomerase, normal lagging strand synthesis presumably makes a complementary copy of all but the 3′ most terminal sequences.

3. **Clinical relevance of telomeres.** The number of telomere repeats varies in the cells of different tissues. This difference in telomere length represents a shortening of telomeres that occurs during the replication in some cells but not in others. This shortening occurs because of the absence of telomerase. There is a correlation in tissue-culture cells of the presence of telomerase and the immortality of the cells. Of potential medical relevance is the fact that cancer cells, which are immortal in culture, have high levels of telomerase.

E. **The cell cycle.** Eukaryotic cell division occurs in four distinct phases, which are collectively called the cell cycle (Figure 8-9).

1. **S phase** is the phase in which DNA is synthesized.
   a. Unlike the prokaryotes, in which a second round of DNA synthesis can begin before cell division takes place, **eukaryotes replicate their DNA only once per cell division cycle.**

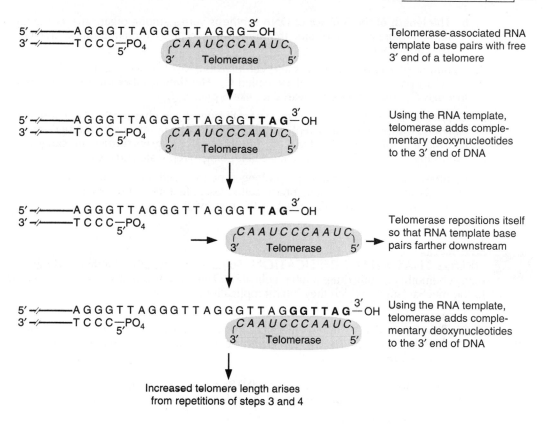

FIGURE 8-8. Model of the mechanism of replication of human telomeres.

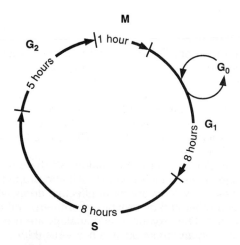

FIGURE 8-9. The human cell cycle. A continuously dividing human cell takes approximately 22 hours to divide. After cell division takes place during mitosis (*M* phase) the cells enter a gap phase (G_1) before beginning DNA synthesis (*S* phase). Following *S* phase, the cells pass through a second gap phase (G_2) before entering *M* phase. Cells not continuously dividing enter a prolonged phase during G_1 called G_0 in which they do not commit to replicate.

    b. The **length of the S phase** of DNA synthesis varies among organisms, but takes an invariable amount of time in any one species (e.g., human S phase always lasts about 8 hours).

  2. G$_2$ and M phase. Before mitosis and cell division, or M phase, can take place, the cell must pass through a **gap phase** called G$_2$. **The time it takes for a cell to pass through G$_2$ and M phase is invariable,** like S phase.

  3. G$_1$ phase. After M phase, the cell must pass through a gap phase called G$_1$ before it can initiate another round of replication in S phase. The normal cellular functions take place in this phase. **The time it takes for a cell to progress through G$_1$ can vary.** Events that occur in G$_1$ determine if a cell is going to replicate and divide.

  4. G$_0$ phase. Many cells go through prolonged periods without dividing. These cells leave G1 and go into a resting phase called G$_0$. A feature of **tumor cells** is that they can no longer enter G$_0$, which is the nondividing state.

IV. DRUGS THAT AFFECT REPLICATION.
Some antibacterial and antiviral drugs and many chemotherapeutic drugs inhibit replication. These drugs can be classified according to the mechanism by which they inhibit replication.

A. **Antimetabolites** reduce or inhibit the production of the substrate for replication (i.e., dNTPs). Without substrate, DNA polymerases cannot make DNA. Examples of this drug class are presented in Chapter 26.

B. **Substrate analogs.** Numerous analogs of dNTPs can be incorporated into DNA by DNA polymerases. Many analogs then inhibit further replication. A few examples are:

  1. Dideoxynucleoside analogs
    a. Structure. All of these drugs lack a 3'-hydroxyl group as well as the 2'-hydroxyl group on the sugar moiety. Examples of these drugs are:
      (1) Zidovudine (azidothymidine, AZT). An azido (N$_3$) group replaces the hydroxyl group on the 3' position of thymidine.
      (2) Didanosine is a dideoxyinosine. Inosine is an intermediate in purine biosynthesis (see Chapter 26).
      (3) Zalcitabine is a dideoxycytidine.
      (4) Stavudine lacks both hydroxyl groups and hydrogen at the 3' and 2' position of thymidine.
    b. Mechanism of action. On incorporation into cells, they become phosphorylated and incorporated into DNA. The lack of a 3'-hydroxyl group makes them unacceptable primers for further DNA synthesis.
      (1) They are effective antiviral drugs because they are **accepted as substrate by viral DNA polymerases better than by the human DNA polymerases.**
      (2) Retroviral DNA polymerase is called **reverse transcriptase** because it uses RNA as a template to synthesize DNA. It is therefore an RNA-dependent DNA polymerase.
      (3) Although dideoxynucleoside analogs all share a common mechanism of action, differences in their pharmacokinetic properties may alter their clinical properties. They often are more effective drugs when used in combination with each other and other types of antiretroviral drugs.
    c. Therapeutic use. Dideoxynucleoside analogs are used to treat retroviral infections such as human immunodeficiency virus (HIV).

  2. Cytarabine (also called **cytosine arabinoside, ara-C**)
    a. Structure. It is considered an analog of 2'-deoxycytidine. It has both 2'- and 3'-hydroxyl groups; however, the 2'-hydroxyl group of the sugar is in the trans configuration. That is, it is on the opposite side of the sugar plane from the 3'-hydroxyl.

b. Mechanism of action. The exact mechanism of action of this drug is unknown. The cell phosphorylates it, and, when incorporated into DNA, it slows the rate of replication. On incorporation into DNA, it is believed to alter the structure of DNA and make it more prone to breakage (and cell death if breakage is extensive).

c. Therapeutic use. Ara-C is a potent acute myelocytic antileukemia drug. An analog, adenine arabinoside (ara-A), exhibits antiviral activity.

C. **Inhibitors that interact directly with DNA**

1. **Intercalators** are drugs, usually with aromatic rings, that insert between adjacent, stacked base pairs.

   a. General mechanism of action. Intercalation causes a physical block as well as a disruption or change in the DNA conformation that inhibits the action of replication enzymes. Many intercalators are mutagenic and induce mistakes in replication, which can cause disease.

   b. Anthracycline glycosides

   (1) **Daunorubicin** and **doxorubicin** are two commonly used anthracycline glycosides. They are antibiotics produced by a strain of *Streptomyces*. The planar tetracycline ring intercalates between the bases of DNA.

   (2) **Therapeutic use.** Daunorubicin is used to treat leukemia. Doxorubicin is used to treat a wide range of cancers. A number of synthetic derivatives of these compounds also show potent anticancer activity.

   c. Actinomycin D is an antibiotic also created from a strain of *Streptomyces*. Its planar phenoxazone ring intercalates between the bases of DNA. It is useful in treating a number of cancers, especially when used with other therapies. For example, actinomycin D is beneficial in treating Wilms' tumor in children when used in combination with surgery, radiotherapy, and other chemotherapeutic drugs.

2. **Drugs that damage DNA**

   a. Alkylating agents. There are many alkylating agents in this class that share the feature of acting as strong electrophiles. These drugs evolved from the sulfur and nitrogen mustard gases of World War I.

   (1) **General mechanism of action.** As strong electrophiles, alkylating agents become linked to many cellular nucleophiles, in particular the seventh nitrogen in the purine ring of guanine in DNA. The alkyl linkage that is formed causes mispairing with guanines during replication, which results in mutations. The alkyl linkage also causes breakage of DNA and cross-linking of the double helix.

   (2) **Therapeutic use.** The numerous alkylating agents are used to treat many different cancers.

   b. Platinum-coordination complexes. A wide array of platinum-containing compounds, such as **cisplatin,** has been made.

   (1) **Mechanism of action.** Platinum-containing compounds react with nucleophiles, such as the seventh nitrogen on the purine ring of guanine, and lead to the formation of cross links between adjacent guanines in DNA.

   (2) **Therapeutic use.** Several of these compounds are effective chemotherapeutic drugs, especially in conjunction with other chemotherapeutic drugs, for testicular and ovarian cancers as well as others. Cisplatin also has been shown to enhance the toxic effect of radiation therapy in cancer cells.

   c. Bleomycins are complex compounds isolated from a strain of *Streptomyces*. They can be made with a wide number of different side groups, which produce related agents with different toxic effects that can be used for different tumors.

   (1) **Mechanism of action.** Bleomycins bind to DNA and interact with oxygen and ferrous iron (Fe^{2+}) to cause DNA breakage.

   (2) **Therapeutic use.** Bleomycin in conjunction with other chemotherapeutic drugs is used to treat testicular and other cancers.

D. **Inhibitors of replicative enzymes**

1. **DNA polymerase inhibitors.** Very few drugs have been found to inhibit DNA polymerases directly, and those that do have shown very limited clinical use.

2. **Topoisomerase inhibitors**
   a. The **quinolones and the fluoroquinolones** inhibit the bacterial topoisomerase DNA gyrase (see II E 2). By inhibiting DNA gyrase, these compounds prevent it from relieving the positive supercoils formed during replication. These drugs are clinically effective in the treatment of urinary tract infections.
   b. **Etoposide (VP-16)** and **teniposide (VM-26)** form a complex with topoisomerase II and DNA that allows topoisomerase II to cut the DNA but inhibits the re-ligation of the cut. These drugs are used to treat a number of different neoplasms.

V. **MUTATIONS** are permanent changes in a DNA sequence. Although germ line mutations are the driving force of evolution, it is undesirable to have a high rate of mutation, especially in somatic cells.

A. **Causes.** Mutations arise by a number of different means.

1. **Errors in replication.** If a base that is noncomplementary to the template base is added during replication, then a mispairing or mismatch occurs. This leads to a mutation during the next round of replication if the error is not repaired.
   a. **Proofreading** is a component activity in replication [see II B 1 c (1)] that reduces the number of misincorporated bases or rare tautomers (i.e., forms of the same chemical structure that differ in proton positions or double bond position) of bases that may become incorporated during replication.
   b. **Postreplicative repair systems** also exist to correct base mispairing that occurs during replication and is not corrected by proofreading.
   c. In both prokaryotes and eukaryotes, mutations that arise from replication errors occur less than once for every 10^9 bases replicated.

2. **Errors that occur during recombination events**
   a. The **DNA of living cells is surprisingly mobile and often is rearranged or recombined.** Examples of this include the following.
      (1) Immunoglobulin gene diversity arises in part from the translocation and rearrangement of immunoglobulin genes (see Chapter 12 VIII C).
      (2) Chromosomes sometimes cross over and recombine during meiosis.
      (3) Many viruses are capable of moving their DNA in and out of their host cell's genomic DNA.
      (4) Some pieces of DNA are mobile and can move to different positions in the genome, and some RNAs occasionally undergo reverse transcription to DNA that is inserted into the genome.
   b. Typically, some of these DNA rearrangements leave no changes or only a few small changes that can be repaired. However, **some of these DNA rearrangements may change the cell's DNA to such a great extent that it cannot be repaired.** This often leads to severe or even lethal mutations.

3. **Chemical mutagens.** Many chemicals alter DNA bases or the structure of DNA. These alterations often lead to mutations if they are not repaired. Types of chemical mutagens are:
   a. **Base analogs** can become incorporated into DNA. Some lead to the inhibition of replication, whereas others are mutagenic because they lead to mispairing.
   b. **Chemical mutagens**
      (1) **Nonalkylating agents.** For example:
         (a) **Formaldehyde** (HCHO) reacts with amine groups and cross-links DNA, RNA, and proteins.

      (b) Hydroxylamine (NH_2OH) specifically reacts with cytosines to form derivatives that pair with adenines instead of guanines. This change leads to a transversion [see V B 1 a (2)].

      (c) Nitrous acid (HNO_2) oxidatively deaminates cytosines, adenines, and guanines to form uracils, hypoxanthines, and xanthines respectively. These changes result in AT-to-GC transitions [see V B 1 a (1)].

    (2) Alkylating agents (see IV C 2 a)

    (3) Intercalating agents. Many intercalating compounds disrupt replication (see IV C 1). Some intercalating agents, such as **acridines,** also tend to cause frameshift mutations. By an unknown mechanism, intercalating agents lead to the insertion of one or two additional base pairs during replication.

4. Irradiation

  a. Ultraviolet (UV) light (200–400 nm) induces dimerization of adjacent pyrimidines, particularly adjacent thymines. This direct mutation of DNA distorts the DNA structure, inhibits transcription, and disrupts replication until it is repaired.

  b. Ionizing radiation, such as roentgen rays (x-rays) and gamma rays (γ-rays), can cause extensive damage to DNA including opening purine rings, which leads to depurination, and breaking phosphodiester bonds.

5. Spontaneous changes. DNA undergoes several spontaneous changes that lead to mutations if they are not repaired before a round of replication.

  a. Deamination of cytosine (C) to form uracil (U) occurs spontaneously. If this is not repaired before a round of replication, an adenine (A) pairs with the template strand containing the uracil instead of a guanine (G).

  b. Spontaneous depurination. Purines are less stable under normal cellular conditions than pyrimidines. The glycosidic bond that links purines to the sugar–phosphate backbone of DNA often is broken. If these purines are not replaced before a round of replication, any base may be added to complement the missing base during replication.

B. **Types of mutations.** Regardless of the method of formation, there are only a limited number of types of mutations.

1. Base substitution

  a. Definition. Base substitutions are the **most common type of mutation,** and they can be classified into **two subtypes:**

    (1) Transitions, in which one purine is replaced by another purine or one pyrimidine is replaced by another pyrimidine

    (2) Transversions, in which a purine is replaced by a pyrimidine or a pyrimidine is replaced by a purine

  b. Missense, nonsense, or silent mutations are possible if base substitutions occur in the coding region of a gene.

    (1) A missense mutation leads to a changed codon and results in an amino acid change in the protein product of that gene.

      (a) Effect. Depending on the amino acid that is changed, missense mutations can have either no effect or very serious consequences.

      (b) Clinical example. Sickle cell anemia is an example of a missense mutation with very serious health consequences [see Chapter 3 II B 4 b (1)].

    (2) A nonsense mutation leads to the conversion of an amino acid codon to a stop codon. Translation of the RNA from a gene with a nonsense mutation is prematurely terminated.

      (a) Effect. The protein products of nonsense mutations are usually nonfunctional.

      (b) Clinical example. Many **thalassemias** are the result of nonsense mutations (see Chapter 3 II B 4 c).

    (3) A silent mutation leads to the formation of a codon synonym (see Chapter 10 I B 1 d) and no change in the amino acid sequence of the gene product.

2. Deletion of one or more base pairs

    a. A **frameshift mutation** results if a deletion of base pairs in a gene occurs that is not a multiple of three. That is, the reading frame of translation changes. This usually results in the production of a nonfunctional gene product.

    b. If a deletion of three (or a multiple of three) base pairs occurs in a gene, then there is no change in the reading frame and only a deletion of one or more amino acids. Such a mutation is likely to be less severe than a frameshift mutation.

3. Insertion of one or more base pairs. As with deletions, insertions of base pairs into genes can lead to severe frameshift mutations (e.g., thalassemias; see Chapter 3 II B 4 c) or less severe additions of codons, depending on whether the insertions are multiples of three.

C. **Mutagenesis and carcinogenesis.** Most mutagens can cause cancer and, therefore, are said to be carcinogenic as well. However, many chemicals are not mutagenic in the form in which they enter the body, yet they are carcinogenic. Because of this apparent paradox, **carcinogens are classified into two types.**

1. Direct carcinogens exist in a mutagenic form when they enter the body. Unless they are rapidly inactivated before they can interact with DNA, they are potentially carcinogenic. Their carcinogenic potential can be estimated by the **Ames test.**

    a. Background. The Ames test assumes there is a relationship between mutagenesis and carcinogenesis.

    b. Procedure

        (1) The Ames test uses a mutant strain of *Salmonella typhimurium,* which requires histidine in the medium to grow.

        (2) This mutant strain of *S. typhimurium* has a low rate of reversion back to the wild type (i.e., normal) that does not require histidine for growth. The rate of **back conversion** (i.e., reversion) to wild type is greatly enhanced by the presence of a mutagen.

        (3) The relative mutagenicity of a substance is correlated with the rate of reversion of the *Salmonella.*

2. Indirect carcinogens are chemicals that are not mutagenic in the form in which they enter the body but are converted to mutagens on metabolism in the body.

    a. The liver has a very active detoxification system that converts many inactive mutagens to active mutagens.

        (1) Many lipophilic chemicals accumulate in the body if they are not made water soluble. In the liver, there are a large number of endoplasmic reticulum (ER)-bound enzymes in the **cytochrome P_{450} oxidase system** that serve this purpose.

        (2) Essentially, these enzymes hydroxylate (or make other chemical modifications to) the lipophilic compounds that convert them to hydrophilic compounds, which are readily excretable.

        (3) Sometimes these modifications convert nonmutagenic compounds to strongly mutagenic compounds.

    b. Indirect carcinogens can be detected in the Ames test if the agar plates on which *Salmonella* are grown are supplemented with liver extracts containing the liver P_{450} detoxification enzymes.

    c. Chemicals shown to be mutagenic by the Ames test usually are found to be carcinogenic when tested in animals.

VI. **DNA REPAIR.** Numerous systems exist in prokaryotes and eukaryotes to repair damaged DNA before mutants become fixed by replication.

A. **Excision repair.** Several repair systems are capable of recognizing and excising damaged DNA. These systems then replace damaged DNA with newly synthesized, properly base-paired DNA.

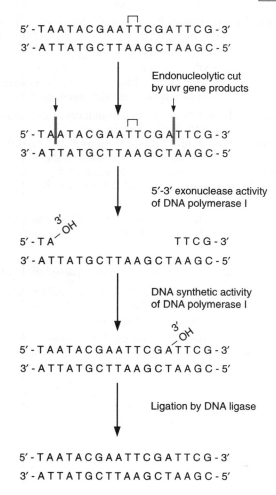

FIGURE 8-10. Excision repair of a thymine–thymine dimer in prokaryotes.

1. **Repair of thymine–thymine dimers** (Figure 8-10)
   a. **In prokaryotes, a multigene family called the *uvr* genes,** recognizes and excises thymine–thymine dimers via the following process.
      (1) The *uvr* gene products **unwind the DNA** in an ATP-dependent manner and **cut the sugar–phosphate backbone** within seven nucleotides on each side of the thymine–thymine dimers.
      (2) The piece of DNA containing the thymine–thymine dimer is removed by **digestion with the 5′ to 3′ exonuclease** (excision–repair) activity of DNA polymerase I (see II B 1 c).
      (3) **DNA polymerase I** then **fills in the gap** left by the excision of the damaged strand of DNA.
      (4) **DNA ligase** (see II D 2 e) **seals the gap** between the newly synthesized segment and the main chain.
   b. **Xeroderma pigmentosum.** Eukaryotes also have an excision–repair system that is called **nucleotide excision repair.** Xeroderma pigmentosum, an autosomal recessive disease that may involve up to nine genes, results in hypersensitivity of the skin to UV light damage.
      (1) **Cause.** Xeroderma pigmentosum is caused by a deficiency in the repair of thymine–thymine dimers. Skin cells from many of these patients do not excise thymine–thymine dimers efficiently.

(2) **Clinical presentation.** Patients with this disease have many skin and eye problems and a high incidence of skin cancer due to exposure to UV light.

2. **Apurinic repair.** If a depurination or a rare depyrimidination occurs, then an **apurinic or apyrimidinic (AP) endonuclease** excises the remaining sugar and phosphate. This leaves a one-nucleotide gap that, in *E. coli,* is repaired by DNA polymerase I and DNA ligase. Eukaryotes have a similar repair pathway.

3. **Removal of uracils** that arise from deamination of cytosines is facilitated by the action of the enzyme **uracil N-glycosylase.**
   a. **Uracil N-glycosylase** recognizes and removes uracils from DNA by cleavage of the N-glycosidic bond that holds the base to the sugar–phosphate backbone.
   b. **AP endonuclease** then removes the sugar and phosphate groups.
   c. In *E. coli,* **DNA polymerase I and DNA ligase** then repair the one-nucleotide gap. Eukaryotes have a similar repair system.

4. Humans also have a **thymine-mismatch DNA glycosylase** that excises thymines when mispaired with guanines. This occurs when methylcytosines (see Chapter 12 V A 4) become deaminated.

B. **Direct repair.** Some base modifications can be repaired directly without excision repair.

1. **Photoreactivation.** An enzyme found in all organisms, except placental mammals, called **DNA photolyase** cleaves the covalent bonds that form thymine–thymine dimers. These enzymes are activated by visible light in the range of 400–600 nm.

2. **Dealkylation of guanines. Guanine alkyltransferases** remove the methyl and ethyl groups from alkylated guanines. The enzymes alkylate themselves in the process and become inactivated. Therefore, it takes one protein to dealkylate one guanine.

C. **Mismatch repair.** Errors in replication or recombination, as well as insertions or deletions may lead to mismatched base pairs or unpaired bases. A mismatch repair system exists in both prokaryotes and eukaryotes that recognizes and repairs the structurally altered DNA that arises from the mismatch.

1. It is not exactly known in eukaryotes how this system distinguishes the strand of DNA that contains the mutant deoxynucleotides from the strand that contains the correct deoxynucleotides.

2. Clinically, people with hereditary nonpolyposis colorectal cancer have been shown to have a mutation in one of the mismatch repair genes.

D. **Recombination repair** provides a method to replicate around a thymine–thymine dimer that is not repaired before replication. Thymine–thymine dimers cannot serve as templates during replication. However, replication can bypass the region containing dimers, and they can be repaired after replication (Figure 8-11).

1. **Repair of strand**
   a. Bypassing the region containing thymine–thymine dimers leaves a **gap** in the newly synthesized strand complementary to the one containing the dimer and a perfect copy of the original complementary strand.
   b. A **recombination event** then occurs. The single strand of the original complement strand of the thymine–thymine dimers exchanges with the newly synthesized complement.
   c. This effectively **moves the newly synthesized strand,** with the gap, across from the newly synthesized strand that does not have thymine–thymine dimers.
   d. This **gap is repaired** because it does not have thymine–thymine dimers.
   e. The **end result** is two DNA duplexes: one with the original thymine–thymine dimer and one without.

2. **Repair of thymine–thymine dimer**
   a. The thymine–thymine dimer can be repaired by **excision repair or DNA photolyase.** Recombination repair provides a mechanism that allows replication to proceed around the dimer and not leave any gaps.

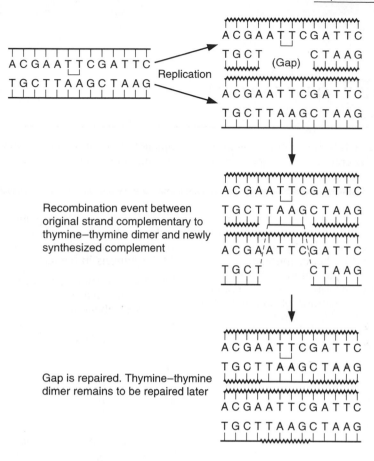

FIGURE 8-11. Recombination repair of a thymine–thymine (*T-T*) dimer. Recombination allows copies of damaged DNA to be made during replication. Repair of the damage is made after replication.

    b. Recombination repair is known to exist in prokaryotes and is **believed to exist in eukaryotes.**

Case 8-1 Revisited

Doxorubicin, fluorouracil, and cisplatin are potent chemotherapeutic drugs that work through the inhibition of DNA replication. Cells that cannot complete DNA replication often undergo cell death. Fluorouracil is an antimetabolite (see IV A). For DNA replication to take place, deoxynucleotide precursors are required. Fluorouracil specifically inhibits the production of deoxythymidine monophosphate (dTMP; see Chapter 26 V A). Doxorubicin inhibits DNA by intercalating into DNA. It causes a physical block to and disruption of active replication (see IV C 1). Cisplatin is a nucleophile that cross-links adjacent guanines in DNA. This leads to mutations and the disruption of DNA synthesis (see IV C 2 b).

    These drugs are not selective for cancer cells, but they are toxic to any actively dividing cell type to which they have intercellular access. This is why patients undergoing chemotherapy often have side effects such as hair loss, gastric distress, and suppression of immune function. Intercalating agents and drugs that modify DNA, such as cisplatin, are also mutagens. As such, they also are potentially carcinogenic.

    Prior to direct animal testing, the Ames test can be used to estimate the carcinogenic potential of chemicals (see V C 1,2). The Ames test measures the mutagenicity of chemicals and assumes that there is a relationship between mutagenesis and carcinogenesis. The Ames test can measure if chemicals are direct carcinogens or, if done in the presence of liver extracts, it can measure if they are indirect carcinogens.

STUDY QUESTIONS

DIRECTIONS: Each of the numbered items or incomplete statements in this section is followed by answers or by completions of the statement. Select the **one** lettered answer or completion that is **best** in each case.

1. *Escherichia coli* cells that had been cultured in a light medium containing ^{14}N-ammonium chloride as the sole nitrogen source were transferred to a heavy medium containing ^{15}N-ammonium chloride. After three generations of growth in the heavy medium, what will be the proportion of dual light (LL) strands, dual heavy (HH) strands, and hybrid light + heavy (LH) strands in the DNA duplexes?

(A) 3 LH to 1 HH
(B) 3 HH to 1 LH
(C) 6 HH to 2 LL
(D) 15 LL to 1 LH
(E) 7 HH to 1 LH

2. Which one of the following DNA polymerases is essential for both the replication and repair of DNA?

(A) DNA polymerase I
(B) DNA polymerase δ
(C) DNA polymerase II
(D) DNA polymerase γ
(E) DNA polymerase III

3. Short chains of nucleic acid can be isolated from cells in which DNA is undergoing replication. These segments, known as Okazaki fragments, have which one of the following properties?

(A) They are double-stranded
(B) They contain covalently linked RNA and DNA
(C) They are DNA–RNA hybrids
(D) They arise from the nicking of the sugar–phosphate backbone of the parental DNA chain
(E) They are removed by nuclease activity

4. Which one of the sequences listed below best describes the order in which the following enzymes participate in lagging strand DNA synthesis in bacteria?

1 = DNA polymerase I (pol I)
2 = 5′-Exonuclease
3 = DNA polymerase III (pol III)
4 = DNA ligase
5 = RNA polymerase (primase)

(A) 5,1,3,2,4
(B) 3,2,1,5,4
(C) 5,3,4,2,1
(D) 5,3,2,1,4
(E) 3,2,5,1,4

5. Which chemotherapeutic drug inhibits replication through intercalation?

(A) Bleomycinic acid
(B) Doxorubicin
(C) Zidovudine (azidothymidine)
(D) Etoposide (VP-16)
(E) Cisplatin

6. All cells do not divide at the same rate. Events in which phase of the cell cycle determine when a cell is going to replicate?

(A) M phase
(B) G_1 phase
(C) S phase
(D) G_2 phase

7. A unique feature of the replication of the ends of eukaryotic chromosomes as compared with the replication of the rest of the genome is

(A) the ends are replicated in a template-independent manner
(B) an RNA molecule associated with telomerase serves as a primer for the synthesis of ends
(C) the ends that are synthesized are short, tandem repeats of ribonucleotides
(D) an RNA molecule serves as the template for the synthesis of ends
(E) telomerase synthesizes both the leading and lagging strands of ends

8. Ionizing radiation such as x-rays causes which one of the following results?

(A) Deamination of cytosines
(B) Formation of thymine-thymine dimers
(C) Cross-linking of DNA
(D) Breaking of phosphodiester bonds
(E) Insertion of additional base pairs into DNA

9. Which mutation of the sequence GATCCT is a transition?

(A) GGTCCT
(B) GTTCCT
(C) GTATCCT
(D) GTCCT
(E) There is insufficient information

10. A mutation that converts an amino acid codon to a stop codon is a

(A) nonsense mutation
(B) transversion
(C) silent mutation
(D) frameshift mutation
(E) missense mutation

11. Which one of the following is most likely to lead to a frameshift mutation?

(A) Ultraviolet light
(B) Intercalation
(C) Spontaneous depurination
(D) Alkylation
(E) Spontaneous deamination

12. The Ames test of mutagenicity is characterized by which one of the following statements?

(A) The mutant bacterial strain used in the Ames test reverts back to the wild type when histidine is removed from the medium
(B) The mutant strain of bacteria requires histidine in the medium to grow and reverts to the wild type, which does not require histidine for growth, at a slow rate
(C) Mutagenicity as determined by the Ames test and carcinogenicity as determined in animal studies are not correlated
(D) The Ames test cannot be used to test indirect carcinogenicity
(E) Mutagens prevent the reversion of the bacterial strain to the wild type

13. Which statement concerning the repair of thymine-thymine dimers is correct?

(A) In recombination repair, thymine-thymine dimers are removed by a recombination event
(B) The photoreactivation of thymine-thymine dimers by DNA photolyase requires an endonucleolytic cut
(C) DNA photolyase is activated by ultraviolet (UV) light (200–400 nm)
(D) In prokaryotes, DNA polymerase I is responsible for the exonucleolytic digestion of the fragment containing the thymine-thymine dimers
(E) In the excision repair of thymine-thymine dimers, an N-glycosidase initially removes the thymine-thymine dimers

14. Which enzyme activity exclusively repairs cytosine (C) deamination but does not repair the alkylation of a guanine (G) by ethylmethane sulfonate (EMS)?

(A) DNA polymerase
(B) Apurinic endonuclease
(C) N-glycosylase
(D) DNA ligase
(E) The repair of each requires the same enzyme activities

DIRECTIONS: The group of items in this section consists of lettered options followed by a set of numbered items. For each item, select the **one** lettered option that is most closely associated with it. Each lettered option may be selected once, more than once, or not at all.

Questions 15-18

Match the following enzymes with the correct description of its action

(A) It alters the supercoil structure of DNA
(B) It hydrolyzes the RNA primers of replication
(C) It catalyzes the formation of phosphodiester bonds between two DNA chains of the double helix
(D) It unwinds the DNA preceding replication forks
(E) It is the primary polymerization enzyme in replication

15. Helicase

16. DNA polymerase I (pol I)

17. Gyrase

18. Ligase

ANSWERS AND EXPLANATIONS

1. The answer is B [I B; Figure 8-1]. The proportion of 3 dual heavy (HH) strands to 1 hybrid light + heavy (LH) strand is the basis of the Meselson-Stahl demonstration that DNA replication in bacteria is semiconservative. However, the order for growing the organism in light and heavy media is reversed from the original study. Semiconservative replication means that at each replicative event the new duplex genome contains one strand of parental DNA (conserved) and one strand of newly synthesized DNA.

2. The answer is A [II B, D 2 d; III B; VI A 1,2,3; Table 8-1, Table 8-2]. Prokaryotic DNA polymerase I (pol I) is essential for lagging strand synthesis and many types of DNA repair. Prokaryotic DNA polymerase II appears to be involved only in DNA repair. Prokaryotic DNA polymerase III (pol III) is the primary replication enzyme and does not appear to be involved in DNA repair. Eukaryotic DNA polymerase δ is essential for both leading and lagging strand synthesis. Eukaryotic DNA polymerase γ is mitochondrial and responsible only for replication of mitochondrial DNA.

3. The answer is B [II D 2 a-d]. Okazaki fragments are made during lagging strand synthesis. Primase makes a small RNA that serves as the primer for the synthesis, by DNA polymerase III (pol III), of the remainder of the Okazaki fragments. This means that the RNA primer and the newly synthesized DNA are covalently linked. The Okazaki fragment is complementary to only the segment of the lagging strand template that directed its synthesis. Neither the RNA primer portion nor the DNA portion of Okazaki fragments are complementary to each other. Therefore, they are not RNA-DNA hybrids nor are they double-stranded. Okazaki fragments arise by discontinuous synthesis, not by fragmentation of the parental DNA chain.

4. The answer is D [II D]. The RNA primer is first laid down on the separated DNA strands, where primase carries out this function on the lagging strand and on the leading strand. Short stretches of DNA (Okazaki fragments) are then formed on the template by the DNA polymerase III (pol III) holoenzyme. The primer RNA is removed from both daughter strands by the 5'-exonuclease activity of DNA polymerase I (pol I) and is replaced with deoxyribonucleotides by its polymerizing activity. Finally, the fragments are joined by the DNA ligase.

5. The answer is B [IV B 1, C 1 b, 2 b-c, D 2 b]. Doxorubicin is an effective chemotherapeutic drug that inhibits replication by intercalation. The bleomycins bind to DNA and lead to its breakage. Zidovudine, or azidothymidine, is a dideoxynucleoside analog that inhibits replication when it is incorporated into DNA because it lacks a 3'-hydroxyl group. Etoposide (VP-16) inhibits replication by forming a complex with topoisomerase II and DNA. This interaction allows topoisomerase II to cut DNA but inhibits the re-ligation of the cut. Cisplatin is a platinum-coordination complex that reacts with the nitrogen in the seventh position of the purine ring of guanine and leads to the cross-linking of adjacent guanines.

6. The answer is B [III E]. The time it takes for cells from a particular species to progress through the S, G_2, and M phases of the cell cycle is invariable. The only phase of the cell cycle that takes a variable time to be completed is G_1. Events that occur in G_1 determine when the cell progresses through S, G_2, and M phases. Cells that enter a prolonged G_1 phase and do not commit to enter S phase are said to be in the G_0 phase of the cell cycle.

7. The answer is D [III D]. Telomerase is responsible for synthesis of the ends of eukaryotic chromosomes. It is a DNA polymerase and as such requires a template and primer. A unique feature of telomerase is that it contains an RNA molecule that serves as the template for the synthesis of ends. The ends that it synthesizes are short, tandem repeats of DNA. Therefore, it is an RNA-dependent DNA polymerase. The free 3'-hydroxyl groups at the end of one of the strands of chromosomal DNA serve as the primer for telomerase-based DNA synthesis of the leading strand. Lagging strand synthesis presumably takes place by the normal replication machinery.

8. The answer is D [V A 3-5] Ionizing radiation causes extensive damage to DNA, including the opening of purine rings, which leads to depurination, and the breaking of phosphodiester bonds. Deamination of cytosines to form uracils is a type of mutation that may occur spontaneously. Thymine–thymine dimers are caused by irradiation of DNA with ultraviolet light. DNA may become crosslinked by reaction with formaldehyde, which reacts with amine groups in the bases. Intercalating agents, such as acridines, often cause insertion of additional bases into DNA.

9. The answer is A [V B 1 a (1)]. A transition is a base substitution mutation in which a purine is replaced by another purine or a pyrimidine is replaced by another pyrimidine. It is a transition regardless of the method of formation. A transversion mutation occurs when a purine is replaced by a pyrimidine or a pyrimidine is replaced by a purine. Therefore, the change of adenine (A) to thymine (T) in the sequence GTTCCT is a transversion. The sequences GTATCCT and GTCCT represent insertions and deletions, respectively.

10. The answer is A [V B 1 a (2), b, 2 a]. A nonsense mutation leads to the conversion of an amino acid codon to a stop codon. Translation of the RNA from a gene with a nonsense mutation is prematurely terminated. The product formed is therefore shorter and often nonfunctional. A silent mutation leads to the formation of a codon synonym and is said to be silent because there is no change in the protein product. A missense mutation leads to a change in a codon such that a codon for another amino acid is formed. The severity of such mutations depends on the importance of the amino acid that is changed in the protein product of the mutated gene. A frameshift mutation occurs if a deletion or insertion of base pairs in a gene occurs that is not a multiple of three. As with nonsense mutations, the product formed from genes with these mutations is often nonfunctional. A transversion is said to take place when a purine base is replaced by a pyrimidine base or vice versa.

11. The answer is B [V A 3-5]. Many intercalating agents, such as the acridines, disrupt replication and, by an unknown mechanism, this may lead to an insertion of additional bases to the replicating DNA. If the inserted bases are in a gene and not a multiple of three, then a frameshift mutation is formed. Ultraviolet light causes dimerization of adjacent pyrimidines (usually thymine–thymine dimers). Cross-linked dimers disrupt replication and transcription but do not cause the insertion or deletion of bases. Likewise, alkylation, and spontaneous depurination or deamination are modifications of DNA that lead to mutations but not to the insertion or deletion of bases.

12. The answer is B [V C 1-2]. The Ames test uses *Salmonella typhimurium,* which requires histidine for growth. It reverts back to the wild type, which does not require histidine for growth, at a slow rate. Mutagens increase the rate of reversion to wild type. If the growth medium is supplemented with liver extracts, the Ames test can be used to detect indirect carcinogens. There is a strong correlation between mutagenicity as determined by the Ames test and carcinogenicity as determined by animal studies.

13. The answer is D [VI A 1 a, B 1, D]. In prokaryotes, the covalent linkage of the fragment containing the thymine–thymine dimers is broken by endonucleolytic cuts by the *uvr* gene products. The 5′ to 3′ exonuclease activity of DNA polymerase I digests this fragment, then its polymerization activity fills in the gap. Recombination repair does not remove thymine–thymine dimers. It allows replication to be completed with the proper complement to the thymine–thymine dimers being formed. The dimers are repaired after replication either by excision repair or by DNA photolyase. DNA photolyase directly reverses the covalent bonds that link the pyrimidine rings and does not require any nucleolytic cuts. DNA photolyase is activated by visible light (400–600 nm). N-glycosidase plays no role in excision repair of thymine-thymine dimers.

14. The answer is C [IV C 2 a; VI A 2, 3]. Deamination of cytosine (C) results in the formation of uracil (U). Uracil is a stable base, and the first step in repairing deaminated cytosine is the removal of uracil by uracil N-glycosylase. Alkylation of a guanine (G) by ethylmethane sulfonate (EMS) results in an unstable N-glycosidic bond that spontaneously hydrolyzes to leave a site without a base. The repair of each of these DNA alterations is identical, except for the initial removal of uracil by the N-glycosylase. After uracil is removed, the repair of sites without bases is the same. An apurinic (AP) endonuclease excises the remaining sugar phosphate, the one-nucleotide gap is filled in by DNA polymerase I (in prokaryotes), and the sugar-phosphate backbone is resealed by DNA ligase.

15-18. The answers are: 15D [II E 1], **16B** [II D 2 d], **17A** [II E 2; IV D 2], **18C** [II D 2 e]. A helicase unwinds the DNA preceding the replication fork to provide single-strand templates for replication. This unwinding of the double helix causes positive supercoils to build up in front of replication forks.

Gyrase, a topoisomerase, relieves these positive supercoils. Therefore, like all topoisomerases, it alters the supercoil structure of DNA.

The 5′ to 3′ exonuclease activity of DNA polymerase I (pol I) removes the RNA primers that are needed to initiate leading strand synthesis and complete lagging strand synthesis. DNA polymerase III (pol III) is the primary polymerization enzyme in DNA replication. It makes all of the leading strand and most of the lagging strand.

DNA ligase joins Okazaki fragments after pol I has removed the RNA primer portion and replaced it with DNA.

Chapter 9

RNA Synthesis and Processing
Donald Sittman

MAJOR CLASSES OF RIBONUCLEIC ACID (RNA). Multiple steps are required to produce functional cellular RNAs. Although some of these steps are common to the production of all RNAs, others depend on the class of RNA being produced. Three functionally distinct classes of RNA are produced in prokaryotes, and four are produced in eukaryotes.

A. **Messenger RNA (mRNA)** carries information from genes to ribosomes, where it is translated into proteins.

1. Prokaryotic mRNA
a. Basic features
(1) Most prokaryotic mRNAs are **polycistronic.** That is, they carry the information for the production of multiple polypeptides.
(2) Not all portions of prokaryotic mRNA code for polypeptides (Figure 9-1A).
  (a) The 5′ ends of mRNA contain sequences that are never translated into protein. They are called **leader sequences** or **5′ untranslated regions (5′ UTR).**
  (b) Likewise, the 3′ ends contain sequences that are never translated into protein. They are called **trailer sequences** or **3′ untranslated regions (3′ UTR).**

A. Prokaryotic mRNA

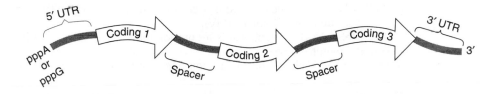

B. Eukaryotic mRNA

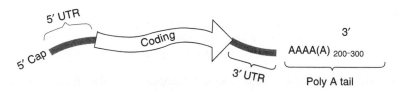

FIGURE 9-1. Schematic representation of typical prokaryotic and eukaryotic messenger RNAs (mRNAs). The coding regions are indicated with *open arrows.* (A) A polycistronic prokaryotic mRNA with three coding regions is shown. The coding regions are separated by noncoding spacer sequences. Flanking the proximal and distal coding sequences are noncoding 5′ and 3′ untranslated regions *(UTRs).* The 5′ end of the mRNA is a purine nucleoside triphosphate. (B) A monocistronic eukaryotic mRNA is shown. The single coding region is flanked by a 5′ and 3′ UTR. The 5′ end has a 7-methylguanylate cap and the 3′ end has a polyadenylate *(poly A)* tail.

        (c) If the mRNA is polycistronic, the sequences between those that code for proteins (i.e., cistrons) are called the **intercistronic regions** or **spacers.**

   b. Abundance. Messenger RNA accounts for only **5%** of the total cellular RNA in prokaryotes.

   c. Stability. The lifetime of prokaryotic mRNA is short. Most mRNAs are stable for just a few minutes.

  2. Eukaryotic mRNA

   a. Basic features (see Figure 9-1B)

    (1) Eukaryotic mRNA is monocistronic; that is, it carries only the information for the production of a single polypeptide.

    (2) Precursor form. Most, but not all, eukaryotic mRNAs arise by extensive post-transcriptional processing of large precursors. This processing occurs during the passage of the sequences that become mRNA from the nucleus to the cytoplasm (see III B 2). These large precursors of mRNA are called **heterogeneous nuclear RNA (hnRNA).**

    (3) Like prokaryotic mRNA, eukaryotic mRNA contains **leader sequences** (5′ UTRs) and **trailer sequences** (3′ UTRs).

    (4) The 5′ ends of eukaryotic mRNAs have a **7-methylguanylate** attached by a 5′ to 5′ triphosphate linkage. This structure is called a **cap** (see III B 2 a).

    (5) Most, but not all, eukaryotic mRNAs have a **polyadenylate (poly A) tail,** which consists of 200–300 adenylate residues at the 3′ end (see III B 2 b).

   b. Abundance. Eukaryotic mRNA accounts for **3%** of the total cellular RNA. Its precursor, hnRNA, accounts for **7%** of the total cellular RNA.

   c. Stability. Compared with prokaryotic mRNA, most eukaryotic mRNAs are relatively stable and exhibit half-lives on the order of hours to days.

B. **Ribosomal RNA (rRNA)** comprises approximately 50% of the mass of ribosomes. The function of rRNA is both structural as well as catalytic.

  1. Prokaryotic rRNA

   a. Basic features

    (1) There are **three kinds of prokaryotic rRNA.**

     (a) 23S[1] rRNA (2904 nucleotides) is a component of the large, 50S ribosomal subunit (see Chapter 10 IV).

     (b) 16S rRNA (1541 nucleotides) is a component of the small, 30S ribosomal subunit.

     (c) 5S rRNA (120 nucleotides) is a component of the large, 50S ribosomal subunit.

    (2) Processing. Prokaryotic rRNAs arise from the processing of a large 30S precursor rRNA (see III A 2).

   b. Abundance. Ribosomal RNAs are the most abundant RNA class. They account for **80%** of the total cellular RNA in prokaryotes.

  2. Eukaryotic rRNA

   a. Basic features

    (1) The rRNAs of eukaryotes are typically bigger than those of prokaryotes. Also, **eukaryotes have four kinds of rRNA.**

     (a) 28S rRNA (4718 nucleotides) is a component of the large, 60S ribosomal subunit.

     (b) 18S rRNA (1874 nucleotides) is a component of the small, 40S ribosomal subunit.

     (c) 5.8S rRNA (160 nucleotides) is a component of the large, 60S ribosomal subunit.

     (d) 5S rRNA (120 nucleotides) is a component of the large, 60S ribosomal subunit.

---

[1] S stands for a Svedberg unit, which is derived from the sedimentation constant (s) and is related to the size and shape of a molecule (see Chapter 2 V B 2 c).

  (2) Processing. Similar to those of prokaryotes, three of the eukaryotic rRNAs arise from the processing of a large (45S) precursor rRNA. The **5S rRNA is the transcription product of a separate gene.**

 b. Abundance. Approximately **4%** of the total eukaryotic cellular RNA is 45S precursor rRNA, and **71%** is fully processed rRNAs.

C. **Transfer RNAs (tRNAs)** serve to transfer amino acids to the ribosomes and to facilitate the incorporation of the amino acids into newly synthesized proteins in a template-dependent manner (see Chapter 10 II). For each amino acid, there is one or more specific tRNA.

 1. Prokaryotic tRNA

  a. Basic features

   (1) Size. Transfer RNAs are small RNAs with an average size of 80 nucleotides.

   (2) Structure. All tRNAs have common structural features that allow them to function in the ribosome. They also have unique structural features that are necessary for recognition by the enzymes that catalyze the attachment of amino acids to tRNAs. The sequences that pair with the appropriate codons in the ribosome are also unique for each tRNA (see Chapter 10 III).

   (3) Processing. All tRNAs arise from the processing of large precursor tRNA (see III A 3).

   (4) Modification. To adopt a functional structure, prokaryotic **tRNAs are heavily modified post-transcriptionally** (see III A 3).

  b. Abundance. The tRNAs account for **15%** of the total cellular RNA in prokaryotes.

 2. Eukaryotic tRNA

  a. Basic features

   (1) Eukaryotic tRNAs are very similar to prokaryotic tRNAs in size and in structural features.

   (2) Eukaryotic tRNAs are also heavily post-transcriptionally processed and modified (see III B 3).

  b. Abundance. The total amount of small RNAs in the eukaryotic cell, of which the tRNAs are the most abundant, is **15%.**

D. **Small RNAs.** In addition to tRNA, eukaryotes have numerous other small RNAs that serve a variety of functions. They are classified into two broad types according to where they are localized.

 1. Small cytoplasmic RNAs (scRNAs). The major scRNA is **7S RNA** (294 nucleotides), which is the RNA component of signal recognition particles (see Chapter 10 VII B 1).

 2. Small nuclear RNAs (snRNAs). Many of the snRNAs are associated with proteins in **small nuclear ribonucleoprotein particles** or **SNRPs.** SNRPs function in the splicing reactions needed to process hnRNA to mRNA (see III B 2 c).

II. **TRANSCRIPTION.** The process of RNA synthesis directed by a DNA template is termed transcription, and it occurs in three phases: initiation, elongation, and termination.

A. **Elongation.** The basic requirements and fundamental mechanism of the elongation phase of RNA synthesis is the **same in prokaryotes and eukaryotes** (Figure 9-2) and must be understood before initiation and termination can be understood.

 1. Template. A single strand of DNA acts as a template to direct the formation of complementary RNA during transcription.

 2. Substrate. The substrates for RNA synthesis are the four ribonucleoside triphos-

A

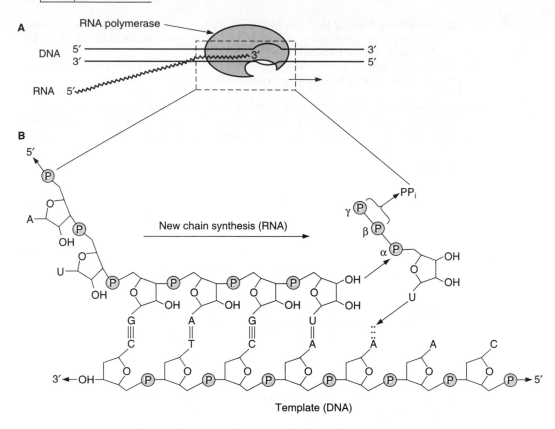

FIGURE 9-2. Features of elongation of transcription. *(A)* The *shaded oval* represents RNA polymerase. At the site of RNA synthesis, the DNA is unwound so that one strand of the DNA can act as a template. New RNA *(squiggly line)* chain growth is in a 5′ to 3′ direction. *(B)* The addition of a single ribonucleotide to the 3′ end of the growing RNA chain is shown. Cleavage of the high-energy phosphate bond between the α and β phosphates of an incoming ribonucleoside triphosphate provides the energy for formation of a phosphodiester bond with the 3′-hydroxyl (OH) of the preceding nucleotide.

phates: adenosine triphosphate (ATP), guanosine triphosphate (GTP), cytidine triphosphate (CTP), and uridine triphosphate (UTP). Cleavage of the high-energy phosphate bond between the α and β phosphates of these nucleoside triphosphates provides the energy for the addition of nucleotides to the growing RNA chain.

3. **Direction of synthesis.** After the first nucleoside triphosphate [see II B 2 a (2) (b)], subsequent nucleotides are added to the 3′-hydroxyl of the preceding nucleotide. **Therefore, RNA chain growth proceeds in the 5′ to 3′ direction.**

4. **Enzyme**
   a. **Prokaryotes** have a single RNA polymerase responsible for all cellular RNA synthesis. The structure of this enzyme is complex.
      (1) A **core enzyme** with the subunit structure α_2 (40,000 MW), β (155,000 MW), and β′ (160,000 MW) is required for the **elongation** steps of RNA synthesis.
      (2) A **holoenzyme,** which is a core enzyme with an additional subunit σ (85,000 MW), is required for proper **initiation** of transcription (see II B 1 b).
   b. **Eukaryotes** have one mitochondrial and three nuclear RNA polymerases. The **nuclear RNA polymerases are distinct enzymes that function to synthesize different RNAs.**

(1) **Structure.** The nuclear RNA polymerases are large enzymes of greater than 500,000 MW. Each has a very complex subunit composition with more than 10 subunit polypeptides.

(2) **Location and function.** The subnuclear localization and the RNA product of each type of RNA polymerase are determined by the RNA polymerase's differential sensitivity to **α-amanitin** (a toxic bicyclic octapeptide from the poisonous mushroom *Amanita phalloides*). These variations are summarized in Table 9-1.

5. **Other enzymatic activities.** Unlike some of the DNA polymerases (see Chapter 8 II B 1 c), **the RNA polymerases have no other associated enzyme activities,** such as proofreading.

B. Initiation of transcription

1. **Promoter sequences.** Unlike the initiation of replication, transcriptional initiation does not require a primer. **Promoter sequences are responsible for directing RNA polymerase to initiate transcription at a particular point.** Promoter sequences differ between prokaryotes and eukaryotes.

   a. **Nomenclature and numbering conventions** are used to avoid confusion in the description of sequences, such as promoter sequences, and their location in genes.

      (1) Because DNA is double-stranded, the **sequence of only one strand is presented.**

      (2) Because RNA synthesis occurs in a 5' to 3' direction, and sequences are written in a 5' to 3' direction (see Chapter 6 I C 3), the sequence of the DNA strand that is **identical to the RNA transcript** is presented.

      (3) For any one gene, the location of particular sequences related to the expression of that gene is given relative to its transcriptional startpoint. Therefore, **position 1 of a gene is the base that is equivalent to the first base of the 5' end of the RNA transcript of that gene.**

      (4) Sequences preceding the first base are numbered negatively and said to be **upstream** of the initiation point. Sequences following the first base are numbered positively and are said to be **downstream** of the initiation point.

   b. **Prokaryotic promoters.** For most prokaryotic genes, there are **conserved sequences** that are necessary to promote accurate initiation of transcription. The **promoters for most prokaryotic genes have three sequence elements** (Figure 9-3A).

      (1) **Initiation site (i.e., startpoint).** Transcription for most genes always starts at the same base (position 1). **The startpoint is usually a purine.**

      (2) **Pribnow box.** For all prokaryotic genes there is a sequence called the Pribnow box that lies 9–18 base pairs upstream of the startpoint.

         (a) The sequence of a typical Pribnow box is either identical to or very similar to the sequence **TATAAT.**

TABLE 9-1. Eukaryotic Nuclear RNA Polymerases

Type	α-Amanitin Sensitivity	Subcellular Localization	RNA Product
I	Insensitive	Nucleolus	45S rRNA
II	Very sensitive to low levels	Nucleoplasm	hnRNA (mRNA) and some snRNAs
III	Sensitive to high levels	Nucleoplasm	tRNA, 5S rRNA, 7S RNA and some snRNAs

hnRNA = heterogeneous nuclear RNA; mRNA = messenger RNA; rRNA = ribosomal RNA; snRNAs = small nuclear RNAs; tRNA = transfer RNA.

A. Prokaryotic promoter

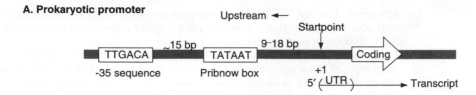

B. Eukaryotic RNA polymerase II promoter

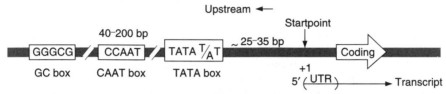

C. Eukaryotic RNA polymerase III promoter 5S rRNA gene

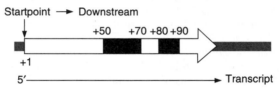

FIGURE 9-3. Sequence features of typical prokaryotic and eukaryotic promoters. Conserved promoter sequence elements *(enclosed boxes)* are shown relative to the startpoint of transcription. *(A)* Prokaryotic promoter. *(B)* A typical eukaryotic RNA polymerase II promoter. For both *(A)* and *(B)*, the startpoint precedes the coding region so that the transcripts have a 5′ untranslated region *(UTR)*. *(C)* The eukaryotic RNA polymerase III promoter elements are downstream of the startpoint and within the transcribed portion of the 5S gene. They are shown as *shaded boxes.*

    (b) The Pribnow box also has been called the **–10 sequence** because it is usually found 10 base pairs upstream of the startpoint.

  (3) The **–35 sequence** is a component of typical prokaryotic promoters. It is a sequence that is either identical to or very similar to the sequence **TTGACA.** It is named the –35 sequence because it is typically found 35 base pairs upstream of the startpoint.

 c. Eukaryotic promoters. Each type of eukaryotic RNA polymerase uses a different promoter. The promoters used by RNA polymerase I and II are similar to the prokaryotic promoter in that they are upstream of the startpoint. However, the promoters used by RNA polymerase III are unique because they are usually downstream of the startpoint.

  (1) Initiation site (i.e., startpoint). The promoters of all the eukaryotic RNA polymerases direct the initiation of transcription to a particular startpoint. As in prokaryotes, the startpoint is usually a purine, although pyrimidine startpoints are not uncommon in eukaryotes.

  (2) Multiple RNA polymerase II promoter sequence elements. Unlike RNA polymerase I promoters, which are all the same, and prokaryotic promoters, which are similar, **there is much diversity among RNA polymerase II pro-**

moters. Several sequence elements are conserved and common to many of these RNA polymerase II promoters (see Figure 9-3B).

   (a) The **TATA box** is a sequence either identical to or very similar to the sequence TATA(T or A)T. It is typically found 25–35 base pairs upstream of the startpoint.

   (b) The **CAAT box** and the **GC box** are sequences similar to CCAAT and GGGCG, respectively, that are found one or more times anywhere from 40–200 base pairs upstream of the startpoint.

(3) The **RNA polymerase III promoters** are of interest because they usually occur downstream of the startpoint.

   (a) The **5S rRNA promoter** is made of two sequence elements; one is the sequence 50–70 base pairs downstream of the startpoint and the other is the sequence 80–90 base pairs downstream of the startpoint. Both are in the transcribed portion of the gene (see Figure 9-3C).

   (b) The **tRNA promoters** are also made of two sequence elements that are downstream of the startpoint and within the transcribed portion of the gene; one is between +8 and +30, and one is between +50 and +70.

(4) Other sequence elements—**response elements and enhancers—affect the rate of initiation of transcription** (see Chapter 12 V B 3 b) but are not strictly promoter elements because they do not have an effect on the accuracy of the initiation of transcription.

2. **Initiation factors** are needed to initiate transcription. In prokaryotes, only a single factor, **sigma (σ),** is needed to initiate transcription. In eukaryotes, multiple factors are required, in part because of the diversity of promoters.

   a. The **prokaryotic σ factor is required for accurate initiation of transcription** (Figure 9-4).

   (1) **Function.** The σ factor enables the RNA polymerase holoenzyme to recognize and bind tightly to the promoter sequences.

   (2) **Process**

   (a) Upon binding, the σ factor facilitates the opening or melting of the DNA double helix.

   (b) The enzyme then catalyzes the formation of a phosphodiester bond between the first two bases. The first base is usually a purine nucleoside triphosphate (pppA or pppG).

   (c) Elongation proceeds after the formation of the first phosphodiester bond. By the time 10 nucleotides have been added, the σ factor dissociates. The core enzyme then continues the elongation of the transcript.

   (d) The released σ factor can combine with free core enzyme to form another holoenzyme that can initiate transcription.

   (3) **Rifampin** is an effective antibacterial drug and one of the few therapeutic drugs that affects only transcription.[2] Actions of rifampin include the following.

   (a) **Rifampin binds to the β subunit of RNA polymerase when the polymerase is in the holoenzyme form.**

   (b) Through binding of the β subunit of the holoenzyme, rifampin **specifically inhibits initiation of transcription** and not elongation.

   (c) Rifampin has **no effect on eukaryotic nuclear RNA polymerases.**

   b. **Eukaryotic initiation factors.** The initiation of transcription in eukaryotes is considerably more complex than in prokaryotes, partly because of the increased complexity of eukaryotic RNA polymerases and partly because of the diversity of their promoters.

   (1) **Multiple factors and RNA polymerase II are needed to initiate transcription from TATA box promoters.** Including RNA polymerase II, more than 40 different polypeptides are needed to initiate transcription.

---

[2] Most drugs that interact directly with DNA, such as intercalators and DNA damaging drugs (see Chapter 8 IV C), also disrupt transcription.

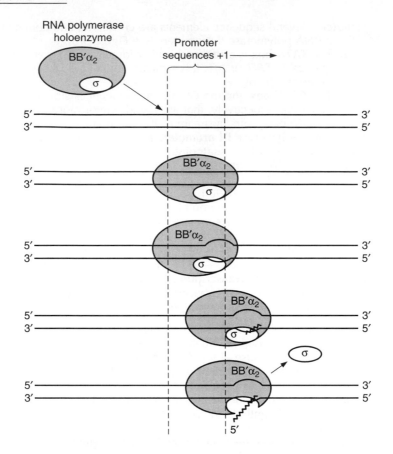

FIGURE 9-4. Sigma (σ) factor mediates initiation of prokaryotic transcription. Sigma factor enables the RNA polymerase holoenzyme to recognize and bind tightly to the promoter, where it facilitates the initiation of transcription. After initiation, the sigma factor dissociates within the time it takes for new chain growth to proceed 10 nucleotides.

     (a) Transcription factor IID (TFIID) recognizes and binds to the TATA box sequences independently of RNA polymerase II.
         (i) The **TATA box-binding protein (TBP)** is the subunit of TFIID that binds to the TATA-box DNA sequence.
         (ii) TFIID is made of eight other subunits called **TBP-associated factors (TAF).**
     (b) Five other transcription factors are required for the proper initiation of transcription by RNA polymerase II (TFIIA, TFIIB, TFIIF, TFIIE, and TFIIH).
   (2) RNA polymerase I and III also need specific transcription factors to initiate transcription from their respective promoters. Other factors are needed for the recognition of response elements and enhancers, which modulate the rate of transcription [see II B 1 c (4); Chapter 12 V B 2].

C.   **Termination.** Prokaryotes and eukaryotes use an identical mechanism of synthesizing RNA and share many similarities in the way that they initiate transcription. They appear, however, to have very little in common in the way they terminate transcription.

   1. Prokaryotes. There are two basic classes of termination events in prokaryotes.
     a. Factor-independent termination. Particular sequences can cause the core enzyme to terminate transcription. These sequences share several common **features** (Figure 9-5).

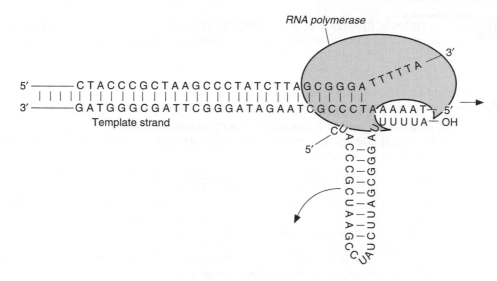

FIGURE 9-5. Rho-independent termination. When transcription pauses at the guanine–cytosine (GC)-rich sequences, a stable stem-loop structure forms in the RNA. This causes displacement—and subsequent termination—while the uracil (U)-rich sequence, which is only weakly base-paired to the template, is being synthesized.

      (1) All of these sequences have a sequence that codes for a self-complementary sequence that **can form a stable stem-loop structure** (see Chapter 6 IV B 2).

      (2) The DNA codes for a **stretch of uracils (Us)** to be formed just after the stem-loop region.

      (3) **Termination becomes favorable** when the transcript forms a stable stem-loop structure. This structure causes the RNA polymerase to slow its synthesis, and the transcript is displaced when the slowed RNA polymerase synthesizes the U-rich segment. Displacement occurs easily because only weak adenine–uracil bonds hold the transcript to the template.

      (4) Because of the nature of this displacement, there is **no specific base where transcription stops** (i.e., different transcripts have a different number of uracil residues on their 3' end).

  b. Factor-dependent termination. Particular sequences act as termination sequences in the presence of factor **rho (ρ).**

      (1) **Rho-dependent termination sequences** do not appear to share common structural features as do the factor-independent termination sequences.

      (2) **Rho binds as a hexamer** to the forming transcript at these unique sequences.

      (3) **Rho is an ATPase.** The exact mechanism that rho uses to terminate transcription is unknown, but it requires the cleavage of ATP by rho.

 2. Eukaryotes. Compared with prokaryotes, very little is known about how eukaryotes terminate transcription.

  a. RNA polymerase I terminates transcription in a factor-dependent manner at a particular sequence.

  b. RNA polymerase III terminates transcription by an unknown mechanism after the synthesis of a series of U residues.

  c. There is no known transcriptional termination signal for **RNA polymerase II.** For most genes, it transcribes up to several thousand base pairs beyond the point of polyadenylation (see III B 2 b).

III. **POST-TRANSCRIPTIONAL RNA PROCESSING.** Once a gene transcript has been synthesized, numerous post-transcriptional modification or processing events may be needed before the transcript is functional.

A. **Prokaryotes.** Post-transcriptional processing of RNA is not as extensive in prokaryotes as in eukaryotes; however, some processing does occur.

1. In prokaryotes, **mRNA is not post-transcriptionally processed.** Prokaryotic mRNA is functional immediately upon synthesis. In fact, its translation often begins before transcription is complete.

2. Seven genes produce **rRNA.** Each gene produces a **30S precursor rRNA** that is processed to discrete, functional rRNAs (Figure 9-6A).
   a. All seven genes contain the sequences that become **23S, 16S, and 5S rRNA.** Within the transcribed portion of these genes are some of the **tRNA genes.** Different rRNA genes contain different tRNA genes.
   b. **Cleavage.** Upon formation of the 30S rRNA precursor, the nonfunctional spacer sequences are removed by a series of specific endonucleolytic cleavages by the enzymes **ribonuclease P** and **ribonuclease III.**
   c. **Base modification.** In addition to the removal of the spacer sequences, some of the bases in the final rRNAs are **methylated.** Methylation is needed for the rRNAs to be functional.

3. The **tRNAs** not formed from processing of the precursor rRNA arise from **large precursor transcripts.**
   a. The tRNA genes are clustered, and each transcript contains sequences for two to seven tRNAs.
   b. **Cleavage.** The portions of the transcript that form functional tRNAs are removed by the enzymes **ribonuclease P** and **ribonuclease D.**
   c. **Addition of the sequence CCA to the 3′ end.** After excision from the precursor, some of the tRNAs are left without the sequence CCA, which is common to all tRNAs, on the 3′ end. This sequence is added to these tRNAs by the enzyme **tRNA nucleotidyl transferase.**
   d. **Base modification.** Many of the bases of the tRNAs are modified. These modifications are various methylations and other more extensive modifications of some of the bases. These modifications are necessary for the tRNAs to adopt their unique, functional conformations (see Chapter 10 II A).

B. **Eukaryotes.** Overall, post-transcriptional processing is more extensive in eukaryotes than in prokaryotes. This partly is due to the presence of a nucleus from which most RNAs must be transported. RNAs are processed during this transport. Processing gives them the characteristics they need to be functional in the cytoplasm, such as an increased stability of mRNAs, as well as allowing for another level of gene regulation (see Chapter 12 VI A, B).

1. **Eukaryotic rRNA processing** is very similar to that of prokaryotes (see Figure 9-6B).
   a. Three of the eukaryotic rRNAs (28S, 18S, and 5.8S) are derived from a **45S precursor rRNA.** (The fourth, 5S rRNA, is produced by the transcription of a 5S gene by RNA polymerase III.) Unlike prokaryotes, there are no tRNA sequences in this precursor.
   b. 45S rRNA is made by the transcription of **hundreds of separate rRNA genes** (see Chapter 6 II E 2 a) in the nucleolus by RNA polymerase I. The processing of the 45S rRNA and formation of the ribosomal subunits begin in the nucleolus.
   c. The 45S rRNA is highly **methylated** before it is cleaved to the functional rRNAs. Most of the bases that are methylated are in sequences that are maintained throughout processing.
   d. As in prokaryotes, the **spacer sequences are removed by endonucleolytic cleavage** of the 45S rRNA by specific endonucleases.

A. Prokaryotes

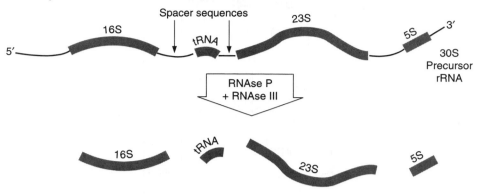

B. Eukaryotes

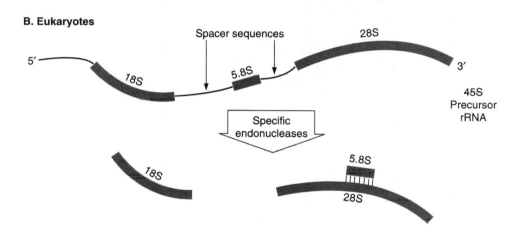

FIGURE 9-6. Processing of ribosomal RNA (rRNA). *(A)* Prokaryotic rRNA formation. The *16S, 23S,* and *5S* rRNA sequences and the sequences of a transfer RNA *(tRNA)* are within the precursor 30S rRNA. The *spacer sequences* separating these rRNA and tRNA sequences are removed by specific endonucleolytic cleavages by ribonuclease P *(RNAse P)* and ribonuclease III *(RNAse III). (B)* Eukaryotic rRNA formation. Three eukaryotic rRNA sequences, *18S, 5.8S,* and *28S,* are within the precursor 45S rRNA. The *spacer sequences* separating these rRNA sequences are removed by specific endonucleolytic cleavages. The 5.8S rRNA base pairs with the 28S rRNA after each is released from the 45S precursor.

  e. The **5.8S rRNA base pairs with the 28S rRNA** during formation of the ribosomal subunits, which is completed before transport from the nucleus.

 2. **Eukaryotic mRNA** is formed from extensive processing of a large precursor called **hnRNA** (see I A 2 a).

  a. **5′ caps.** Unlike prokaryotes, which have an unmodified pppA or pppG on the 5′ end of their mRNAs, eukaryotes have a cap structure on the 5′ ends of their mRNAs.

   (1) **Structure** (Figure 9-7). A **7-methylguanylate** is linked to the 5′ end of mRNAs by a 5′ to 5′ triphosphate linkage. Three cap structures are possible, depending on the presence or absence of additional methyl groups on the two nucleotides adjacent to the 7-methylguanylate.

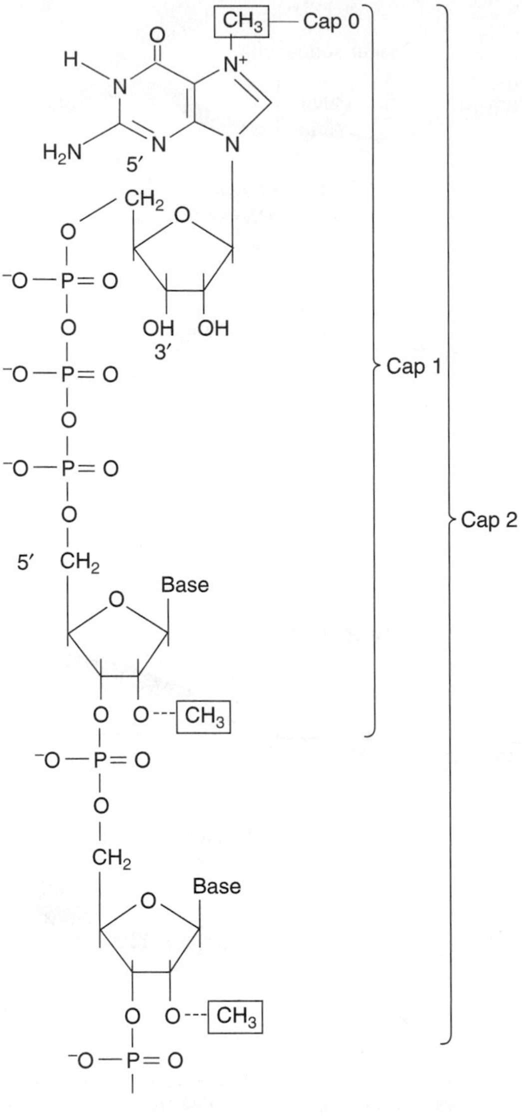

FIGURE 9-7. The cap structure on the 5′ end of eukaryotic messenger RNA (mRNA). The fundamental cap structure is a 5′ to 5′-pyrophosphate linkage on the 5′ end of eukaryotic mRNA to 7-methylguanylate. There are three subtypes of cap structures: cap 0, cap 1, and cap 2. A *cap 0* has only a 7-methylguanylate. If the first ribose from the end is also methylated, it is a *cap 1*. If the first and second riboses are methylated, it is a *cap 2*.

     (2) **Cap formation.** All mRNAs are capped. Cap formation is a multistep process that begins during transcription or immediately after.
     (3) **Functions.** Caps serve two functions.
        (a) The mRNAs with caps are **translated more efficiently** (see Chapter 10 VI A 2 b).
        (b) Caps help **stabilize mRNAs** by protecting them from digestion by ribonucleases that degrade RNAs from their 5′ end (e.g., 5′-exonucleases).
   b. Polyadenylation. The 3′ ends of most mRNAs are polyadenylated (poly A).
     (1) **Structure. Poly A tails** are polymers of 200–300 adenylate residues linked with phosphodiester bonds.
     (2) **Formation** (Figure 9-8). Polyadenylation is template independent.

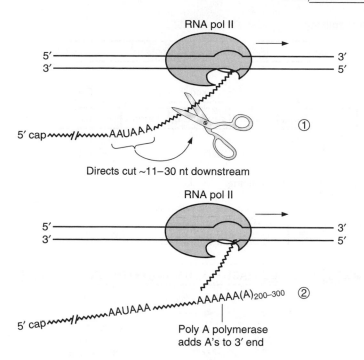

FIGURE 9-8. Polyadenylation. First the sequence AAUAAA directs a cleavage of the RNA being transcribed to a point 11–30 nucleotides *(nt)* downstream. Then poly A polymerase adds several hundred adenylate residues to the free 3′ end of the RNA formed from the cleavage reaction.

(a) **The signal that identifies the site of polyadenylation lies within the RNA.** Termination of transcription occurs downstream of the polyadenylation site.

(b) The sequence AAUAAA is an essential component of what is called the **cleavage/polyadenylation signal.** A complex of proteins called the **cleavage and polyadenylation specificity factor** recognizes and binds to the cleavage/polyadenylation signal. This complex directs an endonucleolytic cut of the RNA to a particular point 11–30 nucleotides downstream.

(c) The enzyme **poly A polymerase** joins the complex and, after the RNA is cut, it catalyzes the polymerization of adenylate residues onto the free 3′ end of the mRNA.

(d) **Polyadenylation occurs after capping and before splicing** (see III B 2 a, c). Polyadenylation is a necessary event for all hnRNAs to be successfully converted to mRNA.

(3) **Function.** Polyadenylation helps **stabilize mRNA.** In the cytoplasm, poly A tails are slowly shortened. When the poly A tail is completely removed, the mRNA is rapidly degraded.

c. **Splicing.** All the sequences necessary to form an mRNA that codes for a protein product are contained in hnRNA. The coding sequences, however, are often split and separated by noncoding sequences. **The process by which noncoding sequences are removed to form a functional mRNA is called splicing** (Figure 9-9).

(1) **Exons** are the transcribed portions of genes that are retained in the processing of hnRNA to mRNA. The term exon stands for the **expressed** portion of genes.

A. General splicing

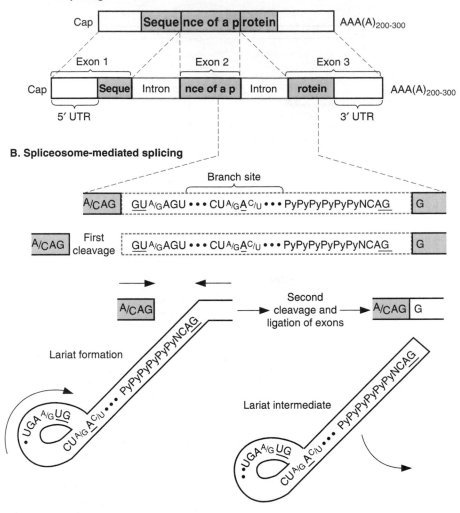

B. Spliceosome-mediated splicing

FIGURE 9-9. Splicing of heterogeneous nuclear RNA (hnRNA) to form messenger RNA (mRNA). *(A)* The *upper panel* shows the net results of the removal of introns by splicing to form mRNA from hnRNA. *(B)* The *lower panel* shows the individual steps of the spliceosome-catalyzed removal of an intron and joining of adjacent exons. The first step is a cleavage at the 5′ intron/exon junction. The 5′ phosphate of the conserved guanylate of the 5′ intron/exon junction is then covalently linked to the 2′-hydroxide of the adenylate located in the branch site. After formation of this intermediate, lariat-like structure, a second cleavage at the 3′ intron/exon junction occurs. The two exons are then ligated; the lariat-like structure is lost and is eventually degraded. *UTR* = untranslated region; *Py* = pyrimidine.

   (2) Introns are the transcribed portions of genes that are removed in the processing of hnRNA to mRNA. The term intron refers to the **intervening** sequences between exons.

   (3) Different genes have different numbers of introns of different sizes. For instance, the β-globin genes have only two introns, whereas the low-density lipoprotein receptor gene has 17 introns. Some genes, like the histone genes, have no introns.

   (4) Intron/exon junctions. A few conserved sequences shared by introns and exons are sufficient to allow recognition by the splicing apparatus of the precise junction between introns and exons.

(a) All hnRNA introns have a **guanine–uracil (GU) sequence** on the 5' border and an **adenine-guanine (AG) sequence** on the 3' border of their intron/exon junctions.

(b) The GU and AG sequences are flanked by sequences that are either identical to or similar in all introns and exons.

(c) Within introns is a conserved sequence, which is called the **branch site** because of an intermediate formed at this site in the splicing reactions.

(5) Mechanism of splicing. Splicing occurs through a multistep process, shown in Figure 9-9, that is catalyzed by a large (50S–60S) ribonucleoprotein complex called a **spliceosome.** Spliceosomes are made of **five SNRPs** (see I D 2) that contain five snRNAs: U1, U2, U4, U5, and U6.

(a) Function of snRNAs. The snRNAs are responsible for recognition of the conserved sequences in introns and the bringing together of RNA sequences into perfect alignment for splicing.

(b) Research involving snRNAs. The role of snRNAs in splicing was elucidated by inhibition studies with antibodies that are specific for individual SNRPs. Interestingly, these antibodies came from patients with the autoimmune disease **systemic lupus erythematosus.** There is increasing evidence that snRNAs are, evolutionarily, the original catalytic component of splicing.

(6) Transport of mRNA from the nucleus to the cytoplasm **is coupled to splicing** and does not occur until all the splicing is complete.

(7) Regulation of gene expression is often at the level of splicing (see Chapter 12 VI A).

3. The tRNAs are formed in eukaryotes similar to the way they are formed in prokaryotes, except that some have introns that are removed.

a. Eukaryotic tRNAs are processed from large precursor RNAs. In eukaryotes, these precursors may contain one or more tRNA sequences.

(1) The tRNA sequences are excised from the precursor by specific endonucleolytic cleavage.

(2) The sequence CCA is added to the 3' end after the tRNA is cleaved from the precursor.

(3) As in prokaryotes, the bases of eukaryotic tRNAs are also extensively modified before the tRNA can adopt its final functional structure.

b. Some, but not all, eukaryotic tRNAs have small (14–50 nucleotide) **introns.**

(1) The introns of different tRNAs have no sequence homology.

(2) The mechanism of tRNA splicing differs from mRNA splicing. The splicing enzymes recognize characteristic structural features of the tRNA to identify the intron/exon junctions.

STUDY QUESTIONS

DIRECTIONS: Each of the numbered items or incomplete statements in this section is followed by answers or by completions of the statement. Select the **one** lettered answer or completion that is **best** in each case.

1. The factor required only for accurate initiation of transcription in prokaryotes is

(A) alpha (α)
(B) beta (β)
(C) transcription factor IID (TFIID)
(D) sigma (σ)
(E) rho (ρ)

2. Which one of the following statements regarding the termination of transcription is correct?

(A) The rho protein binds tightly to RNA polymerase and inactivates the polymerization activity
(B) DNA sequences that can terminate transcription by the core RNA polymerase contain a self-complementary sequence that results in the RNA transcript adopting a stem-loop structure
(C) Each termination site contains a unique base where transcription stops
(D) All prokaryote termination sites contain a stem-loop-forming sequence and require the participation of the rho protein to halt RNA synthesis

3. The colinearity of gene and product clearly seen in prokaryote systems is obscured in eukaryotes because

(A) the DNA sequence coding for a protein is interrupted by noncoding sequences that are not transcribed
(B) the sequence of bases in the messenger RNA (mRNA) is modified in the cytoplasm before interaction with the ribosomes
(C) ribosomes in eukaryotes translate only exon regions of the mRNA
(D) the coding sequence in DNA is interrupted by DNA sequences that are transcribed and then spliced out of the mRNA
(E) the protein product is modified after leaving the ribosome

4. The level of which RNA is reduced first by treatment of cells with low levels of α-amanitin?

(A) 28S ribosomal RNA (rRNA)
(B) Messenger RNA (mRNA)
(C) Transfer RNA (tRNA)
(D) 5S rRNA
(E) 7S RNA

5. Which one of the following statements best describes the action of introns?

(A) They are excised upon processing of heterogeneous nuclear RNA (hnRNA) to messenger RNA (mRNA)
(B) They are retained upon processing of ribosomal RNA (rRNA)
(C) They are spacer sequences
(D) They are added to mRNAs during the splicing reactions

6. Which one of the following is a component of the splicing reactions necessary to convert heterogeneous nuclear RNA (hnRNA) to messenger RNA (mRNA) in eukaryotes?

(A) A 7-methylguanylate cap
(B) The sequence AAUAAA within the intron
(C) Ribonuclease P
(D) The sequences guanine-uracil and adenosine-thymine spanning the intron/exon borders
(E) Small nuclear ribonucleic acid (snRNA) U1

7. A comparison of prokaryotic and eukaryotic RNAs reveals which one of the following?

(A) Both the spacer sequences of polycistronic prokaryotic messenger RNA (mRNA) and introns of eukaryotic heterogeneous nuclear RNA (hnRNA) must be removed to form functional mRNA
(B) All of the ribosomal RNAs (rRNAs) of both prokaryotes and eukaryotes arise from the processing of large precursor rRNAs
(C) Both prokaryotic and eukaryotic mRNAs account for more than 70% of the total cellular RNA
(D) Both prokaryotic and eukaryotic small nuclear RNAs (snRNAs) are involved in post-transcriptional processing
(E) All of the transfer RNAs (tRNAs) of both prokaryotes and eukaryotes arise from the processing of large precursor RNAs

8. Which one of the following statements best describes eukaryotic transcriptional promoters?

(A) They require sigma (σ) factor to be recognized by RNA polymerase II
(B) They are different for each type of RNA polymerase
(C) They direct initiation to a diversity of startpoints
(D) They are all the same for RNA polymerase II genes
(E) They are all upstream of the startpoint of transcription

9. A post-transcriptional processing event that occurs in the formation of both messenger RNA (mRNA) and transfer RNA (tRNA) in eukaryotes is

(A) the addition of the sequence CCA to their 3′ ends
(B) the removal of introns by splicing
(C) the addition of a 7-methylguanylate cap to their 5′ ends
(D) the modification of some of their bases
(E) a cleavage event before polyadenylation

10. Eukaryotic messenger RNAs (mRNAs) differ from prokaryotic mRNAs in that

(A) they do not have a 5′ untranslated region (UTR)
(B) their coding regions are separated by spacers
(C) they do not have a 3′ UTR
(D) they have a free 3′ hydroxyl group on each of their ends
(E) they have poly A sequences on their 3′ ends that are coded for by the genes for each mRNA

ANSWERS AND EXPLANATIONS

1. The answer is D [II A 4 a, B 2 a, b (1), C 1 b]. The sigma (σ) factor enables the RNA polymerase holoenzyme to recognize and bind tightly to the promoter sequences. It then facilitates the promoter-directed initiation of transcription. The σ factor is released after transcription has progressed beyond 10 nucleotides. Factors α and β are subunits of prokaryotic RNA polymerase. The core RNA polymerase, which is all that is needed for the elongation of transcription, is comprised of two α, one β, and a β' subunit. Transcription factor IID (TFIID) is one of at least four factors required by eukaryotic RNA polymerase II to use the TATA box promoter element to initiate transcription. The rho (ρ) factor is required for termination of transcription in prokaryotes at rho-dependent termination sequences.

2. The answer is B [II C 1]. There are two basic classes of termination events in prokaryotes: factor-independent and factor-dependent. A feature of the factor-independent sequences is that the DNA sequence is self complementary. When transcribed, this sequence forms a stem-loop structure that leads to a displacement of the transcript and termination of transcription. Factor-dependent termination requires the protein rho. Rho binds as a hexamer to particular sequences in the RNA, cleaves adenosine triphosphate (ATP), and, by a mechanism that is poorly understood, it facilitates termination of transcription.

3. The answer is D [III B 2 c]. In eukaryote genomes, unique DNA sequences coding for cellular proteins are interrupted by regions that are transcribed but not translated. These noncoding intron regions are spliced out of the messenger RNA (mRNA) during its processing in the nucleus. The sequence of bases in the coding region of the mature mRNA and the gene product are colinear.

4. The answer is B [II A 4 b (2); Table 9-1]. The type of RNA produced by the three different eukaryotic RNA polymerases was determined by their differential sensitivity to the toxin α-amanitin, which is found in poisonous mushrooms. The activity of RNA polymerase II is most sensitive to α-amanitin. Upon treatment of cells with very low levels of α-amanitin, the production of heterogeneous nuclear RNA (hnRNA) and concomitantly messenger RNA (mRNA) is quickly stopped. This indicates that RNA polymerase II is responsible for the transcription of the genes that code for proteins (i.e., that produce mRNA). If cells are treated with high levels of α-amanitin, the RNAs produced by RNA polymerase III [i.e., transfer RNAs (tRNAs), 5S ribosomal RNA (rRNA), and 7S RNA] would be stopped, as well as those RNAs produced by RNA polymerase II. RNA polymerase I is not inhibited by α-amanitin and, therefore, the production of 45S rRNA (the precursor of 18S, 28S, and 5.8S rRNA) would continue at least for a short time. After a prolonged treatment with even low levels of α-amanitin, all RNA levels would drop because continuous mRNA production is required to sustain life.

5. The answer is A [III B 2 c (2)]. Introns are the transcribed portions of genes that are removed in the processing of heterogeneous nuclear RNA (hnRNA) to messenger RNA (mRNA). Exons are the transcribed portions of genes that are retained in the processing of hnRNA to mRNA. Spacer sequences are the transcribed nontranslated sequences between cistrons in prokaryotic polycistronic mRNA. The sequences in ribosomal RNA (rRNA) precursors that are removed during processing of rRNAs are also called spacer sequences. The only sequences added to mRNAs during processing are the adenylate residues in the formation of polyadenylate (poly A) tails.

6. The answer is E [III B 2 c (5)]. Spliceosomes are made of five small nuclear ribonucleoprotein particles (SNRPs) that contain the small nuclear ribonucleic acids (snRNAs) U1, U2, U4, U5, and U6. The snRNAs are essential in splicing because they are responsible for the recognition of splicing signals in introns and their alignment in the splicing reactions. Caps are added to all messenger RNAs (mRNAs) during post-transcriptional processing, but this is not a component of the splicing reactions. The sequence AAUAAA is an essential component of the cleavage/polyadenylation signal. Ribonuclease P is an endoribonuclease that participates in the processing of prokaryotic ribosomal RNAs (rRNAs). The sequences guanine-uracil and adenosine-guanine (not adenosine-thymine; thymine is not a component of RNA) are components of splicing, but they are found within introns adjacent to intron/exon junctions.

7. The answer is E [I A 1, 2, B, C, D; III A 3, B 2]. Transfer RNAs are formed in eukaryotes from large precursor RNAs similar to the way they are formed in prokaryotes, except that some have introns that are removed. Unlike introns, the spacer sequences of polycistronic messenger RNA (mRNA) are not removed. In prokaryotes, all of the ribosomal RNAs (rRNAs) are processed from a large precursor. In eukaryotes, only the 28S, 18S, and 5.8S rRNAs are processed from a large precursor rRNA. The 5S rRNA is the transcription product of a separate gene. Prokaryotic mRNA and eukaryotic mRNA are both low-abundance RNAs, 5% and 7% respectively. Prokaryotes do not have small nuclear RNA (snRNA).

8. The answer is B [II B]. Each type of eukaryotic RNA polymerase uses a different promoter. They all direct initiation of transcription to a discrete startpoint. The promoters for RNA polymerase I are all the same but the promoters for RNA polymerases II and III differ, even within each class. The promoters for RNA polymerase I and II lie upstream of the startpoint; however, the promoters for RNA polymerase III genes lie downstream of the startpoint. Initiation factors are needed for promoter recognition and initiation of transcription. Prokaryotes use a single factor, sigma,

whereas eukaryotes utilize multiple factors, in part because of the diversity of their promoters.

9. The answer is B [III B]. Both eukaryotic messenger RNA (mRNA) and transfer RNA (tRNA) precursors may contain introns that are removed by splicing, although the mechanism of tRNA splicing differs from that of mRNA splicing. The 3' ends of tRNAs have the sequence CCA added post-transcriptionally, whereas mRNAs are post-transcriptionally polyadenylated on their 3' ends. The 5' ends of tRNAs remain unmodified, whereas the 5' ends of mRNAs have a 7-methylguanylate cap added. Only tRNAs have their bases heavily modified. These modifications are required for the tRNAs to adopt their unique functional conformations.

10. The answer is D [I A 1; III B 2]. Eukaryotic messenger RNAs (mRNAs) have a 7-methylguanylate cap on their 5' ends that prokaryotic mRNAs do not have. 7-Methylguanylate caps are linked to the 5' ends of mRNAs by a 5' to 5' triphosphate linkage. This means that the 3' hydroxyl group of the 7-methylguanylate cap is free. Both prokaryotic and eukaryotic mRNAs have both 5' and 3' untranslated regions (UTRs). Prokaryotic mRNAs are often polycistronic and have spacers separating the different coding regions. Eukaryotic mRNAs are monocistronic and have no spacer sequence. Their precursor heterogeneous nuclear RNAs (hnRNAs) have introns that are spliced out to form a functional mRNA. Eukaryotic mRNAs have poly A sequences on their 3' ends, but these sequences are added post-transcriptionally. They are not coded for by the genes for each mRNA.

Chapter 10

Translation of mRNA: Protein Synthesis
Donald Sittman

Case 10-1

During a mission trip to West Africa, a physician examines a 10-year-old boy in a clinic. He has a fever and difficulty breathing. The child has had a very sore throat that has made it difficult to swallow for approximately 1 week. A physical examination reveals a swollen neck, and the child's throat is covered with a gray, thick membrane. The child's heart sounds are all normal. The physician suspects the child may have diphtheria because the diagnosis is consistent with his symptoms and because the incidence of diphtheria in the tropics is high. However, because of the primitive environment of the clinic, the physician cannot confirm the diagnosis with laboratory tests and culture, and it is advised not to delay treatment while tests are being run. Immediately after a skin test reveals the absence of an allergic response to diphtheria antitoxin, the physician begins administering antitoxin to the patient. The physician follows the diphtheria antitoxin treatment with a treatment of erythromycin and the best nursing care that can be provided in the clinic.

- What organism produces diphtheria toxin?
- What is the mechanism of action of diphtheria toxin?
- Why is the physician concerned about the patient's heart sounds?
- Why is immediate inactivation of diphtheria toxin by diphtheria antitoxin important?
- What is the mechanism of action of erythromycin?

I. INTRODUCTION

A. **Translation** is the process by which ribosomes convert the information carried by **messenger RNA (mRNA)** to the synthesis of new proteins.

B. **Genetic code** (Table 10-1). The information needed to direct the synthesis of proteins is contained in the mRNA in the form of a genetic code. The genetic code is the system of RNA sequences that designate particular amino acids in the process of translation.

1. The genetic code is in the form of **codons.** Codons are groups of **three adjacent bases** that specify the amino acids of protein.
   a. **Number of codon sequences.** Because mRNAs are composed of four bases [adenine (A), uracil (U), guanine (G), and cytosine (C)] and each codon is three bases, there are 4^3 or **64 possible codon sequences.**
   b. **Stop codons.** Of the 64 codons, 61 specify the 20 amino acids. The remaining three codons—**UAA, UAG, and UGA**—are called stop codons or termination codons. These codons facilitate, or code for, the termination of translation.
   c. **Unambiguous codons; degenerate code.** A given codon either designates a single amino acid or is a stop codon. However, more than one codon can specify the same amino acid, so the genetic code is said to be degenerate.
   d. **Synonyms.** Different amino acids are specified by different numbers of codons. For instance, the amino acids methionine and tryptophan are both specified by a single codon, whereas leucine, serine, and arginine are both specified by six codons. Codons that designate the same amino acid are called synonyms, and synonymous codons usually differ only in the third base of the codon (see Table 10-1).

TABLE 10-1. The Genetic Code

First Position	Second Position				Third Position
	U	**C**	**A**	**G**	
U	Phe	Ser	Tyr	Cys	U
	Phe	Ser	Tyr	Cys	C
	Leu	Ser	STOP	STOP	A
	Leu	Ser	STOP	Trp	G
C	Leu	Pro	His	Arg	U
	Leu	Pro	His	Arg	C
	Leu	Pro	Gln	Arg	A
	Leu	Pro	Gln	Arg	G
A	Ile	Thr	Asn	Ser	U
	Ile	Thr	Asn	Ser	C
	Ile	Thr	Lys	Arg	A
	Met	Thr	Lys	Arg	G
G	Val	Ala	Asp	Gly	U
	Val	Ala	Asp	Gly	C
	Val	Ala	Glu	Gly	A
	Val	Ala	Glu	Gly	G

To find the codon for a given amino acid, it is necessary to read the first base (*left-hand column*) for the amino acid, then the second base (*middle columns*), and then the third base (*right-hand column*). Codons are referred to as written in the 5' to 3' direction. Most amino acids are coded for by more than one codon. The codons called stop codons indicate to the RNA polymerase that it is the end of the message.

Ala = alanine; Arg = arginine; Asn = asparagine; Asp = aspartic acid; Cys = cysteine; Gln = glutamine; Glu = glutamic acid; Gly = glycine; His = histidine; Ile = isoleucine; Leu = leucine; Lys = lysine; Met = methionine; Phe = phenylalanine; Pro = proline; Ser = serine; Thr = threonine; Trp = tryptophan, Tyr = tyrosine; Val = valine.

2. **The code does not overlap.** During translation, the code is read sequentially, one codon after another without spacer bases, from a fixed starting point.

3. **The genetic code is nearly universal.** With only a few exceptions, the genetic code is universal. The genetic code of mitochondria may differ by a few codons from the genetic code of nuclear DNA both within an organism and between organisms. A very small number of variations in the genetic code of nuclear DNA between organisms also has been identified.

C. **Overlapping genes.** Some viruses code for more proteins than would be predicted from their nucleotide content. DNA sequencing revealed that some of the expressed portions of viral genomes overlap and code for multiple products in different reading frames.

II. **ACTIVATION OF AMINO ACIDS: FORMATION OF AMINOACYL-TRANSFER RNAs (tRNAs)**

A. **Adaptor molecules.** In a ribosome, the message is carried by mRNA and is read or translated to produce a protein. The linkage between the message to protein is made by adaptor molecules, which are **aminoacylated tRNAs** (also called charged tRNAs). Aminoacylated tRNAs are tRNAs to which a specific amino acid has been covalently attached.

1. tRNAs are a family of RNAs, all of which have a similar, common structure (Figure 10-1; see Chapter 6 IV C 2).

2. Each type of tRNA has sufficiently unique structural features that only the appropriate amino acid may be attached to it.

B. **Aminoacyl-tRNA synthetases** are enzymes that activate amino acids and attach them to the 3′ terminal adenosine of their cognate tRNA. There is at least one, and occasionally two, specific tRNA synthetases for each amino acid.

1. **Structure.** The tRNA synthetases vary in molecular weight, number of subunits, and amino acid composition.

2. **Specificity.** The tRNA synthetases are very specific in their attachment of the correct amino acid to the correct tRNA. Because the codon recognition is entirely related to the tRNA and not to the attached amino acid, the fidelity of protein synthesis depends largely on the high specificity of tRNA synthetases.

3. **Aminoacylation reaction.** The attachment of an amino acid to its appropriate tRNA, which is catalyzed by tRNA synthetases, requires adenosine triphosphate (ATP) and proceeds by the formation of an **activated aminoacyl intermediate.** This is a three-step process.
   a. **Formation of an aminoacyl-adenylate complex** is the first step of the reaction and is expressed as:

$$\text{Amino acid} + \text{ATP} \leftrightarrow \text{Aminoacyl-AMP} + \text{PP}_i$$

   where PP_i is pyrophosphate and AMP is adenosine monophosphate.
   b. **Transfer of the aminoacyl group to the 2′- or 3′-hydroxyl group of the 3′ adenosine** of the appropriate tRNA is the second step. It is expressed as:

$$\text{Aminoacyl-AMP} + \text{tRNA} \leftrightarrow \text{Aminoacyl-tRNA} + \text{AMP}$$

   The sum of the activation and transfer steps is expressed as:

$$\text{Amino acid} + \text{ATP} + \text{tRNA} \leftrightarrow \text{Aminoacyl-tRNA} + \text{PP}_i + \text{AMP}$$

   c. **PP_i is then hydrolyzed** to form two free phosphates. This final reaction makes the overall reaction irreversible. A total of two high-energy phosphate bonds of ATP are expended in the formation of a single aminoacyl-tRNA.

III. CODON–ANTICODON RECOGNITION

A. **Antiparallel relationship.** The tRNA anticodons base pair in the ribosome in a normal, antiparallel fashion, with their complementary codons in the mRNA. However, to compensate for the degeneracy of the genetic code, some tRNAs base pair with more than one codon. The advantage of compensating for degeneracy in this way is that otherwise a different tRNA would have to evolve for each codon.

1. The **first two bases of the codon** and the **last two bases of the anticodon** base pair by normal guanine–cytosine and adenine–uridine base pairing (see Chapter 6 IV B).

2. The pairing of the **third base of the codon with the first base of the anticodon** follows less rigid requirements than the first two bases. This allows some tRNAs to base pair with more than one codon.

B. **The wobble hypothesis** proposed that the third base position of codons could form alternate base pairs with the first base position of tRNAs. Unusual base pairs can form partly because of flexibility of the bases in the anticodon loop of the tRNA. The rules that govern base pairing of the codons' third base position are shown in Figure 10-2.

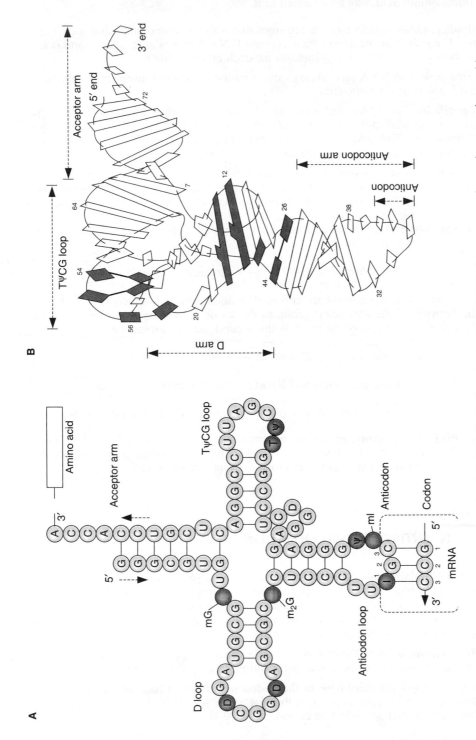

FIGURE 10–1. Structure of yeast alanine transfer RNA (tRNA). (A) Cloverleaf model of tRNA showing normal complementary base pairing. The darker *shaded* nucleotides are post-transcriptionally modified. (B) The structure of yeast alanine tRNA as determined by x-ray crystallography. A number of nonstandard molecular interactions (*shaded*) help stabilize the L-shaped molecule. ψ = pseudouridine, D = dihydrouridine, I = inosine; TψCG = a sequence on the loop of an arm of all tRNA molecules. (Reprinted with permission from Lodish H, Baltimore D, Berk A, et al: *Molecular Cell Biology*, 3rd ed. New York, Scientific American Books, 1995, p 124.)

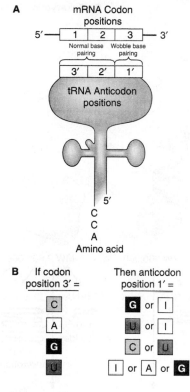

A

mRNA Codon
positions

5' ── | 1 | 2 | 3 | ── 3'

Normal base   Wobble base
pairing   pairing

| 3' | 2' | 1' |

tRNA Anticodon
positions

5'
C
C
A
Amino acid

B   If codon
position 3' =

Then anticodon
position 1' =

C		G or I
A		U or I
G		C or U
U		I or A or G

FIGURE 10-2. Alternative base pairings that may occur between the third base position of the codon and the first base position of the anticodon. *(A)* Depiction of antiparallel relationship of the codon and anticodon. *(B)* For the four possible bases that may be in the third position of the codon, the bases in the first base position of the anticodon are shown that can base pair with them. *A* = adenine; *C* = cytosine; *G* = guanine; *I* = inosine; *mRNA* = messenger RNA; *tRNA* = transfer RNA; *U* = uracil.

IV. STRUCTURE OF RIBOSOMES

A. Prokaryotic ribosomes

1. In *Escherichia coli,* the ribosome is approximately **65% RNA and 35% protein.**
2. The prokaryotic ribosome is a large structure with a sedimentation coefficient of 70S (Figure 10-3A).[1]
3. The ribosome is made of two subunits: the **50S large subunit** and the **30S small subunit.**
   a. The 50S subunit is made of 34 large subunit proteins and a 23S and 5S ribosomal RNA (rRNA; see Chapter 9 I B 1).
   b. The 30S subunit is made of 21 small subunit proteins and a 16S rRNA.
   c. Most ribosomal proteins are small, basic proteins. Their basic charge reflects their ability to interact with negatively charged RNA.
   d. The rRNA molecules have defined secondary structures and interact with ribosomal proteins in a defined manner.

B. Eukaryotic ribosomes are larger than prokaryotic ribosomes and have a sedimentation coefficient of 80S (see Figure 10-3B).

1. The eukaryotic ribosome is made of two subunits: a **60S large subunit** and a **40S small subunit.**

---

[1] S stands for a Svedberg unit, which is derived from the sedimentation constant (s) and is related to the size and shape of a molecule [see Chapter 2 V B 2 c (2)].

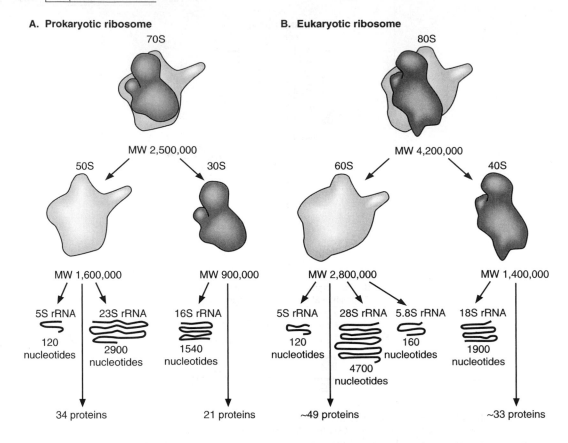

FIGURE 10-3. Structure and composition of *(A)* prokaryotic and *(B)* eukaryotic ribosomes. *MW* = molecular weight; *rRNA* = ribosomal RNA; *S* = Svedberg unit. (Reprinted with permission from Alberts B, Bray D, Lewis J, et al: *Molecular Biology of the Cell,* 3rd ed. New York, Garland Publishing, 1994, p 233.)

    a. The 60S subunit is made of 49 proteins and three rRNAs: 28S, 5.8S, and 5S.
    b. The 40S subunit is made of 33 proteins and an 18S rRNA.

  2. Mitochondria and chloroplasts have their own ribosomes. These ribosomes resemble those of prokaryotes, both in structure and in their sensitivity to antibiotic inhibitors of translation.

V. **PROTEIN SYNTHESIS IN PROKARYOTES** is well described and occurs by a mechanism that is prototypical of protein synthesis in all organisms. Protein synthesis occurs in three stages: initiation, elongation, and termination. Figure 10-4 summarizes all the steps of protein synthesis in both prokaryotes and eukaryotes.

A. **Initiation**

  1. The **formation of a 30S initiation complex** is the first event in protein synthesis. The formation of the 30S initiation complex requires the following:
    a. A strand of **mRNA**
    b. The **initiation factors** (IF-1, IF-2, IF-3) **and guanosine triphosphate (GTP)**
    c. A **30S ribosomal subunit**
    d. **Formylmethionine-tRNA$_f$ (fmet-tRNA$_f$)**

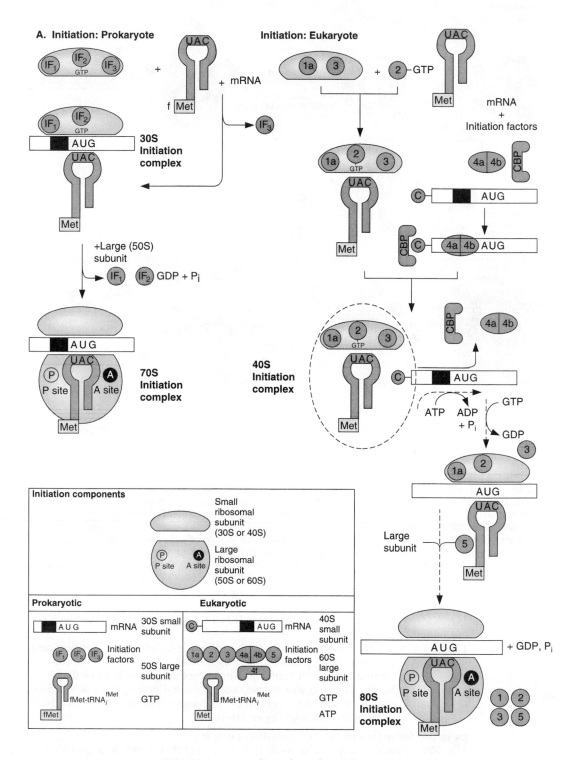

FIGURE 10-4. See figure legend on following page.

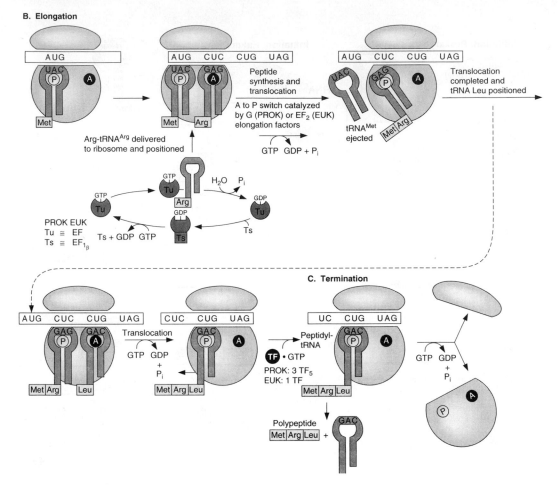

FIGURE 10-4. Translation in prokaryotes and eukaryotes. There are three stages in translation: *(A)* initiation, *(B)* elongation, and *(C)* termination. The mechanism of protein synthesis in eukaryotes and prokaryotes is similar. In general, eukaryotes require more factors. *ADP* = adenosine diphosphate; *Arg* = arginine; *ATP* = adenosine triphosphate; *CBP* = cap-binding protein; *EF* = elongation factor; *GDP* = guanosine diphosphate; *GTP* = guanosine triphosphate; *IF* = initiation factor (eukaryotic IFs are preceded by *e*); *Leu* = leucine; *Met* = methionine; *mRNA* = messenger RNA; P_i = inorganic phosphate; *TF* = release factor; *tRNA* = transfer RNA. (Reprinted with permission from Lodish H, Baltimore D, Berk A, et al: *Molecular Cell Biology,* 3rd ed. New York, Scientific American Books, 1995, pp 134–135.)

    (1) A specific tRNA, called the **initiator tRNA (tRNA$_f$),** brings fmet to the 30S initiation complex.

    (2) The tRNA$_f$ has a different sequence than the tRNA that inserts methionine in internal positions of the peptide chain (i.e., tRNA$_m$).

    (3) The same aminoacyl-tRNA synthetase links methionine to both of these tRNAs. The enzyme, **transformylase,** adds a formyl group, from N^{10}-formyl-tetrahydrofolate, to the amino group of methionine that is attached to the tRNA$_f$ to form N-fmet-tRNA$_f$ (Figure 10-5).

  2. Steps in the formation of the 30S initiation complex

    a. The **30S subunit,** in association with IF-1, IF-2, and IF-3, binds to a specific site on mRNA.

      (1) This purine-rich sequence (the **Shine-Dalgarno sequence**), which is either identical with or similar to the sequence AGGAGGU, base pairs with a pyrimidine sequence in the 16S rRNA.

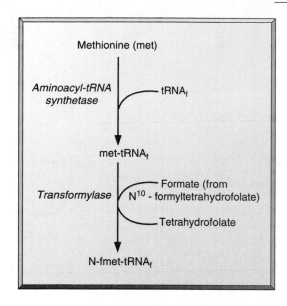

FIGURE 10-5. Outline of the pathway for the formation of N-formylmethionine-transfer RNA$_f$ (N-fmet-tRNA$_f$).

      (2) The Shine-Dalgarno sequence lies within 10 nucleotides of the initiator codon, AUG. It places the initiator codon in the appropriate position in the 30S subunit to bind to the initiator tRNA, fmet-tRNA$_f$.

    b. To complete **formation of the 30S initiation complex,** fmet-tRNA$_f$ binds to the 30S particle.

  3. IF-3 dissociates from the 30S initiation complex upon the binding of fmet-tRNA$_f$. This allows the 50S subunit to bind to the 30S initiation complex to form the **70S initiation complex.**

    a. GTP is hydrolyzed to guanosine diphosphate (GDP) and Inorganic phosphate (P$_i$) upon formation of the 70S initiation complex.

    b. IF-1, IF-2, and the GDP and P$_i$ are all released from the 70S initiation complex.

    c. There are two sites on the 70S ribosome that can be occupied by aminoacylated tRNAs: the **peptide (P) site** and the **amino (A) site.**

    d. The P site is occupied by fmet-tRNA$_f$.

B.   **Elongation**

  1. The **aminoacylated tRNA** that is complementary to the codon adjacent to the initiator codon (i.e., AUG) is **inserted in the A site,** starting the process of elongation.

    a. Three **elongation factors** (EF) are required for elongation: EF-Tu, EF-Ts, and EF-G. They are abundant proteins and are present in the cell at levels of 5%–10% of all proteins.

    b. Delivery of an aminoacyl-tRNA to the empty A site on the ribosome is effected by EF-Tu, EF-Ts, and GTP (see Figure 10-4). This process delivers all aminoacyl-tRNAs except fmet-tRNA$_f$ to the A site.

  2. Peptide bond formation

    a. The activated amino acid attached to the tRNA in the P site is transferred to the amino group of the aminoacyl-tRNA in the A site (Figure 10-6).

    b. This formation of a peptide bond is catalyzed by **peptidyl transferase.** Interestingly, peptidyl transferase appears to be the 23S rRNA.

    c. This reaction results in two amino acids being attached to the tRNA (dipeptidyl-tRNA) in the A site and leaves an uncharged tRNA in the P site.

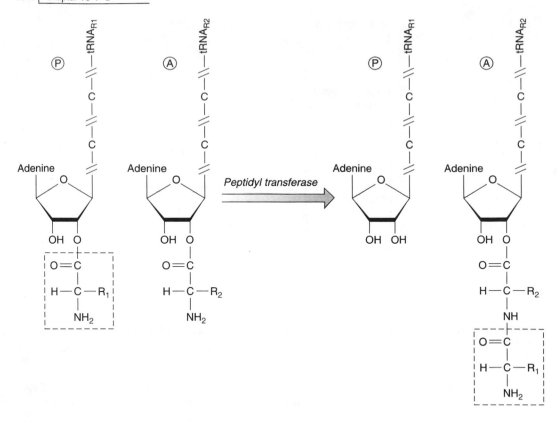

FIGURE 10-6. Peptidyl transferase catalyzes the transfer of the amino acid or peptide attached to the transfer RNA *(tRNA$_{R1}$)* in the peptide *(P)* site to the amino group of the aminoacyl-tRNA in the amino *(A)* site *(tRNA$_{R2}$)*.

3. **Translocation**
   a. The ribosome is moved three nucleotides in a 5′ to 3′ direction along the mRNA. This movement results in the following:
      (1) Release of the uncharged tRNA from the P site
      (2) Movement of the dipeptidyl-tRNA to the P site
      (3) An unoccupied A site
   b. This translocation is catalyzed by EF-G and requires the hydrolysis of GTP to GDP.

C. **Termination.** Elongation continues until a termination codon is encountered.

1. **Release factors**
   a. No tRNAs pair with stop codons. Instead, the stop codons are recognized by the protein release factors RF-1 or RF-2.
      (1) **RF-1** recognizes UAA and UAG.
      (2) **RF-2** recognizes UAA and UGA.
   b. A third release factor, **RF-3,** in association with GTP, promotes termination.

2. The **binding of release factors** induces peptidyl transferase to release the polypeptide from the tRNA in the P site by hydrolysis. The tRNA is also released from the P site.

3. The **ribosomal subunits then separate** in a GTP hydrolysis-dependent manner. The 30S subunit may move along the mRNA until another Shine-Dalgarno sequence is encountered and translation resumes, or it may completely dissociate from the mRNA.

D. **High-energy requirements for protein synthesis.** Each peptide bond requires the cleavage of at least four high-energy phosphate bonds for its formation. This high-energy requirement of protein synthesis serves the following functions:

1. **High fidelity of translation.** Protein synthesis in *E. coli* has an error frequency of less than one misincorporation per 2000 amino acids coupled. This low error rate is a consequence of a high-energy expenditure.
   a. The **accuracy of aminoacylation of tRNA** requires the cleavage of two high-energy phosphate bonds in ATP.
   b. **Codon–anticodon recognition.** Genetic and biochemical evidence suggests that GTP hydrolysis is coupled to a proofreading function that "tests" a codon–anticodon interaction for a mismatch.

2. **High rate of translation.** Protein synthesis is rapid and, therefore, requires a high-energy input.
   a. In *E. coli,* a single ribosome can couple 15 amino acids per second.
   b. Once an initiation event occurs and the ribosome moves along the mRNA, nothing precludes a further reinitiation event by another ribosome. An abundance of ribosomes that are actively synthesizing proteins can be attached to a single mRNA. An mRNA with many ribosomes attached is called a **polyribosome.**

VI. **PROTEIN SYNTHESIS IN EUKARYOTES.** The mechanism of protein synthesis in eukaryotes is similar to that of prokaryotes (see Figure 10-4). The differences are a consequence of the more complex cellular organization of the eukaryotic cell.

A. **Initiation.** Although initiation in eukaryotes is considerably more complex than in prokaryotes, the same basic events occur.

1. Initiation of translation in eukaryotes begins with the formation of a **40S initiation complex,** which requires the following:
   a. A strand of **mRNA**
      (1) Eukaryotic mRNAs are monocistronic.
      (2) Eukaryotic mRNAs do not use a Shine-Dalgarno sequence to direct initiation to the initiator codon. However, less rigidly defined sequences are known to be involved in this process.
      (3) Eukaryotic mRNAs have a 7-methylguanylate cap on their 5′ ends that plays a role in initiation of translation.
   b. **Initiation factors.** Eukaryotes use at least 10 initiation factors, which are labeled eIF with distinguishing numbers and a letter appended.
   c. **40S ribosomal subunit**
   d. **met-tRNA$_i$**
      (1) The initiator tRNA (tRNA$_i$) in eukaryotes carries an unmodified methionine to the 40S initiation complex.
      (2) Eukaryotes contain two structurally different tRNAs that recognize AUG codons. The initiator codon tRNA is recognized by tRNA$_i$. Internal, noninitiator methionine codons are recognized by tRNA$_m$.
      (3) The same enzyme, methionyl-tRNA synthetase, is responsible for adding a methionine residue to either tRNA$_i$ or tRNA$_m$.
   e. **Energy requirements.** Both GTP and ATP are required for initiation in eukaryotes, whereas only GTP is required in prokaryotes.

2. **Steps in the formation of the 40S initiation complex**
   a. **Formation of a preinitiation complex.** A **ternary complex** formed between eIF-2, GTP, and met-tRNA$_i$ binds to the 40S subunit to form a preinitiation complex.
   b. **mRNA binds to the preinitiation complex of the ribosome** by a considerably more complex process in eukaryotes than in prokaryotes.

(1) The cap structure on the 5' end on mRNA plays a role in the formation of the 40S initiation complex.

(2) Eukaryotic initiation factor 4A (eIF-4A) is a complex factor that includes a subunit that acts as a **cap-binding protein (CBP).**

    (a) **CBP may initiate mRNA binding** by interacting with the 5' cap structure.

    (b) The **importance of the cap** in initiation is indicated by the fact that the cap analog 7-methylguanosine monophosphate is a potent initiation inhibitor.

(3) **ATP is hydrolyzed and bound by eIF-4A,** an action that results in the unwinding of secondary structure in the 5' untranslated region of the mRNA.

c. Recognition of the initiation codon. The 5' untranslated region of eukaryotic mRNA is of variable length (usually 40–80 nucleotides), although regions longer than 700 nucleotides are known to occur. No Shine-Dalgarno sequence is present, although less rigidly defined sequences are known to be involved in the process of initiator codon selection.

(1) **Initiation occurs at the first AUG codon from the 5' end** in more than 90% of the eukaryotic mRNAs.

(2) The **most common sequence** around the initiation codon is AXXAUGGG, where X is any base. If the first AUG is **not** used, it usually occurs in the sequence YXXAUGY, where Y is a pyrimidine (uracil or cytosine).

(3) It is postulated that the **40S ribosomal subunit binds near the 5' end of the mRNA and scans the mRNA** in the 3' direction until it finds the first AUG in the proper sequence context. ATP hydrolysis may be essential for this scanning process.

3. Formation of the 80S initiation complex. The joining of the 60S subunit to the 40S initiation complex to form the 80S initiation complex requires the action of eIF-5 and eIF-4C. By completion of the formation of the 80S initiation complex, all initiation factors are removed.

B. **Elongation** occurs by a very similar mechanism in eukaryotes as in prokaryotes.

1. The necessary components, which are analogous to those required by prokaryotes, include the following:

    a. The 80S initiation complex

    b. Aminoacyl-tRNA

    c. GTP

    d. Eukaryotic elongation factors: eEF-1$_\alpha$, eEF-1$_\beta$, and eEF-2

2. Aminoacyl-tRNAs are bound to the P site as ternary complexes (eEF-1$_\alpha$·GTP·aminoacyl-tRNA). The GTP is hydrolyzed to GDP in this process.

3. Prokaryotic EF-Tu is analogous to eEF-1$_\alpha$, and eEF-1$_\beta$ is analogous to prokaryotic EF-Ts. The eEF-1$_\beta$ catalyzes the GDP to GTP exchange on eEF-1$_\alpha$.

4. Peptide bond formation occurs by the same mechanism in eukaryotes as in prokaryotes (see V B 2).

5. Translocation requires the eEF-2–GTP complex and hydrolysis of GTP. This is analogous to translocation in prokaryotes mediated by the EF-G–GTP complex.

C. **Termination** occurs by a mechanism in eukaryotes that is similar to that in prokaryotes.

1. A **single release factor** with an associated GTP recognizes all three termination codons.

2. When the release factor binds to the ribosome, termination is effected by the **peptidyl transferase activity** of the ribosome.

3. **GTP hydrolysis** is required for termination and dissociation of the ribosomal subunits.

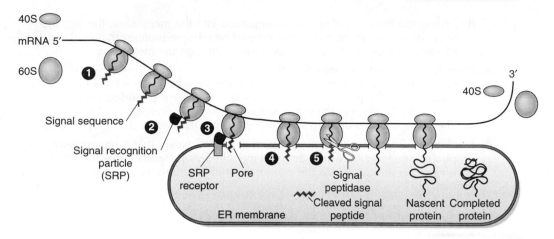

FIGURE 10-7. Signal hypothesis model of protein synthesis showing how the synthesis of a protein is directed to the endoplasmic reticulum *(ER)*. Translation begins in the cytoplasm *(1)*. The signal recognition particle *(SRP)* recognizes and binds to the signal sequence, as it emerges from the ribosome, and to the ribosome itself *(2)*. This binding arrests further translation. The SRP–ribosome complex binds to the SRP receptor on the ER *(3)*. The SRP and SRP receptor dissociate from the ribosome and protein synthesis resumes with newly synthesized protein being passed through the membrane into the lumen of the ER *(4)*. A signal peptidase cleaves the signal sequence from the protein *(5)*. (Adapted with permission from Marks DB, Marks AD, Smith CM: *Basic Medical Biochemistry: A Clinical Approach.* Baltimore, Williams & Wilkins, 1996, p 211.)

VII. PROTEIN SYNTHESIS ON THE ENDOPLASMIC RETICULUM

A. **Introduction.** In eukaryotic cells, most protein synthesis occurs in the cytoplasm. The remainder of the protein synthesis, such as that of proteins to be secreted, occurs on the **rough endoplasmic reticulum (ER).** Proteins synthesized on the rough ER require transport across a membrane before they reach their final destination.

B. **Protein synthesis on membrane-bound ribosomes.** Proteins synthesized on the ER are made in a precursor form that is processed before they reach their final destination. The **signal hypothesis** describes how protein synthesis is directed to the ER. Proteins to be made on the ER have a very characteristic **leader or signal sequence** on their amino-terminal end that directs their synthesis to the ER. The leader sequence is usually 15–30 amino acids long and contains a stretch of hydrophobic amino acids. The steps involved in recognition of this signal sequence and direction of protein synthesis from the cytoplasm to the ER are described below and shown in Figure 10-7.

1. **Recognition of the signal sequence by the signal recognition particle (SRP).** The SRP is an elongated complex of six nonidentical proteins and a 7S small cytoplasmic RNA (scRNA; see Chapter 9 I D 1). The SRP recognizes and binds to the signal sequence and ribosome and arrests further translation.

2. **Binding of the SRP–ribosome complex to the ER and continuation of protein synthesis into the lumen of the ER.** The translation-arrested SRP–ribosome complex next interacts with an **SRP receptor** on the ER.
   a. The SRP receptor is made of two dissimilar, integral membrane proteins.
   b. The interaction of the SRP–ribosome complex and the SRP receptor results in an **insertion of the signal sequence** into the membrane and a **resumption of protein synthesis.**
   c. Just before the resumption of protein synthesis, the SRP receptor cleaves GTP and causes the SRP and SRP receptor to dissociate from the ribosome.

    d. During the insertion of the signal sequence into the membrane, the signal sequence may associate with other integral membrane proteins that facilitate the translocation of newly synthesized protein through the membrane.

3. **Completion of synthesis into the ER**
    a. While the signal sequence is attached to the signal sequence receptor and the remainder of the protein is being synthesized, a **signal peptidase** on the luminal side of the ER cleaves the signal sequence from the protein.
    b. The protein passes through the membrane into the lumen during synthesis.

4. **Synthesis of integral membrane proteins** is similar except that a sequence of hydrophobic amino acids within the protein, called **stop-transfer signals,** halts the transfer of the protein across the membrane and functions as a membrane-binding sequence.

VIII. DRUGS AND INHIBITORS OF PROTEIN SYNTHESIS IN EUKARYOTES

A. **Therapeutic drugs.** A number of antibiotics that inhibit protein synthesis have proved to be effective antibacterial drugs.

1. **Streptomycin** is an aminoglycoside often used to treat heart infections. It acts by inhibiting the initiation of protein synthesis by preventing the binding of fmet-tRNA$_f$ to the P site of the initiation complex. Its effect has been localized to the S12 protein of the 30S ribosomal subunit. It also causes misreading of the mRNA sequence. The effects, at concentrations used, are solely on the bacteria.

2. **Tetracycline** is a wide-range antibiotic that binds to the 30S ribosomal subunit of bacteria and inhibits the binding of aminoacyl-tRNAs.

3. **Chloramphenicol** is a wide-range antibiotic that binds to the 50S ribosomal subunit and blocks the peptidyl transferase reaction.

4. **Erythromycin** is an antibacterial drug that inhibits the translocation reaction by binding to the 50S ribosomal subunit.

B. **Inhibitors.** Other antibiotics inhibit protein synthesis and are used for research purposes but have not proved to be good therapeutic drugs.

1. **Cycloheximide** inhibits protein synthesis in eukaryotes by binding to the 60S ribosomal subunit and inhibiting the peptidyl transferase reaction.

2. **Puromycin** is an analog of the aminoacyl-adenosine moiety of aminoacyl-tRNA and leads to premature termination of translation in both prokaryotes and eukaryotes. It competes with aminoacyl-tRNAs for binding to the A site. In the A site, peptidyl transferase links its amino group to the carboxyl group of the peptidyl-tRNA in the P site. This linkage causes premature termination.

C. **Toxins.** The mechanism of action of several potent toxins is through the inhibition of protein synthesis.

1. **Diphtheria toxin**
    a. **Source.** Diphtheria toxin is produced by a lysogenic bacteriophage that infects *Corynebacterium diphtheriae,* which can infect the nasopharynx region of the respiratory tract.
    b. **Mechanism of action.** Diphtheria toxin catalyzes the transfer of adenosine diphosphate ribose (ADP-ribose) from oxidized nicotinamide adenine dinucleotide (NAD^+) to an already post-translationally modified histidine in eEF-2. This **ADP ribosylation** inactivates eEF-2 and inhibits the translocation step of elongation. Because diphtheria toxin is catalytic, only small amounts are needed to be toxic to the cell.
    c. **Clinical aspects.** Infected patients start out with a sore throat that can progress to severe edema and blockage of the airways. It may progress to heart infections

and often results in death. In third-world countries, diphtheria is a serious health problem. However, because of an effective childhood immunization program, death due to diphtheria is not a problem in the United States.

2. **Ricin**
    a. **Source.** Ricin is a protein produced by castor beans.
    b. **Mechanism of action.** The ricin toxin is an N-glycosidase that removes a single adenine from 28S rRNA. This depurination inhibits protein synthesis in eukaryotes.
    c. **Clinical aspects.** Ricin is the protein component of castor oil, a distasteful laxative sometimes given to children. Because ricin is extremely toxic, castor oil should not be administered over long periods of time. In fact, castor oil is considered to be too strong for treating common constipation. Long-term use of castor oil can lead to persistent diarrhea and the subsequent loss of intestinal function, which may be fatal.

3. **rRNA specific nucleases.** Other toxins inhibit protein synthesis by the specific cleavage of rRNAs.
    a. **α-Sarcin** is a fungal toxin that cleaves 28S rRNA. This specific cleavage leads to the inhibition of aminoacyl-tRNA binding.
    b. **Colicin E3** is secreted by some strains of *E. coli* and inhibits protein synthesis in other bacteria. It does this by specifically cleaving 16S rRNA, which leads to the inhibition of initiation.

Case 10-1 Revisited

Diphtheria toxin is produced by a lysogenic bacteriophage that infects *C. diphtheriae,* which can infect the nasopharynx region of the respiratory tract.

Diphtheria toxin is a secreted protein that may enter the bloodstream as well as affect mucosal and epithelial tissues on which *C. diphtheriae* may grow. The toxin is comprised of two regions. One region facilitates its entry into cells, and the second portion is an enzyme that catalyzes the transfer of ADP-ribose from NAD^+ to an already post-translationally modified histidine in eEF-2. This ADP ribosylation inactivates eEF-2 and inhibits the translocation step of elongation. Because diphtheria toxin is catalytic, even small amounts are toxic to cells.

When in the bloodstream, diphtheria toxin can be taken up by tissues removed from the primary site of infection. The heart is particularly sensitive to diphtheria toxin; a large number of deaths are attributed to its toxic effects on the myocardium of the heart. Because it is such a potent toxin, it is important to inactivate diphtheria toxin as soon as possible.

Erythromycin is administered to kill the host bacterium and to make the patient less contagious. It inhibits the translocation reaction of translation through binding to the 50S ribosomal subunit.

STUDY QUESTIONS

DIRECTIONS: Each of the numbered items or incomplete statements in this section is followed by answers or by completions of the statement. Select the **one** lettered answer or completion that is **best** in each case.

1. The genetic code refers to which one of the following?

(A) The number of chromosomes in the diploid cells of a species
(B) The nucleotide sequences that correspond to common amino acids
(C) The amino acid sequence of cellular proteins
(D) The ratios of mendelian inheritance
(E) The hierarchy of DNA, RNA, and protein

2. The translation of messenger RNA (mRNA) into the amino acid sequence of a polypeptide in prokaryotes is terminated at the end of the message by one of three chain termination codons in the mRNA. The stop codon is recognized by

(A) a specific uncharged transfer RNA (tRNA)
(B) a specific aminoacyl-tRNA
(C) a specific ribosomal RNA (rRNA)
(D) a specific protein
(E) a specific ribosomal subunit

3. The "wobble" hypothesis refers to the less stringent base-pairing specificity of the

(A) 5'-end base of the codon
(B) 3'-end base of the anticodon
(C) middle base of the anticodon
(D) 5'-end base of the anticodon
(E) middle base of the codon

4. The formation of peptide bonds by the ribosome-messenger RNA (mRNA) complex continues until

(A) the ribosome reaches the 5' end of the mRNA
(B) a tRNA with an anticodon for UAA, UAG, or UGA interacts with the amino (A) site on the ribosome
(C) formylmethionine-transfer RNA_f or tRNA_i interacts with the A site on the ribosome
(D) a stop codon on mRNA is reached
(E) the ribosome dissociates into large and small subunits

5. A protein to be secreted has which one of the following characteristics?

(A) It has a signal sequence on its carboxyl-terminal end that is recognized by the signal sequence receptor on the endoplasmic reticulum (ER)
(B) It is synthesized by a subset of ribosomes, which are different from free ribosomes, and are bound to the ER
(C) It is modified by signal peptidase in the cytoplasm
(D) It is recognized by free ribosomes and transferred to the ER after undergoing N-linked glycosylation
(E) It has a signal sequence on its amino-terminal end that is recognized by a signal recognition particle (SRP) in the cytoplasm

6. Which therapeutic antibiotic blocks the peptidyl transferase reaction of protein synthesis?

(A) Chloramphenicol
(B) Erythromycin
(C) Tetracycline
(D) Streptomycin
(E) Puromycin

7. Degeneracy of the genetic code means that

(A) a given base triplet can code for more than one amino acid
(B) there is no punctuation in the code sequences
(C) the third base in a codon is not important in coding
(D) a given amino acid can be coded for by more than one base triplet
(E) codons are not ambiguous

8. Which one of the following toxins inhibits eukaryotic protein synthesis through the depurination of a single adenine residue in 28S ribosomal RNA (rRNA)?

(A) Diphtheria toxin
(B) Ricin
(C) α-Sarcin
(D) Colicin E3
(E) Cycloheximide

9. In the formation of aminoacyl-transfer RNAs (tRNAs) by the aminoacyl-tRNA synthetases

(A) the appropriate amino acid is attached to the 5′ end of the appropriate tRNA
(B) the amino acid is first attached to adenosine monophosphate (AMP)
(C) the accuracy of the aminoacyl-tRNA formation is achieved by the full reversibility of all of the steps in the aminoacylation reactions
(D) the activation step requires the hydrolysis of the terminal phosphate group of guanosine triphosphate (GTP)
(E) only one kind of tRNA will serve as a substrate for each amino acid

10. Eukaryotic ribosomes are bigger than prokaryotic ribosomes. This increased size is due to more subunit proteins and to larger sized ribosomal RNAs (rRNAs). Which component of a eukaryotic ribosome has no smaller or equal-sized equivalent in the prokaryotic ribosome?

(A) 40S ribosomal subunit
(B) 28S rRNA
(C) 60S ribosomal subunit
(D) 18S rRNA
(E) 5.8S rRNA

11. Cell-free protein-synthesizing systems from *Escherichia coli* that translate synthetic polyribonucleotides can be prepared. They do not require a Shine-Dalgarno sequence or an initiator codon, and they translate the polyribonucleotide in all three reading frames. Such systems were used to determine the genetic code. Translation of the repeating sequence CAA in a cell-free protein-synthesizing system produced three homopolypeptides: polyglutamine, polyasparagine, and polythreonine. If the codons for glutamine and asparagine are CAA and AAC, respectively, which one of the following triplets is a codon for threonine?

(A) AAC
(B) CAC
(C) CCA
(D) ACA
(E) There is insufficient information to determine the codon for threonine

---

DIRECTIONS: Each group of items in this section consists of lettered options followed by a set of numbered items. For each item, select the **one** lettered option that is most closely associated with it. Each lettered option may be selected once, more than once, or not at all.

Questions 12-14

Match the factor or enzyme with the stage of protein synthesis in which the factor is required in prokaryotes.

(A) EF-Tu
(B) RF-2
(C) Formylmethionine-transfer RNA$_f$ (tRNA$_f$)
(D) Cap-binding protein
(E) tRNA synthetase

12. Initiation

13. Elongation

14. Termination

ANSWERS AND EXPLANATIONS

1. The answer is B [I B]. The genetic code refers to the nucleotide triplet sequences in messenger RNA (mRNA) that code for the 20 common amino acids found in proteins and that react in an antiparallel manner with triplet nucleotide sequences on transfer RNAs (tRNAs). The amino acid sequence of any protein is encoded in a gene in the form of nucleotide triplets. The genetic code refers to these sequences and not to the amino acid sequences in the protein. The genetic code does not refer to chromosome number or behavior during cell division. The hierarchy of DNA, RNA, and protein was an early assumption in the development of molecular genetics, which has now been modified by the finding of RNA-directed DNA synthesis in certain viruses by the enzyme reverse transcriptase.

2. The answer is D [V C]. In prokaryotes, the three chain termination codons—UAA, UAG, and UGA—do not specify amino acids, and there are no transfer RNAs (tRNAs) whose anticodon recognizes them. They are recognized by the protein release factors, RF-1 and RF-2, which bind to the termination codons. RF-1 recognizes UAA or UAG, and RF-2 recognizes UAA or UGA. The binding of the release factors initiates the hydrolysis of the link between the polypeptide and the tRNA.

3. The answer is D [III A-B; Figure 10-2]. The codon-anticodon interaction is due to complementary base pairing between the two triplets, which line up antiparallel to one another. The base pairing between the 5'-end base of the codon and the 3'-end base of the anticodon is the usual Watson-Crick base pairing; that is, adenine (A) with uracil (U) and guanine (G) with cytosine (C), as is the base pairing of the middle base of the triplet. The base pairing of the 3'-end base of the codon and the 5'-end base of the anticodon shows more latitude. When the 5'-end base (first base) of the anticodon is C or A, the base pairing with the codon is regular; that is, the base in the codon is G or U. If the first base of the anticodon is U, then the 3'-end base (third base) of the codon can be either G or A. If the first base of the anticodon is G, then the third base of the codon can be U or C. If the first base of the anticodon is I (inosine), then the third base of the codon can be A, C, or U, but it cannot be G.

4. The answer is D [V C]. The genetic code contains three stop codons—UAA, UAG, and UGA—for which there are no corresponding transfer RNA (tRNA) molecules. In prokaryotes, these codons are recognized by two protein release factors, one of which recognizes UAA or UGA, the other recognizing UAA or UAG. The binding of these factors to the stop codons in conjunction with a third release factor, RF-3, and guanosine triphosphate (GTP) promotes the hydrolysis of the bond between the polypeptide and the tRNA.

5. The answer is E [VII B 1]. Proteins to be secreted are synthesized on the endoplasmic reticulum (ER) and have a signal sequence on their amino-terminal end that directs their synthesis to the ER. All protein synthesis begins on free ribosomes in the cytoplasm. There is no difference between the ribosomes that produce secretory proteins and those that produce cytoplasmic proteins. The signal recognition particle (SRP) binds to the signal sequence when it emerges from the ribosome and halts further protein synthesis until the SRP-ribosome complex interacts with an SRP receptor on the ER, and the SRP is removed. The signal peptidase removes the signal sequence from the newly synthesized secretory protein on the luminal side of the ER.

6. The answer is A [VIII A, B]. Chloramphenicol is a wide-range antibiotic that binds to the 50S ribosomal subunit of the bacteria and blocks the peptidyl transferase reaction. Erythromycin inhibits the translocation reaction of protein synthesis. Tetracycline binds to the 30S ribosomal subunit and inhibits the binding of aminoacyl-transfer RNA (tRNA). Streptomycin inhibits the initiation of protein synthesis by preventing the binding of fmet-tRNA$_f$ to the P site of the initiation complex. Puromycin is a nontherapeutic drug that is an analog of the aminoacyl-adenosine moiety of an aminoacyl-tRNA. It binds at the amino (A) site on the ribosome, and its amino group forms a peptide bond with the carboxyl group of the peptidyl-tRNA on the peptide (P) site. The resulting peptide with a C-terminal puromycin group leaves the ribosome.

7. The answer is D [I B; III B]. Of the 20 common amino acids, 18 are coded for by more than one base triplet (codon), which is the reason for calling the code degenerate. However, the code is not ambiguous; that is, a given codon specifies only one amino acid. The third base in a codon (i.e., the 3'-end base) has less stringent pairing requirements than the other two bases. Many, but not all, of the multiple codons for an amino acid differ only in the 3' base. This latitude has been termed "wobble."

8. The answer is B [VIII C 2]. Ricin is an N-glycosidase from castor beans. It depurinates a single adenine residue in 28S ribosomal RNA (rRNA). This depurination is sufficient to inhibit protein synthesis in eukaryotes. Diphtheria toxin is produced by a lysogenic bacteriophage that infects *Corynebacterium diphtheriae,* which can infect the nasopharynx region of the respiratory tract. It results in the adenosine diphosphate (ADP) ribosylation of eukaryotic elongation factor-2 (eEF-2), which inhibits the translocation step of protein synthesis in eukaryotes. α-Sarcin is a fungal toxin that specifically cleaves 28S rRNA. This cleavage inhibits the binding of aminoacyl-transfer RNAs. Colicin E3 is produced by some strains of *Escherichia coli,* and it cleaves 16S rRNA. This cleavage inhibits initiation of translation in other bacteria.

9. The answer is B [II B; V A 1 d (3); VI A 1 d (3)]. The attachment of amino acids to their appropriate transfer RNAs (tRNAs) is catalyzed by the tRNA synthetases. These reactions all occur in a three-step process. In the first step the amino acid is attached to AMP forming an aminoacyl-adenylate complex. In the second step of the reaction the amino acid is transferred to the 2'- or 3'-hydroxyl group of the 3' adenosine of the appropriate tRNA. In the third step of the reaction, the pyrophosphate generated in the first step of the reaction is hydrolyzed to form two free phosphates. This makes the overall reaction irreversible. Formation of aminoacyl-tRNAs requires only adenosine triphosphate (ATP) as an energy source to drive the reactions. Methionyl-tRNA synthetases can attach methionine to either the initiator tRNA (tRNA$_f$ in prokaryotes or tRNA$_i$ in eukaryotes) or to the tRNA used to recognize the AUG codon during elongation (i.e., tRNA$_{met}$).

10. The answer is E [IV A, B]. Both prokaryotes and eukaryotes have large subunits (60S and 50S, respectively) and small subunits (40S and 30S, respectively). The small subunits each contain a single ribosomal RNA (rRNA) that is larger in eukaryotes (18S) than in prokaryotes (16S). The large subunit of eukaryotes has three rRNA constituents (28S, 5.8S, and 5S), whereas the large subunit of prokaryotes has two rRNA constituents (23S and 5S). The 28S and 5S rRNA of eukaryotes are equivalent to the 23S and 5S rRNAs of prokaryotes. The 5.8S rRNA is unique to the large subunit of eukaryotes.

11. The answer is D [I B 1; Table 10-1]. The synthetic polyribonucleotide sequence of CAACAACAACAA ... is read in an in vitro protein-synthesizing system starting at the first C, the first A, or the second A. Once translation begins, the triplet codons are read sequentially without spacer bases. The first triplet codon and all subsequent codons would be CAA, which codes for glutamine. The second triplet codon and all subsequent codons would be AAC, which codes for asparagine. The last triplet codon and all subsequent codons would be ACA, which would have to be a codon for threonine.

12–14. The answers are: 12-C [V A 1 d], **13-A** [V B 1 a], **14-B** [V C 1 a]. A specific transfer RNA (tRNA) is required for initiation of translation—the initiator tRNA (tRNA$_f$). It brings a modified methionine, formylmethionine (fmet), to the 30S initiation complex.

Three elongation factors (EF) are required for elongation: EF-Tu, EF-Ts, and EF-G. Delivery of an aminoacyl-tRNA to the empty A site on the ribosome is effected by EF-Tu, EF-Ts, and GTP. This process delivers all aminoacyl-tRNAs except fmet-tRNA$_f$ to the A site. Elongation continues until a termination (stop) codon is encountered. No tRNAs pair with stop codons. Instead, the stop codons are recognized by the release factors RF-1 or RF-2. A third release factor, RF-3, in association with GTP, promotes termination.

Cap-binding protein is important for initiation of translation in eukaryotes. It is a subunit of initiation factor 4a and may initiate mRNA binding by interacting with the 5'-cap structure of eukaryotic mRNAs.

Aminoacyl-tRNA synthetase activity is required prior to translation. Aminoacyl-tRNA synthetases are enzymes that activate amino acids and attach them to the 3'-terminal adenosine of their cognate tRNA.

Chapter 11

Recombinant DNA
Donald Sittman

Case 11-1

A female infant initially presents 2 days after birth with an infection. She suffers recurrent infections and poor growth until 26 months of age, when she is diagnosed with severe combined immunodeficiency disease (SCID) and adenosine deaminase (ADA) deficiency. The patient receives two haploidentical bone marrow transplants, 1 year apart. Although she initially does well after each transplantation, her immune function declines to pretransplantation levels within 3–4 months after each transplantation. The patient is then treated with regular intramuscular injections of ADA coupled to polyethylene glycol (PEG-ADA). She is now entered into a gene therapy trial to correct her ADA deficiency.

A retroviral vector carrying a human ADA complementary DNA (cDNA) clone under the control of the human ADA promoter was used to transfect, *ex vivo,* samples of the patient's bone marrow (BM) and peripheral blood lymphocytes (PBLs). The clone also carries a selectable marker coding for the neomycin resistance gene. The patient receives nine intravenous injections of transfected lymphocytes and bone marrow progenitor cells over a 2-year period. The patient remains under PEG-ADA therapy throughout and after the course of her gene therapy. Administration of the genetically modified cells rapidly restores full immune function to the patient. One year after the completion of the patient's gene therapy, transfected PBL- and BM-derived lymphocytes could be found in her blood plasma. It is also noted that T cells derived from transfected PBL cells are being replaced by T cells from transfected bone marrow cells.

- Why was a retroviral vector used?
- Why was an ADA cDNA clone used rather than the ADA gene? What sequences are needed for expression of ADA?
- Why was the neomycin resistance gene part of the ADA-retroviral vector construct?
- What techniques could be used to detect the presence or absence of each vector in different cell types?

I. INTRODUCTION

A. **Definition.** Recombinant DNA basically refers to techniques that are used to manipulate, move, recombine, and propagate DNA.

B. **Impact on modern medicine.** Recombinant DNA technology is beginning to have a tremendous impact on medicine. It is rapidly increasing our knowledge of gene expression and the cause of many diseases. It is also leading to new approaches for the diagnosis and treatment of many diseases.

II. TOOLS OF RECOMBINANT DNA.
At the heart of recombinant DNA are the **nucleic acid enzymes.** They have become tools that allow DNA and RNA to be manipulated. Knowledge of their specific enzymatic activities is essential for their use.

A. **Restriction enzymes.** No single group of enzymes has had as great an impact on recombinant DNA as restriction enzymes. In fact, recombinant DNA technology developed primarily as a result of the discovery of restriction enzymes.

1. **Source.** Restriction enzymes are isolated from bacteria and are named for the bacteria from which they are derived.
   a. **Restriction–modification systems.** Many bacteria have a restriction–modification system that functions as a defense against bacteriophage infections. As the name implies, there are two components to restriction–modification systems.
      (1) **Restriction system.** Bacteria contain enzymes that restrict the ability of the bacteriophage to infect them. These enzymes are **highly specific endonucleases** that digest bacteriophage DNA that has never been propagated within the bacterium.
      (2) **Modification system.** Bacteria also contain enzymes that modify their own DNA to protect it from being digested by their own restriction enzymes.
         (a) The modifications are **sequence-specific methylations.**
         (b) These methylation enzymes are specific for the same sequences as the host's restriction enzymes.
         (c) Methylated sequences are not digested by the host's restriction enzymes.
   b. There are different types of restriction–modification systems in bacteria. Only the type II restriction enzymes are widely used as tools of recombinant DNA.

2. **Enzymatic activity of type II restriction enzymes.** Restriction enzymes recognize specific sequences in double-stranded DNA and make two sequence-specific cuts, one in each strand. These cuts generate 3'-hydroxyl and 5'-phosphate ends.
   a. The **recognition site** for each enzyme from each bacterial strain is usually unique. Hundreds of different restriction enzymes have been isolated that cleave at different recognition sites.
      (1) Restriction enzyme recognition sites are short. They are usually four, five, or six base pairs, although a few are eight base pairs in length.
      (2) Restriction enzyme recognition sites typically exhibit **twofold rotational** or **dyad symmetry** (Figure 11-1A).
      (3) They are also **palindromic** in nature; that is, the sequence of each strand is the same when each strand is read in a 5' to 3' direction.
   b. Restriction enzymes **require no additional energy** from adenosine triphosphate (ATP) or other energy source for cleavage.
   c. **Restriction enzyme cuts** are symmetrical and usually within the sequence, but they are not necessarily along the axis of symmetry (see Figure 11-1B).
      (1) If the cuts are along the axis of symmetry, they are said to produce **blunt ends.**
      (2) If the cuts are not along the axis of symmetry, they are said to produce **cohesive** or **sticky ends.**
         (a) The cohesive ends produced by a restriction enzyme cut are **complementary** and can base pair.
         (b) This concept of complementary, cohesive ends is important in the generation of recombinant DNA molecules for cloning purposes (see III A 1 b).

B. **Other nucleic acid enzyme tools.** Many other nucleic acid enzymes are routinely used as tools in recombinant DNA research. However, for the procedures discussed in this chapter, knowledge of only one other specific enzyme and one class of enzymes besides restriction endonucleases is needed.

1. **DNA polymerases.** Different DNA polymerases with different activities and characteristics have been of great use in recombinant DNA research.
   a. **DNA-dependent DNA polymerases** (see Chapter 8 II B). These enzymes make complementary copies of DNA templates and are **useful in a number of procedures.**
      (1) **Production of labeled probes.** If radioisotopically or appropriately[1] chemically labeled deoxynucleoside triphosphates (dNTPs) are used as substrates,

---

[1] An appropriate label is one that can be incorporated into DNA in nucleotides, does not significantly alter the physical characteristics of the DNA, and can be detected by an analytical procedure. A number of such labels are commercially available

A

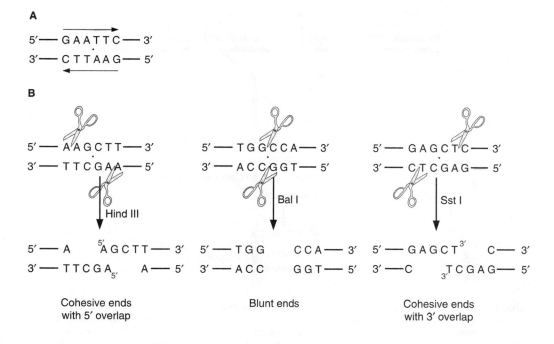

B

FIGURE 11-1. *(A)* Restriction enzyme recognition sites are palindromes and exhibit twofold rotational (dyad) symmetry. *(B)* Examples of types of cuts made by various restriction enzymes. Some restriction enzymes can generate cohesive ends that have either 5′ (e.g., *Hind III*) or 3′ (e.g., *Sst I*) overlaps. Other restriction enzymes (e.g., *Bal I*) cut in the center of the symmetrical recognition sequence and generate ends with no overlapping cohesive sequences but blunt ends. Scissors indicate the cut positions for the enzymes shown.

then they are incorporated into the DNA synthesized by most of these enzymes. Labeled DNA is useful in a number of procedures, the most important of which is hybridization [see III A 3 b (1)].

  (2) DNA sequencing (see IV E). The predominant method of sequencing DNA uses DNA polymerases.

  (3) DNA amplification. DNA-dependent DNA polymerases from thermophilic organisms have allowed the development of an automated method of amplifying segments of DNA that is called the **polymerase chain reaction** (**PCR;** see IV F).

 b. RNA-dependent DNA polymerase. Reverse transcriptase is an RNA-dependent DNA polymerase derived from RNA tumor viruses that makes cDNA copies of RNA templates. This enzyme is particularly useful in cloning DNA sequences that are complementary to messenger RNA (mRNA; see III C 2).

 2. DNA ligase (see Chapter 8 II D 2 e) catalyzes the formation of a phosphodiester bond between adjacent 3′-hydroxyl and 5′-phosphate ends of DNA. It is an essential tool in the formation of recombinant DNA clones (see III A 1 b).

III. **CLONING.** In a biologic sense, a clone refers to cells with an identical genotype. As used in recombinant DNA, a clone refers to identical host cells that carry an identical recombinant DNA molecule.

A. **Basic strategy of cloning.** The basic concepts of cloning are essentially the same for any host cell, vector (see III B), or strategy that is used (Figure 11-2).

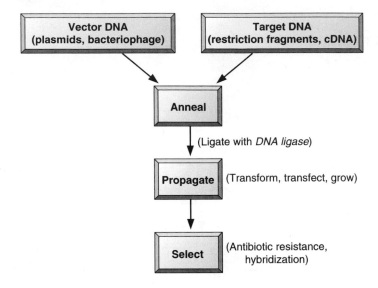

FIGURE 11-2. Basic cloning strategy. A recombinant DNA is made from vector and target DNAs by *annealing* and *ligation*. The recombinant DNA molecule is introduced into the host cell by transformation or transfection. *Propagation* of the molecule takes place in the host cell. The presence of a vector is typically detected by the antibiotic resistance that is conferred to the host cell. The *target DNA* is specifically *selected* by hybridization. *cDNA* = complementary DNA.

1. **Formation of recombinant molecules.** The first step of cloning is to make a recombinant molecule that is to be inserted or "cloned" into an appropriate host. A recombinant molecule refers to one formed by the covalent linkage of two pieces of DNA from different sources.
   a. Recombinant DNA molecules are typically formed by the **covalent joining** of:
      (1) A piece of **vector DNA,** which is required to "carry" another piece of DNA into a host cell and allow its presence to be easily detected
      (2) A piece of **target DNA,** which is the "foreign" piece of DNA that is being inserted into the host cell
   b. **Linkage of vector and target DNA molecules** (Figure 11-3). If two pieces of DNA from different sources are cut with the same restriction enzyme, then they will have complementary, cohesive ends.
      (1) Cohesive ends anneal at low temperatures (see Chapter 6 II D 2).
      (2) The annealed molecules are covalently linked by the action of **DNA ligase,** which forms phosphodiester bonds between adjacent 3'-hydroxyl groups and 5'-phosphate groups.

2. **Insertion into and propagation of recombinant DNA in host cells.** Techniques are available that allow DNA to be put into almost any type of bacterial, plant, or animal cell.
   a. Once inside the cell, or cell nucleus in eukaryotes, an appropriate vector is replicated and propagated.
   b. **Bacteria** that have a selectable marker as a result of taking up a piece of recombinant DNA are said to be **transformed.**
   c. **Eukaryotic cells** that have a selectable marker as a result of taking up a piece of recombinant DNA are said to be **transfected.**

3. **Selection** for transformants or transfectants is done at two levels: The first level is the selection for all cells that are transformed or transfected, and the second level is the selection for only those cells that have taken up a recombinant DNA containing a specific target DNA.
   a. **Selection of all transformants or transfectants**

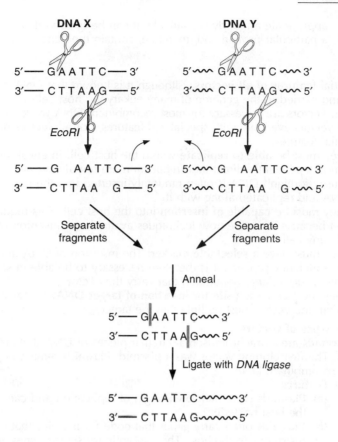

FIGURE 11-3. Formation of a recombinant DNA molecule. Restriction fragments of DNA from two different sources (*X* and *Y*) can be separated after the DNA is cleaved with the restriction enzyme *EcoRI*. Because the restriction fragments from X and Y were generated by the same restriction enzyme, their ends are complementary and may be annealed at a low temperature and covalently linked with *DNA ligase.*

      (1) Most vectors contain genes for **selectable markers.** These genes usually code for resistance to an antibiotic or drug that kills the host cell if a vector expressing resistance is not present.

      (2) **Bacteriophage vectors** (see III B 2 b) are selectable because they can be grown lytically, which means they cause the host cell to break open and die. This is an easily selectable feature.

      (3) Because the actual formation of recombinant DNA molecules is not 100% efficient, many new vectors have selectable markers that can distinguish between vectors carrying a piece of target DNA from those not carrying any target DNA (see III C 1 a).

   b. **Selection for a particular piece of target DNA from a mixture of many.** This is particularly important in isolating clones of particular genes from genomic libraries (see III D). There are **two major approaches:**

      (1) **Hybridization** (see Chapter 6 II D 2 c) generally entails the extraction or removal of DNA from the cells containing recombinant DNA and its hybridization or annealing with complementary labeled DNA probes.

      (2) **Antibody screening.** If the target DNA is placed in the appropriate position in a vector containing a transcriptional promoter sequence and a translational initiation sequence that both function in the host cell, then it is possible for a protein to be produced that is coded for by the target DNA. If an appropriate antibody is available, it can be used to detect cells that produce a particular protein and, therefore, contain the gene for that protein.

B. **Vectors**

1. **Essential features of all vectors.** Although it is known that DNA can be inserted into and carried in the genome of many eukaryotic host cells in the absence of a vector, vectors are necessary for most recombinant DNA work. There are now many vectors available with specialized features, but all vectors have the following essential features.
   a. They must be **able to replicate** within the host cell. In eukaryotes, vectors that can independently direct their replication are not always necessary. This is because "foreign" DNA is often randomly inserted into the host cell's genomic DNA and replicated along with it.
   b. They must be **capable of insertion** into the host cell. This requirement is easily met because there are now techniques available for insertion of DNA into virtually any cell.
   c. They must have a **selectable marker.** The insertion of DNA into cells is often a low-efficiency process. It is therefore necessary to be able to select for the few cells within a large population that carry the vector.
   d. They must **contain a site for insertion of target DNA.** To carry target DNA into a cell, the vector must be linked to the target.

2. **Major types of vectors**
   a. **Plasmids** are extrachromosomal circular pieces of DNA that are found in bacteria. The first cloning vector was a plasmid. Plasmids remain key cloning vectors in recombinant DNA.
      (1) **Features**
         (a) Plasmids carry their own origin of replication and can replicate within the host bacterium.
         (b) Plasmids often carry genes that code for proteins that confer antibiotic resistance to the host. The antibiotic-resistance genes are selectable markers.
      (2) **Major uses of plasmids in cloning** (see III C)
         (a) Cloning of small pieces of DNA, which are typically less than 10 kilobases (kb)
         (b) Cloning of cDNA
   b. **Bacteriophages** are viruses that infect bacteria. The DNA of the bacteriophage can be used as vectors.
      (1) **Features**
         (a) Because they are live, bacteriophages **can replicate** in the appropriate host.
         (b) They **can be propagated** to high copy numbers—several hundred per cell.
         (c) They **can grow in a lytic phase,** in which they cause the host cells to lyse or break open.
         (d) They can very efficiently **infect their host cells.**
         (e) Some types of bacteriophages are single stranded for much of the replication cycle.
      (2) **Major uses of bacteriophages in cloning**
         (a) Cloning of large pieces of DNA, up to 20 kb (see III D)
         (b) Construction of genomic libraries (see III D)
         (c) cDNA libraries (see III C 2)
         (d) Production of single-stranded DNA for DNA sequencing (see IV E)

C. **Plasmid cloning**

1. **General DNA cloning.** An example of the insertion of a DNA fragment with EcoRI (named after the RY13 strain of *Escherichia coli*) cohesive ends into an EcoRI site within a plasmid, and its cloning in *E. coli,* is shown in Figure 11-4.

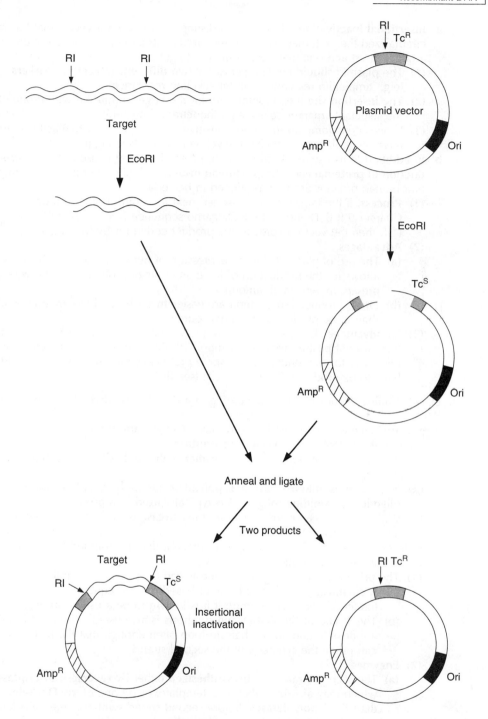

FIGURE 11-4. Cloning of an *EcoRI target* fragment into the EcoRI site of a *plasmid vector.* This vector contains two genes: one that codes for tetracycline resistance *(Tc^R),* which contains the EcoRI cloning site, and one that codes for ampicillin resistance *(Amp^R).* It also contains an origin of replication *(Ori).* After annealing and ligation of a mix of vector and target DNAs, the vector may or may not contain a target DNA insert. Host cells transformed with a vector containing an insert are resistant to ampicillin but sensitive to tetracycline *(Tc^S)* because the coding sequence for tetracycline resistance is disrupted by the presence of the target DNA *(insertional inactivation).* Host cells transformed with a vector that recircularizes without a target insert are resistant to both ampicillin and tetracycline.

a. Insertional inactivation allows one to distinguish between a vector that has re-circularized (i.e., returned to its normal circular structure) and does not contain a target insert and one that does contain a target insert.

(1) The plasmid should contain **genes for two different selectable markers** (e.g., ampicillin resistance and tetracycline resistance).

(2) The **insertion site** (i.e., cloning site) for the target should be within one of the selectable marker genes (e.g., the tetracycline gene).

(3) Clones containing an insert are sensitive to tetracycline, whereas those that have recircularized remain tetracycline resistant (see Figure 11-4).

b. In addition to its usefulness in research, plasmid cloning is useful for the **production of proteinaceous drugs. Human insulin** and other therapeutically important human proteins are now produced in bacteria.

(1) Process. If the target DNA is inserted next to a transcriptional promoter (see Chapter 9 II B 1) and a Shine-Dalgarno sequence [see Chapter 10 V A 2 a (1)], then the vector expresses the product coded for by the target.

(2) Advantages

(a) The use of plasmids for the expression of human proteins in bacteria allows for the production of large amounts of protein that otherwise are present in very small amounts.

(b) Drugs produced in bacteria are **easier to purify** and **less immunogenic** than those produced in animal sources.

(3) Disadvantage. The disadvantage of producing some drugs in bacteria is that they are not post-translationally modified. Post-translational modification is necessary for the functioning of some proteins, which means they would have to be produced in animal cells (see III E 1).

2. cDNA cloning (Figure 11-5) is the cloning of a double-stranded DNA copy of an RNA.

a. The **first step** of cDNA cloning is to make a single-strand complementary DNA copy of the mRNA with **reverse transcriptase.**

(1) As with all DNA polymerases, a **primer** with a 3'-hydroxyl group is required.

(2) Because most mRNAs have a 3' polyadenylate (poly A) tail, a short-chain **oligodeoxythymidine (oligo dT)** is typically used as a primer.

(3) With oligo dT as a primer, reverse transcriptase uses mRNA as a template and synthesizes DNA.

b. The **second step** of cDNA cloning is to make a double-stranded DNA copy so that it can be inserted into the DNA vector.

(1) The **primer** for second-strand synthesis can be either of the following.

(a) A **chemically synthesized** primer based on the sequence of the mRNA (preferably near the 5' end), if it is known to be a useful primer.

(b) The **3' end of the first-strand synthesis** is also useful. The ends of DNA are flexible and form a hairpin loop often enough that the first strand can prime the synthesis of the second strand.

(2) Enzymes

(a) The second strand can be **synthesized** either **by reverse transcriptase,** which may also use DNA as a template, or by one of the **DNA-dependent DNA polymerases.** Before second-strand synthesis, the mRNA is removed by heat denaturation or alkaline hydrolysis.

(b) Another enzyme, **S1-nuclease,** which is a single-strand nuclease used to remove the hairpin loop that forms between the first and second strands if a second primer is not used, creates **blunt ends.**

(3) By a procedure called **blunt-end ligation,** small (approximately 10 base pairs), chemically synthesized, double-stranded pieces of DNA containing restriction enzyme sites, called **linkers,** are ligated to the ends of the blunt-ended, double-stranded DNA with **DNA ligase.**

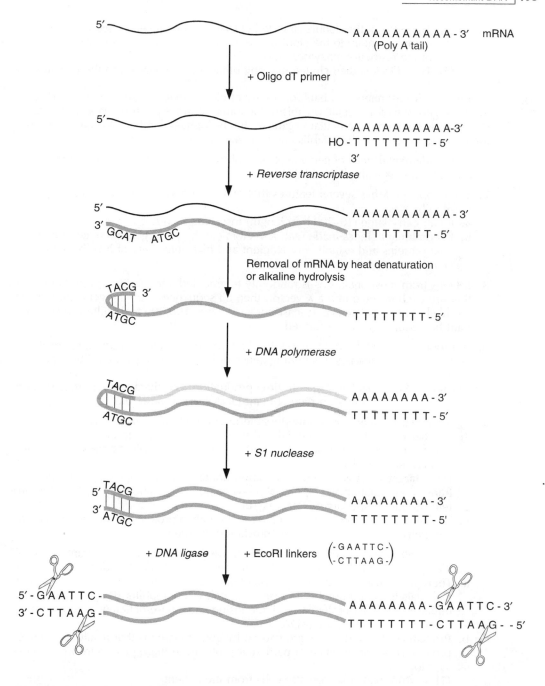

FIGURE 11-5. Formation of a double-stranded DNA copy of a strand of messenger RNA (mRNA) that can be inserted into a vector containing an EcoRI cloning site. An oligodeoxythymidine *(oligo dT) primer* primes first-strand synthesis from all mRNAs with a polyadenylate *(poly A) tail.* The RNA, which is from the RNA–DNA duplex that is formed after the first round of synthesis, is removed by heat denaturation or hydrolysis of the mRNA with an alkali. The second-strand synthesis as shown is primed by the 3' end of the first strand, when it forms a *hairpin loop.* Either *DNA polymerase* or *reverse transcriptase* can be used to synthesize the second strand. The hairpin loop is removed by the single-strand nuclease, *S1 nuclease.* The product of this reaction is duplex complementary DNA (cDNA) with blunt ends. Chemically synthesized, double-stranded *linkers* containing an EcoRI recognition site are covalently linked to the cDNA with *DNA ligase.* EcoRI cohesive ends are generated by cleavage with EcoRI. The cDNA may be inserted into a vector with an EcoRI cloning site, as shown in Figure 11-4.

       (4) The ends of the double-stranded cDNA are then given **cohesive termini** complementary to the cloning site in the vector by digestion with the appropriate restriction enzyme.

       (5) The cDNA is then **cloned** like any other piece of DNA into the plasmid.

D. A **genomic library** refers to a bank or library of clones that contains every sequence from the genome of a specific organism. Genomic libraries are used as a source for clones of genes from a particular organism. **Bacteriophage lambda (λ)** has become the preferred vector for the establishment of genomic libraries.

    1. The fundamental steps of generating recombinant DNA with λ DNA as a vector are the same as with plasmid DNA.

    2. Bacteriophage λ has several features that make it a good vector for making genomic libraries.

      a. It can carry large (10–20 kb in length) insert fragments.

      b. Recombinant clones made with λ vectors can be packaged in bacteriophage λ coat proteins and exhibit very efficient and high infectivity of host bacterial cells.

    3. If DNA from most organisms is randomly fragmented into 10–20 kb pieces of DNA that are each inserted into a λ vector, then all sequences carrying genes of interest are likely to be represented at least once for every 100,000 to 1 million recombinant bacteriophage clones formed.

    4. Appropriate protocols are available to allow for the selection of unique, specific recombinant bacteriophage-containing genes of interest from genomic libraries.

E. **Eukaryotic cell cloning.** For research, drug production, and therapeutic purposes, transfection of eukaryotic cells with recombinant DNA is often desirable.

    1. Somatic cell transfection is now possible in cultured eukaryotic cells.

      a. The **basic principles** of bacterial cell transformation apply to eukaryotic cell transfection. A number of vectors with genes for selectable markers in eukaryotes are now available.

      b. If the **target DNA** is cloned in the appropriate position relative to a promoter, a translation initiation signal, and a cleavage/polyadenylation signal, then the protein product of the target DNA may be expressed.

      c. Unlike proteins produced in bacteria, mammalian proteins produced in mammalian cells are appropriately **post-translationally modified.**

    2. Somatic cell gene therapy is in use now and will likely become a common therapeutic approach for the treatment of a number of metabolic disorders.

      a. Therapeutic use. Somatic cell transfection protocols have been approved in clinical trials to treat a number of diseases, such as hemophilia B, cystic fibrosis, familial hypercholesterolemia, and adenosine deaminase-deficient severe combined immunodeficiency (ADA-SCID).

      b. Procedure. These diseases are caused by gene mutations that result in inactive proteins or in the absence of particular proteins. In these procedures, it is necessary to:

        (1) Culture particular somatic cells from the patient

        (2) Transfect somatic cells with genes in vectors that lead to the production of normal protein that functions in place of the mutated protein

        (3) Reintroduce the transfected cells that produce the normal protein into the patient

    3. Transgenic animals. Transfection is not limited to somatic cells. Germline cells of most animals can be made to take up recombinant DNA, which then becomes heritable DNA.

      a. Recombinant DNA can be microinjected into the pronucleus of a fertilized egg or early embryonic cells, which have yet to enter a committed line of development, and may be transfected with recombinant DNA.

    b. These **eggs or cells can be implanted** into pseudopregnant females, where they continue normal fetal development. Upon birth, newborns may carry the transfected genes in their germline cells as well as in their somatic cells.

    c. These **first generation animals** are heterozygous for the transfected DNA but can be crossed with other first generation animals to form homozygous animals.

    d. Uses of transgenic animals

        (1) Drug production. Animals can be made to produce proteins from human genes.

            (a) These proteins are appropriately post-translationally modified.

            (b) Some animals can be made to secrete protein in their milk, from which it is easily harvested (Figure 11-6).

        (2) Research. Animals can be created that have particular human diseases or cancers. Various therapies or drugs may then be tested on these animals to see if a cure can be found.

IV. MAJOR ANALYTIC TECHNIQUES. Recombinant DNA-based analytic techniques are used with increasing frequency in the medical sciences.

A. **Southern blot analysis** is a diagnostic technique used to detect specific sequences contained on a DNA fragment. The fragment is generated by restriction enzyme digestion within a mixture of all of the restriction enzyme fragments of a genome. The principles of Southern blot analysis form the basis of a number of other diagnostic techniques (Figure 11-7).

    1. Procedure. In this technique, genomic DNA is isolated and cut with a **restriction enzyme** and separated according to size by **agarose gel electrophoresis.**

        a. After electrophoresis, the DNA is visualized by **staining** with a nucleic acid-specific stain, such as the intercalator ethidium bromide (EtBr).

        b. If **human DNA** is cut with a restriction enzyme and subjected to agarose gel electrophoresis, it appears as a **"smear"** when stained.

            (1) A 6–base-pair recognition site statistically occurs every 4096 base pairs if the DNA sequence is random.

            (2) The human genome is approximately 3.3×10^9 base pairs; therefore approximately 800,000 ($3.3 \times 10^9 \div 4096$) fragments might be generated upon digestion with a restriction enzyme with a 6–base-pair recognition site.

            (3) This large number of bands cannot be resolved by agarose gel electrophoresis and therefore appears as a smear.

        c. The DNA is **denatured** with an alkaline buffer within the gel.

        d. The denatured DNA is **transferred** from the gel to a piece of nitrocellulose paper by a blotting technique known as Southern transfer. The DNA becomes bound to the paper in the relative position to which it migrated upon electrophoresis.

        e. The DNA is then **hybridized** with a specific labeled probe.

        f. The nitrocellulose paper is **exposed** to a sheet of radiographic film, and only the DNA fragment or fragments that formed a hybrid with the probe appear as an exposed band.

    2. Uses of Southern blot analysis include:

        a. Identifying the number of genes in the genome

        b. Forming the **basis of restriction fragment length polymorphism (RFLP;** see IV C) **and DNA fingerprint analysis** (see IV D)

B. **Northern blot analysis** is procedurally similar to Southern blot analysis, the difference being that Northern blot analysis **detects RNA.**

    1. Procedure. In Northern blot analysis, RNA is **isolated** and **separated** by electrophoresis in a denaturing agarose gel.

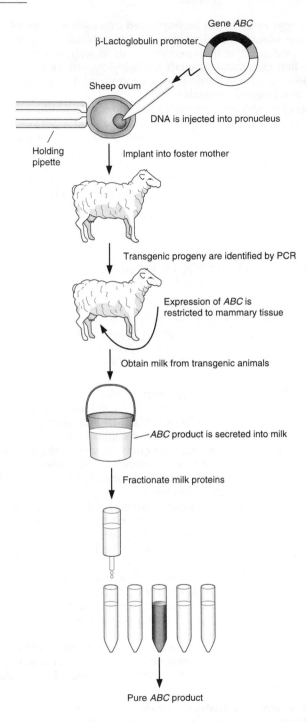

FIGURE 11-6. Formation of a transgenic sheep that produces the protein product of *gene ABC* in its milk. The ABC gene is inserted into a vector so that its expression is under the control of the promoter of the gene that produces the milk protein, β-lactoglobulin. This recombinant DNA is microinjected into the pronucleus of a fertilized egg, which is then implanted into a foster mother. DNA from small amounts of tissue are tested for the presence of the vector and ABC gene insert by polymerase chain reaction (PCR) analysis (see IV F). The product of the recombinant vector is produced in the milk from which it is easily harvested and purified. (Reprinted with permission from Watson J, Gilman M, Witkowski J, et al: *Recombinant DNA,* 2nd ed. New York, WH Freeman, 1992, p 480.)

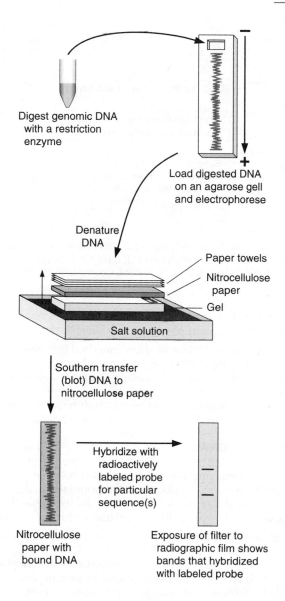

Digest genomic DNA
with a restriction
enzyme

Load digested DNA
on an agarose gell
and electrophorese

Denature
DNA

Paper towels

Nitrocellulose
paper

Gel

Salt solution

Southern transfer
(blot) DNA to
nitrocellulose paper

Hybridize with
radioactively
labeled probe
for particular
sequence(s)

Nitrocellulose
paper with
bound DNA

Exposure of filter to
radiographic film shows
bands that hybridized
with labeled probe

FIGURE 11-7. Restriction fragments complementary to a particular probe can be identified within a mix of restriction fragments from total genomic DNA by Southern blot analysis. Genomic DNA is cut with a restriction enzyme and separated according to size by agarose gel electrophoresis. The DNA is denatured within the gel and transferred or blotted to a piece of nitrocellulose. It is then hybridized with a radioactively labeled probe. Hybrids are detected by exposure of the nitrocellulose paper to a piece of radiographic film.

    a. A **denaturant** is used in the gel so that the RNA separates according to its size upon electrophoresis. Without a denaturant, the RNA forms a secondary structure and cannot be separated by size.

    b. As in Southern blot analysis, the electrophoretically separated RNA is **transferred** from the gel to a piece of nitrocellulose paper. It is then **hybridized** with a specific labeled probe and **exposed** to a piece of radiographic film to detect the hybrid.

2. Uses of Northern blot analysis. Northern blot analysis is primarily used to detect and quantitate specific mRNAs from different tissues.

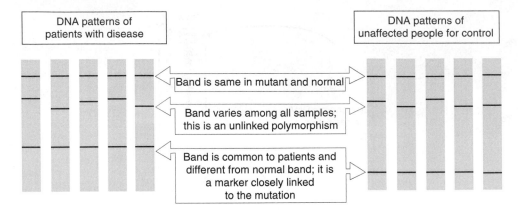

FIGURE 11-8. A restriction fragment length polymorphism (RFLP) may show a close genetic linkage or coin-heritance with an inherited disease. This occurs if the RFLP is physically close to the gene causing the disease. (Reprinted with permission from Lewin B: *Genes IV.* Oxford, Oxford University Press, 1990, p 97.)

C.   **RFLP linkage analysis** is a technique in which restriction fragment markers that demonstrate tight linkage to a mutant phenotype are identified.

    1. Any region of genomic DNA can show inherited (genotypic) variations in sequences within the population (i.e., **polymorphism**).

        a. Some polymorphisms occur in **coding sequences** and lead to genetic variation or disease states within the population.

        b. **Noncoding DNA sequences** can be polymorphic and show no phenotypic variation in the population. However, some of these polymorphisms can still be detected.

            (1) A **change in DNA sequence** may lead to a gain or a loss of a restriction enzyme recognition site (a restriction enzyme site polymorphism).

            (2) **Restriction enzyme site polymorphisms** result in different size restriction fragments among individuals in the population. They may be detected by Southern blot analysis if there is a probe available that detects the fragment whose size changes with the addition or loss of a restriction site.

    2. In **human genome mapping** experiments, thousands of probes have been used to map the chromosomal position of anonymous DNA fragments. Many of these probes have been shown to **detect restriction enzyme fragment length polymorphisms.** These RFLPs are particularly **useful in genetic linkage analysis.**

        a. Some RFLPs show a tight linkage to inherited disorders; that is, people with a particular inherited disease may often coinherit a particular RFLP (Figure 11-8).

        b. If a gene for a disease and an RFLP are frequently coinherited, then they are genetically linked and physically close.

    3. **Uses of RFLP linkage analysis**

        a. The demonstration of a linkage between an RFLP and an inherited disease can lead to the **cloning of the mutant gene** that causes the disease.

        b. RFLPs that are known to be linked to a genetic disease can be used in genetic counseling to **determine the probability of occurrence** of the genetic disease in the offspring of two individuals.

D.   **DNA fingerprinting** is a variation of RFLP analysis in which the probe hybridizes to sequences between restriction enzyme sites that are highly polymorphic (Figure 11-9).

    1. These highly polymorphic sites are called **hypervariable regions (HVRs).**

        a. HVRs are made up of tandem repeats of short sequences (i.e., 11–60 base pairs).

        b. The number of repeats may vary considerably between individuals and often are called **variable number of tandem repeats (VNTR).**

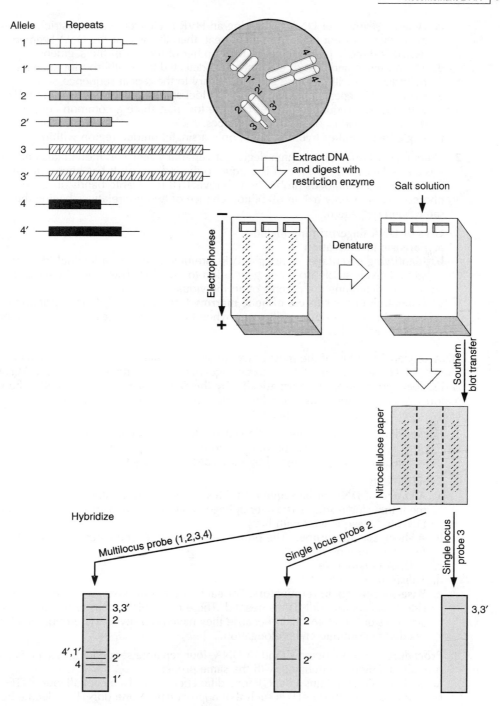

FIGURE 11-9. DNA fingerprinting. Various alleles within the human genome contain hypervariable regions (HVRs) made up of a variable number of tandem repeats. The number of repeats may be different for each allele. The sequence of each repeat may be unique and detected by a single locus probe or have core regions common to many other HVRs that may be detected by a multilocus probe. The hybridization pattern detected by a Southern blot analysis with different probes may be specific to an individual. The more HVRs that are detected, the more likely the pattern is completely specific to an individual.

    c. When a segment of DNA containing an HVR is cleaved with a restriction enzyme that does not cut within the repeat, then the size of the DNA segment released is directly proportional to the number of repeats in the segment.

    d. The presence and size of the repeat are detected by Southern blot analysis and hybridization with a probe complementary to the repeat sequence.

    e. Many of the repeats from different HVR loci share a high degree of homology within a core sequence. Probes to these loci that share a common core sequence are said to be **multilocus probes.**

    f. **Single locus probes** hybridize with only a single, unique region within an HVR.

2. Uniqueness. HVRs show a high degree of variability between individuals and can serve as a DNA fingerprint that is unique to the individual. It has been estimated that using two multilocus probes, which reveal 18 resolvable bands on gel electrophoresis, there is only a 1 in 69 billion chance of two nonrelatives having the same banding pattern.

3. Uses of DNA fingerprinting include:

    a. Forensic identification

    b. Identifying parentage. Although HVRs are unique for an individual, they are still relatively stable from one generation to the next. They can, therefore, be used to determine the parents of an individual.

    c. Evaluation of the success of bone marrow transplants. DNA fingerprinting can be used to detect donor cells, even when they constitute less than one percent of the host's cells.

E. **DNA sequencing.** One of the most powerful and informative DNA analytical techniques is DNA sequencing. DNA can be sequenced either **chemically, by the Maxam and Gilbert procedure, or enzymatically, by the Sanger procedure.** Presently, the vast majority of DNA sequencing is by the Sanger procedure, as it is easier and qualitatively superior to the chemical procedure.

1. Background. Fundamentally, the **Sanger method** of DNA sequencing, as shown in Figure 11-10, is the replication of a strand of DNA from a precise startpoint with the replication being interrupted by base-specific termination.

2. Requirements

    a. A strand of DNA to be sequenced. This can come from either a cloned fragment in a single-stranded bacteriophage or simply by denaturing the piece of DNA to be sequenced with heat.

    b. A short, specific primer. The primer ensures that all sequence reactions start from the same point.

    c. A DNA polymerase

    d. Substrate (i.e., dNTPs)

    e. Base-specific chain terminators. For each of the four bases, a **dideoxynucleoside triphosphate** (ddNTP) is needed. These molecules act as terminators of the synthesis of the DNA chain because they have no 3'-hydroxyl group, which is needed to continue chain elongation.

3. Procedure. To sequence a strand of DNA, four separate sequencing reactions are run, all of which are initiated with the same primer.

    a. Each reaction contains a ddNTP for a different base and a mix of all four dNTPs.

    b. The ratio of each ddNTP is such that approximately one ddNTP molecule becomes incorporated for every chain synthesized.

    c. For each reaction, a population of DNA chains is synthesized that terminate at each base complementary to the particular ddNTP used in the reaction.

    d. The DNA chains from each reaction are separated by high-resolution acrylamide gel electrophoresis under denaturing conditions. The four reactions are run in adjacent lanes.

    e. The gel is exposed to radiographic film, and bands appear for each primed synthesis.

    f. The sequence is read from bottom to top, as shown in Figure 11-10.

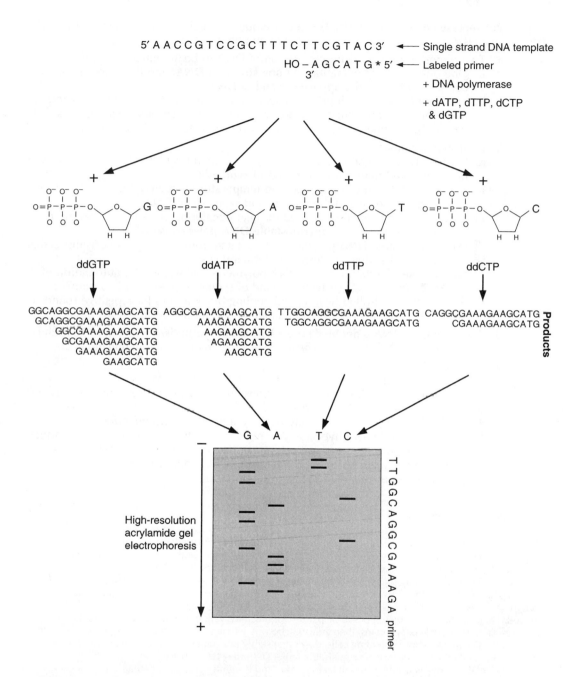

FIGURE 11-10. The Sanger method of DNA sequencing. A labeled primer is used to prime DNA synthesis by DNA polymerase in four separate reactions, each in the presence of a low level of one of the four di-deoxynucleoside triphosphates (ddNTPs). A mixture of product DNAs is synthesized. The products represent different termination events that occur whenever a particular dideoxynucleotide is incorporated instead of a deoxynucleotide. The products of each reaction are separated by high-resolution denaturing acrylamide gel electrophoresis. Bands appear upon exposure of the gel to a piece of radiographic film or other medium. A band should appear at every position in the sequence.

F. **Polymerase chain reaction (PCR)** is a technique in which repetitive rounds of DNA synthesis between two primers are used to amplify DNA (Figure 11-11).

1. **Two opposing primers** define the region of DNA to be amplified.
   a. One primer is **complementary to one strand of DNA,** and the other primer is **complementary to the opposite strand** of DNA.
   b. The **orientation** of each primer is such that when they base pair to their respective strands of DNA, their 3'-hydroxyl group faces each other. This assures that the synthesis initiated from each primer proceeds toward the opposing primer.

2. **Heat denaturation**
   a. Because DNA synthesis requires a single-stranded template, the DNA must be heat denatured **between each round of synthesis.**
   b. After the DNA is heat denatured, the **temperature is lowered** to one that is optimal for the annealing of the primers and synthesis of DNA.
   c. Because the temperature required for heat denaturing DNA inactivates the *E. coli* DNA polymerases, a **thermostable DNA polymerase** is used.
      (1) Thermostable DNA polymerase is isolated from thermophilic organisms that live in hot springs or deep sea thermal vents.
      (2) The use of a thermostable DNA polymerase allows for the **automation of PCR,** which is fast. A typical round of synthesis takes only 2–3 minutes.
   d. A computer-controlled heating and cooling block allows for repetitive rounds of synthesis, denaturation, primer annealing, and further synthesis.

3. **The amount of DNA is doubled for each round of synthesis.** Therefore, in 30 rounds, more than 1.0×10^9 copies may be made of a region of DNA from one molecule.

4. **Uses of PCR**
   a. **Diagnostic uses**
      (1) Genes in which particular mutations are known to cause a **disease** may be quickly amplified and sequenced.
      (2) PCR may be used to quickly detect **bacterial or viral infections.**
   b. **Forensic uses.** Known hypervariable regions in both nuclear and mitochondrial DNA obtained from the blood, semen, or hair of a victim or suspect may be amplified and sequenced. Enough DNA can be obtained from just one hair to amplify and sequence.

Case 11-1 Revisited

A number of different viruses are being developed as vectors for somatic cell gene therapy. Viruses may be engineered to become vectors by removing the genes that are required for their replication. In this manner, they are not infectious and will not cause harm to the patient. They have the advantage that, if their DNA is recombined with target DNA of interest and packaged into the viral protein coats, then they are taken up efficiently into the cells that they naturally infect. Retroviruses are one of the major vectors used in clinical trials to date. They have been engineered to have the genes needed for their replication removed. They can then carry up to 8000 base pairs of target DNA. When recombinant retroviral DNA is packaged into retroviral coat proteins, then they may be very efficiently taken up by a large number of different cells. When taken up by dividing cells, they often stably integrate into the host cell's genomic DNA. When integrated with the appropriate signals, the target DNA may be expressed.

An ADA cDNA clone is used because it lacks introns and is significantly smaller than the ADA gene itself. Only 8000 base pairs of target DNA may be carried in the retroviral vector. For expression, the ADA cDNA needs a eukaryotic promoter. In this case, the native ADA promoter was used. All other signals for full expression of a gene in a eukaryote are also needed: signals for efficient initiation of translation, initiation, and termination codons between the proper open reading frame for ADA; an intron; and a cleavage polyadenylation signal. The intron and cleavage polyadenylation signal are typically provided in the vector itself and are derived from another virus [e.g., simian virus (SV-40)].

The neomycin resistance gene is a selectable marker. In the presence of neomycin, only cells that have taken up the vector/ADA construct survive. The presence of the vector/ADA construct can be detected in different cell types either by a Southern transfer and hybridization with a labeled ADA cDNA or by PCR with appropriate primers specific for sequences contained only in the vector/ADA construct.

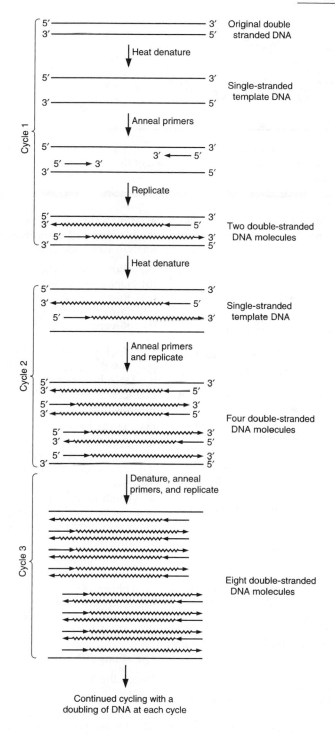

FIGURE 11-11. A region of DNA between two opposing primers may be amplified by the polymerase chain reaction (PCR). For each cycle, the DNA is first denatured with heat, the temperature is then lowered so that the primers (which are present at a very high concentration) may anneal to their complementary sequence, and thermostable DNA polymerase then initiates synthesis from each primer. After a short period of time, the synthesis passes the position of the opposing primer. The two duplexes formed are denatured with heat, and another cycle of DNA synthesis is begun. The process is automated, and the amount of DNA between each primer is doubled after each synthetic cycle.

▮ STUDY QUESTIONS

DIRECTIONS: Each of the numbered items or incomplete statements in this section is followed by answers or by completions of the statement. Select the **one** lettered answer or completion that is **best** in each case.

1. Which one of the following sequences is most likely to be a restriction enzyme recognition site?

(A) CGGC
(B) CGC
(C) GTAATG
(D) GTCGAC
(E) There is insufficient information

2. Restriction enzymes are best described by which one of the following statements?

(A) They ligate termini of recombinant DNA molecules
(B) They confer a selective advantage on invading bacteriophage
(C) They are enzymes that recognize and methylate specific DNA sequences
(D) They make sequence-specific cuts in both strands of duplex DNA
(E) They cleave 5'-terminal nucleotides from duplex DNA molecules

3. Insertional inactivation refers to which one of the following actions?

(A) The repression of a gene after it has been transformed and propagated in a host cell
(B) The killing of nontransformed host cells (i.e., those not containing a vector) by antibiotics
(C) The inactivation of a gene for a selectable marker after its coding sequence has been disrupted by the insertion of a target
(D) The inhibition of a gene's expression by an intercalator

4. Which step is first in the formation of a double-stranded complementary DNA (cDNA) target for cloning?

(A) Blunt-end ligation
(B) DNA-dependent DNA synthesis
(C) Restriction enzyme cleavage
(D) Primer annealing
(E) Reverse transcription

5. Which primers should be paired to amplify, by the polymerase chain reaction (PCR), the DNA between the two indicated sequences?

5'-GGAATTCGT---//---AATGCTACC-3'

(A) ACGAATTCC and AATCGTACC
(B) AATGCTACC and GGAATTCGT
(C) GGTAGCATT and GGAATTCGT
(D) ACGAATTCC and GGTAGCATT

6. Which method is used only to detect RNA and can be used to measure differences in levels of specific messenger RNAs (mRNAs) in different tissues?

(A) DNA fingerprint analysis
(B) Restriction fragment length polymorphism (RFLP) linkage analysis
(C) Southern blot analysis
(D) Polymerase chain reaction (PCR)
(E) Northern blot analysis

Questions 7-9

Match the following procedures to the proper element employed by the procedure.

(A) Bacteriophage lambda
(B) Dideoxynucleoside triphosphates
(C) Plasmids
(D) Ligase
(E) Reverse transcriptase

7. DNA sequencing
8. Creation of recombinant DNA molecules
9. Creation of genomic libraries

ANSWERS AND EXPLANATIONS

1. The answer is D [II A 2 a (3)]. Restriction enzyme recognition sequences are usually four, five, six, or occasionally eight base pairs in length. They typically exhibit twofold rotational (dyad) symmetry and are palindromic. Although the sequences CGGC and GTAATG are symmetrical, they are not palindromes. The sequences of their complement strands are GCCG and CATTAC, respectively. Both strands of GTCGAC are the same sequence when read in the 5′ to 3′ direction.

2. The answer is D [II A]. Restriction enzymes make sequence-specific cuts in both strands of duplex DNA. The cuts are usually made within the recognition sequence. This means that restriction enzymes are endonucleases and not exonucleases; therefore, they cannot cleave 5′-terminal nucleotides from duplex DNA molecules. Restriction enzymes evolved to restrict or prevent bacteriophage infection. They are not methylases. However, restriction enzymes associate with methylases that methylate a base within the same recognition site. This methylation protects the host cell's DNA from digestion by its own restriction enzyme. Restriction enzymes have no detectable reverse reaction, so they cannot ligate cohesive termini. Ligating cohesive termini is done by DNA ligase.

3. The answer is C [III C 1 a]. Insertional inactivation allows one to distinguish between a vector that has recircularized (i.e., returned to its normal circular structure) and does not contain a target insert and one that does contain a target insert.

4. The answer is D [III C 2]. The first step of complementary DNA (cDNA) cloning is to make a single-strand DNA copy of the messenger RNA (mRNA). This is done by first annealing a primer, usually oligodeoxythymidine (oligo dT), to the mRNA. With a primer annealed to the mRNA, reverse transcriptase uses the mRNA as a template and synthesizes DNA. The second strand is often synthesized by a DNA-dependent DNA polymerase. After blunt ends are formed by the action of a single-strand nuclease (e.g., S1 nuclease), linker DNA containing a restriction enzyme recognition site may be added by blunt-end ligation. After the linkers have been attached to the double-stranded cDNA, they are made into cohesive termini for cloning by cleavage with the appropriate restriction enzyme.

5. The answer is C [IV F 1]. The polymerase chain reaction (PCR) is a technique in which repetitive rounds of DNA synthesis between two primers are used to amplify DNA. Two opposing primers define the region of DNA to be amplified. One primer is complementary to one strand of DNA, and the other primer is complementary to the opposite strand of DNA. The orientation of each primer is such that when they base pair to their respective strands of DNA, their 3′-hydroxyl group faces each other. This assures that the synthesis initiated from each primer proceeds toward the opposing primer. The only primers that meet these conditions are GGTAGCATT and GGAATTCGT. (All sequences are written in the standard nucleic acid notation of 5′ to 3′.)

6. The answer is E [IV B]. A Northern blot analysis by definition detects RNA. Northern blot analysis is used primarily to detect and quantitate specific messenger RNAs (mRNAs) from different tissues. In Northern blot analysis, RNA is isolated and separated by electrophoresis in a denaturing agarose gel. Electrophoretically separated RNA is transferred from the gel to a piece of nitrocellulose paper. It is then hybridized with a specific labeled probe and exposed to a piece of radiographic film to detect the hybrid. A Southern blot analysis is a diagnostic technique used to detect specific sequences contained on a DNA fragment. The fragment is generated by restriction enzyme digestion within a mixture of all restriction enzyme fragments of a genome. DNA fingerprint analysis and restriction fragment length polymorphism (RFLP) are really Southern blot analyses that use specialized probes. In DNA fingerprint analysis, the probes detect individual specific, hypervariable regions that are made of variable number tandem repeats. RFLP probes detect restriction sites that are polymorphic. The polymerase chain reaction (PCR) is a technique in which repetitive rounds of DNA synthesis between two primers are used to amplify DNA. It also may be used to amplify mRNA if the first round of synthesis (cDNA) uses reverse transcriptase. All subsequent rounds of amplification can use DNA-dependent DNA polymerase.

7-9. The answers are: 7B [IV E 2 e], **8D** [III A 1 b (2)], **9A** [III B 2 b, D]. Dideoxynucleoside triphosphates (ddNTPs) are key elements of the Sanger or enzymatic method of DNA sequencing. A ddNTP corresponding to each base is used in each of four different reactions. A population of DNA chains is synthesized that terminates at each complementary base to the particular ddNTP used in the reaction, thus revealing a sequence.

A recombinant molecule refers to one formed by the covalent linkage of two pieces of DNA from different sources. DNA from different sources is covalently linked by DNA ligase.

Bacteriophage lambda has become the preferred vector for the establishment of genomic libraries.

Chapter 12

Regulation of Gene Expression
Donald Sittman

Case 12-1

A 61-year-old white man with no previous major medical problems is diagnosed with acute myeloid leukemia and referred to a hospital clinic for chemotherapy. The patient is initially treated with an intensive 7-day chemotherapy protocol using daunorubicin, cytarabine, and thioguanine. Although analysis of the patient's blood and bone marrow indicates no further detectable signs of acute myeloid leukemia (complete remission), the patient remains in remission for only 3 months. The patient is then treated with a postremission chemotherapy protocol of daunorubicin, cytarabine, and etoposide. The patient shows no further remission and dies within 1 month of his final therapy.

- What are the mechanisms of action of these chemotherapeutic drugs (see Chapters 8 and 27)?

- Why was the cancer resistant to the second round of chemotherapy even when another mechanistically unrelated drug was introduced into the protocol?

- What are possible explanations for the failure of some patients with cancers such as acute myeloid leukemia to respond to chemotherapy?

I. PROKARYOTES: THE OPERON MODEL FOR THE REGULATION OF GENE EXPRESSION

A. **Induction.** Based on genetic studies of the production of the enzymes involved in lactose metabolism, Jacob and Monod[1] proposed the operon model to explain gene induction in prokaryotes. Although there are many operons in bacterial cells, the lactose *(lac)* operon (see I C) discovered by Jacob and Monod is the classic example of all operons. Among the observations that led to their model was the finding that there were two kinds of genes.

1. **Inducible genes.** Some proteins are said to be inducible because they are produced only in significant amounts when a specific inducing substance (i.e., an **inducer**) is present. For example, the production of the enzyme β-galactosidase is induced by the presence of its substrate, lactose, in the medium.

2. **Constitutive genes** refer to prokaryotic genes whose **expression is not regulated.** The products of these genes are produced at a constant, often low, rate. Such genes are called constitutive genes, and their expression is said to be constitutive.

B. **Lactose metabolism in *Escherichia coli*.** In the absence of glucose, *E. coli* can use lactose, if present, as a source of carbon and energy.

1. **β-Galactosidase** is the key enzyme in the metabolism of lactose by *E. coli*. It catalyzes the following reaction:

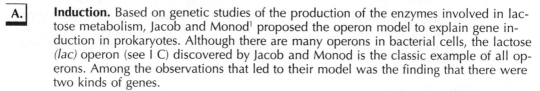

---

[1] Jacob F, Monod J: Genetic regulatory mechanisms in the synthesis of proteins. J Mol Biol 3:318–356, 1961.

Lactose   Galactose   Glucose

2. **Induction of β-galactosidase by lactose**
   a. In the **absence of lactose,** there are fewer than 10 molecules of β-galactosidase per cell.
   b. In the **presence of lactose,** and no other energy source, the number of β-galactosidase molecules can increase to 5000 molecules per cell within several minutes.

3. **Induction of associated enzymes.** As the level of β-galactosidase increases in the presence of lactose, the levels of two other enzymes coordinately increase as well (i.e., coordinate expression).
   a. **Galactoside permease** is a membrane-bound enzyme that transports lactose and other galactosides into the cell.
   b. **Thiogalactoside transacetylase** is an enzyme that catalyzes the transfer of an acetyl group from acetyl coenzyme A (acetyl CoA) to the hydroxyl group on the sixth carbon of a thiogalactoside in vitro. However, the function of thiogalactoside transacetylase in vivo is unknown.

4. **Inducer of β-galactosidase.** Because the addition of lactose to the medium induces the synthesis of β-galactosidase, galactoside permease, and thiogalactoside transacetylase, lactose was originally thought to be the inducer. However, the natural inducer turned out to be **allolactose.** Allolactose is a transglycosylated form of lactose produced as an intermediate in the hydrolysis of lactose by the few β-galactosidase molecules present in the cell during the noninduced state.

5. **Gratuitous inducers.** Some galactosides, such as **isopropylthiogalactoside (IPTG),** are strong inducers of β-galactosidase but do not act as substrates for the enzyme. Such substances are known as **gratuitous inducers** (also called **nonmetabolizable inducers**).

C. **Lactose *(lac)* operon**
   1. **Definition.** An operon is a group of coordinately regulated genes, the products of which typically catalyze a multi-enzyme metabolic pathway and their controlling elements. The purpose of the *lac* operon is to make the enzymes necessary to metabolize lactose (i.e., β-galactosidase and galactoside permease). **Two classes** of genes are needed to make a functional operon.
      a. The products of operons are produced by **structural genes.** Structural genes code for products that may be enzymes or, in fact, truly structural in nature, such as transfer RNA (tRNA), ribosomal RNA (rRNA), or ribosomal proteins. Structural gene products are essential for the life of the cell.
      b. **Regulatory genes** code for products that regulate the level of expression of structural genes. Although regulatory genes often are not considered part of operons because they can be located at sites remote from the structural genes they regulate, they are key elements of operons.
   2. **Structure of the *lac* operon** (Figure 12-1A). The *lac* operon is a region of DNA in the genome that contains the following (Figure 12-1).
      a. **Three linked, structural genes**
         (1) The *lacZ* gene codes for β-galactosidase.

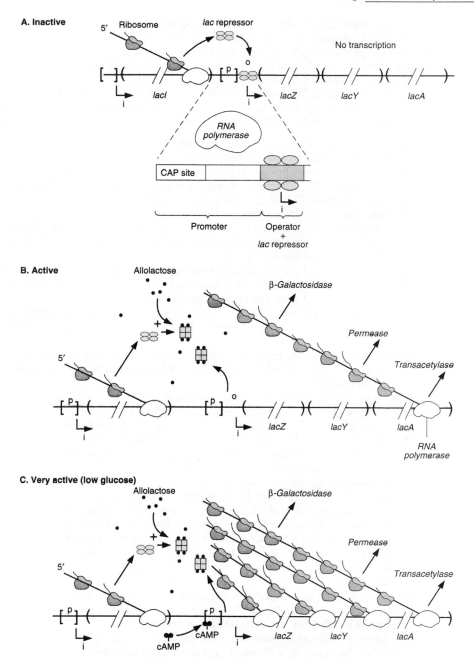

FIGURE 12-1. Diagram of an inactive, active, and very active lactose *(lac)* operon. The structural genes *(lacZ, lacY,* and *lacA),* the regulatory *lacI* gene, the promoter ([*p*]) region, and the operator *(o)* region are indicated. The initiation sites *(i)* of transcription are indicated with a *bent arrow. (A)* An expanded view of the control elements of the *lac* operon is shown for the inactive operon. The operator region spans the initiation site. The *lac* repressor binds to the operator and prevents RNA polymerase from binding to the promoter and initiating transcription. The CAP-binding site, labeled *CAP site,* is shown within the *lac* promoter. *(B)* In the active *lac* operon the inducer, allolactose, binds to the *lac* repressor, releasing it from the operator. RNA polymerase makes a polycistronic messenger RNA (mRNA), which is translated to form β-galactosidase, galactoside permease, and thiogalactoside transacetylase. *(C)* In the very active *lac* operon, the frequency of initiation of transcription events is increased over those shown in (B) by the interaction of a cAMP–CAP complex (which becomes abundant as glucose levels decline) with the CAP site within the promoter. *cAMP* = cyclic adenosine monophosphate; *CAP* = catabolite activator protein.

       (2) The *lacY* **gene** codes for galactoside permease.

       (3) The *lacA* **gene** codes for thiogalactoside transacetylase.

  b. A single **promoter** (see Chapter 9 II B 1) directs proper initiation of transcription. The *lacZ, lacY,* and *lacA* genes are expressed as a polycistronic message from this common promoter.

  c. An **operator** region lies adjacent to the promoter and spans the transcriptional initiation site. A regulatory protein called the *lac* **repressor** (see I C 3) binds to this site and blocks initiation of transcription.

3. Basic regulation of *lac* operon expression (see Figure 12-1A,B)

  a. Negative regulation by the *lac* repressor. In the absence of lactose, the cell has no need for the production of β-galactosidase and galactoside permease. A regulatory molecule, the *lac* repressor, **prevents expression of the *lac* operon in the absence of lactose.** This is an example of negative regulation.

    (1) Structure of the *lac* repressor. The *lac* repressor is a tetrameric protein, with each subunit having a binding site for an inducer. The *lac* repressor is a diffusible product of the regulatory *lacI* gene.

      (a) Structure of the *lacI* gene

        (i) The *lacI* gene is **adjacent to the *lac* operon.** Most regulatory genes of many operons are remote from the structural genes they regulate.

        (ii) The *lacI* gene has its own **promoter.**

      (b) Function of the *lacI* gene. The *lacI* gene is **constitutively expressed.** It maintains the very low level of *lac* repressor needed for the regulation of the *lac* operon.

    (2) Function of the *lac* repressor. In the absence of an inducer, the *lac* repressor binds tightly to the operator, which **blocks initiation of transcription of the structural genes.**

  b. Induction of expression. The presence of inducer—either IPTG or allolactose—relieves the negative regulation by the *lac* repressor.

    (1) Upon **binding of the inducer** to the *lac* repressor, the repressor undergoes a conformational change to a shape that no longer binds the operator tightly. With the repressor no longer blocking the initiation site, **RNA polymerase initiates transcription.**

    (2) Because prokaryotes do not have a nucleus, there is no physical structure such as a nuclear membrane to separate translation and transcription. Therefore, transcription and translation are coupled in prokaryotes. Ribosomes bind to the polycistronic *lac* messenger RNA (*lac* mRNA) and initiate **translation** even before transcription of the *lac* operon is complete.

    (3) The *lacZ, lacY,* and *lacA* cistrons are each translated independently; each has its own Shine-Dalgarno sequence (see Chapter 10 V A 2 a) and termination codon.

    (4) As long as lactose is present, then inducer is present, and transcription of the *lac* operon continues. The result is the continued **production of the enzymes needed for the metabolism of lactose.**

    (5) After the **inducer is removed,** expression of the *lac* operon stops quickly. This is because, as with most prokaryotic mRNAs, the *lac* mRNA is unstable and decays within minutes.

II.   **GENERAL CONTROL OF OPERONS.** The *lac* operon, as described, is said to be **inducible** and **negatively controlled.** The *lac* operon and other operons can be **positively controlled** as well; that is, a regulatory protein can act to promote or enhance transcription. Other operons are **repressible:** In repressible operons, a metabolite produced by the action of the gene products of the operon inhibits further expression of the operon by acting as a **corepressor.**

[Glucose]

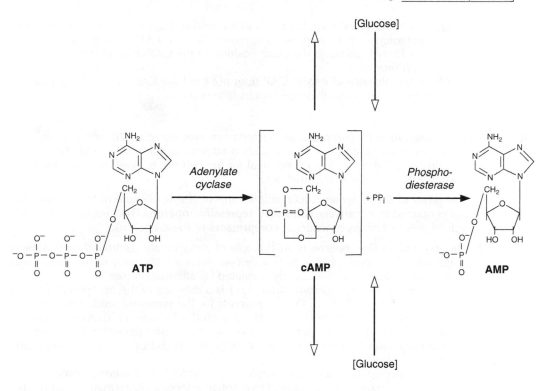

FIGURE 12-2. Formation of cyclic adenosine monophosphate (cAMP) by adenylate cyclase and its breakdown to AMP by phosphodiesterase. The formation and breakdown of cAMP in bacteria are linked to glucose levels. As the glucose concentration [*glucose*] increases, the cAMP level decreases and vice versa. *ATP* = adenosine triphosphate; *PP$_i$* = inorganic pyrophosphate.

A. **Positive control by catabolite repression.** Catabolic enzymes, such as β-galactosidase, galactokinase, and arabinose kinase, are expressed at very low levels when cells are grown in the presence of the preferred fuel source, glucose. This phenomenon is known as **catabolite repression.** The presence of glucose does not so much repress the expression of the operons of these catabolic enzymes as the absence of glucose tremendously enhances their expression.

1. **Cyclic adenosine monophosphate (cAMP)** is the intracellular signal that links the levels of glucose to the expression of catabolic operons.
   a. **Formation of cAMP.** cAMP is made from adenosine triphosphate (ATP) by **adenylate cyclase** and is degraded to AMP by **phosphodiesterase** (Figure 12-2; see also Chapter 15 II D 1).
   b. By a mechanism that is not entirely clear, the **levels of cAMP are inversely linked to the levels of glucose.**
      (1) As glucose levels increase, cAMP levels decrease.
      (2) As glucose levels decrease, cAMP levels increase.

2. **The catabolite activator protein (CAP) and cAMP stimulate transcription of catabolic operons** (see Figure 12-1C).
   a. **Structure of CAP.** CAP is a dimer with two identical 22.5-kdal subunits.
   b. **Function of CAP.** CAP [also called **cyclic AMP receptor protein (CRP)**] is a positive regulatory factor.
      (1) **In the presence of cAMP,** a cAMP–CAP–DNA complex forms that greatly enhances initiation of transcription at CAP-responsive promoters.

(2) The cAMP–CAP complex binds to a conserved sequence within or near the promoters of each responsive operon called the **CAP-binding site** (see Figure 12-1A), although the exact position of the CAP-binding site differs for each promoter.

(3) **In the absence of cAMP,** CAP does not bind the CAP site, and initiation of transcription from these promoters is very low.

B. **Negative regulation by corepression.** Bacteria can synthesize all 20 amino acids. However, bacterial synthesis of amino acids is often a complex time- and energy-consuming process. Therefore, it is economical for the cell not to synthesize an amino acid when it is available in the medium.

1. The **genes of the enzymes** responsible for the synthesis of many of the amino acids are contained in **negatively controlled repressible operons.** The amino acid products of these enzymes function as **corepressors** of these operons.

2. The **tryptophan (trp) operon** is an example of a negatively controlled repressible operon in which tryptophan acts as a corepressor. As with many of the amino acid biosynthetic operons, it also can be regulated by attenuation (see III).
   a. **Structure of the *trp* operon.** Figure 12-3 is a diagram of the *trp* operon. Five structural genes—A, B, C, D, and E—code for the enzymes needed to synthesize tryptophan from chorismic acid. As with the *lac* operon, there is an **operator sequence** in the *trp* operon that overlaps the transcriptional initiation site.
   b. A ***trp* repressor** is coded for by the ***trpR* gene,** which lies at a site remote from the *trp* operon.
      (1) The *trp* repressor forms a complex with tryptophan, the corepressor.
      (2) The *trp* repressor with bound tryptophan adopts a conformation that binds tightly to the *trp* operator causing the inhibition of initiation.
      (3) In the absence of tryptophan, the *trp* repressor does not bind to the *trp* operator, and transcription can proceed.
      (4) Therefore, the level of tryptophan determines the amount of tryptophan that is synthesized, by acting as a corepressor of the *trp* operon.

III. **CONTROL BY ATTENUATION.** The *trp* operon and other amino acid biosynthetic operons have another method of regulation that again couples their expression to the amount of amino acid product available. This method of regulation is called **attenuation,** and it can take place only in prokaryotes because of the coupling of transcription and translation.

A. The **fundamental feature** of attenuation as exemplified by the *trp* operon is that, at low tryptophan concentrations, the operon makes full-length mRNA; but, at high tryptophan concentrations, transcription is prematurely terminated.

B. The **position of the ribosome,** which attaches to the mRNA just after transcription has begun, determines whether or not a termination stem-loop structure (see Chapter 9 II C 1 a) forms before transcription proceeds into the structural genes (Figure 12-4).

1. Preceding the five structural genes is a **leader peptide sequence.** There are **two adjacent tryptophan codons** within this sequence.
   a. The **leader sequence** codes for a small, nonfunctional peptide. Leader sequences are common to all of the amino acid biosynthetic operons that regulate by attenuation.
   b. Leader sequences typically have more codons for the regulating amino acid than does the *trp* operon. For instance, there are seven adjacent histidine codons in the leader peptide sequence of the histidine operon.

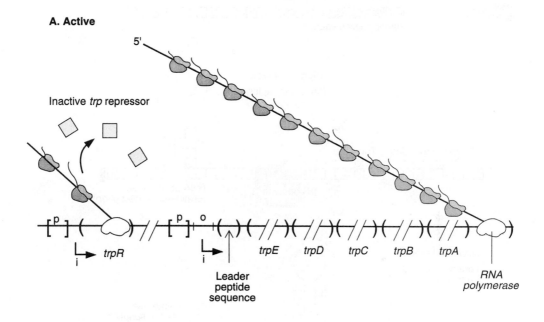

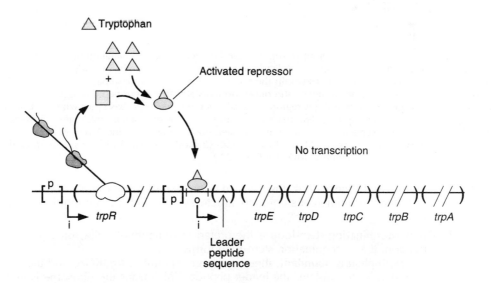

FIGURE 12-3. Diagram of an active and an inactive tryptophan (*trp*) operon. The five structural genes coding for the synthesis of the enzymes that synthesize tryptophan are labeled *trp A–E*. The promoter (*p*) and operator (*o*) regions are as indicated. The initiation sites of transcription are indicated with a *bent arrow*. The gene *trpR*, which produces the *trp* repressor, is remote from the site of the operon. When the *trp* repressor is inactive (▨), the operon is actively transcribed. In the presence of tryptophan (△), the repressor becomes active (⟁), binds to the operator, and blocks the initiation of transcription.

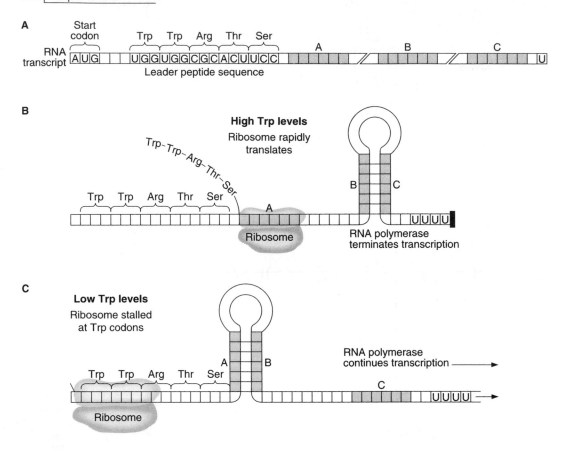

FIGURE 12-4. Regulation of the tryptophan (*trp*) operon by attenuation. *(A)* Diagram of the messenger RNA (mRNA) produced by the *trp* operon. A leader peptide sequence contains two adjacent tryptophan codons. Just downstream are sequences within the mRNA (A,B,C) that can base pair and form stem-loops (A-B or B-C). *(B)* At high tryptophan levels, the ribosome translates the leader peptide sequence rapidly and overlaps the sequences within the A region. This allows the B region to base pair with the C region. The B-C stem-loop is a transcriptional termination codon. *(C)* At low tryptophan levels, the ribosome stalls within the leader peptide sequence. A nonterminating stem-loop forms when the A region base pairs with the B region. (Adapted from Marks D, Marks A, and Smith C: *Basic Medical Biochemistry: a clinical approach.* Williams & Wilkins, Baltimore, MD, 1996, p 222.)

2. The **mRNA sequences** just downstream of the leader peptide sequence can base pair to form two different stem-loop structures; one of these can terminate transcription.

3. The **nonterminating stem-loop** is the preferred structure. If a ribosome blocks its formation, then a termination stem-loop forms.

   a. **If tryptophan is abundant,** there is a large amount of *trp* tRNA, and the ribosome quickly translates the leader peptide. This means the ribosome is near the RNA polymerase. This positioning of the ribosome makes the mRNA favor the formation of a stem-loop that terminates transcription.

   b. **If tryptophan is not abundant,** there are low levels of *trp* tRNA, and translation of the leader sequence stalls. Because the ribosome is not farther along the mRNA, an alternate, nonterminating stem-loop forms in the mRNA. When the ribosome moves forward, the nonterminating stem-loop allows transcription to proceed beyond the point that it can be terminated.

   c. In the **absence of premature termination,** the ribosome translates, albeit at a slower rate, the whole polycistronic mRNA and produces the enzymes needed to synthesize more tryptophan.

IV. INTRODUCTION TO REGULATION OF GENE EXPRESSION IN EUKARYOTES

A. **Complexity of eukaryotes.** Eukaryotes, and particularly mammals, are considerably more complex than prokaryotes. To maintain this complexity, there is a **need for greater gene regulatory capacity.**

1. The **structure of eukaryotic cells** is considerably more complex than that of prokaryotes.
   a. Mammals, in particular, have many cell types that differ considerably in both structure and function.
   b. Although they may differ considerably, all cells contain identical DNA sequences and arise from cells with identical DNA sequences.

2. The **increased cellular complexity** of eukaryotes is reflected in an **increased genetic capacity** (see Chapter 6 II E). For instance, humans have considerably more DNA per haploid cell (3.3×10^9 base pairs) than does *E. coli* (4.2×10^6). The increased cell complexity and increased complexity of cellular processes means there are more levels at which gene regulation can be exerted.

B. As a consequence of the increased complexity of gene regulation in eukaryotes, there is an **increased number of regulatory sites** where disruption can lead to disease or medical problems. Advances in recombinant DNA technology (see Chapter 11) have greatly increased the ability to diagnose disease processes that affect various levels of gene expression and to design therapeutic strategies to treat many genetic diseases.

V. TRANSCRIPTIONAL REGULATION. The major method of regulation in eukaryotes is transcriptional regulation, which is **manifested at two levels** in eukaryotes.

A. **Chromosome packaging** (see Chapter 6 III B). Eukaryotic cells are able to regulate a large area of chromosomes containing many genes (as opposed to individual genes) through chromosome packaging. Few details are known about the signals that regulate chromosome packaging.

1. **Accessibility of transcription.** Whole chromosomes or regions of chromosomes can be made inaccessible to the transcription "machinery" and regulatory factors (see V B 1–2) through the formation of inactive **heterochromatin** (see Chapter 6 III B 4). Likewise, whole regions of chromosomes can be made accessible to transcription through the formation of active **euchromatin** (see Chapter 6 III B 4).

2. **Barr bodies.** A dramatic example of gene inactivation through the tight packaging of DNA into heterochromatin is seen with the formation of Barr bodies.
   a. **Dosage compensation.** In all cells of human females, one of the X chromosomes is made transcriptionally inactive through heterochromatinization (Lyon hypothesis).
   b. **Appearance of Barr bodies.** The inactive X chromosomes are called Barr bodies, and they are small, darkly staining structures near the nuclear membrane.

3. **Maintenance specific to cell types.** Although the process is much less dramatic than the heterochromatinization of a whole chromosome, different regions of different chromosomes may be maintained as transcriptionally inactive heterochromatin in a cell-specific manner. An example of this is the globin genes in pre- and nonerythroid cell lines.

4. **Methylation of eukaryotic DNA** may play a role in the maintenance of inactive heterochromatin.
   a. In eukaryotes, the cytosines on both strands of cytosine–guanine (CG) doublets may be methylated (Figure 12-5).

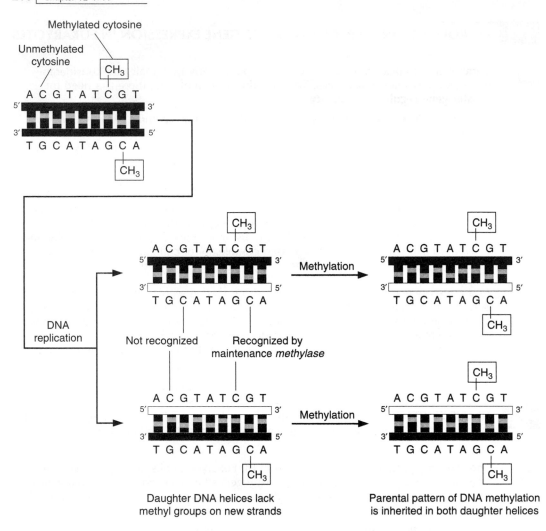

FIGURE 12-5. Maintenance of methylated cytosines in cytosine–guanine (CG) doublets in eukaryotes. (Reprinted with permission from Alberts B, Bray D, Lewis J, et al: *Molecular Biology of the Cell,* 3rd ed. New York, Garland Publishing, 1994, p 450.)

   b. A **maintenance methylase** assures that the methylation pattern of DNA is maintained during replication.
   c. Evidence that methylation plays a role in the maintenance of inactive heterochromatin:
      (1) Correlative evidence
         (a) CG doublets in inactive heterochromatin are often methylated.
         (b) CG doublets in active euchromatin are often unmethylated.
      (2) Experimental evidence
         (a) A drug that inhibits the action of maintenance methylase causes the activation of previously inactive genes.
         (b) Genes on Barr bodies can be reactivated by inhibiting the maintenance methylase during replication.

B. **Individual gene regulation.** The transcriptional regulation of individual genes in eukaryotes is fundamentally similar to the transcriptional regulation of operons in prokaryotes. The major difference is that in eukaryotes the number of DNA sequence elements and regulatory factors is considerably larger than in prokaryotes.

1. **General requirements for transcriptional initiation.** All eukaryotic genes require **promoter elements** (see Chapter 9 II B 1 c) and **transcription factors** (see Chapter 9 II B 2 b) to initiate transcription. Although availability of these general factors affects transcription, they are not regulatory factors for individual genes.

2. **Regulatory factors.** More than 100 different proteins have been identified that either interact with specific DNA regulatory sequences or that have been shown to play a direct role in the regulation of gene transcription. These proteins have one or more structural domains where each domain plays a different role in the regulation of transcription.

   a. **The DNA-binding domains** are responsible for recognizing and binding the regulatory factors to specific DNA regulatory sequences (see V B 3).

      (1) DNA-binding domains often share common structural features, although they differ in amino acid sequence so they can recognize different DNA-binding sequences.

      (2) DNA-binding domains are often dimeric and bind DNA regulatory sequences that exhibit dyad symmetry.

   b. **Transcription-activating domains** interact with other proteins in the transcription complex to enhance transcription. A few of these domains share structural features that allow them to associate with the activating domains of other regulatory factors or to interact with general transcription factors and RNA polymerase.

   c. **Antirepressor.** Nucleosomes (see Chapter 6 III B 2) exhibit an inhibitory effect on transcription, presumably by blocking access of various transcription factors to the DNA. Antirepressor domains of some regulatory factors interact with histones to remove this inhibitory effect.

   d. **Ligand-binding domains.** Steroid and thyroid hormones (see Chapter 15 III C) as well as retinoic acid are known to activate transcription. They bind to the ligand-binding domains of specific regulatory factors, which are also known as **intracellular receptors.**

      (1) These receptors also have DNA sequence-specific binding domains and transcription-activating domains.

      (2) The binding of the ligand induces the receptor to become a positive regulatory factor.

3. **Gene regulatory sequences.** At some point in the transcriptional regulation of genes, the regulatory factors must interact with specific DNA regulatory sequences.

   a. **Regulatory sequences are not promoters,** because they do not affect the accuracy of initiation. In conjunction with the appropriate regulatory factors, they affect the rate of transcription.

   b. Gene regulatory sequences can be classified into **two types,** although the two types share many features, and some sequences fall between the two types.

      (1) **Enhancers** were so named because they were initially observed to be required for an increase in the rate of transcription of many genes. **Common features** of enhancers include the following.

         (a) **Structure.** Enhancers consist of multiple elements within a several hundred base pair region. These elements within enhancers are often short sequences in the range of 10–20 base pairs long. Many of these enhancer elements exhibit **dyad symmetry** [see Chapter 11 II A 2 a (2)].

         (b) **Function**

            (i) Enhancers are functional either **upstream or downstream**—and even at **great distances** (up to 50 kb)—from the initiation site.

            (ii) They are *cis*-acting (i.e., they must be linked to the gene).

            (iii) Their activity is **independent** of their orientation relative to the gene.

            (iv) Although they are called enhancers, some have been found to **lead to a repression** of transcription.

      (2) **Response elements** are regulatory sequences that are common to a group of genes. They coordinate the regulation of these genes. These sequences share many of the features of enhancers, except that they are usually found within 250 base pairs upstream of the initiation site. Because of their rela-

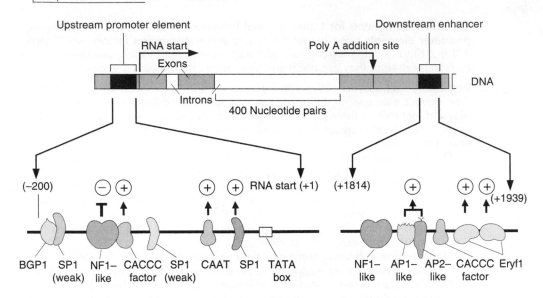

FIGURE 12-6. The regulatory factors and sequence elements involved in the regulation of the expression of the chicken β-globin gene. *Poly A* = polyadenylate. (Reprinted with permission from Alberts B, Bray D, Lewis J, et al: *Molecular Biology of the Cell,* 2nd ed. New York, Garland Publishing, 1989, p 567.)

tive closeness to promoters, response elements also may be called **promoter-proximal elements.** Some genes regulated by response elements are:

    (a) Steroid hormone-regulated genes. Particular steroids, and their receptors, interact with specific steroid hormone response elements to coordinately regulate the expression of all genes that have the specific hormone response element.

    (b) Heat shock response genes. A heat shock transcription factor is activated, upon heat shock or another cellular stress, to induce transcription of a group of genes by interacting with their heat shock response element.

  4. Mechanism of eukaryotic transcriptional regulation. The mechanism of transcriptional regulation of eukaryotic genes is not understood to the same extent as for prokaryotic genes. However, two generalizations about eukaryotic gene regulation can be made.

    a. Many regulatory factors and sequence elements are involved in the regulation of any one gene (Figure 12-6).

      (1) Many of the factors and sequence elements are common to multiple genes. However, many of the factors are known to **work in combination.** The combination of factors and sequences used to regulate any one gene may be unique to that gene.

      (2) Some factors **work as heterodimers.** That is, one part from each of two separate dimeric regulatory factors may work in conjunction to effectively form a new **regulatory factor.**

    b. Because of the distance of many regulatory sequences from the promoter, **DNA bending** is likely a component of eukaryotic transcriptional regulation (Figure 12-7).

VI.   **POST-TRANSCRIPTIONAL REGULATION** is a major type of regulation in eukaryotes. Post-transcriptional processing of mRNA is much more extensive in eukaryotes than in prokaryotes (see Chapter 9 III B 2). There are two major levels at which post-transcriptional regulation takes place.

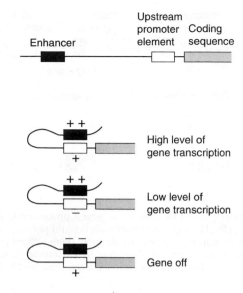

FIGURE 12-7. Regulation of a hypothetical eukaryotic gene by the interaction of different regulatory factors with upstream regulatory and promoter elements. Positive (+) and negative (−) regulatory factors work in combination to modulate the expression of a gene. Proteins bound to distant sites interact with each other. This is likely made possible by the bending of DNA between the different sites. (Reprinted with permission from Alberts B, Bray D, Lewis J, et al: *Molecular Biology of the Cell,* 2nd ed. New York, Garland Publishing, 1989, p 566.)

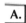 **Alternative splicing.** Many eukaryotic genes are known to be able to produce varied products by the process of alternative splicing.

1. **Isoforms.** Depending on which exons are retained in splicing, the same gene can produce related but different proteins in different cell types. These related products are often called isoforms.

2. An **example of alternative splicing** producing a different product in different cell types is shown in Figure 12-8.
   a. In the thyroid gland, the calcitonin gene produces a transcript that codes for the hormone **calcitonin,** which is involved in calcium regulation.
   b. The same gene is expressed in neurons and produces a transcript that codes for **calcitonin gene-related peptide,** which plays a role in taste.
   c. The **mRNAs** coding for these two products have the same first two coding exons. They differ in which codon is used in the third coding exon position.
   d. As shown in Figure 12-8, the **polyadenylation (poly A) site** may differ as well.

3. The **mechanism** through which alternative splicing is regulated is unknown.

B. **Regulation of RNA stability.** Alterations in RNA stability may make a considerable contribution to gene regulation in eukaryotes. Regulation of RNA stability may operate in either the **nucleus** or the **cytoplasm.**

1. **Nucleus.** Some genes are known to produce heterogeneous nuclear RNA (hnRNA), which, in some cells, is never processed to mRNA and transported to the cytoplasm. These transcripts are degraded in the nucleus before they can be processed.

2. **Cytoplasm.** The stability of the mRNA can control the availability of the mRNA for translation in the cytoplasm.
   a. **Variations in mRNA stability.** The mRNAs of different genes may vary considerably in their half-lives.

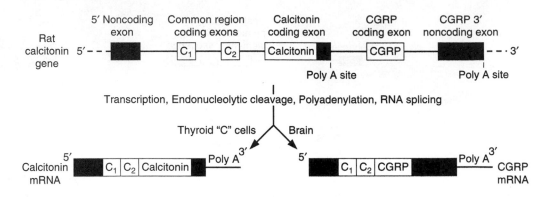

FIGURE 12-8. The primary transcript from the calcitonin gene is processed to produce a message that codes for calcitonin in thyroid cells. Through alternative splicing and polyadenylation (poly A), the same primary transcript is processed in neurons to produce calcitonin gene-related protein (*CGRP*). *mRNA* = messenger RNA. (Reprinted with permission from Rosenfeld MG, Mermod JJ, Amara SG, et al: Production of a novel neuropeptide encoded by the calcitonin gene via tissue-specific RNA processing. *Nature* 304:129–135, 1983.)

    (1) Some genes that code for an **abundant product with a long duration of action,** such as the β-globin gene, may produce mRNA that has a **long half-life.** (The half-life of β-globin mRNA is approximately 10 hours.)

    (2) Other genes that code for a **product with a short duration of action,** such as those of the growth factors, may produce mRNA that has a **short half-life.** (Many growth factor mRNAs have half-lives of less than 1 hour.)

    (3) Sequences within the 3′ untranslated region of unstable mRNAs that are responsible for their rapid degradation have been identified.

    (4) There is also a strong correlation between the length of the poly A tail and the half-life of an mRNA: The longer the poly A tail, the longer the half-life of the mRNA.

  b. Examples of gene regulation by changes in the stability of the mRNA

    (1) **Histone mRNA stability** varies considerably depending on whether the cells are in the S phase of the cell cycle (see Chapter 8 III E). Histone gene expression is under dual control. The rate of transcription of the histone genes changes during the cell cycle as well.

      (a) **During S phase,** histones are abundantly produced to package the newly synthesized DNA into nucleosomes. Histone mRNA is stable in the S phase for several hours.

      (b) **After S phase,** when DNA is not being synthesized, cells produce only small amounts of histones, because they are not needed for packaging DNA. When there is no DNA synthesis, histone mRNA has a half-life of only 10–15 minutes.

    (2) **Iron-dependent regulation of transferrin receptor (TfR) mRNA levels.** Transferrin is a bloodborne iron carrier protein. If iron levels within a cell are low, the cell produces more TfRs that facilitate the uptake of iron into the cell. TfR levels are regulated at the level of stability of their mRNA (Figure 12-9 A).

      (a) TfR mRNA has some stem-loop structures, called **iron response elements (IREs),** within its 3′ untranslated region (see Chapter 6 IV B 2) that signal the mRNA to be rapidly degraded.

      (b) A protein called **iron response element binding protein (IRE-BP)** binds to IREs. When bound to the TfR IREs, this protein prevents the rapid degradation of the TfR mRNA.

*Level of
regulation*

A. mRNA Stability

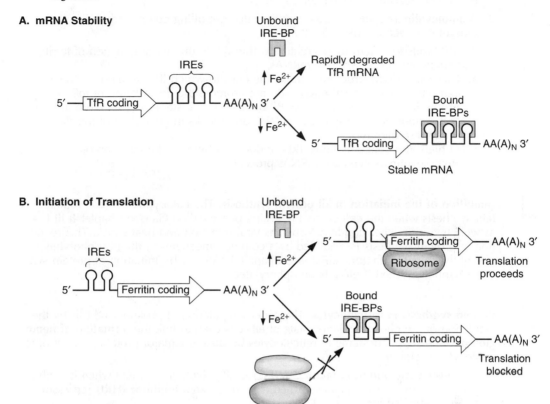

B. Initiation of Translation

FIGURE 12-9. Regulation by the iron response element binding protein (IRE-BP). (*A*) Transferrin messenger RNA (mRNA) stability. At low cytoplasmic levels of iron the IRE-BPs bind to the iron response elements (IREs) in the 3′ ends of transferrin receptor (TfR) mRNA. This binding prevents the TfR mRNA from the rapid degradation signaled by the unbound (high iron levels) IREs in the 3′ end of TfR mRNA. (*B*) Initiation of translation. At low iron levels IRE-BP binds to IREs in the 5′ end of ferritin mRNA. The presence of bound IRE-BP at the 5′ end of ferritin mRNA prevents the initiation of translation of this mRNA. When unbound (high iron levels), the 5′ IREs have no effect on the initiation of translation of ferritin mRNA.

      (c) Iron regulates whether IRE-BP binds to mRNA.
         (i) At low iron concentrations IRE-BP binds and stabilizes TfR mRNA. This leads to the production of more TfR, which leads to an increase in the intracellular iron levels.
        (ii) At high iron concentrations IRE-BP does not bind TfR mRNA. TfR mRNA is degraded, and the iron levels decrease as TfR levels decrease.

VII.   **TRANSLATIONAL REGULATION.** Although it is not a major method of regulation in eukaryotes, translational regulation is known to occur.

A.   **Inhibition of the translation of specific mRNAs.** Interestingly, the IRE-BP [see VI B 2 b (2) (b)] also regulates the levels of two other mRNAs whose products play a role in iron metabolism (Figure 12-9 B).

1. Free Fe^{3+} is toxic to the cell. It is therefore stored in the cell in combination with the protein **ferritin** (see Chapter 25 VII C).

2. **Aminolevulinate synthase** catalyzes the rate-controlling committed step in heme biosynthesis (see Chapter 25 VII A 1).

3. IRE-BP binds to a stem-loop structure within the 5′ untranslated region of ferritin and aminolevulinate synthase mRNAs.

   a. These stem-loop structures, unlike the ones to which IRE-BP binds in the 3′ untranslated region of TfR mRNA, do not promote the degradation of mRNA.

   b. At low iron concentrations, IRE-BP binds to the 5′ stem-loop structure in ferritin and aminolevulinate synthase mRNAs and blocks the initiation of translation from these mRNAs.

   c. At high iron concentrations, IRE-BP does not bind, and translation of ferritin and aminolevulinate synthase mRNAs proceeds.

B. **Inhibition of the initiation of all protein synthesis.** The eukaryotic cell can reduce protein synthesis when the cell enters the resting phase called G_O (see Chapter 8 III E 4) as well as during other conditions such as viral infection and heat shock. This reduction in protein synthesis is mediated by a common mechanism, the phosphorylation of one of the initiation factors, eIF-2 (see Chapter 10 VI A 1 b). Initiation of protein synthesis cannot proceed if eIF-2 is phosphorylated.

C. **Protein synthesis in reticulocytes.** The general regulation of protein synthesis by the regulation of the phosphorylation state of eIF-2 is used to link the **formation of hemoglobin** to the supply of heme in reticulocytes because the major protein product of reticulocytes is globin.

1. The **eukaryotic initiation factor 2 (eIF-2)** is effectively inactivated when it is phosphorylated by a protein kinase called **heme-regulated inhibitor (HRI) repressor** or **heme-controlled inhibitor (HCI).**

2. In the absence of an adequate supply of heme to justify the production of globin, HRI is active and phosphorylates eIF-2, therefore causing the inhibition of protein synthesis.

3. When present, heme prevents the activation of HRI so eIF-2 is not phosphorylated. Protein synthesis then proceeds in reticulocytes, and globin is synthesized as long as heme is abundant.

D. Because of the nuclear membrane and the consequent separation of transcription from translation into different cellular compartments, **there is no regulation by attenuation in eukaryotes** (see Chapter 12 III).

VIII. **ALTERATIONS IN GENE CONTENT OR POSITION.** The eukaryotic genome shows a high degree of plasticity (i.e., it is not a fixed, immobile structure; it can move, be amplified, and be lost), which may play a role in the regulation of some genes, as well as increase genetic diversity. The plasticity of the human genome also plays a role in the development of some cancers and drug resistance.

A. **Gene amplification.** A regulatory approach that eukaryotic cells may use in some circumstances to increase production of a gene product is to increase the number of genes coding for that product. Many genes with products that are often needed in large amounts, such as histones and rRNAs, are present in all cells in a permanently amplified state (see Chapter 6 II E 2 a). However, some genes that normally exist in a low copy number are able, in some cells such as highly mutable cancer cells, to undergo selective gene amplification.

1. This amplification can be either fragments of DNA containing a gene outside of the genome (these **extrachromosomal pieces of DNA** are often called **double minute chromosomes**) or multiple tandem duplications of genes within the chromosome.

2. **Size of amplified region.** The region of DNA that becomes amplified is typically much larger than the gene it contains. It can be in the range of 100–1000 kb in size. Thousand-fold amplifications of genes have been observed.

3. **More than 20 genes** can be amplified. For example:
   a. **Dihydrofolate reductase (DHFR) gene.** Methotrexate is an antifolate drug that inhibits DHFR (see Chapter 26 V B) and is used to treat leukemia and some tumors. After prolonged treatment, some cells become resistant to methotrexate by amplifying their DHFR genes and producing more DHFR than can be inhibited by methotrexate.
   b. **Metallothionein gene.** Metallothionein is a low-molecular-weight protein that binds heavy metals such as copper, mercury, zinc, and cadmium.
      (1) The binding of heavy metals to metallothionein **protects cells from heavy metal toxicity.**
      (2) In response to increasing amounts of heavy metals, some cells amplify their metallothionein genes.
   c. **Multidrug resistance gene.** This gene produces a large membrane-bound glycoprotein that confers resistance to many antineoplastic drugs by pumping them out of the cell in an adenosine triphosphate (ATP)-dependent manner.
      (1) Some cells can become resistant to many unrelated antineoplastic drugs by amplifying this gene.
      (2) Because this gene confers resistance to multiple drugs, a particular chemotherapeutic treatment may lead to resistance to a drug that has never been used on the patient.

B. **Diminution** is a rare form of regulation that completely inactivates genes by removing them from the genome. An extreme example of diminution is the loss of all genes in a red blood cell precursor through the loss of the nucleus during red blood cell development.

1. The amplification of genes (see VIII A) is **unstable** and may be lost in succeeding generations. Double minute chromosomes are particularly unstable from one generation to the next. Double minute chromosomes do not undergo equal mitotic separation as do whole chromosomes. Therefore, if they are not selected for, they can be lost due to unequal dilution or separation during mitosis.

2. The **loss of DNA** is coupled to the gene rearrangements that generate new antibody genes (see VIII C). In particular, the deletion of switch sites [see VIII C 4 c (2) (b)] may ensure that a certain lymphocyte always produces a specific immunoglobulin class.

C. **Gene rearrangements.** Effective cellular immunity requires the production of a large number of antibodies with different antigenic specificities. There is an insufficient number of genes to account for the diversity of antibodies produced by B cells. **Gene rearrangement is a mechanism that plays a major role in the generation of antibody diversity.** [Before reading this section, it is important to review the structure and action of antibodies (see Chapter 3 IV).]

1. **Overview of the organization of immunoglobulin genes.** Immunoglobulin genes are arranged in three different families with each family consisting of a complex of genes. **Each gene family is located at a distinct genetic locus on different chromosomes.** The immunoglobulin genes within each locus are actually partial genes that rearrange to form a complete gene.
   a. **Light-chain (L) gene families.** Light chains can be formed from one of two light-chain gene families.
      (1) **The kappa light-chain (L_κ) gene family** is found in a locus on chromosome 2.

    (2) The lambda light-chain (L$_\lambda$) gene family is found in a locus on chromosome 22.

  b. All of the heavy-chain (H) immunoglobulin gene classes are found in one locus on chromosome 14.

  c. Separation of genomic information. In each of the loci, the DNA that codes for the majority of the variable (V) domains is very far removed from the sequences coding for the rest of the immunoglobulin chain.

2. Light chain formation. A complete gene coding for an L$_\kappa$ is created in a single DNA rearrangement event (Figure 12-10).

  a. Organization of the genes for the L$_\kappa$

    (1) Variable (V) regions. There are approximately **300 partial, variable kappa light-chain (V$_\kappa$) genes.**

      (a) Each of the 300 partial V$_\kappa$ genes codes for the signal peptide sequence that directs protein synthesis of the light chain endoplasmic reticulum (see Chapter 10 VII B) and a unique sequence for the first 95 amino acids of the variable portion of the light chain, which has 108 amino acids.

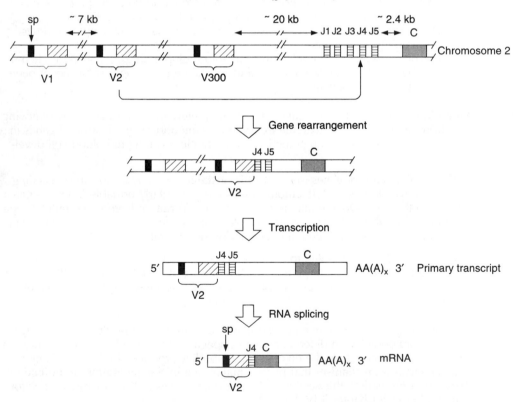

FIGURE 12-10. Example of the formation of a kappa light-chain (L$_\kappa$) immunoglobulin gene. A single DNA rearrangement moves one of the partial, variable light-chain genes *(V2)* immediately upstream of one of the joining regions of the kappa light-chain (J$_\kappa$) genes *(J4)*. Each of the partial variable light-chain genes contains an exon that codes for a signal peptide *(sp)*. Splicing of the primary transcript of this newly formed light-chain gene removes the intervening sequence (i.e., intron), which includes the sequences that code for J5 from V2 to J4 and the exon that codes for the constant *(C)* domain. The intron between the exon that codes for the signal peptide and the exon that codes for the variable light-chain domain is also removed by splicing. Translation of this mRNA is directed to the endoplasmic reticulum. *mRNA = messenger RNA.*

(b) Each of the partial genes is separated by about 7 kb of DNA.

(2) The remaining 13 amino acid codons of the V_κ genes are in any one of 5 different genes for the joining regions of the kappa light-chain **(J_κ) genes** located 20 kb away from the cluster of 300 partial V_κ genes.

(3) The J_κ genes are separated by a 2.4-kb intron from the exon coding for the constant (C) portion of the light chain.

b. V-J joining. A **recombination event** moves one of the partial V_κ genes immediately upstream of any one of the J_κ genes by a mechanism that is not entirely understood. This event is called V-J joining, and it **creates a complete exon for the variable region of a light chain.**

c. The **complete V_κ exon** is separated by the large 2.4-kb intron from the exon that codes for the constant portion of the light chain.

d. Imprecision of V-J joining increases variable light-chain diversity.

(1) When V-J joining occurs, imprecise joining of the 95th codon to the 96th codon leads to a 96th codon that can specify any one of three different amino acids.

(2) Unfortunately, imprecise joining means that two out of three V-J joining events leads to a frameshift mutation (see Chapter 8 V B 2 a). Cells that produce a nonfunctional light chain, because of a frameshift mutation, are lost from the cell population because they cannot become activated (see VIII C 4 b).

e. A total of **4500 different sequence combinations** can result from the single DNA rearrangement event that forms the variable light-chain exon (i.e., 1 of 300 partial V_κ genes combined with 1 of 5 J_κ genes and the generation of a codon that can specify 1 of 3 amino acids; $300 \times 5 \times 3 = 4500$).

f. A similar DNA rearrangement event generates the many L_λ found in humans.

3. **Heavy chain formation.** Greater diversity is generated in the formation of immunoglobulin heavy chains than in light chain formation. Two DNA rearrangement events, between three partial variable heavy-chain genes, generate a single variable heavy-chain (V_H) exon (Figure 12-11).

a. Organization of the genes for the variable exon of the heavy chain

(1) Much like the partial V_κ genes, there are approximately 300 partial V_H genes in humans located in a cluster separate from the genes coding for the remainder of the heavy-chain sequences.

(2) These partial V_H genes all code for a signal peptide sequence and a unique sequence of fewer than 100 amino acids of the V_H domain.

(3) Similar to the V_κ genes, there are 4 J_H genes that code for 4–6 amino acids of the V_H domain.

(4) Between the V_H and J_H genes is an additional cluster of approximately 30 partial genes that code for 2–13 amino acids of the V_H domain. These genes are called **D (diversity) genes.**

b. V_H-D-J_H joining. A joining of one partial gene from each of these three regions, called V_H-D-J_H joining, forms a complete exon that codes for the V_H domain of the heavy chain. **V_H-D-J_H joining takes place in two steps.**

(1) The **first recombination event** moves a single D gene immediately upstream of a J_H gene.

(2) A **second recombination event** then moves a V_H gene immediately upstream of the newly formed D-J_H gene.

c. Imprecision in V_H-D-J_H joining also generates different codons, as in V_κ-J_κ joining.

(1) **Further diversity** arises from the addition of up to 30 random nucleotides to the D-J_H junction or the V_H-D junction upon V_H-D-J_H joining. These additions are catalyzed by an enzyme called **terminal deoxynucleotidyl transferase.**

(a) This event allows the addition of up to 10 new codons.

(b) Frameshift mutations may occur by the random addition of these nucleotides.

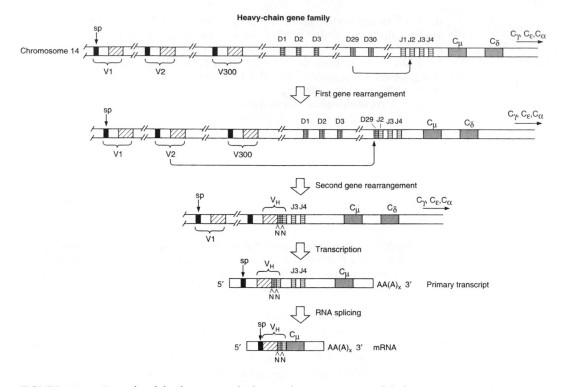

FIGURE 12-11. Example of the formation of a heavy-chain (H) immunoglobulin gene. Heavy-chain gene formation takes place by joining a partial variable region of the heavy (V_H) chain, the diversity (D) region, and the joining region of the heavy chain (J_H), which requires two DNA rearrangements. In the *first gene rearrangement,* one of approximately 30 D segments (*D29*) is moved immediately upstream of one of four J_H genes (*J2*). The *second gene rearrangement* moves one of approximately 300 partial V_H genes (*V2*) immediately upstream of the newly joined D and J segments (*D29-J2*) to form a complete exon that codes for the V_H domain. During these DNA rearrangements, up to 30 nucleotides (*N*) may be added between the V and D and the D and J segments by terminal deoxynucleotidyl transferase. Splicing of the primary transcript of this newly formed heavy-chain gene removes the intron between the V_H exon and the exon that codes for the constant (*C*) domain for immunoglobulin M (i.e., C_μ). The intron between the exon that codes for the signal peptide (*sp*) and the V_H exon also is removed by splicing. Translation of this messenger RNA (*mRNA*) is directed to the endoplasmic reticulum (*ER*).

> **(2)** It is estimated that **more than 2×10^7 possible sequence combinations** can result from V_H-D-J_H joining.
>
> **d.** The **complete V_H exon** formed from V_H-D-J_H joining is separated by a long intron from an exon coding for the constant portion of an M class (i.e., isotype) antibody (C_μ exon).
>
> **e. Splicing of the transcript** (see Figure 12-11) of this newly formed gene combines the sequence for the signal peptide, the sequence for the V_H domain, and the sequence for the C_μ domain. The heavy chain produced is an immunoglobulin M **(IgM)** class antibody.

4. B-cell maturation. B cells continually arise from stem cells in the bone marrow.

  a. Cells that are committed to become B cells undergo a **series of transitions** (Figure 12-12).

    (1) They differentiate to a stage called the **pre–B-cell,** in which they form and produce H_μ chains but no light chains.

    (2) Pre–B-cells become **virgin B cells** when they form a complete light-chain gene and start to synthesize light chains. A complete IgM attaches to the membrane of the virgin B cell.

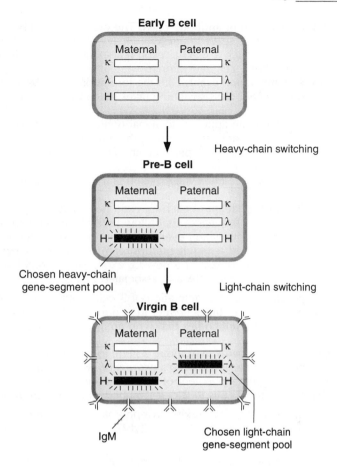

FIGURE 12-12. Formation of virgin B cells. Early B cells become pre-B cells when they undergo heavy chain (H) formation and make H_μ chains but no light chains (L). Pre-B cells become virgin B cells when they undergo light-chain formation and produce membrane-bound immunoglobulin M (IgM). (Adapted with permission from Alberts B, Bray D, Lewis J, et al: *Molecular Biology of the Cell,* 3rd ed. New York, Garland Publishing, 1994, p 1225.)

   b. Activation. A virgin B cell dies within days if it does not encounter an antigen. An encounter with an antigen is necessary for the B cell, in conjunction with a helper T cell, to become activated. Activated B cells develop into two different cell types.
      (1) Plasma cells are enlarged cells that are specialized to produce large amounts of antibody.
      (2) Memory B cells are long-lived cells that circulate in the bloodstream. Upon stimulation by antigen binding, they rapidly divide and produce more plasma cells. **Memory B cells form the basis of immunization.**
   c. Activated B cells are versatile. They can produce membrane-bound or secreted forms of IgM, or they can produce other classes of antibodies.
      (1) Alternative splicing of the heavy-chain RNA primary transcript (see VI A) enables an activated B cell to switch from making plasma membrane-bound IgM antibody to a secreted form of IgM. **Two forms of heavy chains** are produced, which differ only in their carboxyl-terminal ends.
         (a) The **membrane-bound** form has a **hydrophobic** carboxyl-terminal end.
         (b) The **secreted** form has a **hydrophilic** carboxyl-terminal end.
      (2) Heavy-chain class switching enables an activated B cell to switch from producing IgM antibody to another class of antibody.

(a) Designation of antibody class. The class of an antibody is designated by the constant heavy chain (C_H). Heavy-chain class switching refers to an event in which a V_H-D-J_H exon reassociates with a different class of C_H exon after B cell activation.

(b) Recombination event. Like the formation of the V_H and V_κ exons, heavy-chain class switching takes place by a recombination event (Figure 12-13).

   (i) Upon an appropriate signal (which ultimately is determined by the type of antigen for which the antibody is specific), an activated B cell switches to produce an antibody with a heavy chain of the appropriate class.

   (ii) Downstream of the C_μ exon is a cluster of different classes of C_H exons.

   (iii) Just upstream of each C_H exon is a **switch site,** which is made of repeated sequences that allow recombination with other switch sites.

   (iv) A recombination event between the switch site upstream of the C_μ exon and a switch site upstream of another C_H exon moves the V_H exon upstream of a new C_H exon. This recombination deletes the intervening DNA and associated exons.

5. Somatic hypermutation. After activation of B cells, mutation occurs in V-J and V-D-J regions at rates of 10^6 times greater than normal. This increases diversity and leads to a selection for antibodies that bind antigen better than the original B cell.

D. **Aberrant gene rearrangements** may move a gene to a new environment that results in the activation or repression of the gene's expression. For example, a chromosomal translocation involving the movement of immunoglobulin genes leads to the activation of a gene that transforms B cells to B-cell lymphomas called **Burkitt's lymphoma.**

1. In **90% of the patients** with Burkitt's lymphoma, there is an exchange of DNA between **chromosomes 8 and 14** (Figure 12-14). Chromosome 14, in humans, bears the genes of the heavy-chain locus.

2. In **10% of the patients** with Burkitt's lymphoma, there is an exchange between

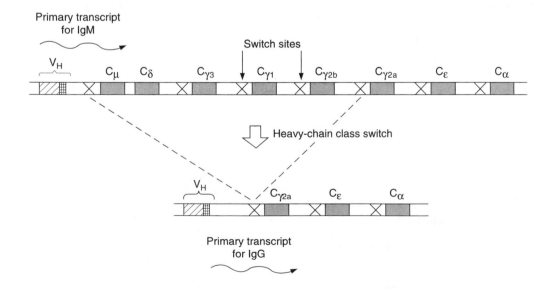

FIGURE 12-13. Example of heavy-chain (H) class switching. A heavy-chain immunoglobulin M (IgM) gene goes through a DNA rearrangement to move the exon that codes for the variable heavy-chain (V_H) domain upstream of an exon that codes for a constant (C_γ) domain. The B cells then switch from producing IgM to producing IgG.

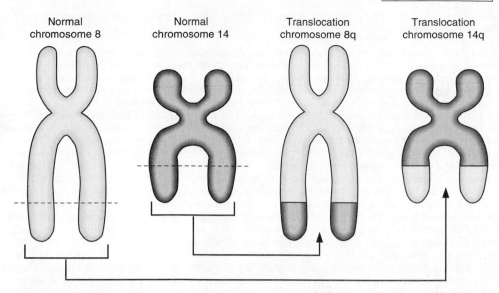

FIGURE 12-14. Chromosome translocation in Burkitt's lymphoma. Chromosomes 8 and 14 exchange portions of their long arms (*q*) to form the abnormal chromosomes 8q and 14q.

chromosomes 8 and 2 or 22, which, in the human genome, carry the kappa and lambda immunoglobulin genes, respectively.

3. The chromosomal breakpoint for chromosome 8 is the site where the **oncogene** *myc* sits.
   a. The **product of *myc*,** which is a normal gene, acts as a nuclear transcription factor that leads to a stimulation of cell division.
      (1) If a mutation causes *myc* to be expressed when it is normally "off" (i.e., not expressed), then it becomes an **oncogene;** that is, its expression can transform cells to unregulated division.
      (2) A normal gene that becomes oncogenic when a mutation causes it to be expressed or activated is called a **proto-oncogene.** More than 60 proto-oncogenes have been identified.
   b. **Translocation** results in the insertion of the *myc* proto-oncogene into the immunoglobulin gene complex, usually in the V-D-J region.
   c. This aberrant gene rearrangement causes *myc* to be expressed, which leads to an **unregulated growth of the B cells** in which the translocation occurred.
   d. It is possible that these translocations occur by a **mechanism** similar to the mechanism of V-J or V-D-J joining. In fact, it may be that a "misuse" of this mechanism results in the chromosomal translocation.

Case 12-1 Revisited

Daunorubicin, cytarabine (cytosine arabinoside), and thioguanine inhibit DNA replication by completely different mechanisms. Daunorubicin is an anthracycline glycoside that inhibits DNA replication through intercalation into the DNA (see Chapter 8). Cytarabine is a dideoxynucleoside analog (see Chapter 8). Upon phosphorylation after cell entry, it becomes incorporated into DNA, where it slows the rate of replication and alters the structure of DNA such that it is more prone to breakage. Thioguanine is an inhibitor of purine metabolism (see Chapter 26). It is converted to a ribonucleotide, 6-thioguanosine monophosphate (6-thioGMP), by hypoxanthine-guanine phosphoribosyltransferase. 6-ThioGMP inhibits conversion of inosine monophosphate (IMP) to GMP, which leads to an inhibition of DNA synthesis by substrate starvation. Etoposide (VP-16) inhibits topoisomerase II, which is a replicative enzyme essential to DNA synthesis (see Chapter 8).

Resistance to chemotherapeutic drugs can arise by many different mechanisms, some known and many unknown. Multi-drug resistance of some cancers is often seen after chemotherapy. Many cases of multi-drug resistance can be linked to expression of the multi-drug resistance gene that codes for a large membrane-bound glycoprotein called P-glycoprotein (Pgp). Pgp confers resistance to many unrelated antineoplastic drugs by pumping them out of the cell in an ATP-dependent manner. Because Pgp confers resistance to multiple drugs, a particular chemotherapeutic treatment may lead to resistance to a drug that has never been used on a patient. Cancer cells may become resistant to mutiple drugs simply through expression or increasing expression of the MDR gene. In some cases, cells increase the production of Pgp through amplification of the MDR gene. The absolute levels of Pgp needed to confer resistance to standard chemotherapeutic regimes are not known. Increased transcription, RNA stability, or other levels of regulation may cause a sufficient increase in Pgp to make cells resistant to multiple drugs.

Pgp is a natural product of many cells. In particular, cancers that derive from cells that are epithelial in origin (e.g., lungs, colon) and bone marrow cells may be resistant to chemotherapeutic drugs prior to treatment, possibly because they express Pgp for their normal functions. It is theorized that prior exposure to other drugs or environmental chemicals may make some cells increase their Pgp levels such that if they mutate to cancer cells, they may already carry multi-drug resistance.

STUDY QUESTIONS

DIRECTIONS: Each of the numbered items or incomplete statements in this section is followed by answers or by completions of the statement. Select the **one** lettered answer or completion that is **best** in each case.

1. Which one of the following compounds is the natural inducer of β-galactosidase in *Escherichia coli?*

(A) Glucose
(B) Allolactose
(C) Isopropylthiogalactoside (IPTG)
(D) Lactose
(E) Galactose

2. An operon is best described by which one of the following phrases?

(A) An unregulated gene system
(B) A coordinately regulated gene system
(C) A gene that produces a monocistronic messenger RNA
(D) The region of DNA to which a repressor binds causing the inhibition of initiation of transcription
(E) A constitutively expressed gene system

3. Cyclic adenosine monophosphate (cAMP) regulates the lactose (*lac*) operon by

(A) binding to the operator to turn on transcription
(B) binding to the *lac* repressor to prevent transcription
(C) combining with the catabolite activator protein (CAP) to form a complex that enhances transcription upon binding to the promoter
(D) combining with the CAP to remove CAP's inhibition of transcription
(E) combining with CAP in the presence of glucose to activate transcription

4. Regulation of gene expression by attenuation is best characterized by which one of the following statements?

(A) It requires a corepressor
(B) It is exerted at the level of transcriptional termination
(C) It is found in both prokaryotes and eukaryotes
(D) It is exerted at the level of translational termination
(E) It requires an operator

5. The absence of which molecule enhances the expression of operons that produce catabolic enzymes?

(A) Allolactose
(B) Catabolite activator protein (CAP)
(C) Glucose
(D) Adenylate cyclase
(E) Cyclic adenosine monophosphate (cAMP)

6. An operator is best defined as

(A) the gene product of a regulatory gene
(B) a constitutively regulated gene that produces operon regulatory proteins
(C) the repressor binding region in operons
(D) the site within an operon to which the catabolite activator protein complexed with cyclic adenosine monophosphate binds
(E) the sequence within an operon that directs the correct site of initiation of transcription

7. Which DNA sequences are functional even at a great distance from either side of the transcriptional initiation site of a gene?

(A) Response elements
(B) Promoters
(C) Enhancers
(D) Operators

8. A B cell is converted to secrete immunoglobulin M (IgM) by which one of the following methods?

(A) Light chain formation
(B) Heavy chain formation
(C) Alternative splicing
(D) Heavy-chain class switching

9. In the presence of low intracellular iron concentrations, the iron response element binding protein (IRE-BP) has which one of the following actions?

(A) It destabilizes transferrin receptor messenger RNA (mRNA)
(B) It allows translation of ferritin mRNA
(C) It stabilizes ferritin mRNA
(D) It blocks translation of transferrin receptor mRNA
(E) It blocks translation of ferritin mRNA

DIRECTIONS: Each group of items in this section consists of lettered options followed by a set of numbered items. For each item, select the **one** lettered option that is most closely associated with it. Each lettered option may be selected once, more than once, or not at all.

Questions 10–12

Match the following formations to the method of gene regulation that is most likely to cause it.

(A) Gene amplification
(B) DNA rearrangement
(C) RNA destabilization
(D) Alternative splicing
(E) DNA packaging

10. Formation of isoforms

11. Formation of antibody diversity

12. Formation of drug resistance

Questions 13–15

Match the following actions with the process or particle with which it is most involved.

(A) Methylation
(B) Ligand-binding domain
(C) DNA amplification
(D) Euchromatin
(E) mRNA stability

13. Transcriptional regulation by steroids

14. Transferrin receptor gene regulation

15. Formation of Barr bodies

ANSWERS AND EXPLANATIONS

1. The answer is B [I B 4]. Allolactose is a transglycosylated form of lactose produced as an intermediate in the hydrolysis of lactose. When lactose is present, the small amounts of β-galactosidase in the cell in the noninduced state form allolactose, which is the natural inducer of the *lac* operon (of which β-galactosidase is a product). Some galactosides, such as isopropylthiogalactoside (IPTG), are strong inducers of β-galactosidase in *Escherichia coli* but do not act as substrates for the enzyme. Such galactosides are known as nonmetabolizable, or gratuitous, inducers. Lactose and allolactose are substrates for β-galactosidase; glucose and galactose are the final products of lactose metabolism by β-galactosidase.

2. The answer is B [I C 1]. An operon is a group of coordinately regulated genes and their controlling elements. Regulatory proteins, such as repressors, interact with operon-associated controlling elements, such as operators, and participate in the control of the operons. The regulatory proteins are produced by regulatory genes that are often expressed constitutively (i.e., in an unregulated fashion).

3. The answer is C [II A 2]. The presence of glucose suppresses the transcription of the structural genes of the lactose (*lac*) operon. It does so by lowering cellular levels of cyclic adenosine monophosphate (cAMP) by an unknown mechanism. In the absence of glucose, cAMP binds to the catabolite activator protein (CAP), and the complex stimulates transcription in several operons, including the *lac* operon, by binding to their promoter sites. In the presence of glucose, cAMP levels are too low for the cAMP–CAP complex to form, and transcription is not activated.

4. The answer is B [III]. Attenuation is a method of regulation described for many of the amino acid biosynthetic operons that requires the coupling of transcription and translation. Therefore, it can occur only in prokaryotes and not in eukaryotes. Attenuation occurs after transcription has been initiated and, therefore, does not involve the action of a corepressor or an operator. The availability of the amino acids produced by the enzyme products of these operons determines the position of the ribosome on the transcript. The position of the ribosome determines whether transcription will be aborted by an early termination event or will be allowed to proceed to completion.

5. The answer is C [II A]. Catabolite repression of operons that produce catabolic enzymes (e.g., β-galactosidase, galactokinase, arabinose kinase) occurs when the preferred fuel source, glucose, is present. The presence of glucose does not so much repress the expression of the operons of these catabolic enzymes as the absence of glucose tremendously enhances their expression. Cyclic adenosine monophosphate (cAMP) is the signaling molecule for the enhancement of expression of the catabolic operons. In bacteria, cAMP levels are inversely linked to glucose levels. Adenylate cyclase makes cAMP from adenosine triphosphate (ATP) when glucose levels are low. Binding of cAMP to the catabolite activator protein (CAP) forms a complex that enhances gene expression of catobolic operons if there is no repressor or if necessary activating factors are present. Therefore, if cAMP or adenylate cyclase or CAP levels are absent, there will be no enhancement of expression from catabolic operons. Allolactose is the positive signaling molecule for expression of only the lactose operon.

6. The answer is C [I C 2 c]. An operator region lies adjacent to the promoter and spans the transcriptional initiation site. Regulatory proteins called repressors bind to operators and block initiation of transcription. Regulatory proteins often are produced from constitutive genes. The CAP–cAMP complex binds to the CAP-binding site, which is within the promoter region. The sequence that directs the correct site of initiation of transcription is the promoter sequence.

7. The answer is C [V B 3 b (1)]. Eukaryotic gene regulatory sequences can be classified into two basic types: enhancers and response elements. Regulatory sequences are not promoters because they do not affect the accuracy of initiation. Enhancers are functional either upstream or downstream and even at great distances from the initiation site.

Response elements usually are found within 250 base pairs upstream of the initiation site (they are also called promoter-proximal elements). An operator is a prokaryotic regulatory sequence that lies adjacent to the promoter and may span the transcriptional initiation site.

8. The answer is C [VIII C 4 c (1)]. An activated B cell switches from making a membrane-bound immunoglobulin M (IgM) to a secreted form of IgM by alternative splicing. An exon that codes for an IgM with a hydrophilic end is used instead of an exon for an IgM with a hydrophobic end. B cells change the class of antibody they produce by a DNA rearrangement event called heavy-chain class switching. Heavy chain and light chain formation are DNA rearrangement events responsible for the formation of the variable domains of both the heavy and light chains.

9. The answer is E [VI B 2 b (2); VII A]. Iron response elements (IREs) are stem-loop structures that may exist in particular messenger RNAs (mRNAs). A protein, the iron response element binding protein (IRE-BP), will bind to these sequences at a low intracellular iron concentration. At high intracellular iron concentrations, the IRE-BP does not bind to IREs. Transferrin receptors facilitate the uptake of transferrin with bound iron into the cell. Transferrin receptor mRNA is inherently unstable. Transferrin receptor mRNA has some IREs in the 3′ untranslated portion of its mRNA. If IRE-BP is bound to these IREs, then the transferrin receptor mRNA becomes stable. More transferrin receptor is synthesized, and this leads to an increase in the intracellular iron levels. Free iron (Fe^{3+}) is toxic to cells. The protein ferritin binds free iron and protects the cell from iron toxicity. Ferritin has some IREs within the 3′ untranslated region portion of its mRNA. When iron concentrations are low (i.e., no need for ferritin), IRE-BP binds to these IREs and prevents their translation. At high iron concentrations, translation proceeds because IRE-BP does not bind to IREs in the presence of high iron concentrations.

10–12. The answers are: 10-D [VI A], **11-B** [VIII C], **12-A** [VIII A 3]. Related but different proteins, called isoforms, can be coded for by the same gene and produced by alternative splicing. A single gene that codes for isoforms has multiple exons that code for different domains of a protein. These genes produce the same primary transcript. Alternative splicing combines different exons, from the primary

transcript, in different cell types, to produce different messenger RNAs.

Antibody diversity arises in part by DNA rearrangement. The coding sequences for the variable domains of either the heavy or light chains exist as clusters of multiple, different copies of partial genes or exons. DNA rearrangement forms a complete exon for the variable domain by combining any one of the partial exons from one cluster with any one of the partial exons from another cluster. The ability to put genes together in different combinations increases diversity tremendously.

Drug resistance may arise by selective gene amplification. The amplified gene may code for a product on which the drug acts or may be a product that inactivates or eliminates the drug.

RNA destabilization and DNA packaging are common forms of gene regulation, but they are not likely to cause the formation of drug resistance, isoforms, or antibody diversity.

13-15. The answers are: 13-B [V B 3 b (2) (a)], **14-E** [VI B 2 b (2)], **15-A** [V A 2, 4]. Steroids regulate genes through their interaction with intracellular steroid receptors. These receptors have ligand-binding domains to which the steroid binds. The binding of the steroid activates the receptor, which then acts as a positive regulatory factor through binding to steroid hormone response elements. Response elements are DNA regulatory sequences that are common to a group of genes.

The transferrin receptor (TfR) genes regulate their gene expression through the modulation of the stability of their mRNA. TfR mRNA is inherently unstable. TfR mRNA has some iron response elements (IREs) in the 3′ untranslated portion of its mRNA. If the iron response element binding protein is bound to these IREs, then the transferrin receptor mRNA becomes stable.

Barr bodies are a dramatic example of gene inactivation through the tight packaging of DNA into heterochromatin. Methylation is known to play a role in the maintenance of Barr bodies. Experiments in which maintenance methylation was inhibited led to the reactivation of Barr body genes.

DNA amplification is not known to be a feature of the regulation of steroid responsive genes or tubulin genes or of the formation of Barr bodies. All active genes are in the euchromatin state and are capable of being transcriptionally regulated. It is necessary for the expression of tubulin genes and steroid hormone responsive genes, but it is not a major feature of their regulation.

METABOLISM

Chapter 13

Introduction to Metabolism
Victor Davidson

I. **METABOLISM** involves the transformation of both **matter** and **energy.** These transformations often involve a number of reactions that are catalyzed by a sequence of enzymes. This **sequence of enzymatic reactions** collectively constitutes a **metabolic pathway.** The product of one enzyme reaction becomes the substrate for the next reaction in the sequence. The successive products of the reactions are known as **metabolites,** or **metabolic intermediates.**

A. **Catabolism** (Figure 13-1) encompasses the **degradative processes,** whereby complex molecules are broken down into simpler ones.

1. **Stage 1.** Complex macromolecules (e.g., starch, protein, triacylglycerols) are broken down into smaller units, such as monosaccharides, amino acids, glycerol, and fatty acids. During this stage, little or no free energy is trapped.
2. **Stage 2.** These smaller molecules are further degraded to a few molecules that can be oxidized to carbon dioxide (CO_2) and water along a common pathway. In this stage, some free energy is trapped as adenosine triphosphate (ATP; see IV).
3. **Stage 3** is the final common pathway by which these molecules are oxidized to CO_2 and water and trap the available free energy as ATP. It consists of:
   a. The citric acid cycle
   b. The electron transport chain
   c. Oxidative phosphorylation

B. **Anabolism** (Figure 13-2) encompasses **biosynthetic pathways** in which metabolic building blocks are converted into complex macromolecules. Anabolic processes require energy inputs, which can be supplied in two ways:

1. By ATP generated during catabolism
2. In some cases, by high-energy electrons in the form of reduced nicotinamide adenine dinucleotide phosphate (NADPH; see V C)

II. **COMPARTMENTALIZATION OF METABOLIC PATHWAYS IN CELLS.** The set of enzymes that catalyze a particular metabolic pathway are often localized in a specific intracellular compartment (Figure 13-3).

A. The **cytosol** is the liquid portion of the cytoplasm that includes macromolecules but not subcellular organelles.

B. **Mitochondria** are called the **"power plants"** of the cell because they convert energy to forms that can be used by the cell. A mitochondrion is a double-membrane organelle. The internal membrane is highly folded, with many **cristae** protruding into the large internal compartment called the **matrix.**

C. In some instances, certain enzymes for a metabolic pathway are contained in the **cytosol,** and others are contained in the **mitochondrial matrix.**

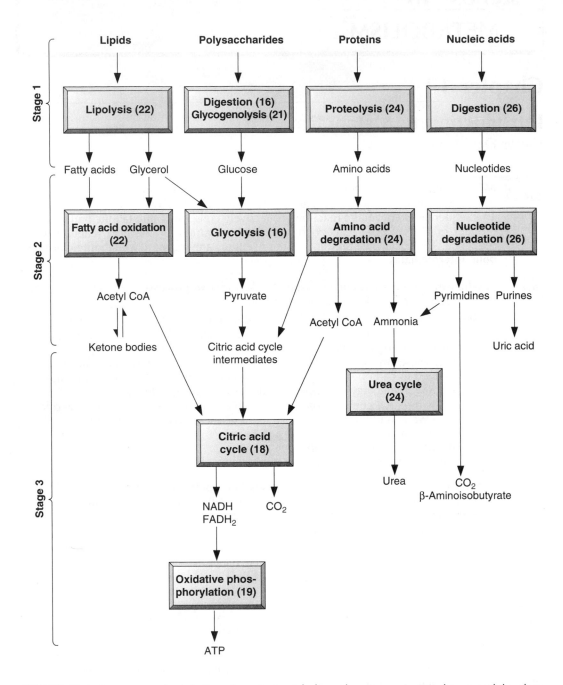

FIGURE 13-1. A summary of catabolism. Important catabolic pathways are given in *boxes,* and the chapters that describe each pathway are given in *parentheses. Acetyl CoA* = acetyl coenzyme A; *ATP* = adenosine triphosphate; CO_2 = carbon dioxide; $FADH_2$ = reduced flavin adenine dinucleotide; *NADH* = reduced nicotinamide adenine dinucleotide.

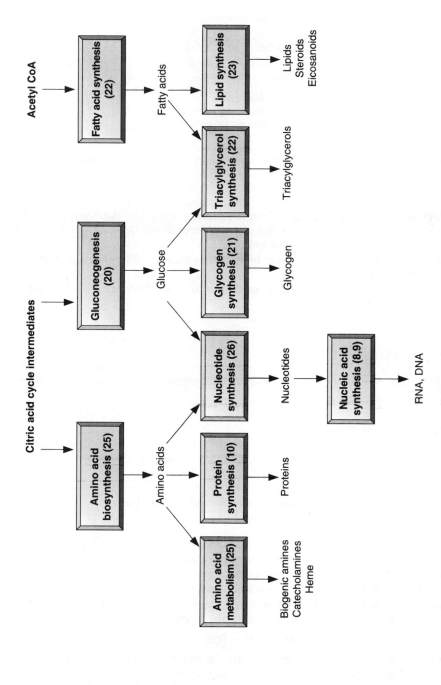

FIGURE 13-2. A summary of anabolism. Important anabolic pathways are given in *boxes*, and the chapters that describe each pathway are given in *parentheses*. *Acetyl CoA* = acetyl coenzyme A; *DNA* = deoxyribonucleic acid; *RNA* = ribonucleic acid.

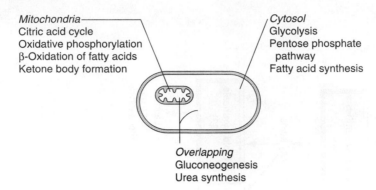

FIGURE 13-3. Compartmentalization of some important metabolic pathways.

D. The **biologic advantage of compartmentalization** of metabolic pathways is that it allows the separation of processes that proceed in opposite directions and may otherwise interfere with one another. For example:
1. The anabolic process of fatty acid **biosynthesis from acetyl coenzyme A (CoA)** is confined to the **cytosol.**
2. The catabolic process of fatty acid **oxidation to acetyl CoA** occurs in the **mitochondrial matrix.**

III. BIOENERGETICS

A. **Standard state.** When considering biochemical systems, a standard state is defined as follows:
1. The pH is 7.
2. The temperature is 25°C (298°K).
3. All solutes are at 1 molar concentration (1 M).
4. All gases are at 1 standard atmosphere (atm) pressure.

B. **Thermodynamic concepts**
1. **Enthalpy (H)** is the **heat content** of a body and is given by

$$H = E + PV \tag{1}$$

where E is the internal energy, and PV is the product of pressure times volume.
2. **Entropy (S)** is the **degree of randomness,** or disorder, of a system. The greater the degree of disorder, the higher the value of S.
3. **Free energy (G)** is the **amount of useful work** that can be obtained from a system.
4. **The change in H, S, or G** (written as **ΔH, ΔS, or ΔG**), rather than absolute values, is usually considered. These parameters are related by:

$$\Delta G = \Delta H - T\Delta S \tag{2}$$

In the standard state, the three functions are written as $\Delta H^{\circ\prime}$, $\Delta S^{\circ\prime}$, and $\Delta G^{\circ\prime}$.
5. **Standard free-energy change** of a reaction can be calculated by:
   a. Subtracting the $\Delta G^{\circ\prime}$ values of reactants from those of the products
   b. Deriving it from the equilibrium constant (K_{eq}) for the reaction
      (1) In the reaction

$$A + B \leftrightarrow C + D$$

the **actual free-energy change (ΔG)** is given by

TABLE 13-1. Free Energies of Hydrolysis of Some Physiologically Relevant Phosphate-Containing Compounds

Compound	$\Delta G^{o\prime}$ (kcal/mol)
Phosphoenolpyruvate (PEP)	−14.8
Carbamoyl phosphate	−12.3
Creatine phosphate	−10.3
Adenosine triphosphate (ATP)	−7.3
Glucose-1-phosphate (G1P)	−5.0
Glucose-6-phosphate (G6P)	−3.3

$\Delta G^{o\prime}$ = change in the standard state of free energy.

$$\Delta G = \Delta G^{o\prime} + RT \ln \frac{[C]\,[D]}{[A]\,[B]} \tag{3}$$

where R is the gas constant (1.987×10^{-3} kcal $\times$ deg^{-1} $\times$ mol^{-1}), T is the temperature in degrees Kelvin (°C + 273), and ln indicates the natural logarithm, which can be converted to $\log_{10}$ by multiplying by 2.303.

(2) **At equilibrium,** when the rate of the forward reaction equals the rate of the backward reaction, there is no change in free energy; that is, **$\Delta G = 0$.** Also, [C][D]/[A][B] is equal to the K_{eq} for the reaction.

(3) **If G$^{o\prime}$ is known,** the actual free-energy change (ΔG) in a reaction can be calculated by substituting the actual temperatures and concentrations of reactants and products in equation (3).

6. **Spontaneity of a reaction** is measured by the value of ΔG.
   a. **Exergonic reaction.** If the change in free energy is less than zero ($\Delta G < 0$), **the reaction can proceed spontaneously with the release of energy.**
   b. **Endergonic reaction.** If the change in free energy is more than zero ($\Delta G > 0$), **the reaction cannot proceed spontaneously unless there is an input of energy** to drive the reaction forward.

C. **Coupled reactions.** A thermodynamically unfavorable reaction can be driven by being coupled to a thermodynamically favorable reaction.

1. For example, the formation of glucose-6-phosphate (G6P) from glucose and inorganic phosphate is an unfavorable endergonic reaction with a $\Delta G^{o\prime}$ of +3.3 kcal/mol. When coupled to the hydrolysis of ATP to adenosine diphosphate (ADP) and inorganic phosphate (P$_i$), this exergonic reaction with a $\Delta G^{o\prime}$ of −7.3 kcal/mol can provide energy for the phosphorylation of glucose.

2. The **coupled reactions** are:
   a. Glucose + P$_i$ → G6P + H$_2$O, with a $\Delta G^{o\prime}$ = +3.3 kcal/mol
   b. ATP + H$_2$O → ADP + P$_i$, with a $\Delta G^{o\prime}$ = −7.3 kcal/mol
   c. The **net reaction** is: Glucose + ATP → G6P + ADP, with a net $\Delta G^{o\prime}$ = −4.0 kcal/mol

IV. **HIGH-ENERGY PHOSPHATE COMPOUNDS**

A. **Group-transfer potential.** High-energy phosphate compounds (Table 13-1) have a large negative $\Delta G^{o\prime}$ for hydrolysis of the phosphate group (i.e., a high group-transfer potential for phosphate).

B. **Adenosine triphosphate (ATP) is the principal donor of free energy in biologic systems.**

1. **Energy is released** when a phosphoanhydride bond is broken by the addition of water. This reaction is highly exergonic because the products of this reaction, ADP and P_i, are more stable than ATP. This can be attributed primarily to two factors.

$$\text{adenine} \quad CH_2-O-\overset{O^-}{\underset{O}{\overset{|}{\underset{\parallel}{P^\alpha}}}}-O-\overset{O^-}{\underset{O}{\overset{|}{\underset{\parallel}{P^\beta}}}}-O-\overset{O^-}{\underset{O}{\overset{|}{\underset{\parallel}{P^\gamma}}}}-O^- + H_2O \rightarrow$$

$$\text{adenine} \quad CH_2-O-\overset{O^-}{\underset{O}{\overset{|}{\underset{\parallel}{P^\alpha}}}}-O-\overset{O^-}{\underset{O}{\overset{|}{\underset{\parallel}{P^\beta}}}}-O^- + ^-O-\overset{O^-}{\underset{O}{\overset{|}{\underset{\parallel}{P}}}}-OH + H^+$$

   a. ADP and P_i exhibit increased resonance stabilization relative to ATP.
   b. Intramolecular electrostatic repulsion is reduced between the negatively charged groups on the β and γ phosphates after hydrolysis.

2. **The free energy of hydrolysis of ATP is intermediate in value** between phosphate-containing compounds of higher and lower group transfer potentials (see Table 13-1). As such, ATP can function as an energy carrier between catabolic pathways (where it is formed) and anabolic pathways (where it is used). Thus, **ATP can act as a "universal currency" for energy in cells.**

3. **Storage forms of high-energy phosphates**
   a. The **turnover rate** for ATP is very high. In humans, an amount of ATP approximately equal to the body weight is formed and broken down every 24 hours. The rapidity of ATP turnover precludes its use as a storage form of energy.
   b. Processes such as muscle activity can require ATP to be hydrolyzed for the release of free energy at a rate much higher than ATP can be resynthesized. High-energy phosphate compounds have evolved that store energy for use during heavy work over limited periods of time.
      (1) **Creatine phosphate** fills this role in muscle.
      (2) During rest periods, creatine phosphate is regenerated at the expense of ATP.

C. **Phosphate pool. Nucleoside triphosphates other than adenine** are also required in some metabolic processes. These are formed in reactions that depend on ATP for their resynthesis and are catalyzed by **nucleoside kinases.**

1. **Guanosine triphosphate (GTP)** is used to supply energy in protein synthesis (as well as act as a modulator of protein conformation).

2. **Cytidine triphosphate (CTP)** supplies energy in lipid synthesis.

3. **Uridine triphosphate (UTP)** supplies energy in polysaccharide synthesis.

V. **OXIDATION–REDUCTION REACTIONS** involve **electron transfers,** and each reaction consists of two coupled half-reactions of the form.

$$\text{A (oxidized)} + \text{B (reduced)} \leftrightarrow \text{B (oxidized)} + \text{A (reduced)} \tag{4}$$

A. **Definitions**
   1. **Oxidation** constitutes a loss of electrons.
   2. **Reduction** constitutes a gain of electrons.

3. In equation 4, A is an electron acceptor when going from its oxidized to reduced form. B is the electron donor on going from its reduced to oxidized form.

B. **Oxidation–reduction potential (redox potential)**

1. Standard reduction potential for the half-reactions is the **electrical potential (E_0')** in volts, measured during the reaction under standard conditions (see III A). The $H_2:H^+$ electrode is used as a reference.

    a. The standard oxidation–reduction potentials for some biologically relevant reactions are given in Table 13-2.

    b. If a reaction proceeds as an oxidation rather than a reduction (i.e., the opposite direction as written in Table 13-2), then the magnitude of the potential remains the same, but the sign is changed from positive to negative or vice versa.

2. Net reaction potential ($\Delta E_0'$) is the difference between the standard reduction potentials. To calculate $\Delta E_0'$, the E_0' of the oxidation half-reaction is added to the E_0' of the reduction half-reaction. For example, consider the following reaction:

$$NADH + H^+ + Pyruvate \rightleftharpoons NAD^+ + Lactate$$

    a. Oxidative half-reaction:

$$NADH \rightleftharpoons NAD^+ + H^+ + 2e^-$$
$$E_0' = +0.32 \text{ volts}$$

    b. Reductive half-reaction:

$$Pyruvate + 2H^+ + 2e^- \rightleftharpoons Lactate$$
$$E_0' = -0.19 \text{ volts}$$

    c. Adding these together gives the net reaction and the $\Delta E_0'$:

$$\Delta E_0' = +0.32 - 0.19 = +0.13 \text{ volts}$$

3. Significance of ΔE

    a. When ΔE is positive, a reaction can proceed spontaneously.

    b. When ΔE is zero, the reaction is at equilibrium.

4. Relationship between oxidation–reduction potential and standard free energy. Knowing the $\Delta E_0'$ of an oxidation-reduction reaction and the number of electrons transferred (n), the standard free-energy change ($\Delta G^{\circ\prime}$) can be calculated by

$$\Delta G^{\circ\prime} = -nF\Delta E_0' \tag{5}$$

where F is the Faraday constant (23.061 kcal × $volt^{-1}$ × $equiv^{-1}$).

C. **Electron carriers.** In aerobic organisms, the ultimate acceptor of electrons derived from fuel molecules is molecular oxygen. The electrons are first transferred from metabolites to specialized electron carriers. The electrons from the carriers reach molecular oxygen via the mitochondrial electron transport system (see Chapter 19 I).

TABLE 13-2. Standard Oxidation–Reduction Potentials for Some Biologically Relevant Reactions

Half-reaction (written as a reduction)	E_0' (volts)
Acetate + $2H^+$ + $2e^-$ $\rightleftharpoons$ Acetaldehyde	−0.60
NAD^+ + $2H^+$ + $2e^-$ $\rightleftharpoons$ NADH + H^+	−0.32
Free FAD + $2H^+$ + $2e^-$ $\rightleftharpoons$ Free $FADH_2$	−0.18
Pyruvate + $2H^+$ + $2e^-$ $\rightleftharpoons$ Lactate	−0.19
Fumarate + $2H^+$ + $2e^-$ $\rightleftharpoons$ Succinate	+0.03
Cytochrome c (Fe^{3+}) + e^- $\rightleftharpoons$ Cytochrome c (Fe^{2+})	+0.25
1/2 O_2 + $2H^+$ + $2e^-$ $\rightleftharpoons$ H_2O	+0.82

H = hydrogen; *e* = electron; *NAD* = nicotinamide adenine dinucleotide; *NADH* = reduced nicotinamide adenine dinucleotide; *FAD* = flavin adenine dinucleotide; *FADH* = reduced flavin adenine dinucleotide; *Fe²⁺* = ferrous iron; *O₂* = oxygen.

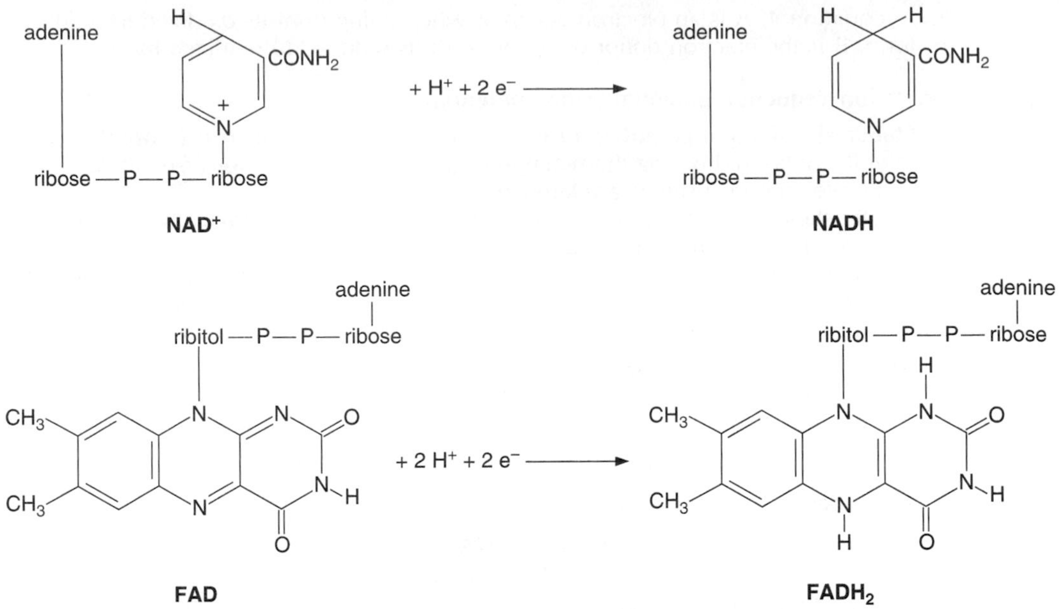

FIGURE 13-4. Conversions of the oxidized form of nicotinamide adenine dinucleotide (NAD$^+$) to the reduced form (NADH) and the oxidized form of flavin adenine dinucleotide (FAD) to the reduced form (FADH$_2$).

1. **Pyridine nucleotides:** Nicotinamide adenine dinucleotide (NAD$^+$) and nicotinamide adenine dinucleotide phosphate (NADP$^+$)
   a. The active portion of NAD$^+$ and NADP$^+$ is the **nicotinamide ring,** which accepts a proton and two electrons (equivalent to a hydride ion, H$^-$) from the substrate to yield the reduced forms, NADH and NADPH (Figure 13-4).
   b. NAD$^+$ and NADP$^+$ are identical except that in NADP$^+$ one of the hydroxyl groups on the ribose bound to adenine is phosphorylated.
   c. NAD$^+$ and NADP$^+$ are usually freely dissociable from enzymes.
   d. **The energy stored in NADH is primarily used to drive the synthesis of ATP.**
   e. **NADPH** serves as an energy source for **reductive biosyntheses,** in which the precursors are more oxidized than the products.

2. **Flavin adenine dinucleotide (FAD) and flavin mononucleotide (FMN)**
   a. The active portion of FAD and FMN is the **isoalloxazine ring,** which accepts two protons and two electrons (equivalent to 2H) from the substrate to yield the reduced forms, FADH$_2$ and FMNH$_2$ (see Figure 13-4).
   b. FMN differs from FAD in that it has only ribitol phosphate bound to the isoalloxazine ring.
   c. In enzymes, using FAD or FMN as an electron acceptor, the cofactor is firmly bound to the enzyme and does not dissociate.

3. NAD$^+$, NADP$^+$, FMN, and FAD are **cofactors** for many dehydrogenase enzymes involved in the oxidation of fuel molecules.

VI. **MONITORING METABOLIC EVENTS IN TISSUES BY MAGNETIC RESONANCE.** In vivo **nuclear magnetic resonance (NMR) spectroscopy,** in conjunction with **magnetic resonance imaging (MRI),** shows promise as a noninvasive method to monitor the metabolic events of intact tissues.

A. **Technique.** NMR spectroscopy is based on the energy absorption of certain atomic nuclei when they are placed in a magnetic field. Atoms that give rise to NMR signals include protons (^1H) and the naturally occurring isotopes of phosphorus (^{31}P) and fluorine (^{19}F).

B. **Uses of NMR**

1. **^1H NMR** has been used to study metabolite levels in tumors.

2. **^{31}P NMR** has been used to study the bioenergetics of several tissues, and it can be used to determine intracellular levels of the following:
   a. Concentration of ATP
   b. Concentrations of phosphocreatine and other high-energy phosphate compounds
   c. Concentrations of P_i and phosphoesters
   d. pH

3. **^{19}F NMR** has been used to study the metabolism of certain drugs (e.g., the anticancer drug 5-fluorouracil).

C. **Clinical example.** In vivo ^{31}P NMR was used to diagnose and differentiate disorders of the liver caused by alcoholic and viral hepatitis, and alcoholic cirrhosis of the liver (Meyerhoff DJ, Karczmar GS, Weiner W: *Invest Radiol* 24:980-984, 1989). This was done by monitoring intracellular pH and concentrations of ATP, Pi, phosphate monoesters (PME), and phosphate diesters (PDE).

1. According to NMR studies, the **normal concentrations** of these metabolites in mmol/kg were ATP = 2, P_i = 2.2, PME = 0.8, and PDE = 5.3. Normal pH was 7.4.

2. **Alcoholic hepatitis.** The level of each metabolite was decreased by 30%–50%, and pH was higher than normal.

3. **Alcoholic cirrhosis.** The PME level was decreased by 18%; levels of the other metabolites were decreased by 30%–50%. The pH was below normal.

4. **Viral hepatitis B.** Metabolite concentrations were normal except for the level of PME, which was 125% higher than normal. The pH level was normal.

D. **MRI uses NMR to create an image** of the distribution of protons in the body, because protons are the most abundant atomic nuclei in the body that exhibit magnetic resonance. With the exception of bone, all tissues have an abundance of protons in water and fat.

1. MRI is an extremely good diagnostic technique in which the abnormal tissue shows a difference in contrast from normal tissue.

2. Diagnostically, MRI has the advantage that it is **noninvasive** and uses no ionizing radiation.

STUDY QUESTIONS

DIRECTIONS: Each of the numbered items or incomplete statements in this section is followed by answers or by completions of the statement. Select the **one** lettered answer or completion that is **best** in each case.

1. If a reaction is at equilibrium, which one of the following statements is correct?

(A) The free-energy change (ΔG) equals zero
(B) ΔG equals $\Delta E_0'$
(C) ΔG equals $\Delta G^{\circ\prime}$
(D) G equals ln K_{eq}
(E) ΔG equals 1

2. The normal concentrations of glucose-6-phosphate (G6P) and fructose-6-phosphate (F6P) in human erythrocytes are 1×10^{-5} M and 1×10^{-6} M, respectively. If the standard free-energy change ($\Delta G^{\circ\prime}$) for the reaction G6P $\rightarrow$ F6P is +0.4 kcal/mol, which one of the following statements is correct?

(A) The equilibrium constant (K_{eq}) for the reaction G6P $\rightarrow$ F6P is 1
(B) The free-energy change (ΔG) is approximately −1.0 kcal/mol
(C) The ΔG for the reverse reaction is −0.4 kcal/mol
(D) The reaction as written cannot occur in the erythrocyte
(E) K_{eq} for the reaction G6P $\rightarrow$ F6P is greater than 1

3. The standard free-energy change ($\Delta G^{\circ\prime}$) for the conversion of compound X to compound Y is +1.4 kcal/mol at 37°C. Which one of the following ratios most closely approximates the equilibrium ratio of the concentration of X to that of Y?

(A) 100:1
(B) 1:100
(C) 10:1
(D) 1:10
(E) 1:1

4. Which one of the following compounds has the highest group transfer potential for phosphate?

(A) Glucose-6-phosphate
(B) Fructose-1,6-diphosphate
(C) Ribose-5-phosphate
(D) 2-Phosphoenolpyruvate
(E) Adenosine triphosphate

5. If an oxidation-reduction reaction with a two-electron transfer has a standard reduction potential of +0.3 volts, what is the free-energy change under standard conditions?

(A) +6.9 kcal/mol
(B) −13.8 kcal/mol
(C) +46.1 kcal/mol
(D) +13.8 kcal/mol
(E) −6.9 kcal/mol

DIRECTIONS: The group of items in this section consists of lettered options followed by a set of numbered items. For each item, select the **one** lettered option that is most closely associated with it. Each lettered option may be selected once, more than once, or not at all.

Questions 6-8

Match the following statements regarding function with the correct subcellular location.

(A) Mitochondria
(B) Cytosol
(C) Both
(D) Neither

6. Contains enzymes that catalyze the final stage (stage 3) of metabolism

7. Contains enzymes that catalyze the formation of glucose from citric acid cycle intermediates

8. Contains the enzymes that catalyze the formation of pyruvate from glucose

Questions 9-11

Match the following statements regarding function with the correct compound.

(A) Adenosine diphosphate (ADP)
(B) Nicotinamide adenine dinucleotide (NAD⁺)
(C) Flavin mononucleotide (FMN)
(D) Flavin adenine dinucleotide (FAD)
(E) Nicotinamide adenine dinucleotide phosphate (NADP⁺)

9. Provides energy for reductive biosynthesis

10. Provides energy for the formation of adenosine triphosphate

11. Is the product of a hydrolysis reaction that can be used to drive thermodynamically unfavorable reactions

ANSWERS AND EXPLANATIONS

1. The answer is A [III B 5; V B 4]. At equilibrium, the free-energy change of a reaction (ΔG) is zero, and the standard free-energy change ($\Delta G^{\circ\prime}$) is equal to $-RT \ln K_{eq}$. For an oxidation-reduction reaction, it is equal to $-nF\Delta E_0{}'$.

2. The answer is B [III B 5]. The free-energy change (ΔG) for the conversion of glucose-6-phosphate (G6P) to fructose-6-phosphate (F6P) can be found from:

$$\Delta G = \Delta G^{\circ} + RT \ln \frac{[F6P]}{[G6P]} = +0.4 + 1.4 \log \frac{10^{-5}}{10^{-6}} = -1$$

The equilibrium constant for the reaction as written (G6P → F6P) can be found from:

$$\Delta G^{\circ\prime} = -1.4 \log K_{eq} \text{ , or, } \log K_{eq} = \frac{-0\cdot4}{1\cdot4}$$

Thus, K_{eq} is less than 1. For the reverse reaction, $\Delta G^{\circ\prime}$ is -0.4 kcal/mol and ΔG is $+1$ kcal/mol. The reaction as written can occur in erythrocytes because the ΔG calculated from the concentration of G6P and F6P is negative.

3. The answer is C [III B 5]. The ratio of the concentration of the product (Y) to the concentration of the reactant (X) at equilibrium is the value for the equilibrium constant (K_{eq}). Given the standard free-energy change ($\Delta G^{\circ\prime}$), the value for the equilibrium constant can be calculated from:

$$\Delta G^{\circ\prime} = -RT \ln K_{eq} \text{ ,}$$
$$\Delta G^{\circ\prime} = -RT \times 2.303 \, \log_{10} K_{eq} \text{ ,}$$
$$\log_{10} K_{eq} = \frac{\Delta G^{\circ\prime}}{-RT \times 2.303}$$

Note that at 25°C to 37°C, the value for RT × 2.303 is approximately 1.4 kcal.

4. The answer is D [IV A; Table 13-1]. The free energy of hydrolysis of 2-phosphoenolpyruvate is -14.8 kcal/mol, giving it a greater group transfer potential than that of adenosine triphosphate, which has a free energy of hydrolysis of -7.3 kcal/mol. None of the other phosphates listed are high-energy phosphate compounds.

5. The answer is B [V B 4]. Given the standard reduction potential change ($\Delta E_0{}'$) for an oxidation-reduction reaction, the standard free-energy change ($\Delta G^{\circ\prime}$) can be calculated from $\Delta G^{\circ\prime} = -nF\Delta E_0{}'$, where n is the number of electrons transferred and F is the Faraday constant (23.061 kcal per volt • equivalents). Thus, $\Delta G^{\circ\prime} = -2 \times 23.061 \times 0.3 = -13.8$ kcal/mol.

6-8. The answers are: 6-A, 7-C, 8-B [I A 3; II; Figures 13-1, 13-2, 13-3]. Stage 3 of metabolism consists of the citric acid cycle, oxidative phosphorylation, and the electron transport chain. The enzymes that comprise these pathways are located in the mitochondria.

The process of formation of glucose from citric acid cycle intermediates is called gluconeogenesis (see Figure 13-2). Certain enzymes that comprise that pathway function in each subcellular location.

The process of formation of pyruvate from glucose is glycolysis (see Figure 13-1). The enzymes that comprise this pathway are located in the cytosol.

9-11. The answers are: 9-E, 10-B, 11-A [IV B 1,2; V C 1,2]. Nicotinamide adenine dinucleotide (NAD^+) and nicotinamide adenine dinucleotide phosphate ($NADP^+$) transfer energy in the form of a proton and two electrons. The energy stored in $NADP^+$ is used primarily for reductive biosynthesis. The energy stored in NAD^+ is used primarily for synthesis of adenosine triphosphate (ATP).

The hydrolysis of ATP to form adenosine diphosphate plus inorganic phosphate exhibits a large negative standard free-energy change. The release of energy from this reaction is often used to drive other thermodynamically unfavorable reactions.

Chapter 14

Vitamins and Minerals
Victor Davidson

Case 14-1

A 6-month-old male infant is admitted to the hospital in a coma. The infant was normal at birth, but his condition has steadily deteriorated, and he is now lethargic and unable to control his head. His weight and head circumference are well below normal. Urinalysis reveals high levels of methylmalonic acid and compounds related to methionine metabolism. His serum level of vitamin B_{12} is 20 pg/ml (normal range = 150–1000 pg/ml). The infant's mother states that she is a strict vegetarian who has eaten no animal products, including milk and eggs, for the past 8 years, and she has taken no vitamin supplements. The infant is being exclusively breast-fed.

- What is the diagnosis?
- What is the treatment?
- What is the basis for abnormal urinalysis results?

Case 14-2

A 50-year-old man exhibits a photosensitive rash, abdominal pain, and diarrhea. He is also experiencing problems with short-term memory and mild impairment of cognitive function. His past medical history reveals a diagnosis several years ago of Crohn's disease. Serum levels of folate and vitamin B_{12} are normal.

- What is the diagnosis?
- What is the treatment?
- What is the significance of the history of Crohn's disease?

I. OVERVIEW

A. **Requirement.** Vitamins and essential minerals are required for normal growth, development, and maintenance of health.

 1. They cannot be synthesized by human tissues but must be included in the diet.

 2. When intake in the diet is below the needed level, deficiency symptoms appear. The time of onset of symptoms depends on the size and the daily flux of body reserves.

B. **Sources**

 1. All vitamins and essential minerals can be supplied by foods, but no single food is a rich source of all vitamins.

 2. Some vitamins also can be synthesized by intestinal microorganisms, but these microorganisms may not provide humans with the total requirement.

C. **Classification.** Vitamins are classified as water soluble or fat soluble.

 1. **Water-soluble vitamins** include B vitamins, folic acid, niacin, pantothenic acid, biotin, and vitamin C.

2. **Fat-soluble vitamins** include vitamins A, D, E, and K.

D. **Enzyme cofactors**

1. Vitamins and their derivatives often serve as cofactors for enzymes. Vitamin cofactors are referred to as **coenzymes.**

2. To be activated, some enzymes depend on conjugation of the protein portion of the enzyme (i.e., the apoenzyme) with a cofactor such that:

Apoenzyme + Cofactor = Holoenzyme

3. Cofactors that remain tightly bound to the enzyme and do not dissociate from it are called **prosthetic groups.**

4. **Minerals,** particularly transition metals (e.g., zinc, iron, copper), may also serve as cofactors. They confer on the enzyme a property that it does not possess in their absence. These metals may:
   a. Play a direct role in catalysis
   b. Serve as a redox reagent
   c. Form complexes with substrates

E. **Deficiency.** With exceptions noted in this chapter, most vitamin and mineral deficiencies present a variety of nonspecific symptoms (e.g., anemia, dermatologic problems, neurologic disorders), which are not easily attributed to a specific vitamin and are not easily distinguished from many other types of metabolic disorders. In the United States and in developed countries, vitamin deficiencies are relatively rare. Causes of deficiency include:

1. **Inadequate dietary intake**

2. **Inadequate absorption,** which may result from:
   a. Biliary obstruction (lack of bile leads to decreased absorption of the fat-soluble vitamins)
   b. Intestinal diseases or disorders
   c. Pernicious anemia, owing to lack of the intrinsic factor (see II C 4 b)

3. **Inadequate use,** which may result from:
   a. Lack of a transport protein for a particular vitamin in the serum
   b. Failure to convert a vitamin to its activated (i.e., coenzyme) form

4. **Increased requirements.** In some instances, an increased caloric requirement can unmask a borderline vitamin deficiency. Increased requirements occur during:
   a. Growth
   b. Pregnancy
   c. Lactation
   d. Wound healing and convalescence

5. **Increased excretion** (e.g., blood loss, diarrhea)

6. **Drug-induced deficiency,** such as:
   a. Loss of microbial vitamin synthesis in the intestine because of antibiotic therapy
   b. **Alcoholism** may increase certain vitamin requirements.
   c. **Drug-nutrient interactions** may increase certain vitamin requirements.

II. **WATER-SOLUBLE VITAMINS.** The water-soluble vitamins are, in most cases, cofactors in enzyme systems or precursors of cofactors. Table 14-1 lists the water-soluble vitamins, the cofactors to which they are converted in the body, some major enzyme systems that require each cofactor, and diseases associated with deficiencies.

A. **Ascorbic acid (vitamin C)**

TABLE 14-1. Water-Soluble Vitamins

Vitamin	Cofactor Form(s)	Some Associated Enzymes	Diseases Caused by Deficiency
Ascorbic acid (C)	Ascorbate	Prolyl and lysyl hydroxylases Dopamine β-hydroxylase	Scurvy
Biotin	Biotin	Carboxylases	Multiple carboxylase deficiency
Cobalamin (B_{12})	5'-Deoxyadenosylcobalamin Methylcobalamin	Methylmalonyl CoA mutase Homocysteine methyltransferase	Pernicious anemia
Folic acid	Tetrahydrofolate	Enzymes that transfer one-carbon units	Megaloblastic anemia
Niacin	NAD^+, $NADP^+$	Dehydrogenases	Pellagra
Pantothenic acid	Coenzyme A	Oxidative decarboxylases Enzymes that transfer acyl groups	
Pyridoxine (B_6)	Pyridoxal phosphate	Glycogen phosphorylase Aminotransferases Enzymes of amino acid metabolism	
Riboflavin (B_2)	FAD, FMN	Dehydrogenases Oxidases Oxygenases	Ariboflavinosis
Thiamine (B_1)	Thiamine pyrophosphate	α-Keto acid decarboxylases Transketolase	Beriberi Wernicke-Korsakoff syndrome

FAD = flavin adenine dinucleotide; FMN = flavin mononucleotide; NAD^+ = nicotinamide adenine dinucleotide; $NADP^+$ = nicotinamide adenine dinucleotide phosphate.

1. **Sources** include citrus fruits and their juices, strawberries, cantaloupes, and raw or minimally cooked vegetables.

2. **Metabolism.** Vitamin C is not metabolized but functions as a cofactor in this form.

3. **Functions**
   a. Vitamin C is required for the hydroxylation of proline and lysine residues during biosynthesis of collagen in fibroblasts (see Chapter 3 V C).
   b. It is required in the syntheses of norepinephrine and epinephrine (see Chapter 25 III A).
   c. Vitamin C is an **antioxidant** that protects cells against free radical damage.
   d. It aids iron absorption.

4. **Deficiency** leads to the condition known as **scurvy** in humans (see Chapter 3 V D).

B. **Biotin**

1. **Sources.** Biotin is synthesized by intestinal microorganisms in sufficient quantities that a dietary source is normally not necessary. Dietary sources include liver and eggs.

2. **Metabolism**
   a. Biotin is not modified but **must be covalently attached to the enzymes** that use it as a prosthetic group.
   b. **Biotin holocarboxylase synthetase** covalently links the free carboxyl group of biotin to a specific lysine residue of the enzyme.
   c. **Biotinidase** catalyzes the removal of biotin from enzymes during protein turnover, which allows biotin to be recycled in the body.

3. **Functions.** Biotin acts as a coenzyme in **carboxylation reactions,** where it is a carrier of carbon dioxide. Four carboxylase enzymes in the body require biotin.

4. **Deficiency**
   a. Biotin deficiency due to inadequate dietary intake is very rare unless accompanied by other factors, such as the following.

  (1) Antibiotics that inhibit the growth of intestinal bacteria eliminate this source of biotin.

  (2) Ingestion of unusually large amounts of **avidin,** a protein present in raw egg whites, prevents biotin absorption because it has a very high affinity for biotin.

 b. **Multiple carboxylase deficiency** results from a biotin deficiency or a defect in biotin holocarboxylase synthetase, which prevents the attachment of biotin to biotin-dependent enzymes (see Chapter 20 IV A). Symptoms include seborrheic dermatitis, anorexia, nausea, and muscular pain.

C. **Cobalamin (vitamin B$_{12}$)**

 1. Sources. Microorganisms are the sole source of cobalamin in nature. Plants are devoid of vitamin B$_{12}$, but it is present in most animal and dairy products.

 2. Metabolism

  a. Structure. Cobalamin is composed in part of a corrin ring with an atom of cobalt present at its active site. In commercial preparations, cyanide serves as a ligand to cobalt. This must be changed to generate the two active cofactor forms of the vitamin, **methylcobalamin** and **5-deoxyadenosylcobalamin.**

  b. Vitamin B$_{12}$ is absorbed in the ileum as a complex with **intrinsic factor,** a glycoprotein formed in the gastric mucosa.

  c. The vitamin is transported in serum bound to globulin and converted to methylcobalamin and 5-deoxyadenosylcobalamin in the liver, bone marrow cells, and reticulocytes.

 3. Functions

  a. Only two human enzymes require cobalamin.

   (1) **Methylmalonyl coenzyme A (methylmalonyl CoA) mutase,** which is involved in the catabolism of isoleucine and valine and in the use of propionyl CoA, **requires 5-deoxyadenosylcobalamin** as its cofactor (see Chapter 24 V E).

   (2) **Homocysteine methyltransferase,** which catalyzes the methylation of homocysteine to methionine, **requires methylcobalamin** as its cofactor (see Chapter 25 II C).

  b. Vitamin B$_{12}$ function is related to folate metabolism; lack of methylcobalamin leads to a deficiency in the folate coenzyme pool (see Chapter 25 II C).

 4. Deficiency

  a. The enterohepatic circulation of vitamin B$_{12}$ provides almost total conservation of the vitamin, and a deficiency would take several years to develop if the vitamin were removed from the diet. However, damage to the stomach or the ileum causes deficiency to occur more rapidly.

  b. **Pernicious anemia** is the consequence of vitamin B$_{12}$ deficiency.

   (1) It is due to an absence of intrinsic factor.

   (2) Consequences include macrocytic anemia, megaloblastosis of bone marrow, degeneration of axis cylinders of spinal cord neurons, lesions of mucous surfaces, glossitis, and methylmalonic aciduria.

  c. A long-term, strict vegetarian diet may also lead to a deficiency of vitamin B$_{12}$.

D. **Folic acid (folate)**

 1. Sources include synthesis by intestinal bacteria, as well as liver and green vegetables in the diet. Folate is easily destroyed by cooking.

 2. Metabolism

  a. Structure. Folic acid is comprised of these connected moieties: a pteridine ring, *p*-aminobenzoate, and glutamic acid.

  b. Folate in food is primarily present in a polyglutamate form. The extra glutamate residues are removed by an intestinal **conjugase** before absorption, primarily in the small intestine.

3. Functions

   a. Folate coenzymes (e.g., tetrahydrofolate) act as carriers of one-carbon fragments at different levels of oxidation (see Chapter 25 II B).

   b. Folate is necessary for proper purine nucleotide and deoxythymidylate synthesis (see Chapter 26 I B).

4. Deficiency. Clinical symptoms of folic acid deficiency include megaloblastosis of bone marrow (megaloblastic anemia).

E. Niacin (nicotinic acid)

1. Sources

   a. Niacin is formed in humans during the catabolism of tryptophan. However, this provides only approximately 10% of the requirement. The remainder must come from the diet.

   b. Dietary sources include cereals, legumes, and meats.

2. Metabolism and function. Niacin is the precursor for biosynthesis of nicotinamide adenine dinucleotide (NAD^+) and its phosphate ($NADP^+$), which are essential cofactors involved in a variety of biologic oxidation–reduction reactions (see Chapter 13 V C).

3. Deficiency of niacin results in pellagra. Clinical symptoms include:

   a. Dermatitis

   b. Diarrhea from chronic inflammation of the intestinal mucosa

   c. Dementia

F. Pantothenic acid (pantothenate)

1. Sources. Pantothenate is widely distributed in foods and is synthesized by some intestinal bacteria.

2. Metabolism and function. Pantothenic acid is a precursor in the biosynthesis of coenzyme A.

3. Deficiency in humans is practically unknown.

G. Pyridoxine (vitamin B₆)

1. Sources include meat, fish, poultry, whole-grain cereals, and certain vegetables. The requirements increase during pregnancy and lactation.

2. Metabolism. Pyridoxine and closely related compounds (i.e., pyridoxamine, pyridoxal) can function as vitamin B_6. However, these compounds must be converted by phosphorylation to the biologically active cofactor, pyridoxal phosphate (PLP).

3. Functions

   a. PLP serves as a cofactor for many enzymes that use amino acids as substrates (see Table 14-1). **PLP enzymes form covalent Schiff-base intermediates** between the aldehyde portion of PLP and the α-amino group of amino acids. A wide range of amino acid transformations are catalyzed by PLP enzymes after formation of this reaction intermediate. These include:

   (1) Transaminations with α-keto acids

   (2) Decarboxylations

   (3) Aldol cleavages

   (4) Racemizations

   (5) Deaminations

   (6) Elimination and replacement reactions at the beta and gamma carbons

   b. PLP also is a cofactor for **glycogen phosphorylase** (see Chapter 21 III A) where it is needed for glycogen metabolism.

4. Deficiency of vitamin B_6 is rare but may occur as a result of interaction with certain drugs, most notably isoniazid, which is used for the treatment of tuberculosis and is an antagonist of PLP. **Clinical symptoms** include:

   a. Lesions of the skin and mucosa

b. Sideroblastic anemia

c. Neuronal dysfunction, including convulsions

H. Riboflavin (vitamin B$_2$)

1. **Sources** include dairy products, meats, vegetables and whole grain foods. The requirement for riboflavin is related to protein use and is increased during growth, pregnancy, lactation, and wound healing.

2. **Metabolism.** Riboflavin is converted to flavin mononucleotide (FMN) in the intestinal mucosal cells and then to flavin adenine dinucleotide (FAD) in the liver.

3. **Functions.** The coenzymes FAD and FMN are required by several oxidative enzymes (see Chapter 13 V C).

4. **Deficiency** of vitamin B$_2$ causes **ariboflavinosis,** which is characterized by vascularization of the cornea; lesions of the lips, mouth, skin, and genitalia, especially angular stomatitis; cheilosis; glossitis; and seborrheic dermatitis.

I. Thiamine (vitamin B$_1$)

1. **Sources** include pork, whole-grain cereals, legumes, and enriched grain products. Storage is limited, and the liver stores can be depleted in 12–14 days.

2. **Metabolism.** Thiamine is the precursor of **thiamine pyrophosphate (TPP),** which is formed by reaction with adenosine triphosphate (ATP).

3. **Functions.** TPP is a cofactor involved in the enzyme complexes that decarboxylate α-keto acids and is also a cofactor for transketolase.

4. **Deficiency** of vitamin B$_1$ can lead to disturbances in carbohydrate metabolism and to decreased transketolase activity, particularly in erythrocytes and leukocytes. Clinically, deficiency can lead to cardiovascular and neurologic lesions, as well as to emotional disturbances.
   a. **"Dry" beriberi** develops when the diet chronically contains slightly less thiamine than required. Symptoms include peripheral neuropathy, fatigue, and impaired capacity to work.
   b. **"Wet" beriberi** develops with a severe deficiency. In addition to neurologic manifestations, cardiovascular symptoms are more apparent, including heart enlargement and tachycardia. Cardiac failure is common after stress, and edema and anorexia are characteristic, as well.
   c. **Wernicke-Korsakoff syndrome** develops in the most acute deficiencies and is seen primarily in alcoholics (see Chapter 17 I C 5 c).

III. FAT-SOLUBLE VITAMINS (Table 14-2)

A. Retinol (vitamin A)

1. **Sources** include green leafy and yellow vegetables, liver, butterfat, and fortified milk.

TABLE 14-2. Fat-Soluble Vitamins

Vitamin	Primary Function	Diseases Caused by Deficiency
A	Role in vision	Blindness
D	Calcium metabolism	Rickets, osteomalacia
E	Free radical scavenger	
K	Role in blood clotting	

2. **Metabolism**
   a. **Carotenoids** (e.g., **beta-carotene**) are provitamins that are converted to retinal and retinol, which are the forms used by the body.
   b. Carotenoids may be directly absorbed, but most are cleaved to retinal and then converted to retinol, which is absorbed.
   c. Retinyl esters are hydrolyzed, and retinol is absorbed in the upper intestine.
   d. In the intestinal mucosal cells, retinol is re-esterified with palmitate and transported to the liver, where 90% of the body's vitamin A is stored.

3. **Functions**
   a. **Role in vision**
      (1) On entering the retina, retinol is esterified to a fatty acid, providing a means of concentrating the retinol within the cell.
      (2) The fatty acid esters are hydrolyzed, and the retinol is oxidized to retinal by a specific NAD^+-linked dehydrogenase.
      (3) The retinal forms complex with proteins called **opsins** in the rods and cones.
      (4) Opsins preferentially bind the 11-*cis* isomer rather than all-*trans* retinal.
      (5) The absorption of light triggers a conformational change in opsin and conversion of the 11-*cis* isomer of retinal to the all-*trans* form, which is only weakly bound to opsin. This results in the generation of an action potential.
   b. Vitamin A also appears necessary for growth of epithelial tissue, reproduction, and bone growth.

4. **Deficiency** may cause the following:
   a. Defects in vision, progressing from night blindness to total blindness
   b. Skin lesions such as follicular hyperkeratosis
   c. Gonadal dysfunction in males and miscarriage in females

B. **Cholecalciferol (vitamin D_3)**

1. **Sources.** Vitamin D is required only as an accessory food factor when humans are deprived of sunlight. It is synthesized in the skin by the action of ultraviolet light. Dietary sources include liver, eggs, and fortified milk.

2. **Metabolism and function.** Cholecalciferol (vitamin D_3), which is formed from 7-dehydrocholesterol, is a precursor of the hormone 1,25-dihydroxycholecalciferol, which is **a regulator of calcium metabolism** (see Chapter 23 IV E).

3. **Deficiency**
   a. In children, vitamin D deficiency leads to a condition known as **rickets,** which manifests as a malformation of the long bones.
   b. In adults, there is an increased radiolucency of bones and tendency for fractures to occur. The condition is known as **osteomalacia.**

C. **Tocopherol (vitamin E)**

1. **Sources** include vegetable and seed oils.

2. **Metabolism.** Vitamin E apparently is unmetabolized in the body.

3. **Function.** Its role appears to be primarily that of a **scavenger of potentially damaging free radicals.** It prevents oxidation and peroxidation of polyunsaturated fatty acids, thus preventing membrane dysfunction and altered lipoprotein metabolism.

4. **Deficiency** of vitamin E in humans is associated with hemolysis of erythrocytes, because of a lack of protection against peroxides, and with creatinuria due to increased muscle breakdown.

D. **Vitamin K**

1. **Sources.** Vitamin K is widely distributed in foods and synthesized by intestinal bacteria.

2. **Metabolism.** There are various forms of vitamin K, which is a lipid, that differ in

the length and degree of unsaturation. The significance of this is unclear.

3. **Functions. Vitamin K plays a role in blood coagulation** (see Chapter 4 VIII). Several enzyme factors involved in the blood-clotting process become active by binding calcium ions. These proenzymes bind calcium ions strongly because their amino-terminal segments contain glutamate residues that have been carboxylated to dicarboxylate forms. Vitamin K acts as a cofactor in these carboxylation reactions.

4. **Deficiency** of vitamin K is rare. It may occur in newborn children, particularly if the gut is sterile, because the placenta is relatively weak in the transmission of lipids.

IV. MINERALS

 Nutritional requirements. Minerals may be categorized based on the extent to which they are required (Table 14-3).

1. **Macrominerals** are required in amounts greater than 100 mg per day.

2. **Microminerals (trace elements)** are required in amounts less than 100 mg per day.

TABLE 14-3. Essential Minerals

Mineral	Primary Functions	Diseases Caused by Deficiency
Macrominerals		
Calcium	Component of bone; nerve and muscle regulation	Rickets, osteoporosis
Chloride	Electrolyte balance; gastric fluid	
Magnesium	Component of bone; enzyme cofactor	
Manganese	Enzyme cofactor	
Phosphorus	Component of bone and metabolites	
Potassium	Electrolyte balance; nerve and muscle regulation	
Sodium	Electrolyte balance; nerve and muscle regulation	
Microminerals		
Chromium	Present in glucose tolerance factor	
Cobalt	Component of vitamin B_{12}	
Copper	Enzyme cofactor	Menkes' syndrome
Iodine	Component of thyroid hormones	Goiter, hypothyroidism
Iron	Component of heme; enzyme cofactor	Anemia
Molybdenum	Enzyme cofactor	
Selenium	Present in glutathione peroxidase	
Zinc	Enzyme cofactor	

B. **Functions.** The functions of specific minerals are summarized in Table 14-3.

C. **Deficiencies** of most minerals are relatively rare and the symptoms are not well defined. Some of the better understood mineral deficiencies include the following.

1. **Calcium** deficiency may cause **rickets** in children and contribute to **osteoporosis** in adults.

2. **Copper. Menkes' syndrome** is caused by an inability to absorb copper from the intestine.

3. **Iodine**
   a. Inadequate dietary intake may cause an enlargement of the thyroid gland **(goiter).**
   b. Chronic deficiency leads to **hypothyroidism,** which is caused by insufficient production of thyroid hormones. In children, this causes cretinism.

4. **Iron** deficiency may cause anemia because iron is a component of hemoglobin.

5. **Zinc** deficiency has been associated with poor wound healing.

Case 14-1 Revisited

The infant's condition is consistent with a deficiency of vitamin B_{12}. Vitamin B_{12} can be obtained only through the diet from animal and dairy products; it is not found in plants. Deficiency of this vitamin is rare because it is highly conserved and stored in the liver. Several years of a diet devoid of the vitamin are required to cause a deficiency. Because the mother has been a strict vegetarian for 8 years, her stores of vitamin B_{12} are not sufficient for her breast milk to contain levels necessary to support the infant.

Because this infant's condition is caused by a deficiency due to inadequate diet, it can be treated simply by administration of the vitamin. The infant is administered a 1 mg/day dose of the vitamin for 4 days, and his condition improves dramatically.

The compounds in the infant's urine are metabolites that are normally processed by the two vitamin B_{12}-dependent human enzymes; that is, methylmalonyl coenzyme A mutase and homocysteine methyltransferase.

Case 14-2 Revisited

The patient exhibits the classic triad of symptoms of pellagra: dermatitis, diarrhea, and dementia. Pellagra is caused by a deficiency of niacin.

The patient is given oral doses of niacin and placed on an adequate diet with vitamin B supplements. Within weeks the rash and diarrhea subside, and within months his mental impairment improves.

Niacin deficiency is very rare in developed countries. In this case, the deficiency is due to chronic malabsorption of the vitamin. Crohn's disease is a gastrointestinal disease, which in this case decreased the efficiency of absorption of the vitamin from the diet.

STUDY QUESTIONS

DIRECTIONS: Each of the numbered items or incomplete statements in this section is followed by answers or by completions of the statement. Select the **one** lettered answer or completion that is **best** in each case.

Questions 1–2

A 50-year-old man presents with impaired cognitive abilities and peripheral neuropathy. He is a chronic alcoholic and has not been eating well for several weeks.

1. In which one of the following vitamins is this patient most likely deficient?

(A) Thiamine (vitamin B_1)
(B) Cobalamin (vitamin B_{12})
(C) Biotin
(D) Vitamin K
(E) Vitamin D

2. What is the most likely diagnosis for the patient's neuologic problems?

(A) Pernicious anemia
(B) Menkes' syndrome
(C) Wernicke-Korsakoff syndrome
(D) Scurvy
(E) Multiple carboxylase deficiency

3. The disease pellagra is due to a deficiency of

(A) vitamin B_6
(B) biotin
(C) pantothenic acid
(D) folic acid
(E) niacin

4. Which one of the following must be modified to serve as a cofactor for enzymes?

(A) Copper
(B) Biotin
(C) Zinc
(D) Pantothenic acid
(E) Ascorbic acid

DIRECTIONS: The group of items in this section consists of lettered options followed by a set of numbered items. For each item, select the **one** lettered option that is most closely associated with it. Each lettered option may be selected once, more than once, or not at all.

Questions 5–11

For each vitamin listed below, select the metabolic process with which it is most likely to be associated.

(A) Degradation of amino acids
(B) Synthesis of DNA
(C) Calcium metabolism
(D) Electron transport
(E) Vision
(F) Blood clotting
(G) Collagen formation

5. Pyridoxine (vitamin B_6)

6. Folic acid

7. Cholecalciferol (vitamin D_3)

8. Niacin

9. Ascorbic acid (vitamin C)

10. Vitamin A

11. Vitamin K

ANSWERS AND EXPLANATIONS

1–2. The answers are: 1-A, 2-C [II I 1, 4 c]. This patient may exhibit multiple nutritional deficiencies. Of the choices, thiamine is most likely. Its storage in the liver is limited. Inadequate diet and malabsorption due to alcohol abuse exacerbate the deficiency. Cobalamin stores in the body last several years. Biotin and vitamin K requirements can be met by synthesis by intestinal microorganisms. Vitamin D is formed by the action of ultraviolet light in the skin.

Dementia and associated neuropathies caused by a deficiency of thiamine is called Wernicke-Korsakoff syndrome. Pernicious anemia is caused by a cobalamin deficiency. Menkes' syndrome is caused by a copper deficiency. Scurvy is caused by a vitamin C deficiency. Multiple carboxylase deficiency results from a biotin deficiency.

3. The answer is E [II E 3]. Pellagra is a disease caused by a deficiency of niacin. The symptoms include dermatitis, diarrhea, and dementia. Niacin is a precursor of nicotinamide adenine dinucleotide and its phosphate, which are cofactors for many oxidoreductases.

4. The answer is D [I D; II F 2; Table 14-1; Table 14-3]. The minerals copper and zinc and the vitamins biotin and ascorbic acid may be considered cofactors, but each associates directly with enzymes without requiring any further modification. Pantothenic acid is a precursor that must be metabolized to form coenzyme A.

5–11. The answers are: 5-A [II G 3], **6-B** [II D 3 b], **7-C** [III B 2], **8-D** [II E 2], **9-G** [II A 3 a], **10-E** [III A 3 a], **11-F** [III D 3]. Phosphorylation of pyridoxine yields the biologically active cofactor pyridoxal phosphate (PLP). PLP serves as a coenzyme for a large number of enzymes, particularly those that catalyze reactions involving metabolism of amino acids (e.g., transamination, deamination, decarboxylation).

The biologically active form of folic acid is tetrahydrofolic acid. This form transfers one-carbon fragments to appropriate metabolites in the synthesis of amino acids, purines, and thymidylic acid, which is a characteristic pyrimidine of DNA.

The active form of vitamin D_3, 1,25-dihydroxycholecalciferol, stimulates the intestinal absorption of calcium and phosphate, increases the mobilization of calcium and phosphate from bone, and promotes the renal reabsorption of calcium and phosphate. These functions in coordination with the activities of other hormones are critical in regulating calcium homeostasis.

The biologically active forms of niacin are nicotinamide adenine dinucleotide (NAD^+) and nicotinamide adenine dinucleotide phosphate ($NADP^+$). These two cofactors serve as coenzymes in oxidation–reduction reactions in which the coenzyme undergoes reduction of the pyridine ring by accepting a hydride ion (hydrogen ion plus one electron). Vitamin C is required as a cofactor for enzymes that catalyze the hydroxylation of proline and lysine residues during collagen biosynthesis.

The *cis* isomer of retinal, which is derived from vitamin A, is preferentially bound by proteins called opsins in the cells of the retina. The absorption of a photon of light by the opsin-*cis*-retinal complex is accompanied by a change in the configuration of the opsin and the conversion of *cis*-retinal to all-*trans*-retinal, which results in the generation of an action potential.

Vitamin K acts as a cofactor in carboxylation reactions that modify enzymes involved in the blood-clotting process. These modifications allow the clotting process to be regulated by calcium binding to these enzymes.

Chapter 15

Mechanisms of Hormone Action
Susan Wellman
Donald Sittman

Case 15-1

A 2-year-old white boy presents with a temperature of 99.5°C and severe, paroxysmal coughing. After coughing 5–15 times in a row, the child makes a whooping sound when he inhales. The coughing episodes sometimes produce a very viscous mucus. The coughing on occasion is severe enough that the child vomits. The parent reports that the child has had cold-like symptoms for longer than 1 week and has been coughing a lot at night.

- What is the likely diagnosis of this patient, and how is it confirmed?
- What is the cause of this disease and its symptoms?
- What is the treatment and prognosis for this patient?

I. **OVERVIEW.** Hormones coordinate metabolism in the body. They are substances that carry information from **sensor cells,** which sense changes in the environment, to **target cells,** which respond to changes. Hormones can be classified by the proximity of their site of synthesis to their site of action, by their chemical structure, and by their degree of water solubility (Table 15-1).

A. **Categorized by site of synthesis**

1. **Endocrine hormones** are synthesized by endocrine glands and transported by the blood to their target cells.

2. **Paracrine hormones** are synthesized near their targets of action.

3. **Autocrine hormones** affect the cells that synthesize them.

TABLE 15-1. Examples of Selected Hormones and Effects

Hormone	Structure	Type	Example of Effect
Epinephrine	Amino acid derivative	Hydrophilic	Increases glycogenolysis
Glucagon	Peptide	Hydrophilic	Increases glycogenolysis
Insulin	Protein	Hydrophilic	Stimulates entry of glucose into cells
Epidermal growth factor	Protein	Hydrophilic	Stimulates cell proliferation
Vasopressin	Peptide	Hydrophilic	Increases water reabsorption in the kidney
Prostaglandin $F_{2\alpha}$	Fatty acid derivative	Hydrophilic	Stimulates smooth muscle contraction
Thyroxine	Amino acid derivative	Lipophilic	Increases metabolic activity of cells
Cortisol	Cholesterol derivative	Lipophilic	Stimulates gluconeogenesis
Estradiol	Cholesterol derivative	Lipophilic	Maintains female secondary sex characteristics

B. **Categorized by chemical structure.** Hormones can be any of the following substances:

1. **Proteins or peptides** (e.g., insulin, glucagon), which are synthesized as larger precursors that undergo processing and secretion

2. **Amino acid derivatives** (e.g., catecholamines, thyroid hormones)

3. **Fatty acid derivatives** (e.g., eicosanoids)

4. **Cholesterol derivatives** (e.g., steroids)

5. **Gases** (e.g., nitric oxide)

C. **Categorized by water solubility.** Except for the gas nitric oxide, which acts as a hormone-like signaling molecule, all hormones fall into two classes of water solubility: hydrophilic and lipophilic. Hormones from different classes elicit their effects on target cells in different ways.

1. **Hydrophilic hormones bind to a receptor molecule on the outer surface of the cell,** with the concomitant initiation of a reaction within the cell that modifies cell function.

2. **Lipophilic hormones bind to intracellular receptors,** with subsequent modulation of gene expression by the hormone-receptor complex. The initial hormone-receptor interaction may occur in the cytoplasm with subsequent transfer to the nucleus, or it may occur initially in the nucleus.

II. **HYDROPHILIC HORMONES.** When hydrophilic hormones interact with receptors on the surface of a cell, they elicit varied responses. These responses depend on the **receptor type,** and, for certain types of receptors, the **receptor subtype.** For example, receptor subtypes exist for epinephrine; the receptor subtypes bind to epinephrine, but the receptors are otherwise different and elicit different effects. Receptor subtypes also exist for many neurotransmitters.

A. **Hormone-receptor interaction**

1. **Structure of receptor molecules.** The receptor molecules for hydrophilic hormones are **large, integral membrane proteins with specificity and high affinity** for a given hormone.

2. The **binding between hormone and receptor is reversible,** and the hormonal action declines as the plasma level of a hormone declines.

3. **Hydrophilic hormones can initiate a response without entering the cell.**

4. **Hydrophilic hormones tend to cause a more rapid response and have a shorter duration of action than do hydrophobic hormones.** Their actions last from seconds to hours.

B. **G proteins mediate the effects of many hormones.** G proteins are associated with hormone receptors on the cytosolic side of the cell membrane.

1. **Nomenclature.** The G protein is so named because it **binds guanine nucleotides.** Either guanosine triphosphate (GTP) or guanosine diphosphate (GDP) may be bound to the G protein.

2. **Structure.** G proteins consist of **three subunits: α, β, and γ.** The α subunit binds GTP or GDP. The β and γ subunits do not bind nucleotides, they bind to the α subunit (see II B 2 b).

   a. The **hormone-receptor complex** catalyzes the exchange of GDP for GTP by the G protein. The receptor alone does not catalyze this exchange.

b. When GDP is exchanged for GTP on the α subunit, G_α-GTP dissociates from $G_{\beta\gamma}$. **G_α-GTP is the active form.**

3. **Types.** The effect of the active form (G_α-GTP) depends on the specific type of G protein. There are several different types of G proteins: **G_s** stimulates the enzyme adenylate cyclase, **G_i** inhibits the enzyme adenylate cyclase, and **G_q** stimulates the enzyme phospholipase C (see II D 1, F).

4. **Function.** The G_α subunit of all G proteins is a **GTPase.** It slowly hydrolyzes its bound GTP to GDP and thereby returns to its inactive, GDP-bound state. G_α then reassociates with $G_{\beta\gamma}$, where it remains until it is reactivated by a hormone-receptor complex.

C. **G-protein–linked receptors.** There are more than 100 different types of G-protein–linked receptors. Although quite varied in the hormones with which they interact and the response that they elicit, their overall structure is similar. Each is made of a single polypeptide that crosses back and forth through the plasma membrane seven times. The amino-terminal end is in contact with the extracellular space, where it can bind to the appropriate hormone. The carboxyl-terminal end is within the cytoplasm, where it can elicit an intracellular response.

D. **Hormone receptors can be linked to G_s proteins.** The G_α-GTP subunit of a G_s protein stimulates adenylate cyclase (Figure 15-1).

1. **Adenylate cyclase** is a large, integral membrane protein.
   a. **Function.** Adenylate cyclase **catalyzes the formation of cyclic adenosine monophosphate (cAMP)** from adenosine triphosphate (ATP; see Chapter 12, Figure 12-2).
      (1) **Second messengers** are a group of compounds that **relay information from certain types of hormone-receptor complexes to molecules within the cell,** where they elicit a response. cAMP is a second messenger.
      (2) **cAMP-dependent protein kinase.** cAMP affects cellular function by **activating a protein kinase,** which through phosphorylation activates specific cellular proteins. The protein kinase is specific for cAMP, and is thus called cAMP-dependent protein kinase.
         (a) **Structure of cAMP-dependent protein kinase.** The cAMP-dependent protein kinase is a tetramer having two types of subunits: two regulatory (R) subunits and two catalytic (C) subunits.
         (b) **The R_2C_2 tetramer is inactive.**
            (i) **Two molecules of cAMP bind to each R subunit,** whereupon the R_2C_2 complex disassociates into an R_2 subunit and two C units that are each catalytically active.
            (ii) The active protein kinase **transfers the γ-phosphate group** from ATP to a specific amino acid of a specific cell protein.
   b. **cAMP-phosphodiesterase activity.** The levels of cAMP are quickly reduced as a result of its hydrolysis to AMP by a cytoplasmic enzyme, **cyclic nucleotide phosphodiesterase (PDEase;** see Chapter 12, Figure 12-2).
   c. **Hormones that activate adenylate cyclase** include glucagon, which is a peptide, and epinephrine, which is an amino acid derivative. This activation occurs at two subtypes of epinephrine receptors: the β_1 and β_2 adrenergic receptors.

2. **Cholera toxin** is an enzyme produced by the bacterium *Vibrio cholerae.*
   a. **Action.** Cholera toxin modifies the α subunit of G_s, which blocks the hydrolysis of GTP to GDP. This prevents the inactivation of G_s by this mechanism (see Figure 15-1).
   b. **Result.** The result is a persistently high level of cAMP, which causes the epithelial cells of the intestine to transport sodium ions and water into the intestinal lumen. This results in severe diarrhea.

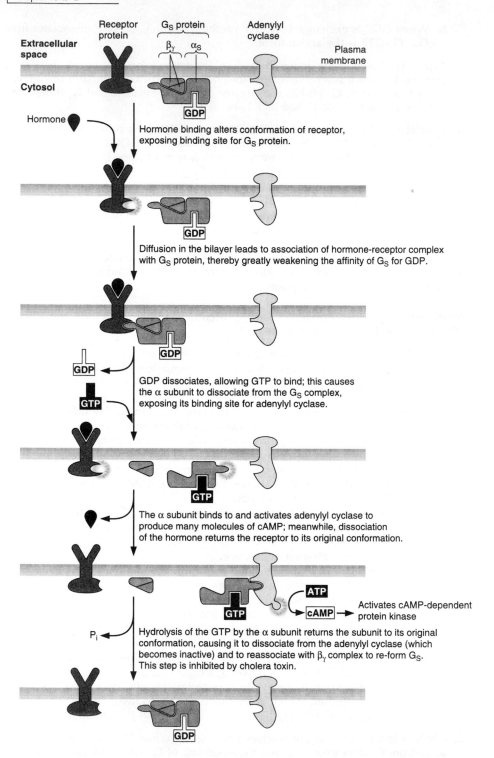

FIGURE 15-1. Activation of adenylate cyclase by a hormone binding to its receptor. The hormone-receptor complex activates G$_s$ protein, which activates adenylate cyclase. *cAMP* = cyclic adenosine monophosphate; *ATP* = adenosine triphosphate; *GDP* = guanosine diphosphate; *GTP* = guanosine triphosphate; *P$_i$* = inorganic phosphate. (Reprinted with permission from Alberts B, Bray D, Lewis J, et al: *Molecular Biology of the Cell,* 3rd ed. New York, Garland Publishing, 1994, p 739.)

E. Hormone receptors can be linked to G_i proteins. The active, G_α-GTP subunits of G_i proteins result in inhibition of adenylate cyclase.

1. **Structure.** The β and γ subunits of G_i and G_s proteins are identical. The α subunits differ.

2. **Function**
   a. The G_α-GTP of the G_i protein inhibits adenylate cyclase. **Also, the $G_{\beta\gamma}$ that is released when the G_α-GTP dissociates from the G_i protein binds to the G_α-GTP of a G_s protein and blocks its activation of adenylate cyclase.**
      (1) An example of a hormone that inhibits adenylate cyclase is **epinephrine** at the α_2 receptor subtype.
      (2) **Pertussis toxin** is an enzyme that modifies the α subunit of G_i. The modification prevents G_i from exchanging GDP for GTP. Therefore, the modified G_i protein is unable to block the activation of adenylate cyclase. Pertussis toxin is produced by *Bordetella pertussis,* the bacterium that causes **whooping cough.**
   b. G_i also serves to activate potassium channels within the plasma membrane.

F. Hormone receptors can be linked to G_q proteins. When activated, G_q proteins stimulate phospholipase C-β (Figure 15-2).

1. **Phospholipase C-β** is a membrane-bound enzyme that hydrolyzes **phosphatidylinositol 4,5-bisphosphate (PIP$_2$),** which is a membrane phospholipid.

2. **Products of hydrolysis** include **inositol 1,4,5-triphosphate (IP$_3$)** and **diacylglycerol (DAG),** both of which are second messengers [see II D 1 a (1)]. In many cells, IP$_3$ and DAG work together to activate protein kinase C.
   a. **IP$_3$,** a water-soluble molecule, diffuses into the cytosol and causes the release of calcium ions from intracellular stores. IP$_3$ is rapidly inactivated by dephosphorylation.

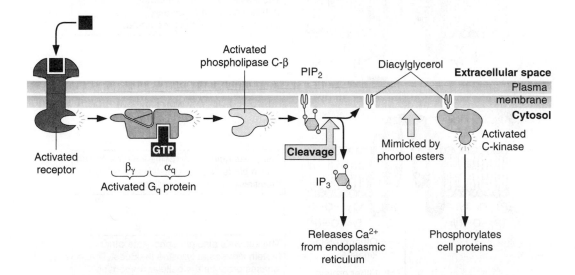

FIGURE 15-2. Activation of phospholipase C-β by a hormone binding to its receptor. The hormone-receptor complex activates a G_q protein, which activates phospholipase C-β. Phospholipase C-β catalyzes the hydrolysis of phosphatidylinositol 4,5-bisphosphate *(PIP$_2$)* to inositol 1,4,5-triphosphate *(IP$_3$)* and diacylglycerol *(DAG).* IP$_3$ causes the release of calcium from intracellular stores. Protein kinase C, which is calcium-dependent, is activated by DAG, so IP$_3$ and DAG can work together to activate protein kinase C. GTP = guanosine triphosphate; ■ = hormone. (Reprinted with permission from Alberts B, Bray D, Lewis J, et al: *Molecular Biology of the Cell,* 3rd ed. New York, Garland Publishing, 1994, p 749.)

b. **DAG,** a lipid-soluble molecule, diffuses laterally in the membrane and **activates protein kinase C, which is calcium-dependent.** DAG is rapidly inactivated by hydrolysis.

c. **Phorbol esters mimic the effects of DAG.** They are **tumor promoters.** Although they do not cause tumors to form, they induce proliferation of cells. Unlike DAG, phorbol esters are not rapidly hydrolyzed. This results in prolonged activation of protein kinase C, which causes cell proliferation.

3. **Example.** A hormone that activates phospholipase C-β is epinephrine at the α_1-adrenergic receptor subtype.

 Hormone receptors may be transmembrane enzymes. Transmembrane enzymes have distinct domains with separate functions. The extracellular domain binds to the hormone; the cytoplasmic domain has enzymatic activity that is stimulated when hormone binds to the extracellular domain (Figure 15-3).

1. One type of receptor is a **transmembrane tyrosine kinase,** which when activated, phosphorylates tyrosine residues.

a. The receptor first phosphorylates itself **(autophosphorylation).** Autophosphorylation usually occurs when two receptors come together, or **dimerize,** upon hormone binding. Each receptor then phosphorylates the other. Autophosphorylated receptors are more active in phosphorylating other proteins.

b. Hormone receptors that are transmembrane tyrosine kinases include receptors for many growth factors such as **epidermal growth factor (EGF)** and **platelet-derived growth factor (PDGF).**

c. **Insulin receptors** are also tyrosine kinases (see Figure 15-3). They are tetrameric in structure, and their two intracellular catalytic domains phosphorylate each other.

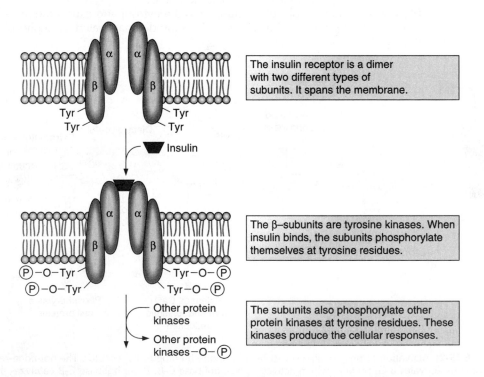

FIGURE 15-3. The insulin receptor is a dimeric transmembrane tyrosine kinase. Upon activation by insulin binding, it phosphorylates itself and other, unidentified cellular proteins. (Adapted with permission from Marks D, Marks A, and Smith C: *Basic Medical Biochemistry, A Clinical Approach.* Philadelphia, Williams & Wilkins, 1996, p 386.)

d. The oncogene *erbB* codes for an altered form of the EGF receptor. The *erbB* protein lacks the hormone-binding domain of the EGF receptor and is always activated. Its unregulated activity leads to unregulated growth and on-cogenesis.

2. **Downstream activation by tyrosine kinases.** A large number of proteins are activated by tyrosine kinases that have been activated by phosphorylation.
   a. These proteins have in common two domains, **SH2 and SH3** (Src homology domains).
      (1) The SH2 domain is responsible for recognition and binding to phosphorylated tyrosine.
      (2) The SH3 domain probably plays a role in binding to other proteins to be activated.
   b. The proteins that bind to activated tyrosine kinases and are activated by phosphorylation are functionally diverse. For example:
      (1) **Signal transduction and activators of transcription (STATs)** dimerize upon phosphorylation and translocate to the nucleus where they activate the transcription of particular genes.
      (2) **Phospholipase C-γ** is activated by the EGF receptor but functions the same as phospholipase C-β (see II F 1).
      (3) **Ras and related proteins** are a family of membrane-bound (cytoplasmic side) monomeric GTPases that are activated like G proteins (see II B) when GDP is exchanged for GTP and inactivated upon GTP hydrolysis. Activated Ras may then induce cell proliferation or differentiation through activation of phosphorylation cascades.

3. **Transmembrane guanylate cyclase.** The receptor for at least one hormone, **atrial natriuretic peptide,** is a transmembrane guanylate cyclase. When this receptor is activated, it catalyzes the formation of cyclic guanosine monophosphate (cGMP) from GTP. cGMP activates cGMP-dependent protein kinase.

H. **Ion channel-linked receptors** (transmitter-gated ion channels). This is a very important class of receptors involved in neurotransmission. They are located at neural synapses and upon interaction with the appropriate neurotransmitters they open or close ion channels.

III. **LIPOPHILIC HORMONES** are carried through the bloodstream by plasma proteins. They enter the cell by diffusion through the cell membrane. Inside the cell, they interact with intracellular receptors. As a result of this interaction, a structural change occurs in the receptor, and the hormone-receptor complex induces a cellular response (Figure 15-4).

A. **Duration of action.** Lipophilic hormones are slower to act and have a longer duration of action than hydrophilic hormones. Their duration of action ranges from hours to days.

B. **Receptors for lipophilic hormones** are proteins that consist of separate domains: One domain is responsible for binding to a specific sequence of DNA, and one domain binds to the specific hormone.

1. **In the absence of the hormone,** some receptors do not bind to their specific DNA sequences; only the hormone-receptor complex binds. Other receptors already may be bound to the DNA but only adopt an activating conformation when the hormone binds.
2. The specific DNA sequence that binds to a hormone-receptor complex is called the **hormone response element (HRE).** For example, the glucocorticoid response element (GRE) is the DNA sequence to which the glucocorticoid hormone-recep-

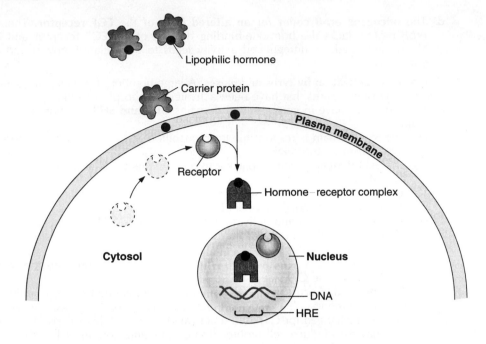

FIGURE 15-4. The carrier protein releases lipophilic hormones into the plasma membrane. Lipophilic hormones then bind to intracellular receptors. The hormone-receptor complex can then bind to a specific sequence of DNA, the hormone response element *(HRE),* and activate transcription of specific genes.

tor complex binds. The response elements for different hormones are similar but sufficiently different to be specific for a particular hormone-receptor complex.

3. **Result.** Binding the hormone-receptor complex to its response element results in the stimulation of transcription of specific genes. The specific genes that are transcribed depend on the target cell, presumably because other cell-type–specific proteins are also required for stimulation of transcription.
   a. The first genes to be activated are called the **primary response genes.**
   b. The primary response gene products may activate other genes—the **secondary response genes.**

 C. **Examples.** The lipophilic hormones that have intracellular receptors include **steroid hormones, thyroid hormones, retinoids, and vitamin D₃.**

Case 15-1 Revisited

The most likely diagnosis is that this patient has whooping cough, a contagious respiratory infection caused by the bacterium *B. pertussis.* The first phase of this disease is the catarrhal stage, in which the patient may have a slight fever and cold-like symptoms that last for approximately 2 weeks. The severe cough phase (paroxysmal phase) then begins and may last for 2 weeks. The patient then enters the final, convalescent phase, in which the symptoms of the paroxysmal phase typically decline over a 2- to 3-week period. Positive diagnosis of this disease requires a laboratory culture and identification of *B. pertussis* from nose or throat specimens. Blood samples also may show an increased number of lymphocytes.

B. pertussis secretes a protein, adhesin, which enables it to attach to a specific glycoprotein receptor on the cilia of respiratory epithelial cells. The bacterium produces a number of toxins that contribute to its ill effects. Pertussis toxin is a hexameric protein that modifies the G_{α} subunit of the G_i protein. The G_i protein normally inhibits the adenylate cyclase activity of cells. Because of this inactivation of G_i, adenylate cyclase is chronically activated. When administered to animals, pertussis toxin alone produces most of the symptoms of whooping cough. The other toxins secreted by *B. pertussis* undoubtedly cause many of the symptoms of the disease, too. Tracheal toxin damages the ciliated cells and therefore destroys the primary mechanical defense barrier of the lungs (the coughing is a reflexive attempt to remove the mucus that ciliated cells normally help remove). Adenylate cyclase toxin or cyclolysin is a bacterial adenylate cyclase that enters the cell and is activated by calmodulin to produce cAMP. This toxin also may lead to cell breakage. Another toxin, heat-labile toxin or dermonecrotic toxin, may also destroy cells.

Whooping cough can occur at any age, but it is usually seen in children younger than 2 years of age. It is a serious disease that may lead to death, especially in infants younger than 6 months of age. Neurologic damage also may occur in some instances, possibly because of hypoxia from the paroxysms of coughing or from the systemic effects of some of the secreted toxins. Depending on the severity of the symptoms, some patients may require hospitalization. Quiet bed rest and maintenance of food and fluid intake usually suffice until the symptoms have abated. Although *B. pertussis* is susceptible to antibiotics, antibiotics may do little to reduce the symptoms of the disease after it has reached the paroxysmal phase.

STUDY QUESTIONS

DIRECTIONS: Each of the numbered items or incomplete statements in this section is followed by answers or by completions of the statement. Select the **one** lettered answer or completion that is **best** in each case.

1. Hydrophilic hormones are best described by which one of the following statements? They

(A) include the thyroid and steroid hormones
(B) bind to cell-surface receptors, which transmit a signal to the interior of the cell
(C) enter the cell, bind to intracellular receptors, and in a complex with the receptor, alter gene expression
(D) bind irreversibly to their receptors
(E) bind to G proteins in the cell membrane

2. The role of G_s protein in the activation of adenylate cyclase is best described by which of the following statements?

(A) G_s protein forms a complex with hormone, and the hormone–G_s protein complex activates adenylate cyclase
(B) Activation of receptor by hormone relieves the inhibition of adenylate cyclase by G_s protein
(C) The G_s protein activates adenylate cyclase in a reaction that is driven by the hydrolysis of guanosine triphosphate (GTP) to guanosine diphosphate (GDP)
(D) The G_α subunit of G_s protein exchanges GDP for GTP, dissociates from the $G_{\beta\gamma}$ subunits, and activates adenylate cyclase

3. Which one of the following statements about cyclic adenosine monophosphate (cAMP) is true?

(A) High levels of cAMP that result from activation of G proteins by hormones are normally prolonged
(B) cAMP is formed by phospholipase C-β and adenylate cyclase
(C) Levels of cAMP quickly decline because it is hydrolyzed by cyclic nucleotide phosphodiesterase (PDEase)
(D) cAMP phosphorylates proteins in the cell

4. Phospholipase C is best described by which one of the following actions?

(A) It exists as a membrane phospholipid
(B) It diffuses into the cytosol and causes the release of calcium ions from intracellular stores
(C) It hydrolyzes phosphatidylinositol 4,5-bis-phosphate (PIP_2) to inositol 1,4,5-triphosphate (IP_3) and diacylglycerol (DAG), which are both second messengers
(D) It directly activates protein kinase C
(E) It dephosphorylates IP_3

5. Which one of the following hormones would have the longest duration of action?

(A) Thyroxine
(B) Insulin
(C) Glucagon
(D) Epinephrine
(E) Epidermal growth factor (EGF)

6. Which one of the following statements best describes the mechanism of action of insulin on target cells?

(A) Insulin binds to cytoplasmic receptor molecules and is transferred as a hormone-receptor complex to the nucleus, where it acts to modulate gene expression
(B) Insulin binds to a receptor molecule on the outer surface of the plasma membrane, and the hormone-receptor complex activates adenylate cyclase through the G_s protein
(C) Insulin binds to a transmembrane receptor at the outer surface of the plasma membrane, which activates the tyrosine kinase that is the cytosolic domain of the receptor
(D) Insulin enters the cell and causes the release of calcium ions from intracellular stores

7. The mechanisms through which the products of the *erbB* oncogene, cholera toxin, and the phorbol esters exert deleterious effects on an organism illustrate which critically important characteristic of hormone-receptor systems?

(A) The appropriate inactivation of the hormonal signal is necessary for normal cell function
(B) Hormone-receptor complexes must form and be internalized for proper cell signaling
(C) Second messengers must be generated for cells to respond to hormones
(D) Gene expression must ultimately be altered for cells to respond to hormones
(E) Covalent modification is not involved in normal cell signaling

8. Which one of the following is true of receptor subtypes?

(A) Subtypes of a specific receptor bind to different hormones
(B) Subtypes of a specific receptor all elicit the same effect
(C) Subtypes of a specific receptor may elicit different effects
(D) No receptor subtypes have been identified
(E) Receptor subtypes for hydrophilic hormones do not exist

9. A hormone response element is best defined by which one of the following statements? It

(A) is a transmembrane protein to which steroid hormones bind
(B) is a DNA sequence to which steroid hormones bind
(C) is the region of a steroid hormone receptor to which the hormone binds
(D) is the DNA sequence to which a specific hormone-receptor complex binds
(E) is the plasma protein that carries a specific lipophilic hormone through the bloodstream

10. Which one of the following inhibits adenylate cyclase?

(A) Phosphodiesterase
(B) G_q
(C) cyclic adenosine monophosphate (cAMP)
(D) G_i
(E) Cholera toxin

11. Which one of the following dimerizes upon phosphorylation by tyrosine kinase and then translocates to the nucleus and directly activates the expression of particular genes?

(A) *erbB*
(B) STATs
(C) Ras
(D) Steroid hormone receptor
(E) Guanylate cyclase

ANSWERS AND EXPLANATIONS

1. The answer is B [I C 1; II A, B]. Hydrophilic hormones do not enter the cell to elicit their effects. They bind to specific receptors on the cell surface, and a signal is transmitted to the interior of the cell as a result. The interaction between hormones and their receptors is reversible. As the hormone levels decline, the hormone action also declines as the hormones dissociate from their receptors. Some hydrophilic hormones bind to G-protein–linked receptors, but they do not bind to the G proteins themselves. Thyroid and steroid hormones are lipophilic, not hydrophilic.

2. The answer is D [II B 2 b, 3, D]. The hormone forms a complex with the receptor, and the hormone-receptor complex stimulates the exchange of guanosine diphosphate (GDP) for guanosine triphosphate (GTP) by the G protein. The G_α-GTP subunit dissociates from the rest of the G protein. The G_α-GTP subunit of a G_s protein activates adenylate cyclase. The G_α subunit is a GTPase and eventually hydrolyzes the GTP that is bound to it. The hydrolysis of GTP inactivates the G_α protein, which then reassociates with $G_{\beta\gamma}$ where it remains until it is reactivated by a hormone-receptor complex.

3. The answer is C [II D 1 b, F 1]. The enzyme cyclic nucleotide phosphodiesterase (PDEase) rapidly reduces the levels of cyclic adenosine monophosphate (cAMP), so the elevated levels are not normally prolonged. Phospholipase C-β cleaves phosphatidylinositol 4,5-bisphosphate (PIP$_2$) to form inositol 1,4,5-triphosphate (IP$_3$) and diacylglycerol (DAG); no cAMP is formed. cAMP does not phosphorylate proteins. It binds to the regulatory (R) subunits of cAMP-dependent protein kinase and causes them to be released from the catalytic (C) subunits. The active C subunits phosphorylate specific proteins in the cell.

4. The answer is C [II F, G 2 b (2)]. Phospholipase C is a type of enzyme that hydrolyzes phosphatidylinositol 4,5-bisphosphate (PIP$_2$), a membrane phospholipid, to inositol 1,4,5-triphosphate (IP$_3$) and diacylglycerol (DAG). Both IP$_3$ and DAG are second messengers, which means that they carry information from the hormone-receptor complex to molecules within the cell. IP$_3$ diffuses into the cytosol, where it causes the release of calcium ions from intracellular stores, and DAG activates protein kinase C. These two second messengers are rapidly inactivated; IP$_3$ by dephosphorylation, and DAG by hydrolysis. There are multiple forms of phospholipase C that have the same enzymatic activities but differ in how they are activated. For instance, phospholipase C-β is a membrane-bound form that is activated by the G_α of the G_q protein, and phospholipase C-γ is activated by the EGF receptor.

5. The answer is A [Table 15-1; II A 4; III A]. Hormones that interact with intracellular receptors, because they affect gene expression, have a longer duration of action than do hydrophilic hormones. Thyroxine, a lipophilic thyroid hormone, interacts with an intracellular receptor. Insulin, glucagon, epinephrine, and epidermal growth factor (EGF) are hydrophilic hormones.

6. The answer is C [II G 1 c]. Insulin binds to transmembrane receptors at the outer surface of the plasma membrane. The cytosolic domain of the receptor is a tyrosine kinase, which is activated by the binding of insulin. The activated tyrosine kinase phosphorylates itself, which leads to the activation by phosphorylation of other proteins. Lipophilic hormones bind to intracellular receptors and lead to the activation of transcription. Some hydrophilic hormones, such as glucagon and epinephrine, lead to the activation of adenylate cyclase through the G_s protein. Because insulin is hydrophilic, it cannot readily diffuse across the cell membrane.

7. The answer is A [II D 2, F 2 c, G 1 d]. The effects of the product of the *erbB* oncogene, the cholera toxin, and the phorbol esters, mimic hormonal signals that are not properly inactivated. The *erbB* oncogene product is an aberrant form of the epidermal growth factor (EGF) that lacks the hormone-binding domain and therefore the regulatory domain. Cholera toxin modifies G_s protein and prevents its inactivation. Phorbol esters mimic the effects of diacylglycerol (DAG) but are not quickly inactivated, as is DAG. Gene expression does not need to be altered for a cell to respond to hydrophilic hormones, and second messengers are not used by hormones that bind to intracellular receptors. Covalent modifications, such as phosphorylation, are important in cell signaling.

8. The answer is C [II]. Subtypes of a specific receptor can bind to the same hormone, but they may elicit different effects. Subtypes of receptors that interact with epinephrine, a hydrophilic hormone, have been identified.

9. The answer is D [III B 2]. Although the hormone response elements have similar sequences, they are specific for particular hormone-receptor complexes. Lipophilic hormones alone do not bind to DNA. Some lipophilic hormone receptors may bind to hormone response elements in the absence of hormones; however, it is only upon binding of hormones that they activate transcription.

10. The answer is D [II B 3, D 1 a–b, 2]. The G proteins mediate the effects of many hormones. The effect of the active form (G_α-GTP) depends on the specific type of G protein: G_i inhibits the enzyme adenylate cyclase, and G_q stimulates the enzyme phospholipase C. Phosphodiesterase converts cyclic adenosine monophosphate (cAMP), the product of adenylate cyclase activity, to AMP. Cholera toxin is an enzyme produced by *Vibrio cholerae* that inhibits the cleavage of guanosine triphosphate (GTP) to guanosine diphosphate (GDP) by G_s. This results in continued stimulation of adenylate cyclase by the G_α subunit of G_s that cannot be inactivated.

11. The answer is B [II G 1 d, 2 b, 3; III C]. STATs are signal transduction and activators of transcription. They are part of the diverse group of proteins that bind to and are activated by phosphorylation by activated tyrosine kinases. STATs dimerize upon phosphorylation and translocate to the nucleus, where they activate the transcription of particular genes. Ras is another protein activated by tyrosine kinase. It is a membrane GTPase and, upon activation, it induces cell proliferation or differentiation through activation of a phosphorylation cascade. *ErbB* is an oncogene that codes for an altered form of the epidermal growth factor (EGF) receptor. It is a permanently activated tyrosine kinase. Guanylate cyclase is a transmembrane protein that forms cyclic GMP (cGMP), which is a second messenger that activates cGMP-dependent protein kinase. Steroid hormone receptors are activated by lipophilic steroid hormones, and their site of action upon activation is the nucleus.

Chapter 16

Glycolysis
Victor Davidson

Case 16-1

A newborn boy is anemic and mildly jaundiced. Blood analysis indicates some variability in red blood cell morphology, below-normal hemoglobin levels, and above-normal levels of reticulocytes relative to total red blood cells. The hemolysate of isolated red blood cells is assayed for the activity of glycolytic enzymes, and pyruvate kinase activity is found to be only approximately 20% of the normal level.

- What is the diagnosis?
- What is the basis for the results of the blood analysis?
- What is the prognosis?

I. OVERVIEW OF GLYCOLYSIS

A. **Definition.** Glycolysis is the process by which glucose molecules are metabolized through a series of enzymatic reactions into two molecules of pyruvate.

B. **Purpose.** Glycolysis results in the net production of adenosine triphosphate (ATP), which fuels the body's cells.

1. **Anaerobic glycolysis** produces 2 moles of ATP per 1 mole of glucose.
2. **Aerobic glycolysis** produces 6–8 moles of ATP per mole of glucose.

II. CARBOHYDRATE DIGESTION produces glucose, as well as galactose and fructose, which also are metabolized in part via glycolysis.

A. **Sources of carbon for glycolysis**

1. **Dietary starch** is a major source of glucose (see Chapter 5 IV D).
2. **Glycogen,** the major form of carbohydrate storage in animals, is a highly branched polymer of glucose (see Chapter 5 IV D).
3. **Sucrose,** a glucose–fructose disaccharide, is the major sugar in our diet.
4. **Lactose,** a disaccharide of **glucose and galactose,** is the major carbohydrate component of milk.
5. **Fructose** is present in fruits and is a component of sucrose.

B. **Enzymes of carbohydrate digestion** present in the digestive tract metabolize carbohydrates into glucose, galactose, and fructose (Figure 16-1).

1. **α-Amylase** hydrolyzes hydrated starch and glycogen. Because starch becomes hydrated (i.e., solubilized) when it is heated, cooking is an important digestive and absorptive aid. Different isozymes are present in saliva and pancreatic juice. α-Amylase produces the following:

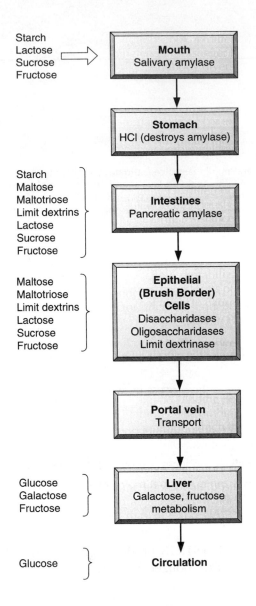

FIGURE 16-1. Pathway for digestion of common dietary carbohydrates.

    a. Maltose, which is α-glucose-(1,4)-glucose
    b. Maltotriose, which is α-glucose-(1,4)-α-glucose-(1,4)-glucose
    c. Limit dextrins, which are highly branched molecules of about eight glucose units joined by one or more α-1,6 bonds

  2. Oligosaccharidases complete the hydrolysis of disaccharides and oligosaccharides on the surface of epithelial cells in the small intestine. These enzymes remove successive units from the nonreducing ends (i.e., the ends opposite the aldehyde or ketone groups).

  3. Disaccharidases, including **α-glucosidases** and **β-galactosidases,** are required for the hydrolysis of sucrose and lactose.

C.   **Active transport.** Glucose, galactose, and fructose are transported into and out of epithelial cells by carrier-mediated processes.

1. **Two transport systems** are involved in the uptake of monosaccharides by the epithelial cells of the intestinal lumen.
   a. **The Na$^+$-dependent monosaccharide cotransport system**
      (1) This system is specific for D-glucose and D-galactose.
      (2) **Phlorhizin,** a plant glycoside, inhibits this system. It also inhibits Na$^+$-dependent monosaccharide transport systems in the renal tubules and other cells and tissues.
   b. **The Na$^+$-independent monosaccharide transport system**
      (1) This system specifically transports D-fructose by facilitated diffusion.
      (2) **Cytochalasin B,** which is derived from molds, inhibits this system. It also inhibits similar Na$^+$-independent monosaccharide transport systems in other cells and tissues.

2. **Transport of monosaccharides out of the epithelial cells** is catalyzed by another distinct Na$^+$-independent transport system that is specific for D-glucose and D-galactose.

III. EMBDEN-MEYERHOF PATHWAY (GLYCOLYSIS) [Figure 16-2]

A. **Glucose to glucose-6-phosphate (G6P).** Glucose is phosphorylated (i.e., a phosphate group is added) immediately on entering the cell and is efficiently trapped inside because phosphorylated intermediates do not readily pass through cell membranes.

1. **Enzyme. Hexokinase** irreversibly catalyzes the phosphorylation of glucose at the expense of one molecule of ATP. Hexokinase is an **allosteric enzyme** (see Chapter 4 V E) that is strongly inhibited by its product, G6P. Several isozymes of hexokinase exhibit different Michaelis constant (K_m) values for glucose and different specificities for hexose substrates.
   a. Most hexokinases have a low K_m for glucose and readily take up glucose and other sugars from the blood. The hexokinase isozyme in the brain has a particularly low K_m for glucose.
   b. In contrast, the liver is unique in that its major enzyme for phosphorylating glucose is **glucokinase.** This enzyme is specific for glucose and has a high K_m, which enables it to handle the high concentration of glucose that is present in the portal venous blood after a meal. It is an inducible enzyme that increases its synthesis in response to insulin secretion and carbohydrate intake.

2. **Product. G6P is an intermediate of pivotal importance.** It is not only an intermediate of glycolysis but also a precursor of:
   a. **Glucose** in gluconeogenic tissues (see Chapter 20 III G)
   b. **Glycogen** via glycogen synthesis (see Chapter 21 II A)
   c. **Ribose-5-phosphate,** which is required for nucleotide synthesis, via the pentose phosphate pathway (see Chapter 17 I C)

3. **G6P is also derived from galactose** (see Chapter 17 IV B), allowing that hexose to be metabolized via glycolysis.

B. **G6P to fructose-6-phosphate (F6P).** This step is **catalyzed by phosphoglucose isomerase.** It is a reversible reaction controlled by substrate–product levels.

C. **F6P to fructose-1,6-bisphosphate (F1,6BP).** This essentially irreversible reaction is **catalyzed by phosphofructokinase (PFK),** which is the **rate-limiting enzyme of glycolysis** in most tissues and the **major regulatory enzyme** of glycolysis.

1. **Activators of PFK**
   a. **Adenosine monophosphate (AMP),** which signals a low energy state

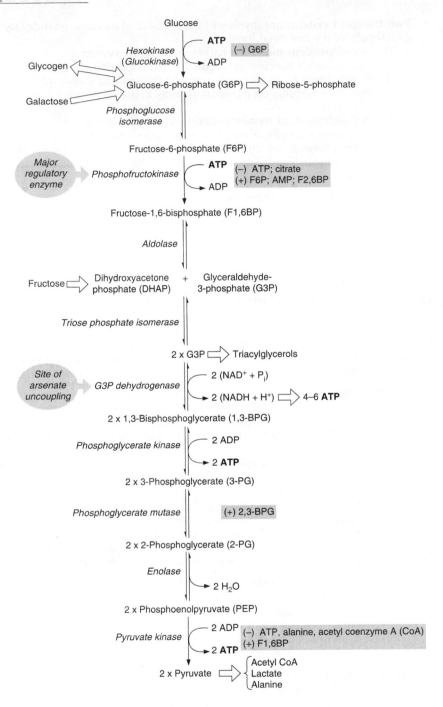

FIGURE 16-2. The pathway of glycolysis. The signs *(+)* and *(–)* indicate the sites of action of allosteric positive and negative modulators of the activities of the key regulatory enzymes. These are shown in boxes with *(+)* = *activators* and *(–)* = *inhibitors*. Enzyme names are in *italic*. *Equilibrium arrows* indicate reversible reactions, and *single arrows* indicate reactions that are essentially irreversible. *Large double arrows* indicate sites of entry of substrates other than glucose into the glycolytic pathway and points at which some glycolytic intermediates may exit the pathway for use as precursors of other metabolites. ATP that is consumed and produced during glycolysis is indicated in *bold type*. *ADP* = adenosine diphosphate; *AMP* = adenosine monophosphate; *ATP* = adenosine triphosphate; *F2,6BP* = fructose-2,6-bisphosphate; *NAD⁺* = oxidized nicotinamide adenine dinucleotide; *NADH* = reduced NAD; *Pᵢ* = inorganic phosphate.

b. **Fructose-2,6-bisphosphate (F2,6BP),** which is formed from F6P when high levels are present, activates PFK **in the liver only.** The kinase that synthesizes F2,6BP, **PFK-2,** is itself a regulatory enzyme.
   (1) PFK-2 is inhibited by citrate and by ATP.
   (2) PFK-2 is also inhibited by phosphorylation of the enzyme by cyclic adenosine monophosphate (cAMP)-dependent protein kinase.

2. **Inhibitors of PFK**
   a. **ATP,** which signals a high energy state
   b. **Citrate** inhibits PFK as well as the synthesis of F2,6BP, thus preventing activation of PFK in the liver. Citrate is formed in the mitochondria during the oxidation of two-carbon fragments from pyruvate (see Chapter 18 III A). When ATP levels are high, citrate is not metabolized further, but instead enters the cytoplasm. This signals a high-energy state, which is a reason to slow down glycolysis.

D. **F1,6BP to dihydroxyacetone phosphate (DHAP) and glyceraldehyde-3-phosphate (G3P)**

1. **Enzyme.** This reaction is catalyzed by **aldolase.** Several tissue-specific isozymes of aldolase exist.

2. **Products.** The triose phosphate products—DHAP and G3P—are not only intermediates in glycolysis, but also precursors for the synthesis of triacylglycerols (see Chapter 22 III A 2).

E. **DHAP to G3P.** This isomerization reaction effectively interconverts the two triose phosphates that were formed in the previous reaction. The reaction is catalyzed by **triose phosphate isomerase.** Although the reaction is reversible, because G3P is used in the subsequent reaction, its removal shifts the equilibrium in the direction of conversion of essentially all of the DHAP to G3P.

F. **G3P to 1,3-bisphosphoglycerate (1,3-BPG).** This reversible reaction requires **nicotinamide adenine dinucleotide (NAD$^+$)** as an electron carrier. Phosphorylation occurs at the expense of inorganic phosphate (P$_i$) and is an example of **substrate-level oxidative phosphorylation.**

$$G3P + NAD^+ + P_i \rightarrow 1,3\text{-}BPG + NADH + H^+$$

1. **Enzyme.** The reaction is catalyzed by **G3P dehydrogenase.**

2. **Products** of this reaction are important high-energy intermediates.
   a. The phosphorylation reaction generates a **high-energy phosphate bond** in 1,3-BPG, which has a high group-transfer potential (see Chapter 13 IV A).
   b. NAD$^+$ is a high-energy compound (see Chapter 13 V C) that can be used to provide energy for ATP synthesis.

3. **Arsenate (AsO$_4^{3-}$)** can uncouple oxidation and phosphorylation at this step.
   a. AsO$_4^{3-}$ can substitute for P$_i$ in the phosphorylation reaction and form an unstable compound, 1-arseno-3-phosphoglycerate, which breaks down to yield 3-phosphoglycerate (3-PG). Energy is lost because the high-energy phosphate bond is not formed (see III F 2 a) and subsequently used to form ATP (see III G).
   b. This is a reason that arsenic-containing compounds are toxic.

G. **1,3-BPG to 3-PG**

1. This is the **first step in glycolysis that generates ATP.**

2. **Enzyme.** The reaction is catalyzed by **phosphoglycerate kinase.**

3. **Energetics**
   a. In the prior step, two molecules of 1,3-BPG were formed from each molecule of glucose. Therefore, two ATP moles are now formed per original mole of glucose.

b. Because up to triose phosphate formation (see III D), two molecules of ATP have been used per molecule of glucose consumed, the balance sheet for ATP use and production is even at this point.

H. 3-PG to 2-PG

1. **Enzyme.** This reversible reaction is catalyzed by **phosphoglycerate mutase.**

2. **Cofactor: 2,3-bisphosphoglycerate (2,3-BPG)**
   a. 2,3-BPG is formed from 1,3-BPG by a mutase and is degraded to 3-PG by a phosphatase.
   b. 2,3-BPG is a strong competitive inhibitor of its own synthesis by the mutase.
   c. 2,3-BPG is present in low concentrations in most cells. However, in red blood cells, the concentration of 2,3-BPG is approximately 4 mM (equal in molarity to hemoglobin). Here it acts as a regulator of oxygen transport, stabilizing the deoxygenated form of hemoglobin (see Chapter 3 II B 3 c).

I. **2-PG to phosphoenolpyruvate (PEP).** This reversible reaction is catalyzed by **enolase.** The phosphoenol bond in PEP is a **high-energy phosphate bond.**

J. PEP to pyruvate

1. This reaction is essentially irreversible under cellular conditions.

2. **Enzyme.** The reaction is catalyzed by **pyruvate kinase,** which is an allosteric enzyme.
   a. The liver isozyme is also an inducible enzyme that increases in concentration with high carbohydrate intake and high insulin levels.
   b. The isozyme of pyruvate kinase that is found in the liver is strongly **activated by F1,6BP.**
   c. Pyruvate kinase is **inhibited by ATP, alanine, fatty acids, and acetyl coenzyme A** (acetyl CoA).
   d. The liver isozyme is also regulated by covalent modification.
      (1) It is inactivated by phosphorylation by cAMP-dependent protein kinase.
      (2) It is activated by dephosphorylation by a phosphatase.

3. **Energetics.** Two molecules of pyruvate are formed per original molecule of glucose. Thus, there is a net production of two ATP molecules per molecule of glucose used in the anaerobic formation of pyruvate (−2+2+2) [see IV A].

IV. ATP PRODUCTION

A. **Anaerobic glycolysis. A net of 2 moles of ATP per mole of glucose** is produced.

1. **Consumed ATP.** Two moles of ATP per mole of glucose are used to form F1,6BP (see III A, C).

2. **Produced ATP**
   a. Two moles of ATP per mole of glucose are produced by the phosphoglycerate kinase reaction (see III G).
   b. Two moles of ATP per mole of glucose are produced by the pyruvate kinase reaction (see III J).

3. **Regeneration of NAD+.** NADH cannot be used to synthesize ATP under anaerobic conditions. To regenerate the NAD+ needed to convert G3P to 1,3-BPG (see III F), NADH is oxidized to NAD+ during the conversion of pyruvate to lactate by lactate dehydrogenase (see VI A).

B. **Aerobic glycolysis.** Overall, **6–8 moles of ATP are formed per mole of glucose.** In addition to the 2 moles of ATP that are formed during anaerobic glycolysis (see IV A), 2–3 moles of ATP are produced from each NADH that is formed on conversion of G3P to 1,3-BPG. However, NADH cannot permeate the inner mitochondrial membrane. To overcome this problem, the NADH produced in the cytosol during glycolysis must be shuttled into the mitochondria to serve as a substrate for ATP production via oxidative phosphorylation (see Chapter 19 II C).

1. **Glycerol-3-phosphate shuttle** (Figure 16-3)
   a. This shuttle functions primarily in skeletal muscle and brain.
   b. It results in **the production of 2 moles of ATP** per mole of NADH.
   c. Cytosolic NADH is used to catalyze the reduction of DHAP to glycerol-3-phosphate.
   d. Glycerol-3-phosphate enters the mitochondrion and is oxidized back to DHAP by a mitochondrial enzyme that uses flavin adenine dinucleotide (FAD) as an electron acceptor.
   e. Reduced FAD ($FADH_2$) formed in the reaction supports the synthesis of 2 moles of ATP via the mitochondrial electron transport chain and oxidative phosphorylation.
   f. The DHAP formed is returned to the cytosol to continue the shuttle.

2. **Malate shuttle** (see Figure 16-3)
   a. This shuttle functions primarily in the heart, kidney, and liver.
   b. It results in the production of **3 moles of ATP** per mole of NADH.

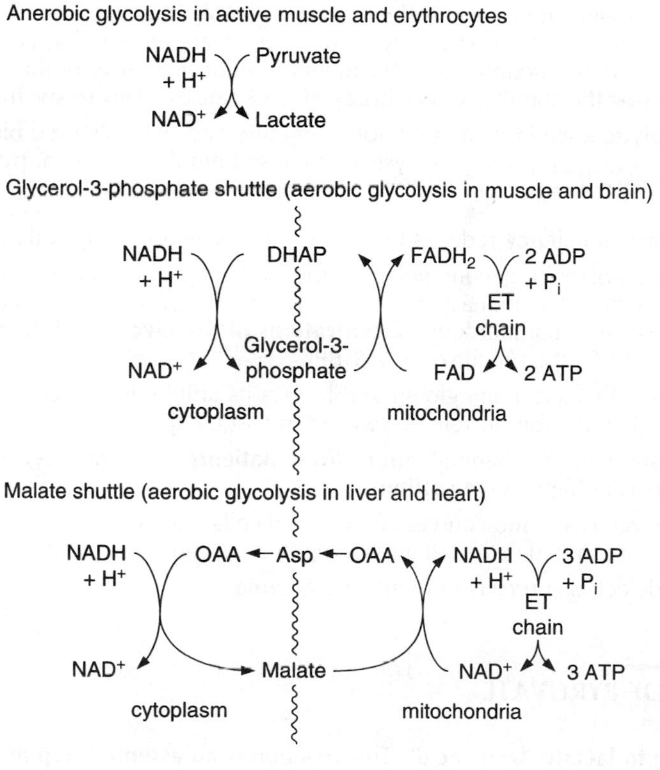

FIGURE 16-3. Mechanisms by which NAD^+ is regenerated for continuation of glycolysis. *Asp* = aspartic acid; *DHAP* = dihydroxyacetone phosphate; *ET* = electron transport; *FAD* = flavin adenine dinucleotide; *FADH₂* = reduced FAD; *NAD⁺* = oxidized nicotinamide adenine dinucleotide; *NADH* = reduced NAD; *OAA* = oxaloacetate; *Pᵢ* = inorganic phosphate.

    c. Cytosolic NADH is used to catalyze the reduction of oxaloacetate (OAA) to malate.

    d. Malate enters the mitochondrion and is oxidized back to OAA by a mitochondrial malate dehydrogenase that uses NAD^+ as an electron acceptor.

    e. Reduced NADH formed in the reaction supports synthesis of 3 moles of ATP via the mitochondrial electron transport chain and oxidative phosphorylation.

    f. OAA is transported across the membrane in the form of aspartate. Aspartate aminotransferase converts OAA to aspartate in the mitochondrion. After transport to the cytosol, another aspartate aminotransferase converts aspartate back to OAA to complete the cycle.

V. DISORDERS ASSOCIATED WITH IMPAIRED GLYCOLYSIS

A. Glycolysis and erythrocyte (red blood cell) metabolism

1. Disorders of glycolysis typically present as disorders of erythrocyte metabolism.

2. Mature erythrocytes contain no mitochondria, so they are totally dependent on glycolysis for ATP production.

3. ATP is required for the activity of the sodium- and potassium-stimulated ATPase–ion transport system, which is necessary to maintain the proper biconcave shape of the erythrocyte membrane.

B. Pyruvate kinase deficiency

1. Pyruvate kinase exists as isozymes (see Chapter 4 VI A), and **genetic defects** in isozyme subunits may selectively affect the glycolytic enzymes of the erythrocyte. Any defect in a glycolytic enzyme (e.g., pyruvate kinase) that does not allow adequate ATP production, and consequently reduces activity of the ATPase–ion pump, **decreases the stability of erythrocytes and causes them to swell and lyse.**

2. **Hemolytic anemia** is the term for premature and excessive red blood cell destruction. Of the defects in glycolysis that cause hemolytic anemia, pyruvate kinase deficiency is the most common.

C. Hexokinase deficiency reduces the amount of oxygen that is available for tissues.

1. Patients possess a genetic defect in the isozyme of hexokinase found in the erythrocyte. Because hexokinase is the first enzyme in glycolysis, the red blood cells of these patients contain **low concentrations of the glycolytic intermediates,** including 1,3-BPG, the precursor of 2,3-BPG.

2. 2,3-BPG binds to hemoglobin and lowers its affinity for oxygen. This normally allows hemoglobin to release oxygen in tissue capillaries.

3. Consequently, the **hemoglobin of these patients** with low levels of 2,3-BPG **has an abnormally high oxygen affinity.**

4. The oxygen saturation curves of red blood cells from a patient with hexokinase deficiency are shifted to the left, indicating that oxygen is less available for the tissues.

5. This defect also results in hemolytic anemia.

VI. FATES OF PYRUVATE

A. Pyruvate to lactate (lactic acid). This reaction is an **essential step in anaerobic glycolysis,** because it is the anaerobic means for reoxidizing the NADH that is formed in the G3P dehydrogenase step. This ensures that the NAD^+ required for the continuation of glycolysis is available.

$$\text{Pyruvate} + \text{NADH} + H^+ \rightarrow \text{Lactate} + NAD^+$$

1. **Enzyme.** This reaction is catalyzed by **lactate dehydrogenase.**

2. **Product.** Lactate is produced in active muscle tissue under anaerobic conditions. This lactate is released into the blood and taken up by the liver, where it is converted back to glucose by the process of gluconeogenesis (see Chapter 20 II A).

B. **Pyruvate to acetyl CoA.** This **irreversible** reaction occurs in the **mitochondria.**

1. **Enzyme.** This reaction is catalyzed by **pyruvate dehydrogenase.**

2. **Product.** Acetyl CoA can enter the **citric acid cycle,** where it is further metabolized to generate additional energy (see Chapter 18 III A), or it may be used as a substrate for the synthesis of fatty acids (see Chapter 22 I B).

C. **Pyruvate to alanine.** This **reversible** reaction links carbohydrate and amino acid metabolism (see Chapter 25 I B 1). This reaction is catalyzed by **alanine aminotransferase.**

VII. LACTIC ACIDOSIS

A. **Blood levels.** Normal blood lactate levels are less than 1.2 mM. With lactic acidosis, the blood lactate level may be 5 mM or more.

1. The high concentration of lactate results in **lowered blood pH and bicarbonate levels.**

2. The high blood lactate levels can result from **increased formation or decreased utilization of lactate.**

B. **Hypoxia,** or lack of oxygen, is a common cause of high blood lactate levels.

1. The shortage of oxygen reduces mitochondrial production of ATP with the consequent activation of PFK, which increases glycolysis and lactate production via pyruvate under anaerobic conditions.

2. **Tissue hypoxia** may occur in conditions that impair blood flow (e.g., shock), in respiratory disorders, and in severe anemia.

Case 16-1 Revisited

The infant suffers from a genetic defect in the isozyme of pyruvate kinase that is present in erythrocytes, and which causes the enzyme to exhibit significantly less-than-normal activity.

Pyruvate kinase deficiency decreases the flow of metabolites through the glycolytic pathway and decreases the production of ATP. Without sufficient ATP, ion pumps that are critical in maintaining the osmotic balance across the red blood cell membrane do not have sufficient energy to function properly. Thus, the erythrocytes are unable to maintain their proper shape, which accounts for the variable morphology. The difficulty in maintaining the correct osmotic balance causes erythrocytes to swell and lyse. This premature and excessive red blood cell death causes anemia and jaundice because of excessive release of heme into the bloodstream (see Chapter 25 VII C 5). Reticulocytes, which are immature erythrocytes, retain their mitochondria. Thus, they are better able to survive than the mature cells, which have lost their mitochondria and rely solely on glycolysis for ATP.

There is no cure for this disorder, but patients often survive well into adulthood, unless complications exacerbate the condition. In severe cases, blood transfusion and removal of the spleen may be necessary. The abnormally fragile cells tend to be destroyed when passing through the spleen, and removal of the spleen may help to reduce the anemia.

This infant's condition improved, and he was discharged after a short stay in the hospital. The physician recommended that the infant be closely monitored for any increase in the severity of the anemia.

STUDY QUESTIONS

DIRECTIONS: Each of the numbered items or incomplete statements in this section is followed by answers or by completions of the statement. Select the **one** lettered answer or completion that is **best** in each case.

1. Which one of the following enzyme-catalyzed reactions generates a high-energy phosphate bond?

(A) The phosphorylation of glucose
(B) 2-Phosphoglycerate to phosphoenolpyruvate
(C) 3-Phosphoglycerate to 2-phosphoglycerate
(D) Dihydroxyacetone phosphate to glyceraldehyde-3-phosphate
(E) Fructose-1,6-bisphosphate to glyceraldehyde-3-phosphate and dihydroxyacetone phosphate

2. The oxidation of 1 mole of glucose by anaerobic glycolysis yields a net of

(A) 2 moles of lactate and 2 moles of adenosine triphosphate (ATP)
(B) 2 moles of pyruvate and 6 moles of ATP
(C) 2 moles of lactate and 6 moles of ATP
(D) 2 moles of pyruvate and 8 moles of ATP
(E) 1 mole each of pyruvate and lactate

3. What is the net production of adenosine triphosphate per glucose during aerobic glycolysis in the brain?

(A) 4 moles
(B) 6 moles
(C) 8 moles
(D) 10 moles
(E) 12 moles

4. Which one of the following sets of glycolytic enzymes is allosterically regulated?

(A) Glucokinase, phosphofructokinase, and pyruvate kinase
(B) Hexokinase, aldolase, and pyruvate kinase
(C) Hexokinase, glyceraldehyde-3-phosphate dehydrogenase, and enolase
(D) Phosphofructokinase, enolase, and pyruvate kinase
(E) Hexokinase, phosphofructokinase, and pyruvate kinase

5. α-Amylase is required for the digestion of which one of the following substances?

(A) Limit dextrins
(B) Hydrated starch
(C) Sucrose
(D) Glucose
(E) Lactose

6. A patient is experiencing tissue hypoxia that reduces mitochondrial adenosine triphosphate (ATP) production and leads to lactic acidosis. Why do low levels of ATP cause increased lactate production?

(A) Low ATP levels increase phosphofructokinase activity
(B) High ATP levels inhibit conversion of pyruvate to lactate by lactate dehydrogenase
(C) Low ATP levels stimulate conversion of pyruvate to phosphoenolpyruvate by pyruvate kinase
(D) High ATP levels inhibit the activity of hexokinase
(E) High ATP levels inhibit the activity of glyceraldehyde-3-phosphate dehydrogenase

Questions 7–8

A patient suffers from a pyruvate kinase deficiency of the red blood cells.

7. Which one of the following substances is likely to be present at abnormally high levels in this patient's red blood cells?

(A) Lactic acid
(B) Alanine
(C) Acetyl CoA
(D) Pyruvate
(E) Phosphoenolpyruvate

8. How will this disorder affect the patient's hemoglobin?

(A) His hemoglobin has an abnormally high affinity for oxygen
(B) His hemoglobin has a normal affinity for oxygen
(C) His hemoglobin has an abnormally low affinity for oxygen

DIRECTIONS: The group of items in this section consists of lettered options followed by a set of numbered items. For each item, select the **one** lettered option that is most closely associated with it. Each lettered option may be selected once, more than once, or not at all.

Questions 9–15

Match the following statements describing enzymes to the proper enzyme.

(A) Phosphofructokinase
(B) Triose phosphate isomerase
(C) Enolase
(D) Glucokinase
(E) Pyruvate kinase
(F) Glyceraldehyde-3-phosphate dehydrogenase
(G) Phosphoglycerate mutase

9. It is the major regulatory enzyme of glycolysis

10. Adenosine monophosphate (AMP) is an activator of this enzyme

11. It has a much higher Michaelis constant (K_m) for glucose than does hexokinase

12. It interconverts dihydroxyacetone phosphate and glyceraldehyde-3-phosphate

13. It catalyzes a reaction that produces a high-energy phosphate bond without the involvement of adenosine diphosphate (ADP), adenosine triphosphate (ATP), or nicotinamide adenine dinucleotide (NAD⁺)

14. It is the site at which arsenate uncouples glycolysis

15. It requires 2,3-bisphosphoglycerate as a cofactor

ANSWERS AND EXPLANATIONS

1. The answer is B [III I]. High-energy phosphate bonds are formed at two points in the glycolytic pathway. The first is during the production of 1,3-bisphosphoglycerate, which is a product of glyceraldehyde-3-phosphate dehydrogenase catalysis. The second is during the production of phosphoenolpyruvate, which is a product of enolase catalysis. The phosphate bonds in glucose-6-phosphate, 2- and 3-phosphoglycerates, glyceraldehyde-3-phosphate, and dihydroxyacetone phosphate are not high-energy phosphate bonds and do not exhibit a large negative free-energy change upon hydrolysis.

2. The answer is A [IV A; Figure 16-3]. Under anaerobic conditions, the pyruvate formed from glucose by glycolysis is converted to lactate at the expense of reduced nicotinamide adenine dinucleotide (NADH), which is formed in the glyceraldehyde-3-phosphate dehydrogenase reaction step. Under these conditions, 1 mole of glucose yields 2 moles of lactate and a net of 2 moles of adenosine triphosphate. In aerobic glycolysis, NADH is oxidized back to NAD^+ by oxidative phosphorylation to yield 2–3 moles of adenosine triphosphate (ATP) per NADH, depending on how the NADH is shuttled into the mitochondria.

3. The answer is B [IV B 1; Figure 16-3]. During aerobic glycolysis in brain and muscle tissue, reduced nicotinamide adenine dinucleotide (NADH) is oxidized by the glycerol-3-phosphate shuttle. In this process, NADH reduces dihydroxyacetone phosphate (DHAP) in the cytoplasm to glycerol-3-phosphate, which enters the mitochondria. Once inside, a flavin adenine dinucleotide (FAD)-linked dehydrogenase converts the glycerol-3-phosphate back to DHAP, which then leaves the mitochondria. The reduced FAD (i.e., $FADH_2$) that is formed supports the formation of 2 moles of adenosine triphosphate (ATP) per mole of DHAP formed, or 4 moles of ATP per mole of glucose used. As the two substrate-level phosphorylations of glycolysis also take place aerobically, a total of 6 moles of ATP are formed per mole of glucose used. In liver and heart

tissue, NADH is transported into mitochondria via the malate shuttle, allowing formation of 3 moles of ATP per NADH.

4. The answer is E [III A 1, C, J 2; Figure 16-2]. There are three allosteric regulatory enzymes in the glycolytic pathway. Hexokinase is inhibited by glucose-6-phosphate; however, the main liver enzyme with the same function, glucokinase, is not a regulatory enzyme. Phosphofructokinase is allosterically inhibited by adenosine triphosphate, citrate, or hydrogen ions, and it is activated by adenosine diphosphate, adenosine monophosphate, or inorganic phosphate. Pyruvate kinase is activated by fructose-1,6-bisphosphate.

5. The answer is B [II B]. α-Amylase hydrolyzes α-1,4-glycosidic linkages of hydrated starch and glycogen, except those of glucose units that serve as branch points. (Cooking enhances the hydration, and thus the digestion, of starch.) Glucose is the major product of the action of α-amylase on starch. Limit dextrins are highly branched molecules composed of approximately eight glucose units joined by one or more α-1,6 bonds. Sucrose and lactose are disaccharides.

6. The answer is A [III C; VII B]. Phosphofructokinase, the major regulatory enzyme of glycolysis, is inhibited by adenosine triphosphate (ATP). Therefore, low levels of ATP stimulate glycolysis. This causes increased production of pyruvate, which is converted to lactate under hypoxic (low-oxygen) conditions. Lactate dehydrogenase, glyceraldehyde-3-phosphate dehydrogenase, and hexokinase are not allosterically regulated by ATP. Pyruvate kinase is also inhibited by ATP and is stimulated under these conditions. However, pyruvate kinase catalyzes the reverse of the reaction listed; that is, the formation of pyruvate from phosphoenolpyruvate.

7–8. The answers are: 7-E, 8-C [III J; V B, C 2; VI]. Pyruvate kinase is the last enzyme in glycolysis. When it is deficient, the intermediates of glycolysis accumulate. Lactate, alanine, and acetyl CoA are all metabolites that can be derived from pyruvate, which is at low levels because it is the product of the deficient enzyme. Phosphoenolpyruvate, which is the substrate for the deficient enzyme, accumulates.

In the red blood cell, 2,3-bisphosphoglycerate (2,3-BPG) is formed from 1,3-BPG, which is a glycolytic intermediate. Therefore, levels of 2,3-BPG increase as well. 2,3-BPG binds to hemoglobin, stabilizing the deoxy form of hemoglobin and promoting the release of oxygen. With high concentrations of 2,3-BPG present, the hemoglobin has an abnormally low affinity for oxygen.

9–15. The answers are: 9-A, 10-A, 11-D, 12-B, 13-C, 14-F, 15-G [III A 1, C, E, F 3, H 2, I; Figure 16-2]. Phosphofructokinase (PFK), an allosteric enzyme, is the major control enzyme of this pathway in most tissues. Adenosine monophosphate (AMP), fructose-6-phosphate, and fructose-2,6-bisphosphate activate PFK. Adenosine triphosphate (ATP) and citrate inhibit PFK.

Glucokinase is an inducible isozyme of hexokinase present in the liver. It specifically acts on glucose, and it has a high Michaelis constant (K_m) value, which enables it to handle large amounts of glucose following a meal.

Triose phosphate isomerase catalyzes the isomerization reaction that maintains an equilibrium mixture of dihydroxyacetone phosphate and glyceraldehyde-3-phosphate.

Enolase catalyzes the reaction that creates phosphoenolpyruvate (PEP) from 2-phosphoglycerate. The phosphoenol bond in PEP is a high-energy phosphate bond. The kinases also can form high-energy phosphate bonds, but they do so in conjunction with the interconversion of adenosine diphosphate (ADP) and ATP. Glyceraldehyde-3-phosphate dehydrogenase also catalyzes a reaction that generates a high-energy phosphate bond in 1,3-bisphosphoglycerate. NAD^+ is required as a co-substrate in this reaction. Arsenate can uncouple oxidative phosphorylation by substituting for inorganic phosphate in this reaction.

2,3-Bisphosphoglycerate is required in trace amounts for glycolysis in all cells. It is a cofactor in the conversion of 3-phosphoglycerate to 2-phosphoglycerate catalyzed by phosphoglycerate mutase.

Chapter 17

Alternative Pathways of Carbohydrate Metabolism
Victor Davidson

Case 17-1

A male infant appears normal at birth but, when fed, exhibits vomiting and diarrhea and an overall failure to thrive. At 5 days of age, he begins to exhibit mild jaundice. Analysis of the infant's urine yields a positive test for reducing sugars, but no glucose is present as indicated by a glucose oxidase assay. The urine and serum are subsequently analyzed for galactose, and high levels are indicated.

- What is the diagnosis?
- How could the diagnosis be confirmed?
- What is the treatment and prognosis?

I. PENTOSE PHOSPHATE PATHWAY (HEXOSE MONOPHOSPHATE SHUNT)

A. Functions

1. Provides a source of **reduced nicotinamide adenine dinuleotide phosphate (NADPH)** for reductive biosyntheses (see I C 1 a, 3)

2. Provides a source of **ribose-5-phosphate** for nucleic acid biosynthesis (see Chapter 26 I A)

3. Provides a route for the **conversion of pentoses** to fructose-6-phosphate (F6P) and glyceraldehyde-3-phosphate (G3P)

4. Erythrocytes depend on the pentose phosphate pathway for NADPH, which is required to maintain glutathione (see Chapter 25 V) in the reduced state. Reduced glutathione is needed to **maintain the integrity of the red blood cell membrane.**

B. Location

1. The pentose phosphate pathway is most active in the **erythrocytes, liver, mammary glands, adipose tissue,** and the **adrenal cortex.**

2. Within the cell, the enzymes of this pathway are located in the **cytoplasm.**

C. Reactions (Figure 17-1)

1. **Glucose-6-phosphate (G6P) to 6-phosphogluconolactone** is catalyzed by **glucose-6-phosphate dehydrogenase (G6PD).**
   a. **Cofactor. Oxidized nicotinamide adenine dinucleotide phosphate (NADP$^+$)** is reduced to NADPH in this reaction.
   b. **G6PD deficiency** can cause the red blood cell disorder **hemolytic anemia** because in erythrocytes, flux through the pentose phosphate pathway is not sufficiently high to maintain reduced glutathione levels.
   (1) G6PD deficiency can be caused by **genetic defects.**
   (2) In people with low G6PD activity, certain drugs and chemicals that act as **oxidizing substances** (e.g., aspirin, the antimalarial primaquine, sulfonamides, and nitrofurans) can cause hemolytic anemia. These compounds reoxidize reduced glutathione and increase the demand for flux through the pentose phosphate pathway.

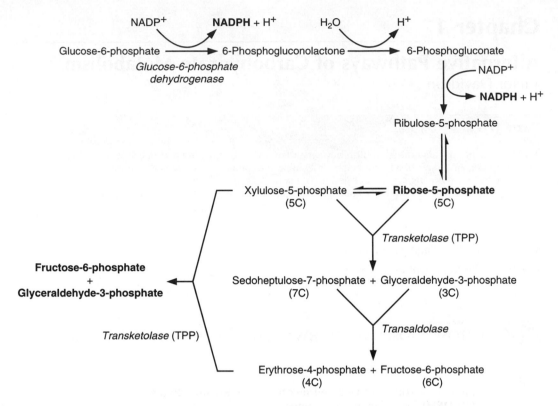

FIGURE 17-1. The pentose phosphate pathway. Key enzymes are indicated in *italics.* Products of the pathway are indicated by *bold type.* The number of carbons (C) in some reaction intermediates are given in parentheses. *NADP⁺* = oxidized nicotinamide adenine dinucleotide phosphate; *NADPH* = reduced NADP; *TPP* = thiamine pyrophosphate.

      (3) G6PD deficiency is particularly prevalent in the African and African-American population. Like the sickle-cell anemia trait, it is thought to have been selected for by resistance to the malaria parasite.

  2. 6-Phosphogluconolactone to 6-phosphogluconate is catalyzed by **lactonase** (gluconolactone hydrolase).

  3. 6-Phosphogluconate to ribulose-5-phosphate and carbon dioxide is catalyzed by **6-phosphogluconate dehydrogenase. NADP⁺ is reduced to NADPH** in this reaction.

  4. Ribulose-5-phosphate to ribose-5-phosphate and xylulose-5-phosphate. These three sugars are isomers that may be interconverted by the enzymes **phosphopentose isomerase** and **phosphopentose epimerase.**

  5. Ribose-5-phosphate and xylulose-5-phosphate to sedoheptulose-7-phosphate and G3P
    a. A two-carbon unit is transferred from xylulose-5-phosphate to ribose-5-phosphate to form a seven- and a three-carbon sugar from two five-carbon sugars.
    b. The reaction is catalyzed by **transketolase,** which requires **thiamine pyrophosphate** (TPP) as a cofactor (see Chapter 14 II I).
    c. Wernicke-Korsakoff syndrome
      (1) This syndrome results from **chronic thiamine deficiency.**
      (2) Patients with this disorder have been shown to have **defective transketolase** that exhibits a reduced affinity for TPP. Thus, in a thiamine-deficient condition, transketolase activity in these individuals is reduced.

        (3) This condition is sometimes seen in patients with chronic alcoholism because of their poor nutrition coupled with impaired absorption of the vitamin.

        (4) Clinical manifestations of the syndrome include weakness or paralysis and impaired mental function.

   6. Sedoheptulose-7-phosphate and G3P to erythrose-4-phosphate and F6P

     a. A three-carbon unit is transferred from sedoheptulose-7-phosphate to G3P to form a four- and a six-carbon sugar from a seven- and a three-carbon sugar.

     b. The reaction is catalyzed by **transaldolase,** which requires no cofactor.

   7. Xylulose-5-phosphate and erythrose-4-phosphate to fructose-6-phosphate and G3P

     a. A two-carbon unit is transferred from a xylulose-5-phosphate to erythrose-4-phosphate to form a six- and a three-carbon sugar from a five- and a four-carbon sugar.

     b. The reaction is also catalyzed by the TPP-dependent transketolase.

D. **Regulation.** The cellular concentration of **NADP⁺ is the major factor** in regulating flux through the pathway. Its availability regulates the rate-limiting G6PD reaction.

II. **URONIC ACID PATHWAY (GLUCURONIC ACID CYCLE).** The reactions of this pathway (Figure 17-2) allow glucose to be used as a precursor for the synthesis of several important metabolites.

A. The pathway is a **source of uridine diphosphate (UDP)-glucose,** which is used for glycogen formation (see Chapter 21 II A).

B. **The formation of glucuronosides for detoxifying the body.** (A glucuronoside is glucuronic acid connected to other compounds by a glycosidic bond.) Many naturally occurring substances, as well as many drugs, are eliminated from the body by the formation of glucuronoside derivatives of the substances, which allows them to be excreted in the bile and urine as water-soluble compounds, also called glucuronides.

   1. Examples of such substances include steroid hormones, bilirubin, morphine, salicylic acid, and menthol.

   2. The **general reaction** is:

$$\text{UDP-glucuronate} + \text{acceptor} \rightarrow \text{glucuronoside} + \text{UDP}$$

C. **The biosynthesis of certain polysaccharides.** UDP-glucuronate is the donor for the glucuronyl moiety in some polysaccharides, such as heparin.

D. **The biosynthesis of chondroitin sulfate,** a glycosaminoglycan (see Chapter 5 V C)

E. The pathway is integral to the **formation of ascorbic acid (vitamin C)** in most animals, with the exception of humans, other primates, guinea pigs, and an East Indian fruit bat.

F. The uronic acid pathway is also necessary for the **formation of pentoses,** which may enter the pentose phosphate pathway and the **metabolism of nonphosphorylated sugar derivatives.**

III. **METABOLISM OF FRUCTOSE**

A. **Sources**

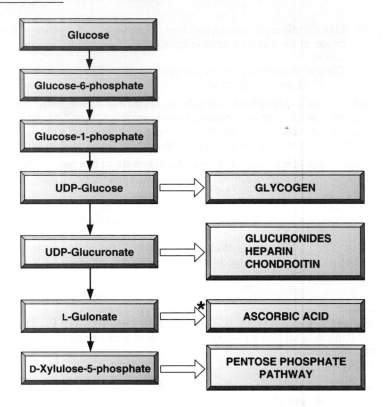

FIGURE 17-2. The uronic acid pathway. Only key intermediates are shown. *Arrows* may represent multiple reaction steps. *Open arrows* indicate important biomolecules that are derived from pathway intermediates and other metabolic pathways that may utilize these intermediates. The *asterisk* indicates that the ability to form ascorbic acid is not present in humans. *UDP* = uridine diphosphate.

1. Fructose is a product of the **hydrolysis of sucrose,** a glucose–fructose disaccharide.

2. Fructose is the major sugar present in plants. Dietary sources include **fruits and honey.**

B. **Major pathway of fructose metabolism** (Figure 17-3)

1. **Fructose and ATP to fructose-1-phosphate and adenosine diphosphate (ADP)**
   a. The reaction is catalyzed by **fructokinase,** which has a very high affinity for fructose, and its activity is not affected by feeding–fasting cycles or by insulin levels.
   b. **Essential fructosuria** is caused by a defect in fructokinase. This condition is not usually serious, because the excess fructose that accumulates is lost in the urine.

2. **Fructose-1-phosphate to dihydroxyacetone phosphate (DHAP) and glyceraldehyde**
   a. This reaction is catalyzed by **phosphofructaldolase** (aldolase B; fructose-1-phosphate aldolase), which is an isozyme of the aldolase of the glycolytic pathway (Chapter 16 III D 1).
   b. **Hereditary fructose intolerance** is caused by a genetic defect leading to phosphofructaldolase deficiency, which causes fructose-1-phosphate to accumulate in cells and leads to liver and kidney damage. This condition is treated by excluding fructose-containing foods from the diet.

3. **Interconversion of DHAP and G3P.** As in glycolysis, DHAP may be converted to G3P by the enzyme **triose phosphate isomerase** (Chapter 16 III E).

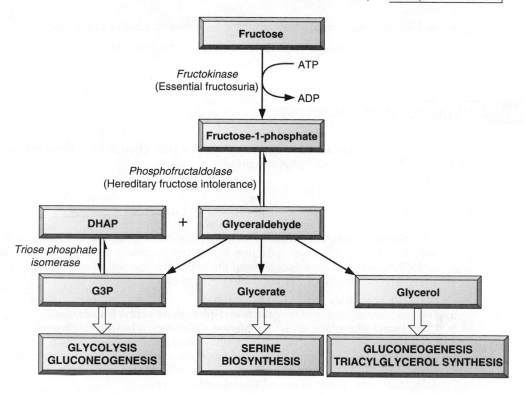

FIGURE 17-3. Metabolism of fructose. Key enzymes are indicated in *italics* and metabolic disorders associated with a deficiency in the enzyme are given in *parentheses*. The intermediates of the pathway are indicated in *capital letters. Open arrows* indicate other metabolic pathways that may utilize products and intermediates. *ADP* = adenosine diphosphate; *ATP* = adenosine triphosphate; *DHAP* = dihydroxyacetone phosphate; *G3P* = glyceraldehyde-3-phosphate.

4. Fates of glyceraldehyde
   a. Phosphorylation to G3P and entry into the pathways of glycolysis or gluconeogenesis
   b. Oxidation to glycerate and conversion to the amino acid serine
   c. Reduction to glycerol and use for gluconeogenesis or triacylglycerol biosynthesis

C. **Regulation of metabolism**

   1. Unlike glucose, fructose uptake by cells is not regulated by insulin.

   2. Because fructose enters the glycolytic pathway as G3P, it bypasses the major regulatory step in glycolysis, which is catalyzed by phosphofructokinase (see Chapter 16 III C).

D. **Fructose metabolism in spermatozoa**

   1. Fructose is the **major energy source for spermatozoa** and is formed from glucose in the seminal vesicle. The fructose concentration of semen may reach 10 mM, most of which is available for the spermatozoa because fructose is used sparingly by the other tissues that come in contact with the seminal fluid.

   2. **Formation.** Glucose is reduced to the sugar alcohol **sorbitol,** which is then oxidized to **fructose.**
   a. **Aldose reductase** catalyzes the conversion of sorbitol to glucose.

$$\text{Glucose} + \text{NADPH} + \text{H}^+ \rightarrow \text{Sorbitol} + \text{NADP}^+$$

b. Sorbitol dehydrogenase catalyzes the conversion of sorbitol to fructose.

$$\text{Sorbitol} + NAD^+ \rightarrow \text{Fructose} + NADH + H^+$$

IV. METABOLISM OF GALACTOSE

A. **Source.** Galactose is derived from lactose, which is a disaccharide of glucose and galactose that is the primary carbohydrate present in milk.

B. **Catabolism of galactose** (Figure 17-4)

1. **Galactose and ATP to galactose-1-phosphate and ADP**
   a. The reaction is catalyzed by **galactokinase.**
   b. **Galactokinase deficiency** leads to an accumulation of galactose in blood and tissues. In the lens of the eye, galactose is reduced by aldose reductase to dulcitol (galacitol), which cannot escape from the cells. This causes an osmotic imbalance, which contributes to the development of **cataracts.**

2. **Galactose-1-phosphate to glucose-1-phosphate**
   a. The reaction is catalyzed by **galactose-1-phosphate uridyl transferase.**
   b. **Galactose-1-phosphate uridyl transferase deficiency (classic galactosemia)** leads to the accumulation of both galactose and galactose-1-phosphate in tissues. Cataracts develop, as in galactokinase deficiency. If not treated, mental retardation and liver cirrhosis may occur because of increased cellular levels of galactose-1-phosphate in neural tissues and liver cells.

3. **UDP-galactose and UDP-glucose are interconverted by UDP-galactose-4-epimerase.**

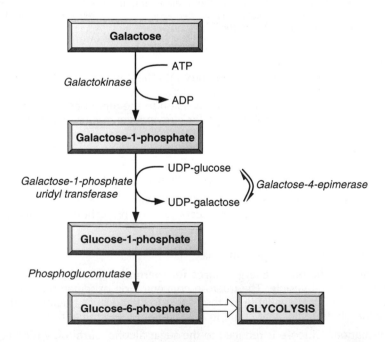

FIGURE 17-4. Metabolism of galactose. Key enzymes are indicated in *italics.* The intermediates of the pathway are indicated in *capital letters. Open arrows* indicate other metabolic pathways that may utilize products and intermediates. *ADP* = adenosine diphosphate; *ATP* = adenosine triphosphate; *UDP* = uridine diphosphate.

C. **Biosynthesis of lactose**

1. In humans, this occurs only in the mammary glands.

2. **Lactose is formed from UDP-galactose and glucose** in a reaction catalyzed by **galactosyl transferase.** This enzyme does not use glucose as a substrate in tissues other than the mammary gland.
    a. **α-Lactalbumin** is a protein that binds to galactosyl transferase and modifies its specificity so that it catalyzes lactose formation. The complex of α-lactalbumin and galactosyl transferase is called lactose synthase. α-Lactalbumin levels in mammary tissue are under hormonal control.
    b. **Prolactin** increases the rate of synthesis of galactosyl transferase and of α-lactalbumin.

D. **Utilization of lactose**

1. **Lactase** hydrolyzes lactose to glucose and galactose in the small intestines.

2. **Lactose intolerance** is often the result of a deficiency of lactase (see Chapter 5, Case 5-1).

V. SORBITOL METABOLISM IN DIABETES

A. The formation of sorbitol from glucose proceeds rapidly in the lens of the eye and in the Schwann cells of the nervous system.

B. Sorbitol cannot pass through the cell membrane, and in people with diabetes, sorbitol levels build up in these cells because the rate of oxidation of sorbitol to fructose is decreased.

C. The elevated sorbitol concentration causes an increase in osmotic pressure, which may be a causative factor in the development of the lens cataracts and the neural dysfunction that occur in patients with diabetes (see Chapter 27 VI C).

VI. FORMATION OF AMINO SUGARS. Glucosamine-6-phosphate is the precursor of all hexosamine residues in glycosaminoglycans (see Chapter 5 VI C). A summary of the reactions of amino sugars leading to glycosaminoglycan and glycoprotein formation is shown in Figure 17-5.

VII. ETHANOL METABOLISM

A. **Oxidation to acetate in the liver**

1. Ethanol is oxidized in the liver by a cytosolic **alcohol dehydrogenase** to acetaldehyde.

$$CH_3CH_2O + NAD^+ \rightarrow CH_3CHO + NADH + 2H^+$$

2. The acetaldehyde is further oxidized to acetate by a mitochondrial **aldehyde dehydrogenase.**

$$CH_3CHO + NAD^+ + H_2O \rightarrow CH_3COO^- + NADH + 2H^+$$

3. Much of the acetate produced from ethanol leaves the liver and is converted to

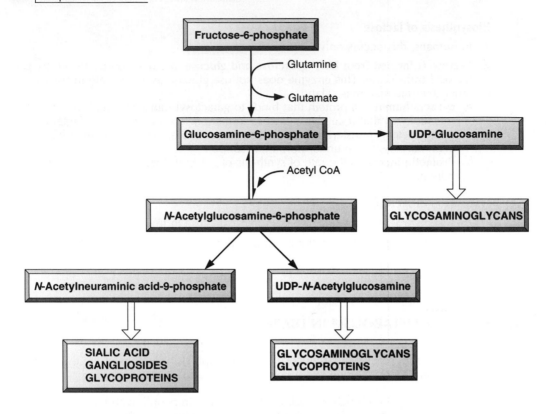

FIGURE 17-5. Metabolism of amino sugars. Only key intermediates are shown. *Arrows* may represent multiple reaction steps. *Open arrows* indicate important biomolecules that are derived from pathway intermediates. *UDP* = uridine diphosphate.

acetyl coenzyme A (acetyl CoA), which can be used to provide energy via the citric acid cycle (see Chapter 18 II D).

4. Acetyl CoA may also be formed in the liver and used as a precursor for lipid biosynthesis.

B. **Mechanism of methanol and ethylene glycol poisoning.** Alcohol dehydrogenase is not a very specific enzyme and also converts methanol to formaldehyde and ethylene glycol to oxalate, both of which are very toxic.

C. Aldehyde dehydrogenase is the enzyme that is inhibited by the drug **disulfiram,** which is given to alcoholics to discourage drinking. It causes acetaldehyde to accumulate, which leads to severe nausea. However, if alcohol consumption is not discouraged, aldehyde levels may become lethal.

D. Ethanol also may be oxidized by a microsomal **cytochrome P$_{450}$ oxidase,** which is induced by ethanol.

Case 17-1 Revisited

The general symptoms exhibited by this newborn could be caused by a wide range of disorders. The mild jaundice indicates the onset of damage to the liver. High levels of a reducing sugar other than glucose in the urine raise the possibility of galactosemia, which is investigated by specifically assaying for galactose levels.

Direct assay of the erythrocytes for the deficient enzyme, galactose-1-phosphate uridyl transferase, may be performed to confirm the diagnosis of galactosemia caused by a deficiency of this enzyme.

Treatment consists of placing the infant on a galactose-free diet. Milk is replaced with a galactose-free formula. When the infant grows older, he will be placed on a diet that excludes milk products and other galactose-containing foods. If this diet is followed, his development should be normal, thanks to early diagnosis and treatment.

STUDY QUESTIONS

DIRECTIONS: Each of the numbered items or incomplete statements in this section is followed by answers or by completions of the statement. Select the **one** lettered answer or completion that is **best** in each case.

1. Ribose-5-phosphate is formed in the pentose phosphate pathway from

(A) isomerization of ribulose-5-phosphate
(B) oxidation of glucose-6-phosphate
(C) reaction of sedoheptulose-7-phosphate and erythrose-4-phosphate
(D) reaction of fructose-6-phosphate and glyceraldehyde-3-phosphate
(E) reaction of xylulose-5-phosphate and erythrose-4-phosphate

2. Which enzyme in the pentose phosphate pathway requires thiamine pyrophosphate (TPP)?

(A) Glucose-6-phosphate dehydrogenase
(B) 6-Phosphogluconate dehydrogenase
(C) Transketolase
(D) Transaldolase
(E) Phosphopentose isomerase

3. Cataracts may result from osmotic imbalance in the lens of the eye caused by the accumulation of

(A) galactose
(B) glucose
(C) sugar alcohols
(D) amino sugars
(E) ethanol

4. Patients suffering from galactosemia are placed on a galactose-free diet. Galactose, however, is required by the body to form brain cerebrosides. How is galactose formed in patients on a galactose-free diet?

(A) Epimerization of uridine diphosphate (UDP)-glucose
(B) Reaction of a 5- and a 4-carbon sugar catalyzed by transketolase
(C) Reaction of a 7- and a 3-carbon sugar catalyzed by transaldolase
(D) Reaction of two 3-carbon sugars catalyzed by aldolase
(E) Oxidation of sorbitol

5. What is the major energy source for spermatozoa in seminal fluid?

(A) Glucose
(B) Fructose
(C) Galactose
(D) Ribose-5-phosphate
(E) Xylulose

6. Hereditary fructose intolerance is a condition caused by a deficiency of

(A) phosphofructokinase
(B) fructokinase
(C) phosphofructaldolase (fructose-1-phosphate aldolase)
(D) fructose-1,6-bisphosphate aldolase
(E) fructose-6-phosphatase

7. Which one of the following substances is metabolized to acetyl CoA?

(A) Galactose
(B) Glucose
(C) Fructose
(D) Sorbitol
(E) Ethanol

Questions 8–10

An otherwise asymptomatic patient exhibits hemolytic anemia after treatment with the antimalarial drug primaquine.

8. What metabolic process is not functioning normally in this patient?

(A) Pentose phosphate pathway
(B) Uronic acid pathway
(C) Metabolism of amino sugars
(D) Galactose metabolism
(E) Fructose metabolism

9. What enzyme is deficient in this patient?

(A) Phosphofructaldolase
(B) Galactose-1-phosphate uridyl transferase
(C) Glucose-6-phosphate dehydrogenase
(D) Lactase
(E) Fructokinase

10. Which one of the following results of this patient's disorder causes the hemolytic anemia?

(A) Low levels of ribose-5-phosphate
(B) Low levels of oxidized nicotinamide adenine dinucleotide phosphate (NADP$^+$)
(C) Low levels of oxidized nicotinamide adenine dinucleotide (NAD$^+$)
(D) Low levels of glyceraldehyde-3-phosphate
(E) Low levels of reduced glutathione

DIRECTIONS: The group of items in this section consists of lettered options followed by a set of numbered items. For each item, select the **one** lettered option that is most closely associated with it. Each lettered option may be selected once, more than once, or not at all.

Questions 11–13

Match the following characteristics or symptoms to the correct disorder.

(A) Glucose-6-phosphate dehydrogenase deficiency
(B) Wernicke-Korsakoff syndrome
(C) Hereditary fructose intolerance
(D) Diabetes mellitus
(E) Classic galactosemia

11. This disorder is treated by a diet devoid of milk products

12. An infant being weaned off breast milk begins to exhibit poor health when fruit juice and sweets are introduced into its diet

13. This disorder may be treated in part by the administration of a vitamin

ANSWERS AND EXPLANATIONS

1. The answer is A [I C 4; Figure 17-1]. Ribose-5-phosphate, required for the synthesis of nucleotides, is formed from isomerization of ribulose-5-phosphate, which arises from glucose-6-phosphate by the sequential action of glucose-6-phosphate dehydrogenase and 6-phosphogluconate dehydrogenase. The reaction of sedoheptulose-7-phosphate and glyceraldehyde-3-phosphate (G3P), catalyzed by transaldolase, produces erythrose-4-phosphate and fructose-6-phosphate. The reaction of fructose-6-phosphate and G3P, catalyzed by transketolase, produces xylulose-5-phosphate and erythrose-4-phosphate.

2. The answer is C [I C 5]. Transketolase is an enzyme that transfers two-carbon units from a ketose to an aldose. It requires a cofactor, thiamine pyrophosphate. Transaldolase, which transfers three-carbon units from a ketose to an aldose, and phosphopentose isomerase do not require a cofactor. The cofactor required by glucose-6-phosphate dehydrogenase and 6-phosphogluconate dehydrogenase is nicotinamide adenine dinucleotide phosphate.

3. The answer is C [IV B 1 b, 2 b; V]. Deficiencies in either galactokinase or galactose-1-phosphate uridyl transferase lead to the accumulation of galactose. In the lens of the eye, galactose is converted to dulcitol, which cannot diffuse out from the cells. The osmotic effects caused by the accumulation of this sugar alcohol contribute to the development of cataracts. In patients with diabetes, a similar effect is seen due to the reduction of glucose to its corresponding sugar alcohol, sorbitol, which may accumulate in the lens of the eye.

4. The answer is A [IV B 3; Figure 17-4]. The interconversion of uridine diphosphate (UDP)-glucose and UDP-galactose is catalyzed by galactose-4-epimerase. UDP-glucose is an intermediate formed from glucose in the uronic acid pathway. The reactions catalyzed by transketolase, transaldolase, and aldolase all form fructose-6-phosphate as a product. Oxidation of sorbitol also yields fructose as a product.

5. The answer is B [III D 1]. Fructose in the seminal vesicle is formed from glucose by reduction to sorbitol, which is then oxidized to fructose. The fructose is used as an energy supply via the glycolytic pathway. This is advantageous for the spermatozoa because fructose is used sparingly by the other tissues that come in contact with the seminal fluid.

6. The answer is C [III B 2 b]. Hereditary fructose intolerance is caused by a deficiency of the aldolase that cleaves fructose-1-phosphate, which is formed from fructose by fructokinase to dihydroxyacetone phosphate and glyceraldehyde. Accumulation of fructose-1-phosphate in cells is believed to underlie the hepatic and renal damage. Fructose-1-phosphate also inhibits several enzyme activities; for example, hepatic glycogen phosphorylase, which causes postprandial hypoglycemia by inhibiting glycogen breakdown, and fructose-1,6-bisphosphate aldolase, which also contributes to the hypoglycemia as gluconeogenesis, are blocked.

7. The answer is E [VII A]. Ethanol in the liver is oxidized to acetate by the sequential actions of alcohol dehydrogenase and aldehyde dehydrogenase. Much of the acetate is converted to acetyl coenzyme A (acetyl CoA) by other tissues and used as an energy source. Glucose, fructose, and galactose are metabolized via glycolysis, the product of which is pyruvate. Sorbitol may be oxidized to fructose in some tissues by sorbitol dehydrogenase.

8–10. The answers are: 8-A, 9-C, 10-E [I A 4, C 1 b]. Erythrocytes depend on the pentose phosphate pathway for reduced nicotinamide adenine dinucleotide phosphate (NADPH), which is used to form reduced glutathione. Glutathione is needed to maintain the integrity of the cell membrane. The oxidizing antimalarial drug can cause hemolytic anemia in individuals with low glucose-6-phosphate dehydrogenase (G6PD) activity because these compounds reoxidize reduced glutathione and increase the demand for flux through the pentose phosphate pathway beyond the capability of cells deficient in G6PD.

Phosphofructaldolase deficiency causes hereditary fructose intolerance. Galactose-1-phosphate uridyl transferase deficiency causes classic galactosemia. Lactase deficiency causes lactose intolerance. Fructokinase deficiency causes essential fructosuria.

G6PD deficiency also may lead to lower-than-normal levels of ribose-5-phosphate and glyceraldehyde-3-phosphate (other products of the pentose phosphate pathway) but this alone would not lead to hemolytic anemia. NADP$^+$ levels will be higher than normal, but levels of NAD$^+$ should not be affected.

11–13. The answers are: 11-E [IV A, B 2 b], **12-C** [III B 2 b], **13-B** [I C 5 c]. Lactose is the primary carbohydrate present in milk. It is hydrolyzed to glucose and galactose. The ill effects of classic galactosemia may be overcome by excluding galactose-containing food, primarily milk products. With infants, the condition is treated by substituting milk with a galactose-free formula.

The major dietary sources of fructose are sucrose and fruits. Hereditary fructose intolerance is caused by a genetic defect in phosphofructaldolase, which leads to the accumulation of fructose-1-phosphate and fructose and a variety of health problems. While being fed milk, an infant's primary source of carbohydrate is lactose, which does not contain fructose, so the infant's carbohydrate metabolism is normal. This disorder may be controlled by excluding fructose-containing foods from the diet.

Patients with Wernicke-Korsakoff syndrome have a defective transketolase, which exhibits a reduced affinity for thiamine pyrophosphate (TPP). The other TPP-dependent enzymes (e.g., pyruvate dehydrogenase) may appear to be normal. If TPP levels in the cell become too low because of vitamin deficiency, the defective transketolase will not function. This can be corrected by administration of sufficient doses of thiamine to raise the cellular TPP levels to overcome the weak affinity of the enzyme for the cofactor.

Chapter 18

Pyruvate Dehydrogenase and Citric Acid Cycle
Victor Davidson

Case 18-1

A male infant is born without complications and appears normal until 1 year of age, when he has trouble standing. By age 2 years, he exhibits severe ataxia and psychomotor retardation. He cannot stand or walk, and he speaks very little. Urinalysis reveals high levels of alanine. Blood tests reveal elevated levels of pyruvate and lactate. Therapeutic doses of thiamine are administered, and within 6 months the boy can walk and speak.

- What is the diagnosis?
- Why did therapeutic doses of thiamine correct this problem?
- What is the long-term prognosis?

I. THE PYRUVATE DEHYDROGENASE (PDH) ENZYME COMPLEX

A. **Function. PDH links glycolysis** (see Chapter 16) **and the citric acid cycle.** PDH oxidizes pyruvate, the product of glycolysis, to CO_2 and acetyl coenzyme A (acetyl CoA), which is the substrate for the citric acid cycle.

B. **Location.** PDH is located within the **mitochondrial matrix** (see Chapter 13 II).

C. The overall reaction requires four distinct enzymatic activities, each of which requires different subunits and cofactors that comprise the PDH enzyme complex (Figure 18-1).

1. **Step 1: Pyruvate decarboxylase activity**
   a. This reaction is catalyzed by the **E_1 subunit** of PDH.
   b. The **cofactor thiamine pyrophosphate** (TPP; see Chapter 14 II I) is required. Carbon dioxide is formed, and the substrate becomes covalently bound to TPP.

2. **Step 2: Transfer of the two-carbon unit from E_1 to E_2**
   a. **E_2 requires the coenzyme lipoic acid,** which is covalently attached to a lysine residue of the protein. This covalently bound form of lipoic acid is called **lipoamide.**

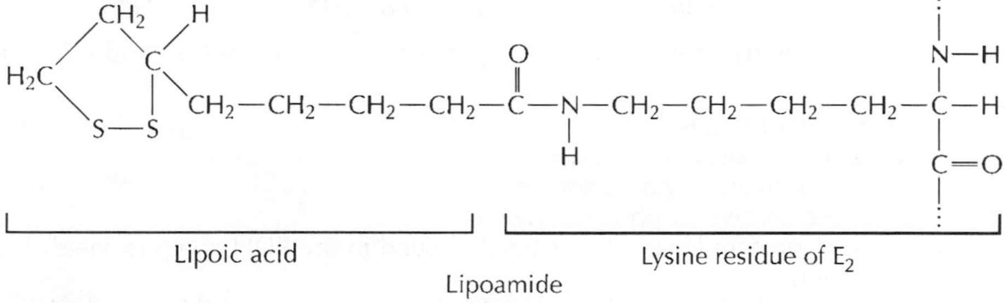

Lipoic acid   Lysine residue of E_2

Lipoamide

   b. In this step, the substrate is simultaneously oxidized to an acetyl group and transferred to the oxidized form of lipoamide. TPP is regenerated in this step.

3. **Step 3: Dihydrolipoyl transacetylase activity**
   a. This reaction is catalyzed by the **E_2 subunit** of PDH.

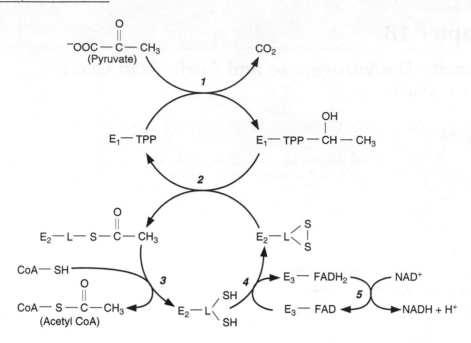

FIGURE 18-1. Summary of the reaction catalyzed by the pyruvate dehydrogenase (PDH) complex. E_1, E_2, and E_3 represent the different subunits of PDH, and L represents lipoamide. The *numbers* indicate the five steps of the overall reaction as described in the text. CoA = coenzyme A; CO_2 = carbon dioxide; FAD = flavin adenine dinucleotide; $FADH_2$ = reduced FAD; NAD^+ = oxidized nicotinamide adenine dinucleotide; $NADH$ = reduced nicotinamide adenine dinucleotide; TPP = thiamine pyrophosphate.

    b. The reaction involves transfer of the acetyl group from lipoamide to coenzyme A to form acetyl CoA. Lipoamide is in the reduced state after this transfer.

4. Step 4: Dihydrolipoyl dehydrogenase activity
    a. This reaction is catalyzed by the **E_3 subunit** of PDH.
    b. Tightly bound flavin adenine dinucleotide (FAD; see Chapter 13 V C 2) is a cofactor for E_3 in this reaction. FAD reoxidizes lipoamide and is reduced to $FADH_2$.

5. Step 5: $FADH_2$ is reoxidized to FAD by nicotinamide adenine dinucleotide (NAD^+; see Chapter 13 V C 1). Reduced NADH and H^+ are produced.

D. **PDH regulation**

1. Product inhibition. Both acetyl CoA and NADH inhibit PDH.

2. Availability of substrates. Adequate concentrations of CoA and NAD^+ must be present.

3. Covalent modification
    a. PDH exists in two forms:
        (1) Inactive, phosphorylated
        (2) Active, dephosphorylated
    b. A **protein kinase** that is tightly bound to the PDH complex yields the inactive form.
        (1) The kinase, which depends on magnesium ion (Mg^{2+}) and adenosine triphosphate (ATP), phosphorylates a serine residue PDH.
        (2) The protein kinase reaction is **stimulated by acetyl CoA and NADH.**
        (3) The protein kinase reaction is **inhibited by free CoA (CoASH), NAD^+, and pyruvate.**

     c. **The complex is reactivated** by dephosphorylation by a **phosphoprotein phosphatase.** It is activated by increasing calcium concentrations in the mitochondria, which occur when ATP levels are low.

     d. **Hormonal regulation**

       (1) Insulin can activate PDH in adipose tissue.

       (2) Catecholamines can activate PDH in cardiac muscle.

  4. The PDH reaction is biologically irreversible. Thus, **it is not possible to make pyruvate from acetyl CoA.**

E. **Genetic defects in PDH**

  1. Results. A defect in any of the protein subunits of PDH can result in a decrease or complete loss of activity. Severe cases are usually fatal.

  2. Symptoms include:

     a. Lactic acidosis

     b. Neurologic disorder

  3. Treatments

     a. Administration of large doses of thiamine may be effective for certain defects in E_1 that reduce the affinity of the enzyme for TPP.

     b. Administration of large doses of lipoic acid may be effective for defects in E_2 with reduced affinity for that compound.

     c. A ketogenic diet high in fat and low in carbohydrate helps to lower the levels of pyruvate and lactate, which is formed from the excess pyruvate.

II. OVERVIEW OF THE CITRIC ACID CYCLE

A. **Description.** The citric acid cycle (also known as the tricarboxylic acid cycle and the Krebs cycle) is a series of enzymatically catalyzed reactions that form a common pathway for the **final oxidation of all metabolic fuels** (i.e., carbohydrates, free fatty acids, ketone bodies, amino acids), which are catabolized to the substrate of the citric acid cycle (acetyl CoA).

B. **Location.** These reactions occur within the **mitochondrial matrix.**

C. **Functions**

  1. The citric acid cycle is involved in both anabolic and catabolic processes.

     a. Anabolic reactions. The intermediates of the citric acid cycle are used as precursors in the **biosynthesis** of many compounds.

     b. Catabolic reactions. The cycle provides a means for the **degradation** of two-carbon acetyl residues, which are derived from carbohydrates, fatty acids, and amino acids.

  2. The citric acid cycle **provides much of the energy for respiration.** Electrons that are generated from the action of this cycle are transferred to the electron transport chain and used in the process of oxidative phosphorylation to generate ATP (see Chapter 19).

D. **Stoichiometry.** The **net reaction of the citric acid cycle** is:

$$\text{Acetyl CoA} + 3\ \text{NAD}^+ + \text{FAD} + \text{GDP} + \text{P}_i + 2\ \text{H}_2\text{O} \rightarrow 2\ \text{CO}_2 + 3\ \text{NADH} + \text{FADH}_2 + \text{GTP} + 2\ \text{H}^+ + \text{CoA}$$

  1. Two carbon atoms enter the cycle as acetyl CoA and leave in the form of carbon dioxide.

  2. Four pairs of electrons are removed from the substrate; three pairs leave in the form of NADH, and one pair leaves as $FADH_2$.

3. One high-energy phosphate bond is generated in the form of guanosine triphosphate (GTP).

4. Although intermediates of the citric acid cycle may be interconverted (see II C 1), the cycle does not consume or produce solely from acetyl CoA any intermediate of the cycle.

E. **Regulation.** There is no single enzyme of the citric acid cycle that serves as a point of regulation. Instead, multiple enzymes are allosterically regulated by the level of ATP (see III), which reflects the energy state of the cell. This type of regulation by ATP levels is referred to as **respiratory control.**

III. REACTIONS OF THE CITRIC ACID CYCLE (Figure 18-2)

A. **Acetyl CoA plus oxaloacetate to citrate and coenzyme A**

1. This initial condensation reaction is catalyzed by **citrate synthase.**

2. **Regulation**
   a. The reaction is inhibited by ATP, NADH, and succinyl CoA.
   b. The reaction is stimulated by adenosine monophosphate (AMP).

B. **Citrate to isocitrate.** This isomerization reaction is catalyzed by **aconitase.**

C. **Isocitrate to α-ketoglutarate and carbon dioxide**

1. This reaction is catalyzed by **isocitrate dehydrogenase.**

2. In this oxidative decarboxylation reaction, **NAD^+ is reduced** to NADH.

3. **Regulation**
   a. This reaction is inhibited by ATP and NADH.
   b. This reaction is stimulated by ADP.

D. **α-Ketoglutarate and CoA to succinyl CoA**

1. This reaction is catalyzed by **α-ketoglutarate dehydrogenase.**
   a. **Prosthetic groups.** α-Ketoglutarate dehydrogenase is a multimeric protein that contains tightly bound TPP, lipoamide, and FAD.
   b. **Structure.** α-Ketoglutarate dehydrogenase is very similar to PDH (see I C). In fact, its **E_3 subunit is identical to that of PDH.**

2. In this oxidative decarboxylation reaction, NAD^+ is reduced to NADH and H^+, and CO_2 is released.

3. The product, succinyl CoA, is an **energy-rich thioester** like acetyl CoA.

4. The reaction is inhibited by ATP, NADH, and succinyl CoA.

E. **Succinyl CoA and GDP and inorganic phosphate (P_i) to succinate and GTP and CoA**

1. This reaction is catalyzed by **succinyl CoA synthetase.**

2. This is a **substrate-level phosphorylation** with energy being conserved in the form of GTP.

F. **Succinate to fumarate**

1. This reaction is catalyzed by **succinate dehydrogenase (SDH).**
   a. **Prosthetic groups.** SDH possesses three different types of **iron–sulfur centers** and **covalently bound FAD.**

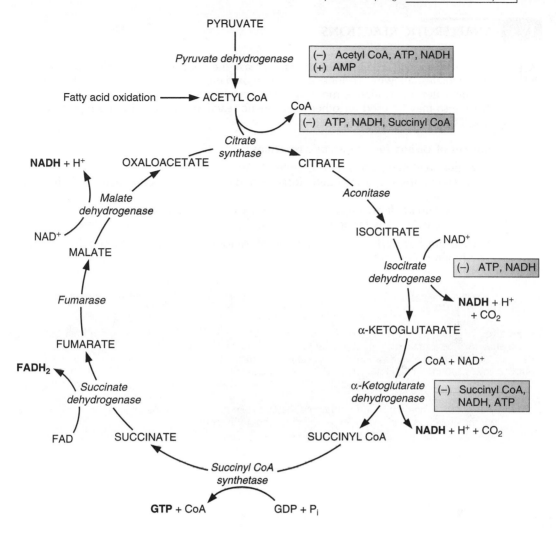

FIGURE 18-2. The reactions of pyruvate dehydrogenase and the citric acid cycle. Enzyme names are indicated in *italic type*. High-energy products of the citric acid cycle are indicated in **bold type**. Inhibitors and activators of regulatory enzymes are indicated by − and +, respectively. *AMP* = adenosine monophosphate; *ATP* = adenosine triphosphate; *CoA* = coenzyme A; *FAD* = flavin adenine dinucleotide; *FADH₂* = reduced FAD; *GDP* = guanosine diphosphate; *GTP* = guanosine triphosphate; *NAD⁺* = oxidized nicotinamide adenine dinucleotide; *NADH* = reduced NAD; *Pᵢ* = inorganic phosphate.

    b. SDH is tightly associated with the **inner mitochondrial membrane.**

  2. This is a dehydrogenation reaction during which **FAD is reduced to FADH₂.** FADH₂ is reoxidized by transferring electrons directly to the electron transport chain of the mitochondrial membrane (see Chapter 19 I D 2).

G. **Fumarate to malate.** This hydration reaction is catalyzed by **fumarase.**

H. **Malate to oxaloacetate**

  1. This reaction is catalyzed by **malate dehydrogenase.**

  2. This is a dehydrogenation reaction during which **NAD⁺ is reduced to NADH.**

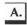 **IV.** **ANAPLEROTIC REACTIONS**

A. **Description.** Anaplerotic reactions can increase the concentration of citric acid cycle intermediates, allowing an increased rate of oxidation of two-carbon units. As more intermediates are available, more moles of acetyl CoA can be processed. The intermediates also may be used for other biosynthetic reactions and need to be replaced (see II C).

B. **Sources of carbon for anaplerotic reactions**

1. **Amino acid metabolism** (see Chapter 24 V)
   a. **Transaminases form α-ketoglutarate and oxaloacetate,** citric acid cycle intermediates.
   b. **Glutamate dehydrogenase** also produces α-ketoglutarate.
   c. **Succinyl CoA** is formed from isoleucine, valine, methionine, and threonine.

2. **Pyruvate carboxylase** (see Chapter 20 III A) forms oxaloacetate from pyruvate. It is a biotin-dependent carboxylase.

Case 18-1 Revisited

High levels of serum pyruvate suggest PDH deficiency. Lactate and alanine levels are also high because they may be formed from pyruvate by the reversible activities of lactate dehydrogenase (see Chapter 20 II A 1) and alanine aminotransferase (see Chapter 24 III A 1). This child's defect is apparently in the E_1 subunit of PDH, which causes a reduced affinity for TPP. This reduced affinity can be overcome by increasing the concentration of TPP, which is achieved by increasing the intake of thiamine, the precursor of TPP.

Symptoms would likely return if the thiamine therapy were discontinued. As long as this therapy is continued, the growth and development of the child should be normal.

▊ STUDY QUESTIONS

DIRECTIONS: Each of the numbered items or incomplete statements in this section is followed by answers or by completions of the statement. Select the **one** lettered answer or completion that is **best** in each case.

1. Which one of the following enzymes is tightly associated with the inner mitochondrial membrane?

(A) Citrate synthase
(B) α-Ketoglutarate dehydrogenase
(C) Succinate dehydrogenase
(D) Fumarase
(E) Malate dehydrogenase

2. A patient is deficient in activities of both pyruvate dehydrogenase (PDH) and α-ketoglutarate dehydrogenase. What is the most likely explanation for this finding?

(A) The patient possesses a genetic defect in the E_1 subunit of PDH
(B) The patient possesses a genetic defect in the E_2 subunit of PDH
(C) The patient possesses a genetic defect in the E_3 subunit of PDH
(D) The decarboxylase component of each enzyme is defective
(E) The dihydrolipoyl transacetylase component of each enzyme is defective

3. Which one of the following compounds is formed directly in one or more reaction(s) of the citric acid cycle?

(A) Reduced nicotinamide adenine dinucleotide (NADH)
(B) Adenosine triphosphate (ATP)
(C) Both
(D) Neither

4. Which one of the following compounds is required for acetyl coenzyme A (acetyl CoA) to enter the citric acid cycle?

(A) Isocitrate
(B) Malate
(C) Oxaloacetate
(D) Pyruvate
(E) Succinate

Questions 5–7

A patient suffers from a genetic defect in the E_2 subunit of the pyruvate dehydrogenase (PDH) complex, which decreases its activity.

5. Which one of the following is a likely symptom of this disorder?

(A) Serum pH greater than 7.4
(B) Above normal levels of serum lactate
(C) Below normal levels of serum alanine
(D) Below normal levels of serum pyruvate

6. Which one of the following treatments is most likely to be beneficial in this case?

(A) Restriction of dietary protein
(B) Restriction of dietary fats
(C) Restriction of dietary carbohydrates

7. Some patients with this genetic defect may respond to therapeutic doses of

(A) thiamine
(B) lipoic acid
(C) riboflavin
(D) niacin
(E) pantothenic acid

DIRECTIONS: The group of items in this section consists of lettered options followed by a set of numbered items. For each item, select the **one** lettered option that is most closely associated with it. Each lettered option may be selected once, more than once, or not at all.

Questions 8-12

Match the following descriptions with the correct enzyme.

(A) Malate dehydrogenase
(B) Succinyl CoA synthetase
(C) Citrate synthase
(D) Pyruvate dehydrogenase
(E) Pyruvate carboxylase

8. The reaction that it catalyzes results in the formation of a high-energy phosphate compound

9. Its activity is regulated by covalent modification

10. It catalyzes an anaplerotic reaction

11. It catalyzes the reduction of nicotinamide adenine dinucleotide

12. It uses acetyl CoA as a substrate

ANSWERS AND EXPLANATIONS

1. The answer is C [II B; III F 1 b]. The enzymes of the citric acid cycle are soluble and located in the mitochondrial matrix (i.e., they are confined within the inner mitochondrial membrane) with the exception of succinate dehydrogenase. This enzyme is embedded in the inner mitochondrial membrane.

2. The answer is C [I C 4, E; III D 1]. Pyruvate dehydrogenase (PDH) and α-ketoglutarate dehydrogenase have similar structures, with each possessing the analogous subunits. Only the E_3 subunit, however, is identical in each enzyme. Therefore, a defect in that subunit affects both enzymes. A defect in the E_1, decarboxylase component or in the E_2, dihydrolipoyl transacetylase component of PDH does not affect the activity of the other enzyme.

3. The answer is A [III C 2, D 2, H 2; Figure 18-2]. Reduced nicotinamide adenine dinucleotide (NADH) is formed from oxidized NAD^+ in reactions catalyzed by three citric acid cycle enzymes, isocitrate dehydrogenase, α-ketoglutarate dehydrogenase, and malate dehydrogenase. The electrons that are transferred to NADH may be used to drive oxidative phosphorylation, which indirectly leads to adenosine triphosphate (ATP) production. However, ATP is not a product of any reaction in the cycle.

4. The answer is C [III A]. Isocitrate, succinate, malate, and oxaloacetate are citric acid cycle intermediates. Oxaloacetate combines with acetyl coenzyme A (acetyl CoA) to form citrate in the initial step in which acetyl CoA enters the cycle. Pyruvate is a major source of acetyl CoA derived from carbohydrate.

5–7. The answers are: 5-B, 6-C, 7-B [I E; Case 18-1]. High levels of serum pyruvate are observed in patients with pyruvate dehydrogenase (PDH) deficiency. Lactate and alanine levels also may be high because they may be formed from pyruvate by the reversible activities of lactate dehydrogenase and alanine transaminase. Because lactate is an acid, high levels of serum lactate can cause acidosis (i.e., pH lower than the normal pH of 7.4).

A ketogenic diet high in fat and low in carbohydrate helps to lower the levels of pyruvate and, consequently, lactate. The acetyl coenzyme A (acetyl CoA) needed to run the citric acid cycle can be derived from fatty acids. Restriction of dietary protein has no benefit because pyruvate is not directly derived from any amino acid except alanine.

Administration of large doses of lipoic acid may be effective in defects on the E_2 subunit, which reduces affinity for this cofactor. Thiamine therapy is beneficial only for PDH deficiencies caused by certain defects in the E_1 subunit. Riboflavin, niacin, and pantothenic acid are precursors of flavin adenine dinucleotide, nicotinamide adenine dinucleotide, and coenzyme A, respectively. Although these are cofactors for PDH, therapeutic doses are not expected to compensate for defects in the E_2 subunit.

8–12. The answers are: 8-B, 9-D, 10-E, 11-A, 12-C [I D 3; III A, E, H; IV B 2]. Only one reaction in the citric acid cycle generates a high-energy phosphate compound, namely, the reaction whereby succinyl coenzyme A (succinyl CoA) is converted to succinate catalyzed by succinyl CoA synthetase. This reaction is coupled to the phosphorylation of guanosine diphosphate (GDP) to the triphosphate (GTP).

Pyruvate dehydrogenase (PDH) exists in two forms: an inactive, phosphorylated form; and an active, dephosphorylated form. The PDH complex is regulated by covalent modification by a protein kinase that generates the phosphorylated form and a protein phosphatase that generates the dephosphorylated form.

Reactions that can increase the concentration of the citric acid cycle intermediates without using other citric acid cycle intermediates are called anaplerotic reactions. One of these anaplerotic reactions is the carboxylation of pyruvate to oxaloacetate (an intermediate of the citric acid cycle), which is catalyzed by pyruvate carboxylase.

Malate dehydrogenase catalyzes the dehydration of malate to form oxaloacetate. During this reaction, nicotinamide adenine dinucleotide (NAD^+) is reduced to NADH.

Citrate synthase catalyzes the initial step of the citric acid cycle in which acetyl CoA combines with oxaloacetate to enter the cycle in the form of citrate.

Chapter 19

Mitochondrial Electron Transport and Oxidative Phosphorylation

Victor Davidson

Case 19-1

A 40-year-old man is brought to the hospital in a coma. An odor similar to that of almonds is noted on the patient's breath. Blood gas analysis indicates severe metabolic acidosis. On questioning a friend, the physician learns that the patient had taken a massive dose of amygdalin, which he obtained in Mexico. Nitrites and thiosulfate are administered. The patient is ventilated on 100% oxygen and given sodium bicarbonate. He recovers and is taken off the ventilator the next day.

- What is the diagnosis?
- Why were nitrites and thiosulfate administered?

I. THE ELECTRON TRANSPORT (RESPIRATORY) CHAIN

A. Function

1. It is the final common pathway in aerobic cells by which electrons derived from various substrates are transferred to oxygen.

2. Different substrates may use this common pathway because they are oxidized by enzymes that use nicotinamide adenine dinucleotide (NAD^+) or flavin adenine dinucleotide (FAD) as electron acceptor cofactors. The reduced NADH and $FADH_2$ then donate the electrons to the electron transport chain.

B. Localization.
The enzymes of the electron transport chain are embedded in the **inner mitochondrial membrane** in association with the enzymes of oxidative phosphorylation.

C. Sources of electrons

1. **NADH** is derived from NAD^+-linked dehydrogenases, including:
   a. The isocitrate, α-ketoglutarate, and malate dehydrogenases of the citric acid cycle
   b. Pyruvate dehydrogenase
   c. L-3-Hydroxylacyl coenzyme A (CoA) dehydrogenase of fatty acid oxidation
   d. Miscellaneous NAD^+-linked dehydrogenases

2. **$FADH_2$** is derived from FAD-linked dehydrogenases, including:
   a. Succinate dehydrogenase of the citric acid cycle
   b. The FAD-linked dehydrogenase of the glycerol-3-phosphate shuttle (see Chapter 16 IV B 1)
   c. Acyl CoA dehydrogenase of fatty acid oxidation
   d. Miscellaneous FAD-linked dehydrogenases

D. ORGANIZATION OF THE ELECTRON TRANSPORT CHAIN (Figure 19-1)

1. **Complex I** is the point of entry into the electron transport chain for electrons from NADH.
   a. This **enzyme complex** is called **NADH–coenzyme Q reductase or NADH dehydrogenase.**

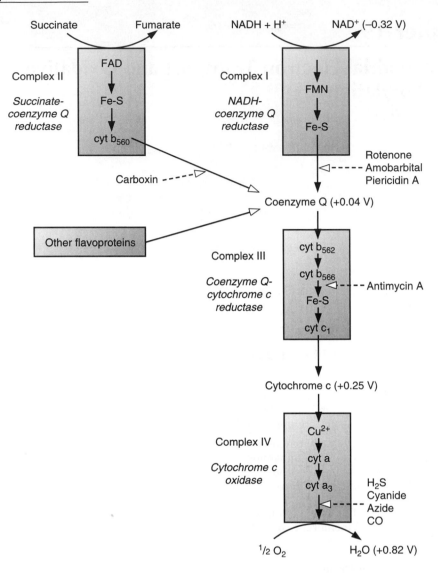

FIGURE 19-1. The mitochondrial electron transport chain. The electron-transferring, oxidation–reduction groups of each complex are *boxed*. The direction of electron flow is indicated by *arrows*. The sites of action of inhibitors are indicated by *dashed lines*. The oxidation–reduction potentials of certain electron carriers are indicated in *parentheses*. Enzymes are *italicized*. CO = carbon monoxide; Cu^{2+} = copper; *cyt* = cytochrome; *FAD* = flavin adenine dinucleotide; *Fe–S* = iron–sulfur; H^+ = protons; H_2O = water; H_2S = hydrogen sulfide; NAD^+ = oxidized nicotinamide adenine dinucleotide; *NADH* = reduced NAD; O_2 = molecular oxygen.

   b. Prosthetic groups
      (1) Flavin mononucleotide (FMN)
      (2) Iron–sulfur (Fe–S) centers
   c. The **electron acceptor** for complex I is **coenzyme Q** (also called ubiquinone or simply Q).
   d. Path of electron transfer. Electrons from NADH are transferred to FAD, then to the Fe–S center, then to coenzyme Q.
   e. Inhibitors of electron transfer from NADH to coenzyme Q include:
      (1) Rotenone, an insecticide
      (2) Barbiturates, such as amobarbital and secobarbital

      (3) Piericidin A, an antibiotic

2. Complex II is the point of entry into the electron transport chain for electrons from succinate.

    a. This **enzyme complex** is called **succinate–coenzyme Q reductase** and includes succinate dehydrogenase, which is the same enzyme that participates in the citric acid cycle (see Chapter 18 III F).

    b. Prosthetic groups include:

        (1) FAD

        (2) Fe–S centers

        (3) Heme (the prosthetic group of cytochrome b_{560})

    c. The **electron acceptor** for complex II is coenzyme Q.

    d. Path of electron transfer. Electrons from succinate are transferred to FAD, then to the Fe–S centers, then to cytochrome b_{560}, and then to coenzyme Q.

    e. Carboxin inhibits complex II.

3. Coenzyme Q is a highly lipid soluble molecule that is **firmly embedded in the membrane.** It accepts electrons from both complex I and complex II and donates electrons to complex III.

                Oxidized form   Reduced form

4. Complex III is the electron acceptor for coenzyme Q.

    a. This **enzyme complex** is called **coenzyme Q–cytochrome c reductase.**

    b. Prosthetic groups in complex III include:

        (1) Heme (b-type cytochromes and cytochrome c_1)

        (2) Fe–S centers

    c. The **electron acceptor** for complex III is cytochrome c.

    d. Path of electron transfer. Electrons from coenzyme Q are transferred to the b-type cytochromes, then to the Fe–S center, then to cytochrome c_1, and then to cytochrome c.

    e. Inhibitors of electron transfer from coenzyme Q to cytochrome c include antimycin A, an antibiotic.

5. Cytochrome c

    a. Unlike the other components of the respiratory chain, cytochrome c is a **soluble protein** that binds to the membrane to perform its electron transfer role.

    b. Function. It mediates the transfer of electrons from complex III to complex IV.

    c. The **prosthetic group** of cytochrome c, as well as the other cytochromes, is heme (see Chapter 25 VII).

6. Complex IV is the electron acceptor for cytochrome c.

    a. This **enzyme complex** is called **cytochrome c oxidase.**

    b. Prosthetic groups in complex IV include:

        (1) Copper (Cu)

        (2) Heme (cytochrome a and cytochrome a_3)

    c. The **electron acceptor** for complex IV is molecular oxygen (O_2), and the **product** of this reaction is water (H_2O).

    d. Path of electron transfer. Electrons from cytochrome c are transferred to Cu^{2+}, then to the a-type cytochromes, and then to O_2.

    e. Inhibitors of electron transfer from cytochrome c to O_2 include:

        (1) Carbon monoxide (CO), which competes with O_2 for its binding site on cytochrome oxidase

        (2) Hydrogen sulfide (H_2S)

(3) Azide (an N_3-containing compound)

(4) Cyanide (CN^-)

II. OXIDATIVE PHOSPHORYLATION

A. Function

1. It is the **main source of energy in aerobic cells.**

2. It is the process whereby the free energy that is released when electrons are transferred along the electron transport chain is coupled to the **formation of adenosine triphosphate (ATP)** from adenosine diphosphate (ADP) and inorganic phosphate (P_i).

B.

Oxidation–reduction potentials. The standard oxidation–reduction potentials (see Chapter 13 V B) of the electron carriers in the respiratory chain become more positive going from the oxidation of NADH to the reduction of molecular oxygen (see Figure 19-1).

1. **Release of energy.** From the difference in potentials between the NAD^+/NADH and O_2/H_2O couples, which is 1.14 volts, it can be calculated that for each electron pair that passes through the chain, approximately 52 kcal of energy are released.

2. **Coupling of free energy.** The energy released for each electron pair passing through the respiratory chain is coupled to the formation of ATP.

C.

Coupling sites for ATP synthesis. The energy released by the electron transfers catalyzed by three coupling sites—complex I, complex III, and complex IV—is sufficient for each to support the formation of approximately 1 mole of ATP.

1. **Electrons that enter the chain from NADH** support the synthesis of approximately 3 moles of ATP.

2. **Electrons that enter the chain from $FADH_2$** bypass complex I and support the synthesis of approximately 2 moles of ATP.

3. The **P:O ratio** is a measure of how many moles of ATP are formed from ADP per gram atom of oxygen for a given substrate. For NAD^+ the P:O ratio is approximately 3:1. For FAD^+ the P:O ratio is approximately 2:1.

D.

The **chemiosmotic theory** of oxidative phosphorylation

1. An **electrochemical gradient of protons** (H^+) across the mitochondrial inner membrane serves to couple the energy flow of electron transport to the formation of ATP.

2. The electron carriers act as pumps, which cause vectorial (directional) **pumping of H^+ across the membrane** (Figure 19-2).

3. Because H^+ is a charged particle, the flow of free energy across the inner membrane is due to the combination of a **concentration gradient** and a **charge gradient.**

4. In the electron transport chain, H^+ is separated from the electron. **As electrons move down the chain, H^+ is transferred from the mitochondrial matrix to the intermembrane space.**

5. The protons in the intermembrane space pass through the inner membrane and back into the matrix via the **ATP synthase** (see Figure 19-2). The dissipation of energy that occurs as the protons pass down the concentration gradient to the matrix drives the phosphorylation of ADP to ATP by the synthase.

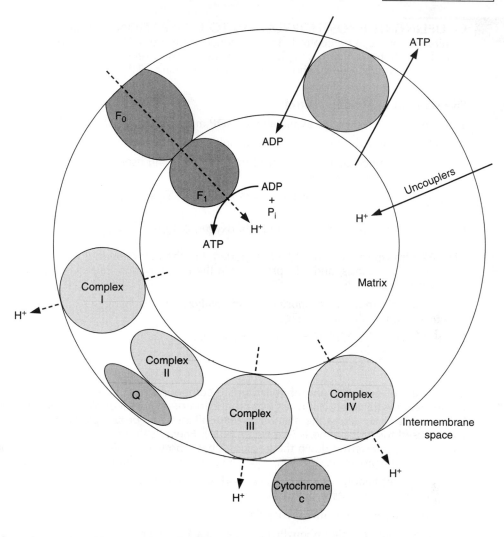

FIGURE 19-2. Schematic diagram of the coupling of electron transport to oxidative phosphorylation. F_0 and F_1 represent the two components of ATP synthase. *ADP* = adenosine diphosphate; *ATP* = adenosine triphosphate; H^+ = protons; P_i = inorganic phosphate; Q = coenzyme Q.

E. The enzyme complex that synthesizes ATP (see Figure 19-2) is called **ATP synthase** and is also known as **H^+–ATPase** or **F_0F_1–ATPase.**
  1. **Composition.** ATP synthase is composed of two units.
     a. **F_0** spans the membrane and is composed of four subunits. It forms a **channel** or path through which protons cross the membrane.
     b. **F_1** is tightly bound to F_0 and sits on the matrix side of the mitochondrial membrane. The F_1 unit is composed of five subunits. It contains the **catalytic site** for ATP synthesis.
  2. **Inhibitors** of ATP synthase include:
     a. Oligomycin, an antibiotic
     b. Dicyclohexylcarbodiimide (DCCD)
  3. **Other enzymes** that can couple ATP synthesis to the transport of ions other than hydrogen down a concentration gradient are found in other parts of the cell.
     a. The **Ca^{2+}–ATPase** of the sarcoplasmic reticulum
     b. The **Na^+K^+–ATPase** of the plasma membrane

III. **COUPLING OF PHOSPHORYLATION TO RESPIRATION.** The rate of respiration of mitochondria can be controlled by the concentration of ADP because **oxidation and phosphorylation are tightly coupled.** That is, as energy is released from oxidation reactions, the energy is used to phosphorylate ADP to create ATP.

A. **Five states of respiratory control**

1. **State 1** is limited by the availability of ADP and substrate (source of electrons).

2. **State 2** is limited by the availability of substrate.

3. **State 3** is limited by the capacity of the electron chain itself, when ADP, oxygen, and substrate are saturating.

4. **State 4** is limited by the availability of ADP only. This is typically the resting state in cells.

5. **State 5** is limited by the availability of oxygen only.

B. **ADP/ATP transport.** ADP must be transported into the mitochondrial matrix to be used for ATP synthesis, and ATP produced in the mitochondria must be transported out for use by the cell.

1. A **membrane-bound transporter** system catalyzes the exchange of ADP and ATP across the membrane (see Figure 19-2).

2. **Inhibitors** of the ADP/ATP transporter include:
   a. Atractyloside
   b. Bongkrekic acid

C. **Uncouplers of oxidative phosphorylation** are compounds that allow normal function of the electron transport chain without production of ATP. Uncouplers **cause leakage or transport of H⁺** across the membrane that collapses the proton gradient before it can be used for ATP synthesis (see Figure 19-2). Energy still may be released as the electrons are transferred down the transport chain; however, this energy is not trapped as ATP but appears instead as heat. Oxidative phosphorylation uncouplers include:

1. **2,4-Dinitrophenol,** which was once used as a weight-loss drug but was discontinued because of its toxicity

2. **Dicumarol,** which is an anticoagulant

3. **Chlorcarbonylcyanide phenylhydrazone (CCCP),** which is a compound that carries protons across the membrane

4. **Bilirubin,** which is a metabolite of heme degradation (see Chapter 25 VII C) but is not normally present in mitochondria in concentrations high enough to affect normal function

IV. **DISORDERS OF MITOCHONDRIAL OXIDATIVE PHOSPHORYLATION**

A. **Genetics**

1. Mitochondria are the only organelles outside the nucleus that contain their own DNA.

2. Some of the proteins that comprise the respiratory chain and oxidative phosphorylation system are encoded by mitochondrial DNA, whereas others are encoded by nuclear DNA.

3. Several disorders of oxidative phosphorylation have been identified (Table 19-1) that are the result of mutations in either nuclear or mitochondrial DNA that is involved in proper biosynthesis of the oxidative phosphorylation system.

TABLE 19-1. Disorders of Mitochondrial Electron Transport and Oxidative Phosphorylation that Result from Genetic Defects

---

Disorders associated with defects in nuclear DNA
Alpers syndrome
Benign infantile myopathy
Fatal infantile myopathy
Leigh syndrome
MNGIE (mitochondrial neuropathy, gastrointestinal disorder, encephalopathy) syndrome

Disorders associated with defects in mitochondrial DNA
Kearns-Sayre syndrome
LHON (Leber hereditary optic neuropathy)
MELAS (mitochondrial encephalomyopathy with lactic acidosis and stroke-like episodes)
MERRF (myoclonic epilepsy and ragged red fibers)
NARP (neuropathy, ataxia, and retinitis pigmentosa)
Pearson syndrome

B. **Clinical manifestations** include muscle cramping and weakness, fatigue, lactic acidosis, central nervous system (CNS) dysfunction, and vision problems.

C. **Treatment** of patients with respiratory chain disorders is difficult and often unsuccessful. In some cases improvement was reported after therapeutic doses of substances that may mediate electron transfer, such as ubiquinone, vitamin C, and menadione.

V. **SUPEROXIDE METABOLISM.** Oxygen is a potentially toxic substance. Toxicity may arise from the partial reduction of molecular oxygen (O_2) to the **superoxide anion free radical (O_2^-).** It is highly reactive and may damage DNA, proteins, and membranes. Superoxide-mediated damage may be a factor in the aging process.

A. **Superoxide formation** may occur in the **mitochondria** by the reactions of O_2 with reduced $FADH_2$ and reduced coenzyme Q. It is formed in **other organelles** by the reaction of O_2 with oxidizing enzymes.

B. **Detoxification of superoxide** is catalyzed enzymatically by **superoxide dismutases** via the reaction:

$$2\ O_2^- + 2H^+ \rightarrow H_2O_2 + O_2$$

C. **Detoxification of hydrogen peroxide (H_2O_2).** This product of the breakdown of superoxide also is a very reactive compound. It is also enzymatically detoxified by **peroxidases** via the reaction:

$$2\ H_2O_2 \rightarrow 2\ H_2O + O_2$$

1. The most widely distributed peroxidase in the body is a heme-containing enzyme, **catalase.**

2. In erythrocytes, **glutathione peroxidase,** a selenium-containing enzyme, catalyzes this reaction with the concomitant oxidation of reduced glutathione.

3. **Vitamin C and vitamin E** also play a role in detoxifying superoxide and other potentially damaging free radicals.

D. **Oxygen can be extremely toxic to premature infants,** who are often ventilated with high concentrations of oxygen to compensate for their immature lung development.

1. Breathing high concentrations of oxygen over a prolonged period of time may lead to **increased production of superoxide** and, in premature infants, their **capacity to produce superoxide dismutase is not fully developed.**

2. One possible consequence of oxygen toxicity to premature infants is **blindness.**

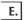 **E.** **Respiratory burst** is an immunologic phenomenon that occurs during phagocytosis.

1. The phagocytic cells of the immune system produce superoxide intentionally to destroy bacteria and viruses. Oxygen consumption increases rapidly and much of the consumed oxygen is converted to superoxide, which destroys the phagocytized material.

2. **Genetic defect. Chronic granulomatous disease** is caused by a genetic defect that reduces the capacity of phagocytic cells to produce superoxide. Patients with this disorder exhibit increased susceptibility to infection.

Case 19-1 Revisited

The diagnosis is cyanide poisoning. The symptoms of cyanide poisoning are nonspecific, and blood cyanide levels are not readily obtainable. The almond odor is a characteristic of gaseous cyanide. This is confirmed by the finding that the patient has used amygdalin, which is a drug that had been purported to cure cancer but is not approved in the United States. Cyanide is a metabolite of amygdalin.

Cyanide binds to the heme of cytochrome oxidase, inhibiting the enzyme and blocking respiration. Nitrites induce the synthesis of methemoglobin and increase serum levels. Cyanide also binds to methemoglobin, which decreases the levels available to react with cytochrome oxidase. Thiosulfate combines with cyanide to produce thiocyanate, which does not react with the free oxidase. This reaction is mediated by the mitochondrial enzyme rhodanese. Using this rationale, cyanide poisoning, although potentially fatal, can be successfully treated if diagnosed early.

STUDY QUESTIONS

DIRECTIONS: Each of the numbered items or incomplete statements in this section is followed by answers or by completions of the statement. Select the **one** lettered answer or completion that is **best** in each case.

1. Electrons derived from many substrates may use the electron transport chain because

(A) each substrate is oxidized in the mitochondria
(B) the substrates are oxidized by enzymes linked to oxidized nicotinamide or flavin adenine dinucleotide
(C) each substrate is oxidized by the same enzyme
(D) electrons from each substrate are transferred to adenosine triphosphate
(E) protons from each substrate are used to form water

2. The mitochondrial electron transport chain carriers are located

(A) in the inner mitochondrial membrane
(B) in the mitochondrial matrix
(C) in the intermembrane space
(D) on the inner surface of the outer mitochondrial membrane
(E) on the outer surface of the outer mitochondrial membrane

3. Which one of the following disorders is characterized by a reduced capacity to produce superoxide?

(A) Leigh syndrome
(B) Alpers syndrome
(C) Pearson syndrome
(D) Chronic granulomatous disease
(E) Benign infantile myopathy

4. When oxidative phosphorylation is uncoupled, which one of the following actions takes place?

(A) Phosphorylation of adenosine diphosphate (ADP) accelerates
(B) Phosphorylation of ADP continues but oxygen uptake stops
(C) Phosphorylation of ADP stops but oxygen uptake continues
(D) Oxygen uptake stops
(E) Both phosphorylation of ADP and oxygen uptake stop

5. The chemiosmotic theory proposes that adenosine triphosphate is formed because of which one of the following reasons?

(A) A change in the permeability of the inner mitochondrial membrane toward adenosine diphosphate (ADP)
(B) The formation of high-energy bonds in mitochondrial proteins
(C) ADP is pumped out of the matrix into the intermembrane space
(D) A proton gradient forms across the inner membrane
(E) Protons are pumped into the mitochondrial matrix

6. A patient is diagnosed with Kearns-Sayre syndrome. Some clinical manifestations of this disorder may respond to therapeutic doses of

(A) 2,4-dinitrophenol
(B) coenzyme Q (ubiquinone)
(C) oligomycin
(D) flavin adenine dinucleotide (FAD)
(E) adenosine diphosphate (ADP)

DIRECTIONS: The group of items in this section consists of lettered options followed by a set of numbered items. For each item, select the **one** lettered option that is most closely associated with it. Each lettered option may be selected once, more than once, or not at all.

Questions 7-13

Match the following descriptions with the correct component of the electron transfer chain or oxidative phosphorylation system.

(A) Complex I
(B) Complex II
(C) Complex III
(D) Complex IV
(E) Adenosine triphosphate (ATP) synthase
(F) Cytochrome c

7. It is the point of entry for electrons from succinate dehydrogenase

8. It is inhibited by rotenone

9. It is inhibited by cyanide

10. It is inhibited by antimycin A

11. It is the point of entry for most of the electrons generated by the action of the citric acid cycle

12. It is inhibited by oligomycin

13. It is the only soluble component of the respiratory chain

ANSWERS AND EXPLANATIONS

1. The answer is B [I A 2]. The electron transport chain acts as a common pathway for the transfer of electrons from a variety of substrates to oxygen because many of the enzymes involved in the oxidation of metabolic fuels are linked to oxidized nicotinamide or flavin adenine dinucleotide (NAD+; FAD). Reduced NADH and FADH$_2$ donate these electrons to the chain, where they are passed on to oxygen.

2. The answer is A [I B]. Mitochondria have two membranes: an outer membrane, which is permeable to most small molecules, and an inner membrane with highly selective permeability. The electron transport chain is localized in the inner membrane along with the enzymes of oxidative phosphorylation. The electron transport chain accepts electrons from nicotinamide adenine dinucleotide–linked dehydrogenases in the mitochondrial matrix. The flavin adenine dinucleotide–linked succinate dehydrogenase, which is common to the citric acid cycle as well as the respiratory chain, is also in the inner mitochondrial membrane.

3. The answer is D [V E 2; Table 19-1]. Respiratory burst is a phenomenon during which phagocytic cells intentionally produce superoxide to destroy bacteria and viruses. Chronic granulomatous disease is due to a genetic defect that reduces the capacity of these cells to produce superoxide. The other disorders are all associated with defects in the electron transport chain and oxidative phosphorylation.

4. The answer is C [III C]. In coupled mitochondria, passage of electrons down the electron transport chain to oxygen is obligatorily tied to the phosphorylation of adenosine diphosphate (ADP) to adenosine triphosphate (ATP). If ADP is limited, then respiration slows down. When oxidative phosphorylation is uncoupled, the respiration rate no longer is governed by the rate of phosphorylation, and the flow of electrons is limited only by the capacity of the system. Thus, oxygen uptake continues, and the phosphorylation of ADP to ATP stops.

5. The answer is D [II D]. The chemiosmotic theory proposes that an electrochemical gradient of protons (H+) is established across the mitochondrial membrane by the functioning of the electron carriers of the electron transport chain. Protons are pumped from the matrix to the intermembrane space to create this gradient. Formation of adenosine triphosphate (ATP) is driven by the free energy released as the protons pass down the concentration gradient via the ATP synthase.

6. The answer is B [IV C]. Treatment of patients with respiratory chain disorders, such as Kearns-Sayre syndrome, is difficult and often unsuccessful. Some improvement may result from therapeutic doses of substances that may mediate electron transfer such as coenzyme Q. 2,4-Dinitrophenol is an uncoupler. Oligomycin is an inhibitor of adenosine triphosphate (ATP) synthase. Oxidized flavin adenine dinucleotide (FAD) is an acceptor of electrons that are donated to the respiratory chain, and adenosine diphosphate (ADP) is phosphorylated during proper function of the respiratory chain.

7–13. The answers are: 7-B [I D 2], **8-A** [I D 1 e], **9-D** [I D 6], **10-C** [I D 4], **11-A** [I D 1], **12-E** [II E 2], **13-F** [I D 5]. Succinate dehydrogenase, which is the only enzyme of the citric acid cycle that is a tightly membrane-bound protein, also is a major component of complex II of the electron transport chain. Electrons from this enzyme are donated to coenzyme Q.

Rotenone, which is used as a fish poison and an insecticide, inhibits respiration by blocking electron transport from reduced nicotinamide adenine dinucleotide (NADH) to coenzyme Q.

The poison cyanide can bind to many heme- and metal-containing proteins. It inhibits respiration by binding tightly to and inhibiting cytochrome oxidase in complex IV.

The antibiotic antimycin A inhibits respiration by blocking the transfer of electrons from coenzyme Q to cytochrome c.

Four pairs of electrons are generated by the action of the citric acid cycle. One pair is transferred to the flavin adenine dinucleotide

(FAD) cofactor of succinate dehydrogenase and enters the respiratory chain at the level of complex II. The other three pairs are used to generate NADH, which donates these electrons to the chain at complex I.

The antibiotic oligomycin inhibits oxidative phosphorylation by binding to and inhibiting adenosine triphosphate (ATP) synthase.

Cytochrome c is the only component of the respiratory chain that is soluble. It binds to the membrane to perform its electron transfer role.

Chapter 20

Gluconeogenesis
Victor Davidson

Case 20-1

A 2-year-old boy is admitted to the hospital with severe lactic acidosis. He has a history of poor growth and development, repeated seizures, ataxia, and persistent metabolic acidosis. Urinalysis indicates high levels of the following organic acids: pyruvate, lactate, β-hydroxybutyrate, β-hydroxypropionate, and β-methylcrotonate. The patient is administered an oral dose of 10 mg of biotin per day. Metabolite levels return to normal within 3 days. The more general symptoms, such as the ataxia, improve over a period of several days following biotin therapy.

- What is the diagnosis and basis for the therapy?
- Will biotin therapy always be effective for this disorder?

I. OVERVIEW OF GLUCONEOGENESIS

A. **Definition.** Gluconeogenesis is the biosynthesis of new glucose.

B. **Substrates** for gluconeogenesis include lactate, pyruvate, glycerol, and glucogenic amino acids.

C. **Location.** Under normal circumstances, the liver is responsible for 85%–95% of the glucose that is made. During starvation or metabolic acidosis, the kidney is capable of making glucose and may contribute up to 50% of the glucose formed because, in these conditions, the amount contributed by the liver is decreased considerably. The only other tissue capable of gluconeogenesis is the epithelial cell of the small intestine, which contributes not more than 5% of the total glucose formation.

D. **Energetics.** The conversion of 2 moles of pyruvate to 1 mole of glucose requires 4 moles of adenosine triphosphate (ATP), 2 moles of guanosine triphosphate (GTP), and 2 moles of reduced nicotinamide adenine dinucleotide (NADH).

E. **Functions**
1. During starvation or periods of limited carbohydrate intake, when the levels of liver glycogen are low (liver glycogen supplies are adequate for 10–24 hours), gluconeogenesis is important in maintaining adequate blood sugar concentrations.
2. During extended exercise, when carbohydrate and lipid reserves are mobilized, gluconeogenesis allows the use of lactate from glycolysis and glycerol from fat breakdown.
3. During metabolic acidosis, gluconeogenesis in the kidney allows the excretion of an increased number of protons.
4. Gluconeogenesis allows the use of dietary protein in carbohydrate pathways.

II. SUBSTRATES FOR GLUCONEOGENESIS

A. **Lactate** (Figure 20-1)

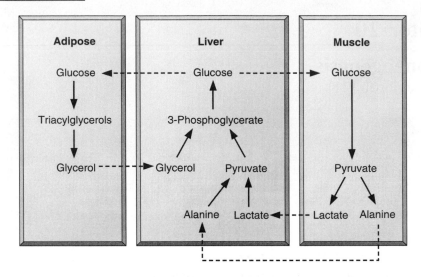

FIGURE 20-1. Interplay between metabolic pathways in different tissues.

1. **Interconversion of lactate and pyruvate** is catalyzed by **lactate dehydrogenase** (LDH), an oxidized nicotinamide adenine dinucleotide (NAD^+)-dependent enzyme.

$$Lactate + NAD^+ \rightleftharpoons pyruvate + NADH + H^+$$

   a. In gluconeogenic tissues (e.g., liver), LDH usually runs this reaction in the direction of pyruvate formation.

   b. In muscle cells and erythrocytes, LDH usually runs this reaction in the direction of lactate formation.

   c. The direction in which the reaction proceeds depends on the following factors.

   (1) The ratios of NAD^+ to NADH and lactate to pyruvate

   (2) The isozyme of LDH that is present

2. **Cori cycle** (see Figure 20-1)

   a. Pyruvate formed from glucose by glycolysis in the muscle cells and erythrocytes is converted to lactate by LDH.

   b. Lactate is released into the blood, taken up by the liver, and converted to pyruvate by LDH.

   c. Pyruvate is converted to glucose via gluconeogenesis in the liver and is released into the blood where it can be used as an energy source for muscle as well as other tissues.

B. **Alanine** (see Figure 20-1)

1. Pyruvate formed from glycolysis in the muscle may be converted to alanine by a transamination reaction (see Chapter 24 III A).

2. Alanine also may be formed in muscle during degradation of protein, which occurs during starvation.

3. Alanine is released by the muscle into the blood, taken up by the liver, and converted back to pyruvate by the reverse of the transamination reaction that occurred in the muscle.

4. Pyruvate is then used to produce glucose via gluconeogenesis.

C. **Glycerol** (see Figure 20-1)

1. Glycerol is formed in adipose tissue by lipolysis of triacylglycerols.

2. Glycerol is released into the blood and taken up by the liver where it is **phosphory-lated to 3-phosphoglycerate,** which is an intermediate in gluconeogenesis.

D. **Amino acids.** Glucogenic amino acids (see Chapter 24 IV B) other than alanine may be converted to citric acid cycle intermediates that are metabolized to oxaloacetate (see Chapter 18 III), an intermediate in gluconeogenesis (see III A).

III. **REACTIONS OF GLUCONEOGENESIS** (Figure 20-2). Gluconeogenesis is essentially the **reversal of the glycolysis** (see Chapter 16), except for **three irreversible steps in glycolysis that must be bypassed.**

A. **Pyruvate to oxaloacetate (OAA)**

1. The hydrolysis of ATP provides energy for the carboxylation of pyruvate.

2. **Pyruvate carboxylase** catalyzes this reaction.
   a. The **prosthetic group** of this enzyme is **biotin** (see Chapter 14 II B).
   b. **Magnesium (Mg^{2+})** and **manganese (Mn^{2+})** are also required for activity.
   c. **Acetyl coenzyme A (acetyl CoA)** is required as an activator and regulates activity in a concentration-dependent manner.

3. This reaction occurs in the **mitochondrial matrix.**

B. **Interconversion of OAA and malate.** OAA cannot permeate the mitochondrial membrane well, and it must be transported across the membrane in the form of malate.

1. **Malate dehydrogenase** catalyzes this reversible reaction.

$$OAA + NADH + H^+ \rightleftharpoons malate + NAD^+$$

   a. **In the mitochondria,** a mitochondrial malate dehydrogenase catalyzes the reaction as written.
   b. **In the cytosol,** a cytosolic malate dehydrogenase catalyzes the reverse reaction, which regenerates OAA.

2. In this process, **malate also transfers reducing equivalents** from the mitochondria to the cytosol.

C. **OAA to phosphoenolpyruvate (PEP).** Hydrolysis of GTP provides the energy for the carboxylation of OAA.

1. **Phosphoenolpyruvate carboxykinase (PEPCK)** catalyzes this reaction, which requires Mn^{2+} for activation.

2. This reaction occurs in the **cytosol.**

3. The two reactions catalyzed by pyruvate carboxylase and PEPCK convert pyruvate to PEP, thus bypassing the irreversible reaction catalyzed by pyruvate kinase during glycolysis.

D. **PEP to fructose-1,6-bisphosphate (F1,6BP).** This conversion occurs by six sequential reactions (see Figure 20-2) that are simply the reverse of those that occur in glycolysis, and they are catalyzed by the same enzymes (see Chapter 16 III).

E. **F1,6BP to fructose-6-phosphate (F6P) and inorganic phosphate (P_i).** This reaction is the reverse of the reaction catalyzed by phosphofructokinase during glycolysis.

1. **Fructose-1,6-bisphosphatase (F1,6BPase)** catalyzes this reaction.

2. F1,6BPase is an allosteric enzyme that is the **major regulatory enzyme in gluconeogenesis.**
   a. **Activator.** F1,6BPase is activated by citrate.

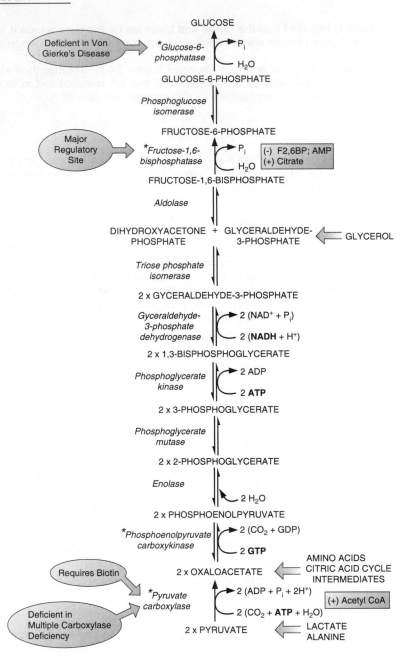

FIGURE 20-2. The gluconeogenic pathway. To facilitate comparison with glycolysis, the sequence of reactions is listed from *bottom to top*. Enzyme names are in *italics*. Enzymes that function in gluconeogenesis but not in glycolysis are indicated with an *asterisk*. The signs *(+)* and *(–)* indicate the sites of action of allosteric positive and negative modulators of the activities of the key regulatory enzymes. These are shown in boxes with (+) = *activators* and (–) = *inhibitors*. *Equilibrium arrows* indicate reversible reactions, and *single arrows* indicate reactions that are essentially irreversible. *Large double arrows* indicate sites of entry of substrates for gluconeogenesis. High energy compounds required for gluconeogenesis are indicated in *bold* type. *ADP* = adenosine diphosphate; *AMP* = adenosine monophosphate; *ATP* = adenosine triphosphate; *CoA* = coenzyme A; *F2,6BP* = fructose-2,6-bisphosphate; *GTP* = guanosine triphosphate; *GDP* = guanosine diphosphate; *NAD+* = oxidized nicotinamide adenine dinucleotide; *NADH* = reduced NAD; *P_i* = inorganic phosphate.

EFFECTIVE OCTOBER 1999. (Supercedes all other licenses.)

Program License Agreement

Read carefully the following terms and conditions before using the Software. Use of the Software indicates you and, if applicable, your Institution's acceptance of the terms and conditions of this License Agreement. If you do not agree with the terms and conditions, you should promptly return this package to the place you purchased it and your payment will be refunded.

DEFINITIONS: As used herein, the following terms shall have the following meanings:

"Software" means the software program contained on the diskette(s), CD-ROM, or preloaded on a workstation and the user documentation, which includes all printed material supplied with the diskette(s).

"Institution" means a nursing or professional school, a single academic organization that does not provide patient care and is located in a single city and has one geographic location/address.

"Geographic location" means a facility at a specific location; geographic locations do not provide for satellite or remote locations that are considered a separate facility.

"Facility" means a health care facility at a specific location that provides patient care and is located in a single city and has one geographic location/address.

"Publisher" means Lippincott Williams & Wilkins, Inc., with its principal office in Philadelphia, Pennsylvania.

"Developer" means the company responsible for developing the software as noted on the product.

LICENSE: You are hereby granted a non-exclusive license to use the Software in the United States. This license is not transferable and does not authorize resale or sublicensing without the written approval or an authorized officer of Publisher.

The Publisher retains all rights and title to all copyrights, patents, trademarks, trade secrets, and other proprietary rights in the Software. You may not remove or obscure the copyright notices in or on the Software. You agree to use reasonable efforts to protect the Software from unauthorized use, reproduction, distribution or publication.

SINGLE-USER LICENSE: If you purchased this Software program at the Single-User License price or a discount of that price, you may use this program on one single-user computer. You may not use the Software in a time-sharing environment or otherwise to provide multiple, simultaneous access. You may not provide or permit access to this program to anyone other than yourself.

INSTITUTIONAL/FACILITY LICENSE: If you purchased the Software at the Institutional or Facility License Price or at a discount of that price, you have purchased the Software for use within your Institution/Facility on a single workstation/computer. You may not provide copies of or remote access to the Software. You may not modify or translate the program or related documentation. You agree to instruct the individuals in your Institution/Facility who will have access to the Software to abide by the terms of this License Agreement. If you or any member of your Institution fail to comply with any of the terms of this License Agreement, this license shall terminate automatically.

NETWORK LICENSE: If you purchased the Software at the Network License Price, you may copy the Software for use within your Institution/Facility on an unlimited number of computers within one geographic location/address. You may not provide remote access to the Software over a value-added network or otherwise. You may not provide copies of or remote access to the Software to individuals or entities who are not members of your Institution/Facility. You may not modify or translate the program or related documentation. You agree to instruct the individuals in your Institution/Facility who will have access to the Software to abide by the terms of this License Agreement. If you or any member of your Institution/Facility fail to comply with any of the terms of this License Agreement, this license shall terminate automatically.

LIMITED WARRANTY: Publisher warrants that the media on which the Software is furnished shall be free from defects in materials and workmanship under normal use for a period of 90 days from the date of delivery to you, as evidenced by your receipt of purchase.

continued

The Software is sold on a 30-day trial basis. If, for whatever reason, you decide not to keep the software, you may return it for a full refund within 30 days of the invoice date or purchase, as evidenced by your receipt of purchase by returning all parts of the Software and packaging in saleable condition with the original invoice, to the place you purchased it. If the Software is not returned in such condition, you will not be entitled to a refund. When returning the Software, we suggest that you insure all packages for their retail value and mail them by a traceable method.

The Software is a computer assisted instruction (CAI) program that is not intended to provide medical consultation regarding the diagnosis or treatment of any specific patient. Except as stated above with respect to the diskette(s), the Software is provided without warranty of any kind, either expressed or implied, including but not limited to, any implied warranty of fitness for a particular purpose of merchantability. Neither Publisher nor Developer warrants that the Software will satisfy your requirements or that the Software is free of program or content errors. Neither Publisher nor Developer warrants, guarantees, or makes any representation regarding the use of the Software in terms of accuracy, reliability or completeness, and you rely on the content of the programs solely at your own risk.

The Publisher is not responsible (as a matter of products liability, negligence or otherwise) for any injury resulting from any material contained herein. This Software contains information relating to general principles of patient care that should not be construed as specific instructions for individual patients. Manufacturers' product information and package inserts should be reviewed for current information, including contraindications, dosages and precautions.

Some states do not allow the exclusion of implied warranties, so the above exclusion may not apply to you. This warranty gives you specific legal rights and you may also have other rights that vary from state to state.

YEAR 2000 COMPLIANCE: Year 2000 compliance of Lippincott Williams & Wilkins, Inc.'s products can be fully utilized only when run on hardware, networks, operating systems, application servers, and desktops that are Year 2000 compliant.

The term "Year 2000 Compliant" means that the product meets the following standard without external intervention, unless such intervention would have been required regardless of the date (e.g., the normal entry of time by some older personal computer software or hardware).

1. General Integrity: The transition of the Year 2000 will not interrupt the product's operation.
2. Date Integrity: Calculations in real time shall not be interrupted, and sequential events from prior dates will be displayed, archived and executed in proper order.
3. Data Integrity: All data will be stored in such a manner as to ensure that relative time is maintained.
4. The Year 2000 is properly treated as a leap year.

LIMITATION OF REMEDIES: The entire liability of Publisher and Developer and your exclusive remedy shall be: (1) the replacement of any diskette(s) which does not meet the limited warranty stated above which is returned to the place you purchased it with your purchase receipt; or (2) if the Publisher or the wholesaler or retailer from whom you purchased the Software is unable to deliver a replacement diskette(s) free from defects in material and workmanship, you may terminate this License Agreement by returning the diskette(s) and your money will be refunded.

In no event will Publisher or Developer be liable for any damages, including any damages for personal injury, lost profits, lost savings or other incidental or consequential damages arising out of the use or inability to use the Software or any error or defect in the Software, whether in the database or in the programming, even if the Publisher, Developer, or an authorized wholesaler or retailer has been advised of the possibility of such damage.

Some states do not allow the limitation or exclusion of liability for incidental or consequential damages. The above limitations and exclusions may not apply to you.

GENERAL: This License Agreement shall be governed by the laws of the State of Maryland without reference to the conflict of laws provisions thereof, and may only be modified in a written statement signed by an authorized officer of the Publisher. By opening and using the Software, you acknowledge that you have read this License Agreement, understand it, and agree to be bound by its terms and conditions. You further agree that it is a complete and exclusive statement of the agreement between the Institution/Facility and the Publisher, which supersedes any proposal or prior agreement, oral or written, and any other communication between you and Publisher or Developer relative to the subject matter of the License Agreement.

NOTE: Attach a paid invoice to the License Agreement as proof of purchase.

b. Inhibitors of F1,6BPase include adenosine monophosphate (AMP) and fructose-2,6-bisphosphate (F2,6BP).

3. **Reciprocal control.** These allosteric effects are exactly the opposite of those observed with phosphofructokinase, the regulatory enzyme in glycolysis. This is an example of reciprocal control of opposing metabolic pathways.

F. **F6P to glucose-6-phosphate (G6P).** This reaction, the reverse of the conversion of G6P to F6P in glycolysis, is catalyzed by the same enzyme, **phosphoglucose isomerase.**

G. **G6P to glucose and P_i.** This is the reverse of the reaction catalyzed by glucokinase and hexokinase during glycolysis. However, in gluconeogenesis this reaction is catalyzed by **glucose-6-phosphatase (G6Pase),** which is present only in gluconeogenic tissues (see I C).

IV. DISEASES ASSOCIATED WITH DEFECTS OF GLUCONEOGENESIS

A. **Multiple carboxylase deficiency**

1. **Causes**
   a. This defect is usually due to a genetic defect in the enzyme **holocarboxylase synthetase,** which is responsible for covalently attaching biotin (see Chapter 14 II B 2) to the following biotin-dependent enzymes, rendering them inactive.

   (1) **Pyruvate carboxylase**
   (2) **Acetyl CoA carboxylase**
   (3) **Propionyl CoA carboxylase**
   (4) **β-Methylcrotonyl CoA carboxylase**

   b. A deficiency in **biotinidase** also can produce this syndrome. Biotinidase removes biotin from proteins during degradation and allows biotin to be recycled for further use (see Chapter 14 II B 2).

2. **Effects.** Symptoms of multiple carboxylase deficiency include developmental retardation, ketoacidosis, hair loss, and erythematous rash.

3. **Treatment.** In some cases in which the defect in holocarboxylase synthetase reduces its affinity for biotin, multiple carboxylase deficiency can be treated with therapeutic doses of biotin. Multiple carboxylase deficiency caused by biotinase deficiency also can be treated with therapeutic biotin supplementation.

B. **Von Gierke's disease** (also called glycogen storage disease type I; see Chapter 21 VI)

1. **Cause.** Von Gierke's disease is caused by a **genetic defect in G6Pase.**

2. **Effect.** The following symptoms occur in people with von Gierke's disease.
   a. **Enlarged liver.** G6P cannot be converted to glucose and released from the liver, causing accumulation of excessive glycogen.
   b. **Hypoglycemia.** Blood glucose levels are low because the liver cannot form glucose from G6P for release into the bloodstream.
   c. **Lacticacidosis.** Because glucose cannot be formed from lactate via pyruvate, blood lactate levels increase and reduce blood pH and alkali reserve.
   d. **Hyperlipidemia.** Reduced glucose production results in the increased mobilization of fat as a metabolic fuel, which increases the level of serum lipids.
   e. **Hyperuricemia** (high serum levels of purine nucleotides). The accumulation of G6P leads to increased activity of the pentose phosphate pathway (see Chapter 17 I), which increases the production of purine nucleotides.

V. CONTROL OF GLUCONEOGENESIS

A. Nonhormonal regulation

1. **Substrate concentration.** The levels of pyruvate, lactate, and alanine are important factors in determining the level of flux through the gluconeogenic pathway.

2. **Allosteric regulation.** Acetyl CoA is a concentration-dependent regulator of the activity of pyruvate carboxylase, the first enzyme of the pathway.

B. Hormonal regulation (see Chapter 27 II C)

1. **Glucagon, epinephrine, and glucocorticoids can each stimulate** the synthesis of enzymes of the gluconeogenic pathway (i.e., PEPCK; F1,6BPase; G6Pase), which are used to bypass the irreversible steps of glycolysis.

2. **Insulin suppresses** the synthesis of these enzymes and stimulates the synthesis of key glycolytic enzymes (i.e., hexokinase, phosphofructokinase, pyruvate kinase).

Case 20-1 Revisited

The organic acids present in the child's urine are all substrates or metabolites of substrates for biotin-dependent carboxylases (see IV A 1 a). This suggests a form of multiple carboxylase deficiency due to a defect in holocarboxylase synthetase or biotinidase.

Therapeutic doses of biotin benefit patients with multiple carboxylase deficiency caused either by biotinidase deficiency or a defect in holocarboxylase synthetase, which reduces its affinity for biotin. In cases caused by a defect in holocarboxylase synthetase, which renders the enzyme inactive for reasons other than affinity for biotin, this therapy is of no benefit. Treatment of these forms of this disorder is much more difficult and less successful.

STUDY QUESTIONS

DIRECTIONS: Each of the numbered items or incomplete statements in this section is followed by answers or by completions of the statement. Select the **one** lettered answer or completion that is **best** in each case.

1. A patient that is diagnosed as having von Gierke's disease is likely to exhibit which one of the following symptoms?

(A) An enlarged liver
(B) Elevated blood pH
(C) Hyperglycemia
(D) Hypolipidemia
(E) Hypouricemia

2. What would be the consequence of a genetic absence of fructose-1,6-bisphosphatase (F1,6BPase)?

(A) Accumulation of fructose phosphates
(B) Failure to metabolize glucose-6-phosphate (G6P) via glycolysis
(C) Inability to produce glucose from lactate
(D) Pentosuria
(E) Von Gierke's disease

3. Which one of the following is a positive allosteric regulator of gluconeogenesis?

(A) Adenosine monophosphate (AMP)
(B) Acetyl coenzyme A (acetyl CoA)
(C) Biotin
(D) Adenosine diphosphate (ADP)
(E) Fructose-2,6-bisphosphate (F2,6BP)

4. A compound that transfers reducing equivalents from mitochondria to the cytosol during gluconeogenesis is

(A) phosphoenolpyruvate
(B) glycerol-3-phosphate
(C) aspartate
(D) malate
(E) oxaloacetate

5. The regulation of the activities of which pair of enzymes provides an example of reciprocal control of opposing metabolic pathways?

(A) Phosphoenolpyruvate carboxykinase (PEPCK) and pyruvate kinase
(B) Fructose-1,6-bisphosphatase (F1,6BPase) and phosphofructokinase
(C) Glucose-6-phosphatase (G6Pase) and glucokinase
(D) G6Pase and hexokinase
(E) Enolase and phosphoglycerate mutase

6. Which enzyme of gluconeogenesis will be affected by a biotin deficiency?

(A) Phosphoenolpyruvate carboxykinase (PEPCK)
(B) Pyruvate carboxylase
(C) Glucose-6-phosphatase (G6Pase)
(D) Fructose-1,6-bisphosphatase (F1,6BPase)
(E) Phosphoglycerate kinase

7. Which one of the following enzymes participates in both gluconeogenesis and glycolysis?

(A) Pyruvate carboxylase
(B) Phosphoglucose isomerase
(C) Phosphoenolpyruvate carboxykinase (PEPCK)
(D) Fructose-1,6-bisphosphatase (F1,6BPase)
(E) Glucose-6-phosphatase (G6Pase)

Questions 8–9

A patient is diagnosed as having a genetic defect specifically in the enzyme pyruvate carboxylase. Other biotin-containing enzymes are functioning normally, so the symptoms are not as severe as in patients with multiple carboxylase deficiency.

8. Which one of the following can be used as a substrate for gluconeogenesis by this patient?

(A)   Pyruvate
(B)   Glycerol
(C)   Lactate
(D)   Alanine
(E)   Acetyl coenzyme A (CoA)

9. When will this patient be most likely to experience the symptoms caused by this defect?

(A)   After a carbohydrate-rich meal
(B)   During a period of extended exercise
(C)   When insulin levels are high
(D)   When epinephrine levels are low
(E)   When glucagon levels are low

DIRECTIONS: The group of items in this section consists of lettered options followed by a set of numbered items. For each item, select the **one** lettered option that is most closely associated with it. Each lettered option may be selected once, more than once, or not at all.

Questions 10–12

Match the following statements about gluconeogenesis with the correct tissue(s).

(A)   Muscle
(B)   Liver
(C)   Brain
(D)   Adipose tissue
(E)   Erythrocytes

10. Glycogen stored in this tissue can be used directly as a source of blood glucose

11. It is a source of alanine, which is used as a substrate for gluconeogenesis

12. It is the primary source of glycerol, which is used as a substrate for gluconeogenesis

ANSWERS AND EXPLANATIONS

1. The answer is A [IV B 2]. Von Gierke's disease is caused by a genetic defect in glucose-6-phosphatase (G6Pase). An enlarged liver results from excessive formation of glycogen from the precursor G6P. Hypoglycemia (low blood glucose levels) results from the inability to form glucose from G6P and release it into the blood. A low blood glucose level causes increased mobilization of fat, which increases the level of serum lipids (hyperlipidemia). Hyperuricemia (high serum levels of purine nucleotides) results from the increased flux of G6P through the pentose phosphate pathway. Because glucose cannot be formed from lactate, its levels increase, which lowers pH.

2. The answer is C [III E; Figure 20-2]. The important consequence of a genetic absence of fructose-1,6-bisphosphatase would be the inability to carry out gluconeogenesis from any substrates, including lactate. Glucose, and fructose phosphates, would still be metabolized via the glycolysis pathway because the reverse of the fructose-1,6-bisphosphate (F1,6BP) reaction is catalyzed by a different enzyme, phosphofructokinase. There would be no increase in the urinary excretion of pentoses (pentosuria). Von Gierke's disease is due to a defect in glucose-6-phosphatase.

3. The answer is B [III A 2, E 2; Figure 20-2]. Pyruvate carboxylase, which catalyzes the carboxylation of pyruvate to form oxaloacetate, is allosterically activated by acetyl coenzyme A. Adenosine monophosphate and fructose-2,6-bisphosphate are negative allosteric regulators of fructose-1,6-bisphosphatase. Biotin is the cofactor involved in the carboxylation reaction. Neither biotin nor adenosine diphosphate allosterically regulates any enzymes of gluconeogenesis.

4. The answer is D [III B]. In mitochondria, oxaloacetate, which cannot cross the mitochondrial inner membrane, is converted to malate by malate dehydrogenase during gluconeogenesis, when the level of reduced nicotinamide adenine dinucleotide (NADH) is high. Malate then crosses the membrane and, in the cytoplasm, is converted back to oxaloacetate and NADH by a cytoplasmic malate de-

hydrogenase. Thus, both oxaloacetate carbon and reducing equivalents are transferred from the mitochondria to the cytosol.

5. The answer is B [III E]. Fructose-1,6-bisphosphatase (F1,6BPase) and phosphofructokinase are the major regulatory enzymes for gluconeogenesis and glycolysis, respectively. F1,6BPase is activated by citrate and is inhibited by adenosine monophosphate and fructose-2,6-bisphosphate. The opposite effects are observed with phosphofructokinase, which is an example of reciprocal control. Glucose-6-phosphatase (G6Pase) catalyzes the reverse reaction that is initially catalyzed by glucokinase and hexokinase. However, all of these are not allosterically controlled enzymes. Phosphoenolpyruvate carboxykinase (PEPCK) and pyruvate carboxylase catalyze the reverse reaction of pyruvate kinase. Although pyruvate carboxylase and pyruvate kinase are affected in opposite ways by acetyl coenzyme A, PEPCK is not. Enolase and phosphoglycerate mutase catalyze different reversible reactions and are common to both glycolysis and gluconeogenesis.

6. The answer is B [III A 2; IV A 1]. Pyruvate carboxylase requires biotin as a cofactor. The enzyme holocarboxylase synthetase is responsible for covalently attaching biotin to pyruvate carboxylase. If insufficient biotin is present in the serum, its activity will be deficient.

7. The answer is B [III; Figure 20-2]. In glycolysis, during which glucose is converted to pyruvate, three reactions are irreversible under cellular conditions. These reactions are catalyzed by glucokinase (or hexokinase), phosphofructokinase, and pyruvate kinase. To bypass these irreversible steps during gluconeogenesis, other enzymes are used. Pyruvate carboxylase and phosphoenolpyruvate carboxykinase catalyze the reverse of the reaction catalyzed by pyruvate kinase. Fructose-1,6-bisphosphatase catalyzes the reverse of the reaction catalyzed by phosphofructokinase. Glucose-6-phosphatase catalyzes the reverse of the reactions catalyzed by glucokinase and hexokinase.

8. The answer is B [II; III A; IV A; Figure 20-2]. Because of this defect, the patient cannot convert pyruvate to oxaloacetate in the initial reaction of gluconeogenesis. To serve as substrates, lactate must be converted to pyruvate by lactate dehydrogenase, and alanine must be converted to pyruvate by an aminotransferase. Thus, they cannot be used as substrates. Glycerol enters gluconeogenesis at the level of glyceraldehyde-3-phosphate, which allows it to bypass the defective first step of the pathway. Acetyl coenzyme A (CoA) is an activator of pyruvate carboxylase, which regulates gluconeogenesis but does not serve as a substrate.

9. The answer is B [I E; V B]. When the patient's blood glucose levels are high, there is no need for gluconeogenesis, and this defect will not pose any serious problems. This will be true after carbohydrate consumption. High levels of insulin, as well as low levels of epinephrine and glucagon, are associated with high serum levels of glucose. During extended exercise, serum glucose and glycogen stores become depleted, necessitating the production of new glucose via glucogenesis. The patient will be unable to do this because of the genetic defect.

10–12. The answers are: 10-B [I E 1], **11-A** [II B], **12-D** [II C]. Glycogen is degraded to glucose-6-phosphate (G6P). The glycogen that is stored in the muscle cannot be directly used for gluconeogenesis because it lacks the enzyme glucose-6-phosphatase (G6Pase). This enzyme is found only in the liver, kidney, and epithelial cells of the small intestine.

Alanine is formed from pyruvate as a result of transamination in muscle cells or protein degradation and released into the blood. It is then taken up by the liver, where it is used as a substrate for gluconeogenesis after conversion back to pyruvate.

Glycerol is formed by lipolysis of triacylglycerols in adipose tissue and released into the blood. It then enters the liver and is converted to 3-phosphoglycerate, which is an intermediate in gluconeogenesis.

Chapter 21

Glycogen Metabolism
Victor Davidson

Case 21-1

A 20-year-old man is admitted to the hospital with painful swelling, cramping, and tightness in his arms. The symptoms began after lifting and carrying heavy objects while moving into a new apartment. Since childhood, he has experienced cramping of muscles after strenuous exercise, and he has routinely experienced weakness of continuously used muscles. No enlargement of the liver is apparent, and blood sugar levels are normal. A muscle biopsy is performed, and histochemical studies reveal excessive deposition of glycogen. Biochemical analysis reveals an absence of glycogen phosphorylase activity.

- What is the diagnosis?
- What is the treatment and long-term prognosis?

I.   **GLYCOGEN** is the **storage form of glucose.** Glycogen stores allow humans to eat intermittently by providing an immediate source of blood glucose for use as a metabolic fuel.

A.   **Structure**

1. Glycogen is a large branched **polymer of glucose molecules** linked by α-1,4-glycosidic linkages; branches arise by α-1,6-glycosidic bonds at approximately every tenth residue.

2. **Glycogen exists in the cytosol as granules,** which also contain the enzymes that catalyze its formation and use.

B.   **Storage.** The polymeric nature of glycogen allows energy to be sequestered without the problems from osmotic effects that glucose would cause.

1. **Sites of glycogen storage** are primarily the **muscle and liver.**
   a. Although the concentration of glycogen is higher in the liver, the much greater mass of skeletal muscle stores a greater total amount of glycogen.
   b. Liver can mobilize its glycogen for the release of glucose to the rest of the body, but muscle can only use its glycogen for its own energy needs.

2. **Duration of glycogen storage.** In humans, liver glycogen stores are typically adequate for up to 12 hours without support from gluconeogenesis (see Chapter 20).

II.   **GLYCOGENESIS (glycogen synthesis)**

A.   **Synthesis of uridine diphosphate glucose (UDP-glucose), the precursor of glycogen**

1. **UDP-glucose,** an activated form of glucose, is formed from uridine triphosphate (UTP) and glucose-1-phosphate (G1P; see Chapter 17 II A).

$$\text{G1P} + \text{UDP} \rightleftharpoons \text{UDP-glucose} + \text{PP}_i$$

2. **UDP-glucose pyrophosphorylase** catalyzes this reaction. Although this is a reversible reaction, the hydrolysis of inorganic pyrophosphate (PP_i) by cellular pyrophosphatases renders it essentially irreversible under cellular conditions.

B. **Formation of the amylose chains** (see Chapter 5 IV D)

1. The synthesis of new glycogen requires the presence of existing glycogen chains and glucosyl residues from UDP-glucose. The residues are successively transferred to the C-4 terminus of an existing glycogen chain in α-1,4-glycosidic linkages.

   UDP-glucose + glycogen(n residues) → UDP + glycogen(n+1 residues)

2. **Glycogen synthase** catalyzes this reaction, which is the **rate-limiting step in glycogen synthesis.**

C. **Formation of branch chains and further growth** (Figure 21-1). Segments of the amylose chain are transferred onto the C-6 hydroxyl of neighboring chains, forming α-1,6 linkages.

1. In **branch formation,** seven-residue segments of the amylose terminal chains are transferred to a C-6 hydroxyl group of a glucosyl residue that is four residues away from an existing branch. A terminal branch must be at least eleven residues in length before a segment is transferred from it.

2. **Glycosyl-4:6-transferase (branching enzyme)** catalyzes this reaction.

3. A **genetic defect** in the branching enzyme causes **type IV glycogen storage disease (Andersen's disease).** Infants born with this disease suffer cirrhosis and failure of the liver as well as hepatosplenomegaly. Most affected infants die by the age of 2 years.

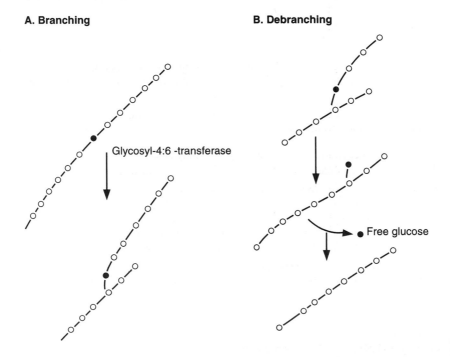

A. Branching **B. Debranching**

Glycosyl-4:6 -transferase

Free glucose

FIGURE 21-1. Formation and removal of branches in glycogen chains. *(A)* During branching, glycosyl-4:6-transferase moves a seven-unit segment of α-1,4 residues from a glycogen chain at least 11 residues long onto a segment of the main chain at a position that is at least four residues from the nearest branch. *(B)* During debranching, a three–glucosyl-residue segment is transferred onto a chain terminus leaving a single residue at the branch point. That residue is then removed to yield free glucose.

III. GLYCOGENOLYSIS (glycogen utilization)

A. Phosphorolytic cleavage of the terminal α-1,4-glycosidic bond

1. This cleavage reaction yields G1P and a glycogen chain that is smaller by one glucose unit.

$$\text{Glycogen(n residues)} + P_i \rightarrow \text{Glycogen(n-1 residues)} + \text{G1P}$$

2. **Glycogen phosphorylase** catalyzes this reaction. It is a dimeric enzyme that utilizes **pyridoxal phosphate** (see Chapter 14 II G) as a prosthetic group. Different isozymes of glycogen phosphorylase are present in different tissues.

3. This reaction is the **rate-limiting step in glycogenolysis.**

4. Disorders caused by genetic defects in glycogen phosphorylase
   a. **Type V glycogen storage disease (McArdle's disease)** is due to a defect in the isozyme of glycogen phosphorylase present in muscle tissue. People with this disease suffer from skeletal muscle cramps, and they demonstrate a low blood lactate level during exercise.
   b. **Type VI glycogen storage disease (Hers' disease)** is due to a defect in the isozyme of glycogen phosphorylase present in liver. Patients with this disease suffer hepatomegaly, moderate hypoglycemia, mild acidosis, and growth retardation.

B. Removal of branch chains (see Figure 21-1)

1. **The debranching enzyme** catalyzes this reaction. This enzyme is a single polypeptide that possesses two enzymatic activities necessary for the removal of branches.
   a. **1,4 → 1,4-glucan transferase (glucosyl transferase).** In this step, three glucosyl residues from a branch are transferred onto a chain terminus, leaving a single residue on C-6.
   b. **α-1,6-Glucosidase (amylo-6-glucosidase).** In this step, a single residue on C-6 is removed to yield a free glucose molecule.

2. In **lysosomes,** a different enzyme, **α-1,4 glucosidase,** is involved in debranching.

3. Disorders due to genetic defects in debranching enzymes
   a. **Type II glycogen storage disease (Pompe's disease)** is due to a defect in the lysosomal α-1,4-glucosidase. Glycogen accumulates and causes problems in the central nervous system (CNS), which leads to psychomotor retardation, an enlarged heart, and eventually failure of the heart and lungs.
   b. **Type III glycogen storage disease (Cori's disease, Forbes' disease)** is due to a defect in the debranching enzyme (see III B 1). This disease also causes heart and lung problems, stunted growth, an enlarged liver, hypoglycemia, and acidosis.

IV. PHOSPHORYLATION CASCADES (Figure 21-2). The enzymes of glycogen metabolism undergo a sequential covalent modification by means of phosphorylation. This process provides a very large amplification of the initial stimulus.

A. Cascade regulation of glycogen synthase activity

1. **Glycogen synthase exists in two forms.**
   a. The **inactive form** is designated **D** because it is dependent.
      (1) The D form is the **phosphorylated** form of the enzyme.
      (2) The D form is an allosteric enzyme form that may be **activated by high concentrations of glucose-6-phosphate (G6P).**

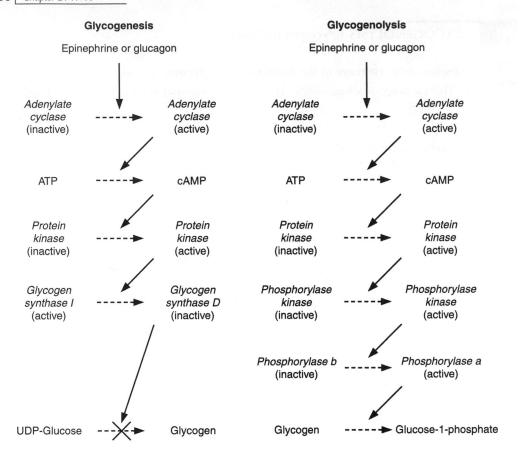

FIGURE 21-2. Cascade regulation of glycogen metabolism. Enzyme names are in *italics. ATP* = adenosine triphosphate; *cAMP* = cyclic adenosine monophosphate; *UDP* = uridine diphosphate.

    b. The **active form** is designated **I** because it is independent.
        (1) The I form of glycogen synthase is the **dephosphorylated** form of the enzyme.
        (2) The I form does not require G6P for activity.

  2. The **interconversion of the D and I forms** of glycogen synthase is catalyzed by a **cyclic adenosine monophosphate (cAMP)-dependent protein kinase.**

  3. Regulatory cascade
    a. Adenylate cyclase regulates the activity of the kinase by regulating the level of cAMP.
    b. Adenylate cyclase is activated by the hormones **epinephrine** and **glucagon,** depending on the tissue.
    c. Only a few molecules of hormone are needed to activate adenylate cyclase, which then produces a large number of cAMP molecules, each of which can activate a cAMP-dependent protein kinase enzyme molecule.
    d. This active enzyme in turn phosphorylates a large number of glycogen synthase molecules, converting each of them to the D form.

B. **Cascade regulation of glycogen phosphorylase activity** (see Figure 21-2)

  1. Glycogen phosphorylase exists in two forms.
    a. Phosphorylase a is the **phosphorylated active form** of the enzyme.

    b. Phosphorylase b is the **dephosphorylated inactive form** of the enzyme.

2. The **interconversion of phosphorylases a and b** is catalyzed by two enzymes.

    a. Phosphorylase kinase phosphorylates a specific serine residue on each subunit of phosphorylase b to convert it to phosphorylase a. The activity of this protein kinase is regulated by adenylate cyclase, which regulates the level of cAMP and consequently is regulated by epinephrine and glucagon.

    b. A **phosphatase** dephosphorylates that serine residue of phosphorylase a to regenerate the b form.

V. REGULATION OF GLYCOGEN METABOLISM

A. **Hormonal regulation**

1. **In muscle**

    a. Epinephrine promotes glycogenolysis and inhibits glycogenesis.

      (1) It stimulates the formation of cAMP by activating adenylate cyclase.

      (2) When epinephrine is released and acts upon the muscle cell membrane, glycogenolysis is activated via the phosphorylation cascade, and simultaneously, glycogenesis is retarded.

    b. Insulin increases glycogenesis and decreases glycogenolysis.

      (1) It heightens the entry of glucose into the muscle cells.

      (2) It reduces cAMP levels, probably by speeding up the destruction of cAMP by phosphodiesterase.

2. **In the liver**

    a. Glucagon activates adenylate cyclase in the liver cell membranes and thus turns on glycogenolysis and reduces glycogenesis.

    b. Insulin increases glycogenesis in the liver by increasing the activity of glycogen synthase by a mechanism that is not yet clear.

    c. The glucagon:insulin ratio appears to be more important than the absolute level of either hormone.

      (1) Insulin domination provides for the storage of glycogen after a meal.

      (2) Glucagon domination favors mobilization of glycogen stores as the blood glucose level declines.

B. **Antithetic effects of covalent modification.** With separate systems for the synthesis and degradation of glycogen, and with G1P acting as a common intermediate, the possibility of **a futile cycling of glycogen** must be considered. The futile cycle is avoided because covalent modification, by phosphorylation, has opposite effects on the enzymes concerned with the synthesis and degradation of glycogen (see Figure 21-2).

VI. GLYCOGEN STORAGE DISEASES are caused by genetic defects that result in deficiencies in certain enzymes of glycogen metabolism. These deficiencies lead to excessive accumulation of glycogen or the inability to use that glycogen as a fuel source.

A. **Deficiencies in phosphofructokinase** in glycolysis (see Chapter 16 III C) and **glucose-6-phosphatase** (G6Pase) in gluconeogenesis (see Chapter 20 III G) each cause an accumulation of G6P, a precursor of G1P, which also results in excessive accumulation of glycogen.

B. The **causes and characteristics** of several glycogen storage diseases are listed in Table 21-1.

TABLE 21-1. Genetic Diseases of Glycogen Metabolism

Type	Disease Name	Defective Enzyme	Glycogen Levels	Glycogen Structure	Principal Tissue Affected
I	von Gierke's disease	Glucose 6-phosphatase (G6Pase)	High	Normal	Liver, kidney
II	Pompe's disease	α-1,4-Glucosidase	Very high	Normal	All organs
III	Cori's, Forbes' disease	Debranching enzyme	High	Short outer branches	Liver, heart, muscle
IV	Andersen's disease	Branching enzyme	Normal	Long outer branches	Liver, spleen, muscle
V	McArdle's disease	Phosphorylase	High	Normal	Muscle
VI	Hers' disease	Phosphorylase	High	Normal	Liver
VII	Tarui disease	Phosphofructokinase	High	Normal	Muscle
VIII	Hepatic phosphorylase kinase deficiency	Phosphorylase kinase	High	Normal	Liver

Case 21-1 Revisited

The findings are consistent with type V glycogen storage disease (McArdle's disease), which results in a defect in phosphorylase that is confined to the muscle. No evidence for abnormal liver function is presented.

There is no cure for this disorder. Treatment is based on using good sense. Strenuous exercise and physical exertion must be avoided when possible. Eating carbohydrate-rich foods prior to anticipated exertion also helps because serum glucose levels are then higher, which decreases the dependence on glycogen for fuel. Type V glycogen storage disease is one of the more benign glycogen storage diseases. The prognosis for long-term survival is good. This is not true of many of the other glycogen storage diseases, which are often fatal within the first few years of life.

STUDY QUESTIONS

DIRECTIONS: Each of the numbered items or incomplete statements in this section is followed by answers or by completions of the statement. Select the **one** lettered answer or completion that is **best** in each case.

1. Which one of the following human tissues contains the greatest amount of body glycogen?

(A) Liver
(B) Kidney
(C) Skeletal muscle
(D) Cardiac muscle
(E) Adipose tissue

2. Glycogen synthase D is allosterically regulated by which one of the following compounds?

(A) Glucose-1-phosphate
(B) Fructose-6-phosphate
(C) Glucose-6-phosphate
(D) Fructose-1,6-bisphosphate
(E) Glucose

3. Which one of the following supports glycogen synthesis?

(A) High cyclic adenosine monophosphate (cAMP) levels
(B) Inactive adenyl cyclase
(C) Active phosphorylase a
(D) Epinephrine
(E) Glucagon

4. The rate-limiting step in glycogenolysis produces which one of the following compounds?

(A) Glucose-1-phosphate
(B) Free glucose
(C) Glucose-6-phosphate
(D) Uridine diphosphate (UDP)-glucose
(E) Three-residue glucose segments

5. Glycogen phosphorylase is best described by which one of the following statements? It

(A) adds glucose-6-phosphate to glycogen
(B) requires pyridoxal phosphate
(C) is deficient in patients with Cori's disease
(D) is deficient in patients with Forbes' disease
(E) is inactivated by phosphorylase kinase

6. A patient who suffers from McArdle's disease is most likely to exhibit which one of the following symptoms?

(A) Hypoglycemia
(B) Hyperglycemia
(C) Enlarged liver
(D) Abnormal glycogen structure
(E) Muscle cramps

DIRECTIONS: Each group of items in this section consists of lettered options followed by a set of numbered items. For each item, select the **one** lettered option that is most closely associated with it. Each lettered option may be selected once, more than once, or not at all.

Questions 7-9

Match the following glycogen storage diseases to the correct symptom(s).

(A) Above normal glycogen levels
(B) Abnormal glycogen structure
(C) Both
(D) Neither

7. Type IV (Andersen's disease), a defect in glycosyl-4:6-transferase

8. Type V (McArdle's disease), a defect in glycogen phosphorylase

9. Type III (Cori's disease), a defect in the debranching enzyme

Questions 10-12

Match the following statements regarding glycogen metabolism with the appropriate tissue.

(A) Liver
(B) Muscle
(C) Both
(D) Neither

10. Epinephrine levels regulate glycogen metabolism in this tissue

11. Insulin levels regulate glycogen metabolism in this tissue

12. Type VI glycogen storage disease (Hers' disease), a defect in phosphorylase, affects this tissue

ANSWERS AND EXPLANATIONS

1. The answer is C [I B 1]. Muscle and liver are major sites for glycogen storage. Although the concentration of glycogen is highest in the liver, the much greater mass of skeletal muscle stores a greater total amount of glycogen. It is important to note that liver glycogen can be mobilized for the release of glucose to the rest of the body, but muscle glycogen is used only to support muscle glycolysis.

2. The answer is C [IV A 1]. Glycogen synthase exists in two forms. The inactive form is glycogen synthase D (dependent), and the active form is glycogen synthase I (independent). Glycogen synthase D is an allosteric enzyme with high concentrations of glucose-6-phosphate (G6P) acting as a positive modulator. In the absence of G6P, the enzyme is inactive. Glycogen synthase I is not an allosterically regulated enzyme and is active in the absence of G6P.

3. The answer is B [IV A; Figure 21-2]. Epinephrine and glucagon activate adenyl cyclase, which generates high levels of cyclic adenosine monophosphate (cAMP). This initiates a phosphorylation cascade that activates phosphorylase, which in turn breaks down glycogen. This same cascade results in the inactivation of glycogen synthase by phosphorylation. When adenylate cyclase is inactive, the phosphorylation cascade does not operate, and glycogen synthase is present in its active form catalyzing glycogenesis.

4. The answer is A [III A]. The rate-limiting step in glycogenolysis, which is catalyzed by glycogen phosphorylase, releases glucose-1-phosphate (G1P) from glycogen. G1P is converted to glucose-6-phosphate by phosphoglucomutase. Uridine diphosphate (UDP)-glucose is the active form of glucose that is used to synthesize glycogen. The debranching enzyme catalyzes the transfer of three glucosyl residues and the release of free glucose, but this step is not rate limiting.

5. The answer is B [III A]. Phosphorylase requires the cofactor pyridoxal phosphate for activity. It is activated by phosphorylase kinase, and it catalyzes the production of glucose-6-phosphate from glycogen. Cori's disease and Forbes' disease are caused by defects in the debranching enzyme.

6. The answer is E [III A 4; Case 21-1]. McArdle's disease is caused by a defect in the isozyme of glycogen phosphorylase that is present in muscle. Because this enzyme is not involved in branching or debranching, the glycogen structure is normal. The liver isozyme functions normally; therefore, normal blood sugar levels may be maintained, and liver glycogen levels are normal. The inability to effectively use muscle glycogen can cause cramping under certain circumstances.

7–9. The answers are: 7-B [II C 3], **8-A** [III A 4 a], **9-C** [III B 3 b; Table 21-1]. Glycosyl-4:6-transferase is the branching enzyme in glycogen synthesis. A deficiency of this enzyme does not affect the levels of glycogen. However, the inability to form branches causes the formation of abnormal glycogen with very long outer chains.

Phosphorylase is required for the first step in glycogenolysis. In the absence of phosphorylase, glycogen is not degraded, and high levels of glycogen accumulate. Because phosphorylase is not involved in glycogen synthesis, the structure of the accumulated glycogen is normal.

Without the debranching enzyme activity, glycogen phosphorylase can cleave only a limited number of glucose residues per chain of glycogen. This results in an accumulation of high levels of glycogen with abnormally short outer chains.

10–12. The answers are: 10-B [V A 1 a], **11-C** [V A 1 b, 2 b], **12-A** [III A 4 b]. The catecholamine hormone epinephrine acts specifically on the muscle. It promotes glycogenolysis and inhibits glycogenesis by stimulating the formation of cyclic adenosine monophosphate (cAMP) and initiating a phosphorylation cascade that regulates the activities of glycogen synthase and glycogen phosphorylase.

The hormone insulin promotes glycogenesis and inhibits glycogenolysis in the muscle and promotes the entry of glucose into muscle cells. In the liver it increases glycogenesis.

Different isozymes of glycogen phosphorylase are present in different tissues. Type V glycogen storage disease (Hers' disease) is caused by a defect in the isozyme of glycogen phosphorylase present in the liver, so only the liver is affected.

Chapter 22

Fatty Acid Metabolism
Victor Davidson

Case 22-1

A 2-year-old boy exhibits increasing irritability and signs of muscle weakness, especially after prolonged exercise. His development is normal, and he eats a normal diet. On examination he is found to have an enlarged heart, and an electrocardiogram is abnormal. A muscle biopsy shows lipid deposition and low carnitine levels. Plasma levels of carnitine are also found to be below normal. After an oral carnitine load, plasma levels rise to nearly normal levels, whereas urinary levels increased to 30 times normal. Treatment is daily therapeutic doses of carnitine. With time, his activity increases, his irritability decreases, his cardiac problems improve, and his strength and exercise tolerance become normal.

- What is the diagnosis?
- If the patient's diet was adequate, why were therapeutic doses of carnitine required?

I. BIOSYNTHESIS OF FATTY ACIDS

A. General features

1. Fatty acids (see Chapter 7 II) may be synthesized from dietary glucose via pyruvate.
2. Fatty acids are the preferred fuel source for the heart and the primary form in which excess fuel is stored in adipose tissue.
3. The major site of fatty acid synthesis is the **liver.**
4. The enzymes that synthesize fatty acids are localized in the **cytosol,** and they are completely different from the mitochondrial enzymes that catalyze fatty acid degradation.
5. The major synthetic pathway involves polymerization of two-carbon units derived from **acetyl coenzyme A (acetyl CoA)** to form a sixteen-carbon saturated fatty acid, palmitic acid.
6. Reduced nicotinamide adenine dinucleotide phosphate **(NADPH)** and adenosine triphosphate **(ATP)** are required for fatty acid synthesis.

B. Sources of acetyl CoA and NADPH

1. **Cytosol**
   a. Acetyl CoA is derived from the oxidation of glucose via glycolysis (see Chapter 16 VI B) and pyruvate dehydrogenase (see Chapter 18 I).
   b. NADPH is generated by the pentose phosphate pathway (see Chapter 17 I).
2. **Mitochondria: The acetyl CoA shuttle system** (Figure 22-1). Acetyl CoA cannot cross the inner mitochondrial membrane and is transported to the cytosol via this shuttle, which also produces NADPH in the cytosol.
   a. Citrate synthetase catalyzes the reaction of acetyl CoA with oxaloacetate to form citrate in the mitochondria.
   b. Citrate is transported into the cytosol by a tricarboxylic acid transport system.
   c. Citrate reacts with CoA in the cytosol to form acetyl CoA and oxaloacetate (OAA).
   d. OAA is converted to malate by an oxidized nicotinamide adenine dinucleotide (NAD$^+$)-dependent cytosolic malate dehydrogenase.

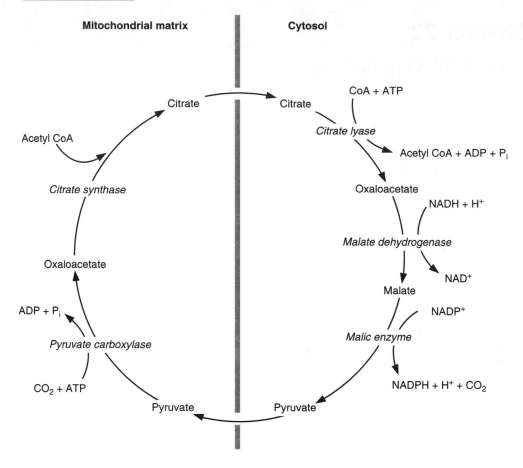

FIGURE 22-1. The acetyl coenzyme A *(acetyl CoA)* shuttle system. Enzyme names are *italicized. ADP* = adenosine diphosphate; *ATP* = adenosine triphosphate; *NAD⁺* = oxidized nicotinamide adenine dinucleotide; *NADH* = reduced nicotinamide adenine dinucleotide; *NADP⁺* = oxidized nicotinamide adenine dinucleotide phosphate; *NADPH* = reduced nicotinamide adenine dinucleotide phosphate; *P_i* = inorganic phosphate.

    e. Malate is decarboxylated to form pyruvate by the malic enzyme, which also forms NADPH from oxidized nicotinamide adenine dinucleotide phosphate ($NADP^+$).

    f. Pyruvate is transported into the mitochondria by an active transport system.

    g. OAA is regenerated from pyruvate by pyruvate carboxylase.

C.   **Pathway of fatty acid synthesis** (Figure 22-2)

    1. Acetyl CoA carboxylase

        a. This enzyme catalyzes the ATP-dependent carboxylation of acetyl CoA to malonyl CoA.

        b. This is the **key regulatory site** for fatty acid synthesis.

            (1) Activators are citrate and insulin.

            (2) Inhibitors are palmitoyl CoA and glucagon.

        c. Biotin is a required cofactor. Acetyl CoA carboxylase is one of the enzymes that is inactive in the condition known as **multiple carboxylase deficiency** (see Chapter 20 IV A), which is due to an inability to utilize biotin.

    2. The **fatty acid synthase enzyme complex** catalyzes several reactions that convert acetyl CoA and malonyl CoA to butyryl CoA (see Figure 22-2).

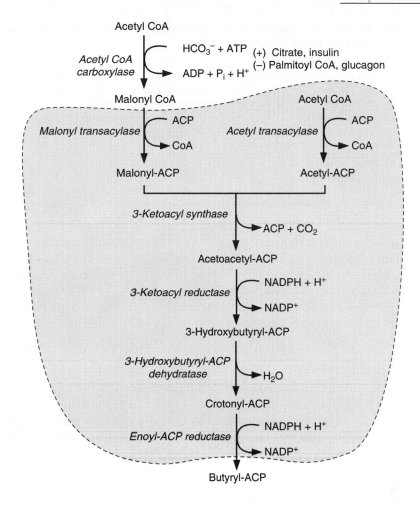

FIGURE 22-2. The principal reactions of fatty acid biosynthesis. Names of enzymes and components of the fatty acid synthase enzyme complex are *italicized*. The multiple reactions catalyzed by the fatty acid synthase enzyme complex are encircled by the *dashed line*. *ACP* = acyl carrier protein; *ADP* = adenosine diphosphate; *ATP* = adenosine triphosphate; *CoA* = coenzyme A; *HCO$_3^-$* = bicarbonate; *NADP$^+$* = oxidized nicotinamide adenine dinucleotide phosphate; *NADPH* = reduced nicotinamide adenine dinucleotide phosphate.

   a. The **acetyl transacylase** component catalyzes the conversion of **acetyl CoA + acyl carrier protein (ACP) → acetyl-ACP + CoA.**

      (1) ACP possesses a **phosphopantetheine prosthetic group,** which is derived from the vitamin pantothenic acid (see Chapter 14 II F) and is identical to that portion of the CoA molecule.

      (2) The acyl groups of the substrate molecules are covalently bound to ACP via a thioester linkage with the terminal sulfhydryl group.

   b. The **malonyl transacylase** component catalyzes the conversion of **malonyl CoA + ACP → malonyl-ACP + CoA.**

   c. The **3-ketoacyl synthase** component catalyzes the conversion of **malonyl-ACP + acetyl-ACP → acetoacetyl-ACP + ACP + CO$_2$.**

   d. The **3-ketoacyl reductase** component catalyzes the NADPH-dependent conversion of **acetoacetyl-ACP → 3-hydroxybutyryl-ACP.**

   e. The **3-hydroxybutyryl-ACP dehydratase** component catalyzes the conversion of **3-hydroxybutyryl-ACP → crotonyl-ACP.**

     f. The **enoyl-ACP reductase** component catalyzes the NADPH-dependent conversion of **crotonyl-ACP** → **butyryl-ACP.**

  3. Formation of palmitic acid
    a. Reaction. Butyryl-ACP (a four-carbon unit) reacts with another malonyl group via the reactions described above (see I C 2 b) to form a six-carbon unit, and the reactions of the fatty acid synthase complex continue.
    b. Reaction repeats. After **seven turns** of this cycle, palmitic-ACP (a 16-carbon unit) is synthesized.
    c. Release. Palmitic acid is released from ACP and the fatty acid synthase complex by **palmitoyl deacylase** (thioesterase).

  4. Stoichiometry of the synthesis of palmitate

$$8 \text{ Acetyl CoA} + 7 \text{ ATP} + 14 \text{ NADPH} + 14 \text{ H}^+ + \text{H}_2\text{O} \rightarrow$$
$$\text{Palmitate} + 7 \text{ ADP} + 7 \text{ P}_i + 8 \text{ CoASH} + 14 \text{ NADP}^+$$

D. **Elongation of fatty acids.** Fatty acids longer than 16 carbons can be formed via one of two **elongation systems** adding 2-carbon units.

  1. The **endoplasmic reticulum system** is the most active. It adds malonyl CoA onto palmitate in a manner similar to the action of fatty acid synthase, except that CoASH is used rather than the ACP. Stearic acid (an 18-carbon unit) is the product.

  2. A **mitochondrial elongation system** uses acetyl CoA units, rather than malonyl CoA units, to elongate fatty acids for the synthesis of structural lipids in this organelle.

E. **Desaturation of fatty acids**

  1. The two most common monounsaturated fatty acids in mammals are palmitoleic acid ($16:1:\Delta^9$) and oleic acid ($18:1:\Delta^9$).

  2. In the endoplasmic reticulum, double bonds are introduced between carbons 9 and 10 by **fatty acid oxygenase,** which requires molecular oxygen (O_2) and NADPH.

II. **FATTY ACID OXIDATION.** Fatty acids are an important energy source. Oxidation of fatty acids generates the high-energy compounds reduced NAD (NADH) and reduced flavin adenine dinucleotide ($FADH_2$) and yields acetyl CoA, which is the substrate for the citric acid cycle (see Chapter 18 II).

A. **β-Oxidation of fatty acids** is the principal pathway. It occurs in the mitochondrial matrix and involves oxidation of the β-carbon to form a β-keto acid.

  1. Activation of free fatty acids. Free fatty acids are taken up from the circulation by cells and are activated by formation of acyl CoA derivatives.
    a. An endoplasmic reticulum acyl CoA synthetase (thiokinase) activates long-chain fatty acids of 12 or more carbons.

$$\text{Fatty acid} + \text{ATP} + \text{CoASH} \rightarrow \text{acyl CoA} + \text{PP}_i + \text{AMP}$$

    b. Inner mitochondrial acyl CoA synthetases activate medium-chain (4–10 carbons) and short-chain (acetate and propionate) fatty acids. These fatty acids enter the mitochondria freely from the cytoplasm, whereas the long-chain fatty acids cannot.

  2. Role of carnitine. Long-chain fatty acyl CoAs cannot freely diffuse across the inner mitochondrial membrane. Carnitine in the inner mitochondrial membrane mediates transfer of fatty acyl groups from the cytosol to the mitochondrial matrix where they are oxidized.

    a. Transfer reaction (Figure 22-3). On the outer surface of the inner mitochondrial membrane, the enzyme **carnitine palmitoyl transferase I (CPT I)** catalyzes the transfer of the acyl group from CoA to carnitine. The fatty acyl group is translocated across the membrane to the inner surface, where the enzyme **carnitine palmitoyl transferase II (CPT II)** catalyzes the transfer of the acyl group to CoA drawn from the matrix CoA pool.

    b. Sources of carnitine

      (1) Dietary sources include red meat and dairy products.

      (2) Synthesis. Carnitine (β-hydroxy-γ-trimethylammonium butyrate) may be synthesized in the body from the amino acid lysine.

    c. Carnitine deficiency in humans may be classified as:

      (1) Systemic, in which levels are reduced in all tissues

      (2) Myopathic, in which levels are reduced only in muscle, including the heart

3. Pathway of β-oxidation. In the mitochondrial matrix, long-chain fatty acyl CoAs are subjected to a **repeated four-step process** that successively removes two-carbon units from the chain until the last two-carbon fragment remains (see Figure 22-3).

    a. Acyl CoA → enoyl CoA

      (1) This **dehydrogenation** reaction is catalyzed by a family of **acyl CoA dehydrogenases** with varying specificity for different length acyl CoA chains.

      (2) The prosthetic group of this enzyme, flavin adenine dinucleotide (FAD), is reduced to $FADH_2$ during this reaction.

      (3) Genetic defects in acyl CoA dehydrogenases (e.g., medium-chain acyl CoA dehydrogenase deficiency) impair β-oxidation.

    b. Enoyl CoA → 3-hydroxyacyl CoA. This **hydration** reaction is catalyzed by **enoyl CoA hydratase.**

    c. 3-Hydroxyacyl CoA → 3-ketoacyl CoA

      (1) This **dehydrogenation** reaction is catalyzed by **3-hydroxyacyl CoA dehydrogenase.**

      (2) NAD^+ is reduced to NADH during this reaction.

    d. 3-Ketoacyl CoA + CoASH → acetyl CoA + tetradecanoyl CoA. This **thiolytic cleavage** reaction is catalyzed by **thiolase** (β-ketothiolase).

4. Stoichiometry of β-oxidation

    a. β-Oxidation of palmitate (16 carbons)

$$\text{Palmitoyl CoA} + 7 \text{ CoASH} + 7 \text{ FAD} + 7 \text{ NAD}^+ + 7 \text{ H}_2\text{O} \rightarrow \tag{1}$$
$$8 \text{ acetyl CoA} + 7 \text{ FADH}_2 + 7 \text{ NADH} + 7 \text{ H}^+$$

A total of 7 moles of $FADH_2$ yields 14 moles of ATP by electron transport and oxidative phosphorylation. A total of 7 moles of NADH yields 21 moles of ATP by electron transport and oxidative phosphorylation. Therefore,

$$\text{Palmitoyl CoA} + 7 \text{ CoASH} + 7 \text{ O}_2 + 35 \text{ ADP} + 35 \text{ P}_i \rightarrow \tag{2}$$
$$8 \text{ acetyl CoA} + 35 \text{ ATP} + 42 \text{ H}_2\text{O}$$

Because it costs 2 moles of ATP to activate the free palmitate, **33 moles of ATP are formed per mole of palmitate via β-oxidation.**

    b. Total oxidation. The acetyl CoA derived from β-oxidation of fatty acyl CoAs may be oxidized to carbon dioxide (CO_2) and water (H_2O) by the citric acid cycle (see Chapter 18 II).

$$8 \text{ Acetyl CoA} + 16 \text{ O}_2 + 96 \text{ ADP} + 96 \text{ P}_i \rightarrow \tag{3}$$
$$8 \text{ CoASH} + 96 \text{ ATP} + 16 \text{ CO}_2 + 104 \text{ H}_2\text{O}$$

The combined yield of ATP is obtained by addition of equations (2) and (3)

$$\text{Palmitoyl CoA} + 23 \text{ O}_2 + 131 \text{ ADP} + 131 \text{ P}_i \rightarrow \tag{4}$$
$$8 \text{ CoASH} + 131 \text{ ATP} + 16 \text{ CO}_2 + 146 \text{ H}_2\text{O}$$

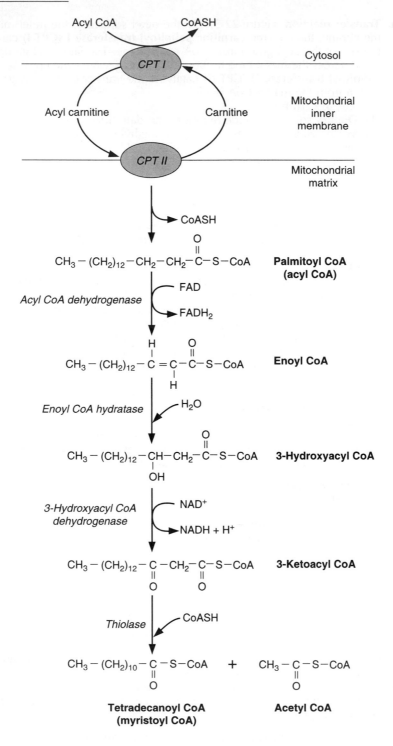

FIGURE 22-3. Transport and β-oxidation of the 16-carbon fatty acyl coenzyme A *(acyl CoA),* palmitoyl CoA. Transport of long-chain fatty acyl groups across the inner mitochondrial membrane is mediated by carnitine and the carnitine palmitoyl transferases I and II *(CPT I* and *CPT II).* Enzyme names are *italicized.* *FAD* = flavin adenine dinucleotide; *FADH₂* = reduced FAD; *NAD⁺* = oxidized nicotinamide adenine dinucleotide; *NADH* = reduced NAD.

After subtraction of 2 moles of ATP for activation of the fatty acyl CoA, **129 moles of ATP are formed by total oxidation of palmitate.**

5. **Respiratory quotient (RQ)** is defined as moles of CO_2 produced, divided by moles of oxygen consumed during complete oxidation of a metabolic fuel to CO_2 and H_2O.

   a. For palmitate, the RQ is given by:

   $$(16 \text{ moles } CO_2 \text{ produced})/(23 \text{ moles } O_2 \text{ consumed}) = 0.7$$

   b. In contrast, the complete oxidation of glucose yields an RQ of 1.0.

B. **Oxidation of fatty acids with an odd number of carbon atoms.** Fatty acids that have an odd number of carbon atoms are a minor species in human tissues.

1. They undergo β-oxidation as acyl CoA derivatives until a three-carbon fragment, propionyl CoA, is formed.

2. Propionyl CoA is carboxylated to methylmalonyl CoA by biotin-dependent **propionyl CoA carboxylase.**

3. Methylmalonyl CoA is converted to succinyl CoA by **methylmalonyl CoA mutase** (see Chapter 24 V E 3).

4. Succinyl CoA can be metabolized via the citric acid cycle, of which it is an intermediate.

C. **Oxidation of unsaturated fatty acids.** In the human body, 50% of the fatty acids are unsaturated. Many unsaturated fatty acids are degraded by the β-oxidation pathway with the help of two additional enzymes.

1. Double bonds in naturally occurring fatty acids are *cis*. The β-oxidation pathway can only process *trans* double bonds using enoyl CoA hydratase (see Figure 22-3).

2. The *cis* double bond is removed by the sequential reactions catalyzed by 2,4-dienoyl CoA reductase and enoyl CoA isomerase to yield a Δ^2-trans enoyl CoA.

D. **α-Oxidation of fatty acids**

1. This **pathway** involves the oxidation of long-chain fatty acids to 2-hydroxy fatty acids, which are constituents of brain lipids, followed by oxidation to a fatty acid with one less carbon. Removal of one carbon from the carboxyl end of a fatty acid has been demonstrated in microsomal fractions from **brain** tissue.

2. **Refsum's disease** (phytanic acid storage disease) is caused by a defect of α-oxidation.

   a. **Phytanic acid** (derived from animal fat and cow's milk and probably originally from chlorophyll) accumulates in affected individuals. Phytanic acid cannot alternatively be oxidized by β-oxidation because the beta position is blocked by a methyl group.

   b. **Symptoms** include retinitis pigmentosa, failing night vision, peripheral neuropathy, and cerebellar ataxia.

E. **ω-Oxidation** involves oxidation of the terminal methyl group to form an ω-hydroxy fatty acid. This is a minor pathway observed with liver microsomal preparations.

III. **TRIACYLGLYCEROLS (TRIGLYCERIDES).** Fatty acids are converted to triacylglycerols for transport to tissues and storage.

A. **Formation** involves the acylation of the three hydroxyl groups of glycerol (see Chapter 7 II D).

1. **Activation of the fatty acid.** Formation of the CoA ester of the fatty acid is catalyzed in the **cytosol** by an ATP-dependent **acyl CoA synthetase.**

    Fatty acid + ATP + CoASH → Acyl CoA + AMP + PP$_i$

2. **Acylation of glycerol**
    a. **First acylation.** There are two routes for the acylation of the first hydroxyl of glycerol.
        (1) One route uses **dihydroxyacetone phosphate (DHAP),** derived from glycolysis (see Chapter 16 III D), as the acceptor of an acyl moiety from a fatty acyl CoA.
            (a) This is followed by reduction, with **NADPH** as the electron acceptor, to form **lysophosphatidate.**
            (b) The fatty acid preferentially introduced to form lysophosphatidate is saturated.
        (2) The second route gives the same product and shows the same preference for a saturated fatty acid, but the order is reversed, and reduction of DHAP to glycerol-3-phosphate occurs before acylation of the C-1 hydroxyl.
    b. **Second acylation.** An unsaturated fatty acyl CoA thioester is introduced to the 2-hydroxyl of lysophosphatidate. An exception occurs in the human mammary gland, where a saturated fatty acyl CoA is used.
    c. **Third acylation.** The phosphate group on C-3 is removed by a phosphatase and either a saturated or unsaturated fatty acid is incorporated at that position.

B. **Storage of triacylglycerols in adipose tissue cells** (adipocytes)

1. The esterification of fatty acids in adipocytes to form triacylglycerols depends on carbohydrate metabolism for the formation of DHAP.

2. Adipocytes lack a glycerol kinase and cannot phosphorylate glycerol to glycerol-3-phosphate. The only source of glycerol-3-phosphate for triacylglycerol synthesis is from DHAP formed during glycolysis.

3. The entry of glucose into adipocytes is insulin dependent. Thus, insulin is an essential requirement for triacylglycerol synthesis in adipocytes.

C. **Lipolysis of triacylglycerols**

1. **Hormonal control of lipolysis in adipocytes**
    a. **Hormone-sensitive lipase** is activated by covalent phosphorylation of the lipase by a cyclic adenosine monophosphate (cAMP)-dependent protein kinase (Figure 22-4).
    b. **Epinephrine** circulating in the blood in response to stress, or **norepinephrine** released by neural connections to adipose tissue, activates the cell membrane adenylate cyclase to produce cAMP. Thus, under conditions of stress or when neural signals indicate low levels of metabolic fuel, the hormone-sensitive lipase is activated.
    c. **Insulin** inhibits lipolysis by two mechanisms.
        (1) It reduces cAMP levels, probably by inhibiting adenylate cyclase activity.
        (2) It increases glucose entry into the adipocytes, so that the formation of DHAP and glycerol-3-phosphate is increased. The availability of these products of glycolysis increases the rate of re-esterification of free fatty acids to triacylglycerols, thus reducing the rate of release of the fatty acids from adipocytes.
    d. **Prostaglandins** (see Chapter 7 V A) inhibit lipolysis by reducing cAMP levels.

2. **Enzymatic steps of lipolysis** (see Figure 22-4)
    a. Three different lipases are required to release the three fatty acids from the triacylglycerols.
        (1) **Hormone-sensitive triacylglycerol lipase** converts triacylglycerol to diacylglycerol plus a fatty acid.

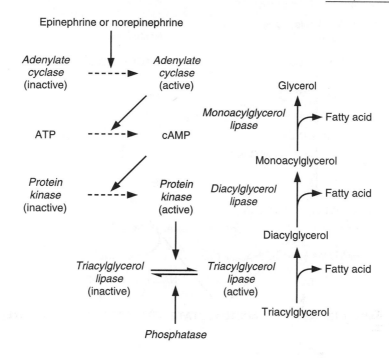

FIGURE 22-4. The cascade system of regulation and enzymatic steps of lipolysis. Enzyme names are *italicized. ATP* = adenosine triphosphate; *cAMP* = cyclic adenosine monophosphate.

    (2) Diacylglycerol lipase converts diacylglycerol to monoacylglycerol plus a fatty acid.

    (3) Monoacylglycerol lipase converts monoacylglycerol to glycerol plus a fatty acid.

  b. The **rate-limiting step of lipolysis in adipocytes** is the reaction catalyzed by the hormone-sensitive triacylglycerol lipase. Diacyl- and monoacylglycerol lipases are present in excess, so that once triacylglycerol lipase is activated, lipolysis of triacylglycerols goes to completion.

3. Lipolysis in other tissues. Triacylglycerols are stored mainly in adipocytes. However, other tissues, including muscle and liver, store small amounts of triacylglycerols as intracellular lipid droplets for their own use. These fat stores appear to be mobilized by hormonal controls similar to those found in adipocytes.

IV. **KETONE BODY METABOLISM.** Ketone bodies (i.e., acetoacetate, β-hydroxybutyrate, acetone; see Chapter 7 II E) are the preferred energy substrates of the heart, skeletal muscle, and kidney during the fasting state (see Chapter 27 II A). If blood levels of β-hydroxybutyrate and acetoacetate increase sufficiently, as they do during starvation, they also become the primary energy substrate for the brain (see Chapter 27 V C).

A. **Biosynthesis of ketone bodies** (Figure 22-5)

1. Thiolase catalyzes the formation of two acetyl CoA molecules from acetoacetyl CoA.

2. 3-Hydroxy-3-methylglutaryl CoA (HMG CoA) synthase catalyzes the addition of another acetyl CoA to acetoacetyl CoA to form HMG CoA.

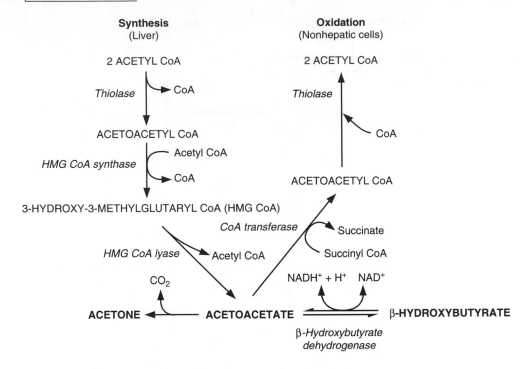

FIGURE 22-5. Ketone body metabolism. Synthesis of acetoacetate from acetyl coenzyme A *(CoA)* occurs in the liver, whereas conversion of acetoacetate back to acetyl CoA occurs in nonhepatic cells. Enzyme names are *italicized*. Ketone bodies are indicated in *bold*. NAD^+ = oxidized nicotinamide adenine dinucleotide; *NADH* = reduced nicotinamide adenine dinucleotide.

   3. HMG CoA lyase catalyzes the cleavage of HMG CoA to **acetoacetate** and acetyl CoA.

   4. β-Hydroxybutyrate dehydrogenase catalyzes the formation of **β-hydroxybutyrate** from acetoacetate when the $NADH/NAD^+$ ratio is high, as it is in the liver during fasting.

   5. Acetone is formed spontaneously from a small fraction of the circulating acetoacetate and is exhaled by the lungs. In patients with untreated diabetes, the odor of acetone is apparent on the patient's breath.

B. Ketone body oxidation

   1. A 3-**keto acid CoA transferase** catalyzes the formation of the CoA thioester of acetoacetate. This is a **nonhepatic enzyme** that prevents ketone bodies from being used as an energy source by the liver.

   2. Thiolase catalyzes the cleavage of acetoacetyl CoA to two acetyl CoA molecules with the use of CoA, providing two-carbon fragments for oxidation by the citric acid cycle.

C. Energy yield from oxidation of ketone bodies

   1. Each mole of acetyl CoA that is formed yields 12 moles of ATP via the citric acid cycle, electron transport, and oxidative phosphorylation.

   2. Conversion of β-hydroxybutyrate to acetoacetate yields an NADH molecule, which in turn yields three more ATP molecules by electron transport and oxidative phosphorylation.

3. The activation reaction requires the equivalent of 1 mole of ATP.

4. Therefore, **oxidation of acetoacetate yields 23 moles of ATP; oxidation of β-hydroxybutyrate yields 26 moles of ATP.**

Case 22-1 Revisited

The below-normal plasma levels of carnitine confirmed a diagnosis of carnitine deficiency. The high level of urinary carnitine and a modest increase in plasma levels after an oral carnitine load suggest that a defect in renal and perhaps gastrointestinal transport of carnitine is responsible for this disorder. This would explain the deficiency despite an adequate diet. The therapeutic doses of carnitine compensate for the defective, inefficient transport system.

STUDY QUESTIONS

DIRECTIONS: Each of the numbered items or incomplete statements in this section is followed by answers or by completions of the statement. Select the **one** lettered answer or completion that is **best** in each case.

Questions 1–2

A patient is suffering from a deficiency in the activity of acetyl coenzyme A (CoA) carboxylase.

1. Which one of the following metabolites is most likely to accumulate in the patient's serum?

(A) Short-chain fatty acids
(B) Long-chain fatty acids
(C) Ketone bodies
(D) Malonyl CoA
(E) Phytanic acid

2. If this patient also exhibited low levels of activity of propionyl CoA carboxylase, therapeutic doses of which one of the following might be beneficial?

(A) Carnitine
(B) Pantothenic acid
(C) Biotin
(D) Riboflavin
(E) Niacin

3. A patient has a defect in carnitine palmitoyl transferase. Which one of the following is most likely to precipitate the symptoms of his disorder?

(A) A diet low in long-chain fatty acids
(B) A diet high in short-chain fatty acids
(C) A diet high in medium-chain fatty acids
(D) Fasting
(E) Inactivity

4. The net yield of high-energy bonds from the complete oxidation of acetoacetate in the brain is

(A) 11
(B) 12
(C) 23
(D) 24
(E) 26

DIRECTIONS: The group of items in this section consists of lettered options followed by a set of numbered items. For each item, select the **one** lettered option that is most closely associated with it. Each lettered option may be selected once, more than once, or not at all.

Questions 5–9

Match the following statements regarding metabolic processes related to fatty acid metabolism with the correct type of metabolism.

(A) Fatty acid biosynthesis
(B) β-Oxidation of fatty acids
(C) Triacylglycerol metabolism
(D) Ketone body metabolism
(E) α-Oxidation of fatty acids

5. Defective in Refsum's disease

6. Regulated by epinephrine

7. Affected in patients with multiple carboxylase deficiency

8. Cannot occur in the absence of carnitine

9. Requires a protein with a covalently bound prosthetic group derived from the vitamin pantothenic acid

ANSWERS AND EXPLANATIONS

1–2. The answers are: 1-A [I C 1], **2-C** [I C 1; II B 2]. Acetyl coenzyme A (acetyl CoA) carboxylase catalyzes the first step in fatty acid biosynthesis: that is, conversion of acetyl CoA to malonyl CoA. Malonyl CoA is required to extend the growing fatty acid chain during biosynthesis. Without it, short-chain fatty acids accumulate. Long-chain fatty acids derived from the diet do not accumulate because fatty acid oxidation is unaffected. Ketone body metabolism is also unaffected. Phytanic acid accumulates in Refsum's disease.

Acetyl CoA carboxylase and propionyl CoA carboxylase are two of four enzymes in humans that require biotin as a cofactor. A defect in the enzyme that attaches biotin to these enzymes will cause the condition multiple carboxylase deficiency, some variants of which are treatable by therapeutic doses of biotin to compensate for the inefficiency of the defective enzyme. Although each of the other nutrients is required for fatty acid metabolism, they are unrelated to this disorder.

3. The answer is D [II A 2; Case 22-1]. The enzymes carnitine palmitoyl transferase (CPT) I and II catalyze the carnitine-mediated transport of long-chain fatty acids, the substrates for β-oxidation, across the inner mitochondrial membrane. Short- and medium-chain fatty acids can freely diffuse across the membrane without CPT. The symptoms of this defect appear when the body must depend on β-oxidation of long-chain fatty acids for energy. This occurs when carbohydrate sources of energy are low, as after prolonged exercise or fasting.

4. The answer is C [IV C 4]. Activation of the ketone body acetoacetate for use as an energy substrate occurs by formation of the coenzyme A (CoA) thioester of acetoacetate. The use of succinyl CoA as a CoA donor bypasses the formation of 1 mole of guanosine triphosphate, which is formed when 1 mole of succinyl CoA is converted to succinate in the citric acid cycle. Thus, this step costs 1 mole of high-energy phosphate bond. Acetoacetyl CoA is cleaved to 2 moles of acetyl CoA, each of which can be oxidized to yield 12 moles of adenosine triphosphate (ATP) via the citric acid cycle, electron transport, and oxidative phosphorylation. Thus, the net yield is $24 - 1 = 23$ moles. The yield for the ketone body β-hydroxybutyrate is 26 moles.

5–9. The answers are: 5-E [II D 2], **6-C** [III C 1 b], **7-A** [I C 1 c], **8-B** [II A 2], **9-A** [I C 2 a]. Refsum's disease (phytanic acid storage disease) is due to a defect of α-oxidation of fatty acids. Phytanic acid accumulates in affected individuals. Phytanic acid cannot alternatively be oxidized by the β-oxidation system because the beta position is blocked by a methyl group.

Epinephrine activates adenyl cyclase, which initiates a cascade mechanism of regulation that activates the hormone-sensitive lipase. This enzyme is required for the first and rate-limiting step in the lipolysis of triacylglycerols. Fatty acid biosynthesis, which occurs in the liver, is also subject to hormonal control. Glucagon, not epinephrine, signals the fasting state to the liver to inhibit fatty acid synthesis.

Acetyl coenzyme A (acetyl CoA) carboxylase, which catalyzes the first step in fatty acid biosynthesis, requires biotin as a cofactor. It is not active in multiple carboxylase deficiency, which is due to an inability to utilize biotin. Another enzyme of fatty acid metabolism, propionyl CoA carboxylase, requires biotin and is affected in this disorder. It is involved in the oxidation of fatty acids with odd-number carbon chains and is not directly involved in the β-oxidation process.

The β-oxidation of fatty acids occurs in the mitochondrial matrix. Carnitine is required for free fatty acids, the substrates for β-oxidation, to enter the mitochondria. This transport across the inner mitochondrial membrane is catalyzed by the enzymes carnitine palmitoyl transferase I and II.

The acyl carrier protein (ACP) is a critical component of the fatty acid synthase enzyme complex, which catalyzes many of the reactions of fatty acid biosynthesis. The prosthetic group of this protein is phosphopantetheine, which is derived from pantothenic acid and is covalently bound to that protein. The phosphopantetheine group is also a part of coenzyme A, but ACP is the only protein possessing this group that is involved in fatty acid metabolism.

Chapter 23

Metabolism of Lipids and Related Compounds
Victor Davidson

Case 23-1

A 30-year-old man presents with evidence of coronary heart disease and xanthomas (i.e., cholesterol deposits) in the tendons. Blood analysis yields serum levels of cholesterol of 420 mg/dl (normal = 150–240 mg/dl) and of triacylglycerols of 75 mg/dl (normal = 35–160 mg/dl). The patient is placed on a diet that restricts cholesterol intake to less than 200 mg/day and calories from saturated fats to fewer than 8% of total calories. He is also administered daily doses of lovastatin and colestipol. After 15 months of this treatment, the patient exhibits normal serum levels of cholesterol.

- What is the diagnosis?
- What is the basis for the treatment?

I. METABOLISM OF PHOSPHOGLYCERIDES

A. **Biosynthesis** (Figure 23-1). The metabolic precursor of phosphoglycerides (see Chapter 7 III) is **lysophosphatidate,** the same as for the triacylglycerols (see Chapter 22 III A 2). Lysophosphatidate initially reacts with a fatty acyl coenzyme A (fatty acyl CoA) molecule to form a **phosphatidate.**

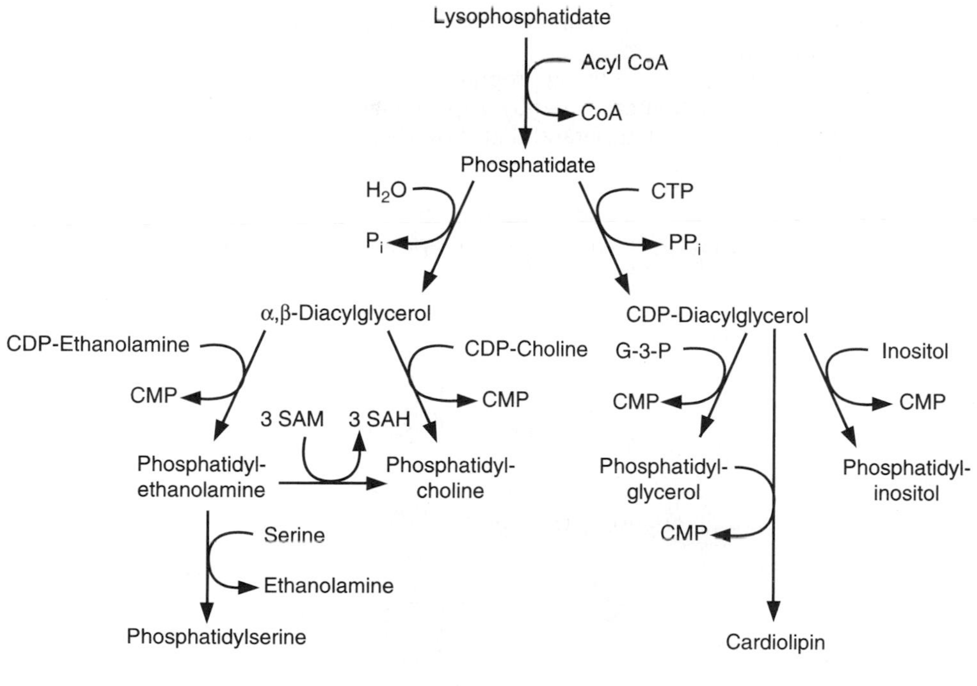

FIGURE 23-1. The biosynthesis of phosphoglycerides. *Acyl CoA* = acyl coenzyme A; *CDP* = cytidine diphosphate; *CMP* = cytidine monophosphate; *CTP* = cytidine triphosphate; *G-3-P* = glycerol-3-phosphate; P_i = inorganic phosphate; *PP$_i$* = inorganic pyrophosphate; *SAH* = S-adenosylhomocysteine; *SAM* = S-adenosylmethionine.

1. The first step in the **biosynthesis of phosphatidylethanolamine, phosphatidylserine, and phosphatidylcholine (lecithin)** is dephosphorylation of phosphatidate to form α,β-diacylglycerol.
   a. α,β-Diacylglycerol reacts with cytidine diphosphate-ethanolamine (CDP-ethanolamine) to form **phosphatidylethanolamine.**
   b. The ethanolamine portion of phosphatidylethanolamine exchanges with serine to form **phosphatidylserine.**
   c. **Phosphatidylcholine** may be formed by two pathways.
      (1) The successive transfer of methyl groups from three moles of S-adenosylmethionine (SAM; see Chapter 25 II C) to phosphatidylethanolamine yields phosphatidylcholine plus three moles of S-adenosylhomocysteine (SAH).
      (2) Cytidine diphosphate-choline (CDP-choline) reacts with α,β-diacylglycerol to form phosphatidylcholine.

2. The first step in the **biosynthesis of phosphatidylinositol and cardiolipin** is the reaction between a phosphatidate and CTP to yield cytidine diphosphate diacylglycerol (CDP-diacylglycerol).
   a. CDP-diacylglycerol reacts with glycerol-3-phosphate to give **phosphatidylglycerol.**
   b. Phosphatidylglycerol reacts with another CDP-diacylglycerol to form **cardiolipin.**
   c. CDP-diacylglycerol also may react with inositol to form **phosphatidylinositol.**

B. **Modification.** Fatty acids found in tissue phospholipids often are modified after insertion by the synthesizing enzymes. Tissues adjust the fatty acid composition of their phospholipids as follows.

1. **Phospholipases** A_1, A_2, C, and D catalyze the removal by hydrolysis of fatty acid substituents of the phosphoglyceride. Each cleaves at a different specific site (Figure 23-2).

2. **Reacylation,** the reintroduction of a fatty acid into the phosphoglyceride, can be one of the following:
   a. Direct acylation with the appropriate fatty acyl CoA
   b. Exchange reaction catalyzed by a specific acyl CoA acyltransferase (e.g., lysolecithin:lecithin acyltransferase) that shows a preference for an unsaturated acyl CoA derivative.

   Acyl CoA + 1-acylglycero-3-phosphocholine (lysolecithin) $\leftrightarrow$
   CoASH + 1,2-diacylglycero-3-phosphocholine (lecithin)

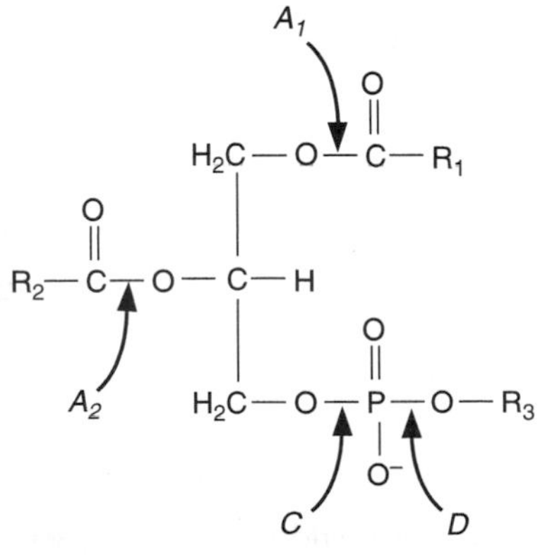

FIGURE 23-2. The specificity of phospholipases. The four phospholipases (A_1, A_2, C, and D) hydrolyze the fatty acid substituents (R_1, R_2, and R_3) at the site on the phosphoglyceride as indicated.

II. METABOLISM OF SPHINGOLIPIDS (see Chapter 7 IV; Figure 23-3)

A. **Sphingosine** is formed from serine and palmitoyl CoA by a process that requires reduced nicotinamide adenine dinucleotide phosphate (NADPH).

B. **Ceramide** (see Chapter 7 IV A 2) is formed from sphingosine by a process that involves addition of a 22-carbon fatty acyl moiety and oxidation by flavin adenine dinucleotide (FAD).

C. **Sphingomyelin** is formed by reaction of ceramide with CDP-choline.

1. Excess sphingomyelin is normally hydrolyzed to ceramide and phosphatidylcholine by the lysosomal enzyme **sphingomyelinase.**

2. **Niemann-Pick disease** is caused by a genetic defect in sphingomyelinase and results in excessive pathologic accumulation of sphingomyelin.

D. **Cerebrosides** (see Chapter 7 IV B 1) are formed by reactions of ceramide with uridine diphosphate (UDP) sugars (e.g., galactocerebroside is formed from UDP-galactose, and glucocerebroside is formed from UDP-glucose).

1. **Gaucher's disease** (see Chapter 7, Case 7-1) is due to a genetic defect in **β-glucocerebrosidase,** a lysosomal enzyme that normally hydrolyzes excess glucocerebroside to glucose and ceramide. This disease causes pathologic accumulation of glucocerebroside.

2. **Krabbe's disease** is due to a genetic defect in **β-galactocerebrosidase,** a lysosomal enzyme that normally hydrolyzes excess galactocerebroside to galactose and ceramide. This disease causes pathologic accumulation of galactocerebroside.

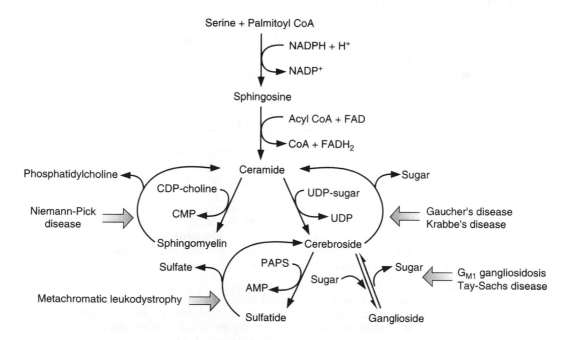

FIGURE 23-3. The metabolism of sphingolipids. *Arrows* may represent multiple reaction steps. *Double arrows* indicate reactions that are blocked in the indicated metabolic disorders. *Acyl CoA* = acyl coenzyme A; *AMP* = adenosine monophosphate; *CDP* = cytidine diphosphate; *CMP* = cytidine monophosphate; *FAD* = flavin adenine dinucleotide; *FADH$_2$* = reduced flavin adenine dinucleotide; *NADP$^+$* = oxidized nicotinamide adenine dinucleotide phosphate; *NADPH* = reduced nicotinamide adenine dinucleotide phosphate; *PAPS* = 3'-phosphoadenosine-5'-phosphosulfate; *UDP* = uridine diphosphate.

E. **Sulfatides** are formed by addition of a sulfate group to cerebrosides.

1. The sulfate group is transferred from **3'-phosphoadenosine-5'-phosphosulfate (PAPS)** by a microsomal transferase.

2. **Metachromatic leukodystrophy** is due to a genetic defect of a lysosomal enzyme that hydrolyzes the sulfate moiety of excess galactocerebroside sulfatide, which leads to its pathologic accumulation.

F. **Gangliosides** (see Chapter 7 IV B 4) are formed from cerebrosides by the stepwise addition of sugar residues.

1. The catabolism of gangliosides occurs by the stepwise hydrolysis of the component moieties to regenerate cerebrosides.

2. Inherited defects involving the lysosomal enzymes that degrade gangliosides have been documented.
   a. G_{M1} **gangliosidosis** is due to a deficiency of **β-galactosidase,** leading to pathologic accumulation of G_{M1} gangliosides, glycoproteins, and the mucopolysaccharide keratan sulfate.
   b. **Tay-Sachs disease** (G_{M2} gangliosidosis) is due to a deficiency of lysosomal **hexosaminidase** A, which hydrolyzes the terminal N-acetylgalactosamine of G_{M2} gangliosides. Its absence leads to pathologic accumulation of the gangliosides in the brain.

III. METABOLISM OF EICOSANOIDS

A. **Mobilization of arachidonic acid.** Arachidonic acid is the precursor of prostaglandins, thromboxanes, and leukotrienes.

1. **Storage.** There is little free arachidonic acid in cells. It is stored almost completely as esters of the 2-position of the glycerol backbone of cell membrane phospholipids.

2. **Regulation.** The synthesis of prostaglandins requires its immediate release from membrane phospholipids.
   a. **Stimulation** of cells by an appropriate agonist causes the release of arachidonic acid. Agonists have specific target cells.
      (1) **Thrombin** causes release of arachidonic acid in platelets and endothelial cells.
      (2) **Bradykinin** acts similarly in renal tubular cells.
   b. **Inhibition.** Release of arachidonate from membrane phospholipids is inhibited by a protein whose synthesis is induced by **glucocorticoid hormones.** This inhibition of arachidonate release accounts for the **anti-inflammatory action of steroids** because prostaglandins play important roles in the inflammatory reaction.

3. **Mechanisms**
   a. Phospholipase A_2 hydrolyzes arachidonate esterified to phospholipids. Kidney and platelet phospholipases cleave only arachidonate or eicosatrienoic acid.
   b. In platelets, phosphatidylinositol is greatly enriched in arachidonate, and arachidonate release is effected by the following pathway:
      (1) A specific phospholipase C cleaves the inositol from phosphatidylinositol to give an α,β-diacylglycerol rich in arachidonate.
      (2) The α,β-diacylglycerol may yield its arachidonate by one of two pathways.
         (a) A specific diacylglycerol lipase hydrolyzes arachidonate from the 2-position.

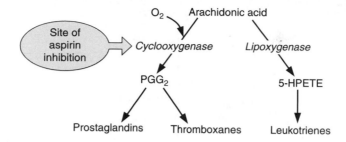

FIGURE 23-4. The biosynthesis of prostaglandins, thromboxanes, and leukotrienes from arachidonic acid. *HPETE* = hydroperoxyeicosatetraenoic acid; PGG_2 = prostaglandin G with two double bonds.

    (b) Phosphatidic acid is formed from α,β-diacylglycerol at the expense of adenosine triphosphate (ATP), and hydrolysis by phospholipase A_2 then yields arachidonate.

B. **Synthesis of prostaglandins, thromboxanes, and leukotrienes** (Figure 23-4). Once arachidonate is released in the cell, it activates both cyclooxygenase and lipoxygenase enzymes.

    1. The **cyclooxygenase system** converts arachidonate (and other C-20 unsaturated fatty acids) to endoperoxides, which are key precursors for thromboxanes and prostaglandins (see Chapter 7 V A, B).

        a. The cyclooxygenase enzyme (prostaglandin synthase) is inhibited by the **nonsteroidal anti-inflammatory agents,** such as aspirin, indomethacin, and ibuprofen.

        b. Inhibition of platelet cyclooxygenase by aspirin is important because it is irreversible and, because platelets cannot synthesize protein, the inactivated enzyme cannot be replaced.

    2. The **lipoxygenase system** converts arachidonic acid to 5-hydroperoxyeicosatetraenoic acid (5-HPETE; see Chapter 7 V C), which is the precursor for the synthesis of **leukotrienes** (see Chapter 7 V D) LTA_4, LTB_4, LTC_4, LTD_4, and LTE_4.

IV. **STEROID METABOLISM** (see Chapter 7 VI)

A. **Biosynthesis of cholesterol** (Figure 23-5). The **liver is the major site** of cholesterol biosynthesis, although other tissues also are active in this regard (e.g., the intestines, adrenal glands, gonads, skin, neural tissue, and aorta). All 27 carbon atoms of cholesterol are derived from the acetate moiety of acetyl CoA, and the enzymes reside in the cytosolic and microsomal fractions.

    1. **3-Hydroxy-3-methylglutaryl CoA (HMG CoA)** is formed in the cytosol from acetyl CoA in two steps by **thiolase** and **HMG CoA synthase.**

    2. HMG CoA is converted to **mevalonate** by **HMG CoA reductase,** an NADPH-dependent enzyme. This is the **key regulatory site** of cholesterol biosynthesis.

        a. This is regarded as the **rate-limiting step in cholesterol biosynthesis.** Although later steps may be affected by a prolonged stimulus (e.g., long-term feeding of cholesterol), their rates never become lower than that of HMG CoA reductase.

        b. The feeding of cholesterol reduces the hepatic biosynthesis of cholesterol by reducing the activity of HMG CoA reductase. Importantly, intestinal cholesterol biosynthesis does not respond to the feeding of high-cholesterol diets.

        c. HMG CoA reductase activity also is reduced by fasting, which limits the availability of acetyl CoA and NADPH for cholesterol biosynthesis.

        d. HMG CoA reductase undergoes reversible phosphorylation–dephosphorylation; the phosphorylated enzyme is less active than the dephosphorylated form.

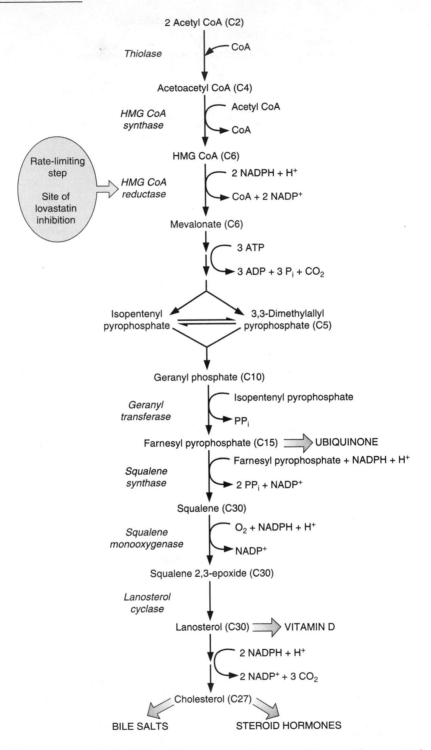

FIGURE 23-5. The biosynthesis of cholesterol. Enzyme names are in *italics. Double arrows* indicate important metabolites that are formed from cholesterol and intermediates in its synthesis. The number of carbon atoms in each intermediate is indicated in *parentheses. Acetyl CoA* = acetyl coenzyme A; *ADP* = adenosine diphosphate; *ATP* = adenosine triphosphate; *HMG CoA* = 3-hydroxy-3-methylglutaryl coenzyme A; *NADP⁺* = oxidized nicotinamide adenine dinucleotide phosphate; *NADPH* = reduced NADP; *Pᵢ* = inorganic phosphate; *PPᵢ* = inorganic pyrophosphate.

   e. **Hormonal effects on cholesterol biosynthesis**
      (1) **Insulin** stimulates HMG CoA reductase activity.
      (2) **Glucagon** antagonizes the effect of insulin.
      (3) **Thyroid hormone** stimulates HMG CoA reductase activity.
   f. The drug **lovastatin,** which is used to treat hypercholesterolemia, blocks endoge-
      nous cholesterol synthesis by inhibiting HMG CoA reductase.

3. Mevalonate is activated with high-energy phosphate bonds and then decarboxylated to form the five-carbon isoprenoid isomers, **3,3-dimethylallyl pyrophosphate**
   and **isopentenyl pyrophosphate.** An isomerase governs an equilibrium between
   these isomers.

4. A molecule of 3,3-dimethylallyl pyrophosphate condenses with a molecule of isopentenyl pyrophosphate to form the 10-carbon compound **geranyl pyrophosphate.**

5. Another molecule of isopentenyl pyrophosphate reacts with geranyl pyrophosphate
   to form the 15-carbon compound **farnesyl pyrophosphate,** which is also a precursor for ubiquinone (see Chapter 19 I D 3).

6. **Squalene synthase** catalyzes the NADPH-dependent conversion of two molecules
   of farnesyl pyrophosphate to **squalene.**

7. Squalene is converted to **squalene 2,3-epoxide** by an NADPH-dependent monooxy-
   genase.

8. A **cyclase** catalyzes the cyclization of squalene to form **lanosterol,** which also is a
   precursor for the synthesis of vitamin D (see IV E).

9. Lanosterol is converted to **cholesterol** by a series of reactions that result in the removal of three methyl groups and rearrangement of double bonds.

B. **Esterification of cholesterol**

1. The bulk of the cholesterol in tissues and approximately 65% of plasma cholesterol
   is esterified with long-chain fatty acids at C-3.

2. The synthesis of cellular cholesterol ester requires ATP to form fatty acyl CoA derivatives, which are then transferred to the 3-β-hydroxyl group of cholesterol.

3. Cholesterol associated with plasma lipoproteins can be esterified by **lecithin:choles-
   terol acyltransferase.**

Phosphatidylcholine + Cholesterol → Lysophosphatidylcholine + Cholesterol fatty acyl ester

C. **Bile acids** (see Chapter 7 VI C)

1. Bile acids are **synthesized** from cholesterol **in the liver** and **stored in the gallbladder.**

2. **Enterohepatic circulation**
   a. After release of bile acids from storage in the gallbladder to the intestine, the
      two primary bile acids—cholic and chenodeoxycholic—are converted in part to
      the secondary bile acids—deoxycholate and lithocholate—by intestinal bacteria.
   b. In the intestine, both primary and secondary bile acids are deconjugated, reab-
      sorbed by the intestinal mucosa, and returned to the liver bound to serum albu-
      min via the portal vein.
   c. The liver takes up the bile acids, reconjugates them with taurine or glycine, and
      secretes them in the bile.

3. Secretion of bile into the intestine is the **main route for the excretion of cholesterol** because the steroid nucleus cannot be oxidized to carbon dioxide and water
   by human tissues.

4. **Solubility of cholesterol in bile**
   a. Bile contains a considerable amount of cholesterol, which would be insoluble
      except for its association with bile salts and phospholipids (chiefly phosphatidyl-
      choline).

b. Despite the presence of these solubilizing agents, an increased concentration of cholesterol in the bile can lead to the formation of **gallstones** in the gallbladder or duct. These are formed if cholesterol is precipitated out of solution around a core of protein and bilirubin (see Chapter 25 VII C), which is a condition known as **cholelithiasis.**

D. **Biosynthesis of steroid hormones** (Figure 23-6; see Chapter 7 VI B)

1. **Adrenocortical hormones**
   a. In the adrenocortical cells, cholesterol is stored in lipid droplets, predominantly as cholesterol esters. It is hydrolyzed to free cholesterol and converted to **progesterone,** a key intermediate in the biosynthesis of adrenal and gonadal hormones.
   b. Progesterone undergoes hydroxylation reactions to form **cortisol.**
   c. **Aldosterone** is formed from **corticosterone** in the zona glomerulosa.

2. **Gonadal steroids**
   a. **Testicular hormones.** Progesterone also is a precursor in the synthesis of **testosterone** in the Leydig cells of the testis. Progesterone is first hydroxylated, and the side chain is then removed to give **androstenedione,** and then reduced to testosterone.
   b. **Ovarian hormones**
      (1) **Progesterone** is formed by the cells of the corpus luteum and by the placenta in pregnancy.
      (2) **17β-Estradiol** is derived from progesterone and formed in the thecal cells of the graafian follicle.

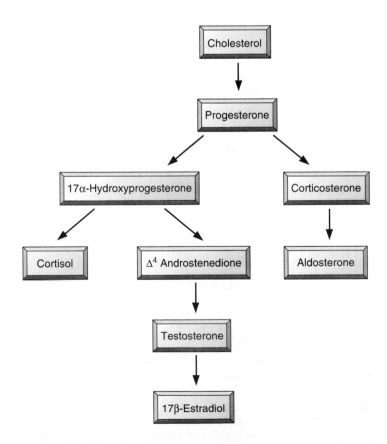

FIGURE 23-6. The biosynthesis of steroid hormones from cholesterol.

3. **Congenital adrenal hyperplasia** refers to any one of a group of disorders of steroid hormone metabolism, which are caused by genetic defects in enzymes involved in the synthetic pathways. The most common disorder is **21-hydroxylase deficiency,** in which the conversion of progesterone to corticosterone is blocked.
   a. **Symptoms** include salt-losing syndrome, hypertension, virilization in females, and precocious puberty in males.
   b. **Treatment** usually includes administration of cortisol or dexamethasone (a synthetic form of cortisol).

E. Vitamin D synthesis

1. 7-Dehydrocholesterol, an intermediate in the synthesis of cholesterol from lanosterol, accumulates in the skin.

2. 7-Dehydrocholesterol is converted to cholecalciferol (vitamin D_3) by ultraviolet light.

3. In the liver, cholecalciferol is hydroxylated by an enzyme that shows strong product inhibition to form 25-hydroxycholecalciferol. This compound is then transported to the kidney, where it is further hydroxylated to form the active compound 1,25-dihydroxycholecalciferol, a regulator of calcium metabolism.

V. LIPOPROTEIN METABOLISM.
Lipoproteins (see Chapter 7 VII), which are composed of a lipid core and a lipid/protein coat, carry lipids through the bloodstream.

A. Digestion of lipids

1. **Triacylglycerol** is the major dietary lipid of nutritional value.

2. **Emulsification**
   a. Digestion of lipids begins in the duodenum, when the entrance of the **acid chyme** from the stomach stimulates secretion of enteric hormones by the duodenal mucosa.
   b. **Bile salts and phosphatidylcholine** act as detergents in the duodenum due to their amphipathic structures. They aid in formation of mixed micelles (which have a large surface area) from fat globules (which have a small surface area).
   c. The micellar associations of lipids are the substrates for hydrolyzing enzymes.

3. **Hydrolysis of triacylglycerols is effected by three enzymes.**
   a. **Pancreatic lipase** cleaves triacylglycerols to 2-monoacylglycerol and two fatty acids.
   b. **Cholesterol esterase** hydrolyzes cholesterol esters to cholesterol plus a fatty acid.
   c. **Phospholipase A_2** hydrolyzes phospholipid (see I B 1).

4. **Formation of chylomicrons**

B. Sites of lipoprotein formation and transport (Figure 23-7)

1. The liver is the formation site of:
   a. **Very low-density lipoproteins (VLDL),** which transport triacylglycerols from the liver to other tissues
   b. **High-density lipoproteins (HDL),** which transport excess cholesterol from other tissues to the liver and are sometimes referred to as "good" cholesterol

2. The **intestine** is the site of **chylomicron formation.** Chylomicrons are triacylglycerols that are given a coat composed of protein, phospholipids, and cholesterol esters.
   a. Chylomicrons are transported in membrane-bound vesicles to membranes of mucosal cells, where they are released by exocytosis into the extracellular space.

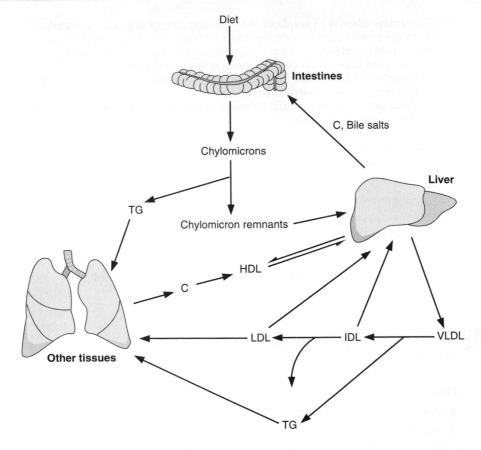

FIGURE 23-7. The metabolism and transport of plasma lipoproteins. *C* = cholesterol; *HDL* = high-density lipoprotein; *IDL* = intermediate-density lipoprotein; *LDL* = low-density lipoprotein; *TG* = triacylglycerols; *VLDL* = very low-density lipoprotein.

Once chylomicrons are in the plasma, most of the lipids contained in the chylomicrons are removed by lipoprotein lipase, forming **chylomicron remnants.**

b. Chylomicron remnants deliver dietary fat to the liver. The chylomicron remnants that remain after delipidation are enriched in cholesterol and cholesterol ester. They are cleared by the liver, where most of the cholesterol is used for bile acid synthesis (see IV C).

3. The **plasma** is the formation site of:
a. Intermediate-density lipoproteins (IDL), which are the initial product of VLDL degradation
b. Low-density lipoproteins (LDL), which transport cholesterol esters
c. Chylomicron remnants (see V B 2 a)

C. Disorders of lipoprotein metabolism
1. Hyperlipidemias (Table 23-1) represent an abnormally high level of plasma lipoproteins. The most serious consequence of hyperlipidemias is increased risk of **atherosclerosis,** an arterial disease that causes heart attacks and stroke.
2. Hypolipidemias are caused by a deficiency of one or more of the plasma lipoproteins.
a. Hypobetalipoproteinemia (abetalipoproteinemia) is a genetic disorder characterized by neurologic symptoms, including ataxia and mental retardation.
(1) Plasma triacylglycerol and cholesterol levels are decreased.

TABLE 23-1. Types of Hyperlipidemias

Type	Generic Classification	Increased Lipoprotein	Increased Lipid
I	Lipoprotein lipase deficiency	Chylomicrons	Triacylglycerols
IIa	Hypercholesterolemia (LDL receptor deficiency)	LDL	Cholesterol
IIb	Combined hyperlipidemia	LDL, VLDL	Triacylglycerols, cholesterol
III	Dysbetalipoproteinemia	β-VLDL	Triacylglycerols, cholesterol
IV	Hypertriglyceridemia	VLDL	Triacylglycerols
V	Mixed hyperlipidemia	VLDL, chylomicrons	Triacylglycerols

LDL = low-density lipoprotein; VLDL = very low-density lipoprotein.

       (2) There is a complete absence of β-lipoproteins (no chylomicrons or VLDLs).
       (3) Absorption of fat is greatly reduced.
  b. **HDL deficiency (Tangier disease)** is characterized by recurrent polyneuropathy, lymphadenopathy, tonsillar hyperplasia, and hepatosplenomegaly (from storage of cholesterol in reticuloendothelial cells).
       (1) Plasma cholesterol levels are low; triacylglycerols are normal or increased.
       (2) There is a marked decrease in plasma HDLs.

Case 23-1 Revisited

High cholesterol and normal triacylglycerol levels are characteristic of the condition broadly described as hypercholesterolemia.

A regimen of diet and combined drug therapy was implemented for this patient. The combined drug treatment is more effective than use of a single drug because each drug affects a different aspect of lipid metabolism. Lovastatin blocks endogenous cholesterol synthesis by inhibiting HMG CoA reductase (see IV A 2), a key enzyme required for the synthesis of cholesterol. Colestipol is an insoluble resin that binds bile acids, thus preventing reabsorption of bile acids by the intestines. Together, the combined effects of these drugs can lower the total serum cholesterol.

STUDY QUESTIONS

DIRECTIONS: Each of the numbered items or incomplete statements in this section is followed by answers or by completions of the statement. Select the **one** lettered answer or completion that is **best** in each case.

1. The release of arachidonate from membrane glycerophospholipids is inhibited by which one of the following compounds?

(A) Aspirin
(B) Linoleic acid
(C) A specific protein induced by glucocorticoids
(D) 2-Acyl lysophosphatidylcholine
(E) Thrombin

2. Which of the following compounds is a precursor of both phosphatidylcholine and sphingomyelin?

(A) Phosphatidylethanolamine
(B) Acetylcholine
(C) Glycerol-3-phosphate
(D) Uridine diphosphate glucose
(E) Cytidine diphosphate choline (CDP-choline)

3. The committed step in the biosynthesis of cholesterol is

(A) formation of acetoacetyl coenzyme A (CoA) from acetyl CoA
(B) formation of 3-hydroxy-3-methylglutaryl CoA (HMG CoA) from acetyl CoA and acetoacetyl CoA
(C) formation of mevalonic acid from HMG CoA
(D) formation of squalene by squalene synthase
(E) cyclization of squalene to lanosterol

4. The synthesis of 1,25-dihydroxycholecalciferol takes place in which one of the following sites?

(A) In the skin under the action of ultraviolet light from 7-dehydrocholesterol
(B) In the liver from cholecalciferol
(C) In the kidney from 25-hydroxycholecalciferol
(D) In the intestine from cholecalciferol
(E) It is not synthesized in mammals

5. Patients with IIa hyperlipidemia (hypercholesterolemia) exhibit

(A) a deficiency of lipoprotein lipase
(B) low serum levels of low-density lipoprotein (LDL)
(C) a deficiency of LDL receptors
(D) normal serum cholesterol levels
(E) elevated serum triacylglycerol levels

6. A common feature of the degradation of sphingolipids, including gangliosides, is

(A) catalysis by lysosomal enzymes
(B) a requirement for high-energy phosphate bonds
(C) regulation by phospholipases
(D) regulation by glucocorticoids
(E) feedback inhibition by cholesterol

7. Which one of the following is a precursor of both gonadal and adrenocortical hormones?

(A) Progesterone
(B) Cortisol
(C) Testosterone
(D) Corticosterone
(E) 17β-Estradiol

DIRECTIONS: The group of items in this section consists of lettered options followed by a set of numbered items. For each item, select the **one** lettered option that is most closely associated with it. Each lettered option may be selected once, more than once, or not at all.

Questions 8-12

Match the following statements to the enzyme to which the statement refers.

(A) Cyclooxygenase
(B) β-Glucocerebrosidase
(C) 3-Hydroxy-3-methylglutaryl coenzyme A (HMG CoA) reductase
(D) Hexosaminidase A
(E) Lecithin:cholesterol acyltransferase

8. Gaucher's disease is caused by a deficiency of this enzyme

9. A deficiency in this enzyme may cause a pathologic accumulation of gangliosides in the brain

10. A drug that inhibits this enzyme may be useful in lowering serum cholesterol levels

11. A drug that inhibits this enzyme may be useful as an anti-inflammatory agent

12. A deficiency in this enzyme may cause abnormalities in lipoprotein structure, because lipoproteins contain abnormally low amounts of cholesterol esters

ANSWERS AND EXPLANATIONS

1. The answer is C [III A 2 b]. The cleavage of the arachidonate moiety from membrane glycerophospholipids by phospholipase A_2 is blocked by an inhibitory protein whose synthesis is induced by glucocorticoids. This is the basis for the suppression of inflammation by glucocorticoids. Aspirin exerts its nonsteroidal anti-inflammatory action by blocking cyclooxygenase, which produces prostaglandins and thromboxanes from arachidonate. Linoleic acid is a precursor of arachidonate, and 2-acyl lysophosphatidylcholine is produced by the action of phospholipase A_1 on phosphatidylcholine. Thrombin causes the release of arachidonate.

2. The answer is E [I A 1 c; II C]. Phosphatidylcholine can be synthesized de novo from phosphatidylethanolamine by three methylation reactions involving S-adenosylmethionine. Phosphatidylcholine also can be formed by salvage reactions, using choline derived either from phospholipid degradation or from the diet. Choline is first converted to choline phosphate, which then reacts with cytidine triphosphate to form cytidine diphosphate choline (CDP-choline). This is the donor of the choline group to α,β-diacylglycerol, forming phosphatidylcholine. CDP-choline also is the choline donor in the formation of sphingomyelin from ceramide. Phosphatidylethanolamine is a precursor of phosphatidylcholine but not of sphingomyelin. Acetylcholine, a neurotransmitter, is not a precursor for either compound. Uridine diphosphate (UDP) glucose is used in carbohydrate polymer biosynthesis. Glycerol-3-phosphate is a precursor of the glycerol moiety of phosphatidylcholine but is not a precursor of sphingomyelin.

3. The answer is C [IV A 2]. The rate-limiting and committed step in cholesterol biosynthesis is the reduction of 3-hydroxy-3-methylglutaryl coenzyme A (HMG CoA) by HMG CoA reductase to form mevalonate. This is the key regulatory site. Hepatic cholesterol synthesis is reduced by the feeding of cholesterol (a feedback effect) or by fasting, which limits the substrates for cholesterol synthesis. Diets high in fat or in carbohydrate increase hepatic cholesterol biosynthesis.

4. The answer is C [IV E 3]. Vitamin D, cholecalciferol, arises from the action of ultraviolet light on 7-dehydrocholesterol in the skin. The latter compound is an intermediate in cholesterol biosynthesis and accumulates in the skin. Cholecalciferol is not active as a vitamin D. In the liver, cholecalciferol is hydroxylated to 25-hydroxycholecalciferol; in the kidney, it is further hydroxylated at C-1 to form the active compound, 1,25-dihydroxycholecalciferol.

5. The answer is C [V C; Table 23-1]. Type IIa hyperlipidemia (hypercholesterolemia) is characterized by a deficiency of functional low-density lipoprotein (LDL) receptors on extrahepatic cell membranes. The serum LDL levels, and, therefore, the serum cholesterol levels, are high, and there is an increased risk of coronary artery disease. Serum triacylglycerol levels are not affected. Lipoprotein lipase deficiency is the cause of type I hyperlipidemia.

6. The answer is A [II C–F]. The degradation (catabolism) of sphingolipids, including gangliosides, is catalyzed by hydrolytic enzymes located in the lysosomes. These reactions do not require an input of energy. Phospholipases degrade phospholipids. Glucocorticoids regulate arachidonic acid metabolism. Cholesterol levels do not affect sphingolipid catabolism.

7. The answer is A [IV D]. In the adrenocortical cells, cholesterol is converted to progesterone, a key intermediate in the biosynthesis of adrenal hormones, cortisol, and corticosterone. Progesterone also is a precursor in the synthesis of testosterone in the testis. The ovarian hormone, 17β-estradiol, is derived from progesterone in the thecal cells of the graafian follicle.

8-12. The answers are: 8-B [II D 1], **9-D** [II F 2 b], **10-C** [IV A 2], **11-A** [III B 1], **12-E** [IV B 3]. A number of inherited diseases are caused by defects of lysosomal enzymes that degrade sphingolipids. The most common of these is

Gaucher's disease. Patients are defective in β-glucocerebrosidase, which causes a pathologic accumulation of β-glucocerebroside in the liver, spleen, and bone marrow.

Tay-Sachs disease is caused by a deficiency of the lysosomal enzyme hexosaminidase A, which causes the accumulation of excess gangliosides in the brain.

3-Hydroxy-3-methylglutaryl coenzyme A (HMG CoA) reductase is the enzyme that catalyzes the rate-limiting step in cholesterol synthesis. It is possible to block the endogenous synthesis of cholesterol by inhibiting HMG CoA reductase. Drugs such as lovastatin are used for this purpose.

Anti-inflammatory drugs such as aspirin and ibuprofen specifically inhibit cyclooxygenase, which converts arachidonate to prostaglandin G_2. It is the precursor for other prostaglandins and thromboxanes, which play a role in a wide range of biologic functions including the inflammatory response.

Cholesterol in association with plasma lipoproteins is esterified to cholesterol esters by lecithin:cholesterol acyltransferase. Cholesterol esters as well as cholesterol are major components of the plasma lipoproteins. A deficiency in this enzyme could explain these symptoms.

Chapter 24

Protein and Amino Acid Degradation
Victor Davidson

Case 24-1

An infant is born without complications but becomes extremely lethargic and begins to hyperventilate beginning 24 hours after birth. Blood analysis indicates a below-normal blood urea nitrogen (BUN) level, a slightly alkaline pH, and a below-normal level of the partial pressure of carbon dioxide (P_{CO_2}). A chest radiograph is normal. Further blood analysis reveals a very high level of ammonia, a high level of glutamine, and no detectable citrulline. Urinalysis reveals extremely high levels of orotic acid. The infant is given a blood transfusion and hemodialysis immediately. This is followed by intravenous administration of sodium benzoate and phenylacetate. The infant is also placed on a low-protein diet supplemented with arginine.

- What is the diagnosis?
- What was the rationale for the treatment?

I. PROTEOLYSIS is the breakdown of protein to free amino acids.

A. Gastrointestinal input

1. Proteins and polypeptides are not absorbed intact but must first be hydrolyzed to free amino acids.

2. Digestion of dietary protein is carried out by **proteases** (proteolytic enzymes; Table 24-1), which are found in gastric and pancreatic juices and on the intestinal cell surface.

   a. Gastric juice
   - **(1)** The **hydrochloric acid** (pH = 2) in gastric juice kills microorganisms, denatures proteins, and provides an acid environment for the action of pepsin.
   - **(2)** The protease **pepsin** works at acid pH. It is secreted into the stomach as the proenzyme **pepsinogen,** which is activated by the autocatalytic removal of 44 N-terminal amino acids at low pH.
   - **(3)** Peptic hydrolysis of proteins yields peptides and some free amino acids.

   b. Pancreatic juice
   - **(1)** Proteases in pancreatic juice also are secreted as proenzymes from the pancreatic acinar cells. Activation of proenzymes occurs by the action of **enteropeptidase** (enterokinase), which is secreted by the duodenal epithelial cells.

TABLE 24-1. Properties of Proteolytic Enzymes

Enzyme	Action Site	Optimum pH	Substrate Specificity
Chymotrypsin	Intestine	7.5–8.5	Aromatic amino acid residues
Elastase	Intestine	7.5–8.5	Small nonpolar amino acid residues
Pepsin	Stomach	1.5–2.5	Most amino acid residues
Trypsin	Intestine	7.5–8.5	Arginine and lysine residues
Aminopeptidase	Intestinal mucosa	7.5–8.5	N-Terminal amino acid residue
Carboxypeptidase	Intestine	7.5–8.5	C-Terminal amino acid residue

TABLE 24-2. Amino Acid Transport Systems and Disorders

Amino Acid Specificity	Disorder Associated with Defective Transport
Small neutral amino acids	. . .
Large neutral and aromatic amino acids	Hartnup's disease
Acidic amino acids	. . .
Basic amino acids and cystine	Cystinuria
Imino acids and glycine	Glycinuria

      (2) Enteropeptidase activates **trypsinogen** by removing six amino acids, and the activated **trypsin** in turn activates the proenzymes of **chymotrypsin, elastase,** and **carboxypeptidases A and B.**

    c. Intestinal proteases

      (1) Aminopeptidases and **dipeptidases** continue the digestion of peptides to free amino acids.

      (2) Di- and tripeptides are usually absorbed as such and digested to free amino acids within the intestinal epithelial cells.

  3. Absorption of free amino acids takes place in the small intestine.

    a. Five major systems (Table 24-2) and a few minor systems have been identified that transport different classes of amino acids from the gut lumen into the intestinal epithelial cell.

    b. Disorders associated with defects in amino acid transport lead to increased levels of those amino acids in the urine **(amino acidurias).**

      (1) Hartnup's disease is due to a defect in the transport system for large neutral and aromatic amino acids.

        (a) Symptoms similar to pellagra are observed in some patients. This is due to a deficiency of niacin (see Chapter 14 II E; Case 14-2), which may be synthesized from tryptophan.

        (b) Treatment. These symptoms can be relieved by administration of niacin.

      (2) Cystinuria is due to a defect in the transport system for basic amino acids, which also transports cystine, the disulfide-linked dimer of cysteine.

        (a) Symptoms. Cystine is relatively insoluble in urine, and its accumulation leads to deposition of crystals, which may cause urinary tract infections and renal stones.

        (b) Treatment to reduce deposition of cystine crystals includes administration of the drug **penicillamine** (β,β-dimethylcysteine), which reacts with cystine to form a soluble cysteine–penicillamine adduct.

      (3) Glycinuria (iminoglycinuria) is due to a defect in the transport system for glycine and the imino acids, proline and hydroxyproline. There are **no clinical abnormalities** other than increased urinary excretion of these amino acids.

B. **Proteolysis of endogenous protein.** Body protein is continuously being broken down to free amino acids, and the rate of degradation for individual proteins varies widely. Some liver enzymes have half-lives of only a few hours, whereas hemoglobin and the red blood cells have a total lifetime of 120 days, and some structural proteins (e.g., collagen) have half-lives too long to be measured.

  1. Factors affecting the rates of protein degradation

    a. Denaturation (i.e., loss of its preferred native configuration) accelerates proteolysis.

    b. Activation of lysosomes increases the rate of intracellular proteolysis.

    c. Glucocorticoids increase protein degradation in muscle tissue.

    d. Excessive thyroid hormones increase protein turnover.

    e. Insulin reduces proteolysis and increases protein synthesis.

2. Purpose

    a. Abnormal, defective, and damaged proteins must be removed because they are of no use to the body, and they may inhibit processes that require the functional proteins.

    b. Inducible enzymes must be removed when their activities are no longer beneficial.

3. Ubiquitin, an 8.5-kilodalton protein in eukaryotic cells, plays an important role in designating the proteins to be degraded. The C-terminal residue of ubiquitin becomes covalently attached to lysine residues of proteins that are then degraded via an **adenosine triphosphate (ATP)-dependent process.**

    a. The protein **E1** catalyzes the formation of an intermediate ubiquitin complex by formation of a thioester bond to a sulfhydryl group of E1.

    b. The protein **E2** receives the ubiquitin molecule from the ubiquitin-E1 complex and transfers it to protein E3.

    c. The protein **E3** couples the ubiquitin molecule to the protein that is to be degraded. Usually, the protein to be degraded becomes conjugated to several molecules of ubiquitin.

II. AMINO ACID POOL (Figure 24-1)

A. **Essential amino acids** are those that cannot be synthesized by humans and are, therefore, essential dietary factors. Nine of the 20 amino acids are essential (Table 24-3).

B. **Inputs to the amino acid pool** are from dietary protein and proteolysis of endogenous cellular protein.

C. **Outputs from the amino acid pool** are for amino acid degradation (catabolism), synthesis of special compounds, and protein synthesis.

D. **Nitrogen balance.** If the **total daily nitrogen losses** in urine, skin, and feces are **equal to the total daily nitrogen intake,** the subject is said to be in nitrogen balance, as a healthy, adequately fed adult should be.

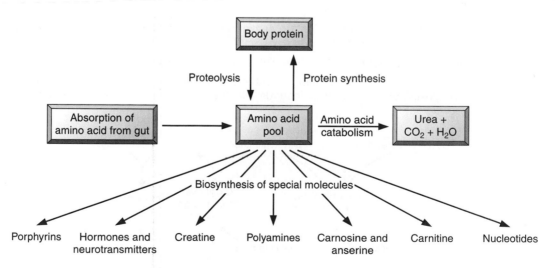

FIGURE 24-1. Sources and fates of the amino acid pool.

TABLE 24-3. The Nine Essential Amino Acids

Histidine	Lysine	Threonine
Isoleucine	Methionine	Tryptophan
Leucine	Phenylalanine	Valine

Note—In growing children, arginine may not be synthesized in amounts adequate to fill the requirements for both protein synthesis and urea formation; under these circumstances, it would be considered an essential amino acid.

1. **Positive nitrogen balance.** If nitrogen losses are *less* than intake, the subject is in positive nitrogen balance, as healthy, growing children and convalescing adults should be.

2. **Negative nitrogen balance.** If nitrogen losses are *greater* than intake, the subject is in negative nitrogen balance, as occurs in people with diseases involving tissue wasting or in those undergoing starvation. Prolonged periods of negative balance are dangerous and can be fatal.

3. **Estimation of muscle protein breakdown.** Some of the histidine residues of the muscle protein complex **actomyosin** are methylated after their incorporation. When actomyosin breaks down, **3-methyl histidine** is liberated and excreted into the urine. The urinary levels provide a measure of muscle protein breakdown.

III. **METABOLIC FLOW OF AMINO ACID NITROGEN** (Figure 24-2). The primary means by which amino acid-derived nitrogen is metabolized is by the sequential action of aminotransferases, glutamate dehydrogenase, and the urea cycle (Figure 24-2).

A. **Transamination** involves the **transfer of an amino group from an amino acid to an α-keto acid** to form a new amino acid and a new α-keto acid.

1. **Aminotransferases (transaminases)** catalyze these reactions. For example, aspartate aminotransferase interconverts the amino acid aspartate plus the α-keto acid α-ketoglutarate, with the amino acid glutamate and the α-keto acid oxaloacetate.

   Aspartate + α-Ketoglutarate ⇋ Oxaloacetate + Glutamate

2. **Pyridoxal phosphate** (see Chapter 14 II G) is an essential cofactor of all aminotransferases.

B. **Oxidative deamination by glutamate dehydrogenase** occurs in the mitochondrial matrix by the following reaction:

   Glutamate + NAD(P)$^+$ + H$_2$O ⇋ α-Ketoglutarate + NAD(P)H + H$^+$ + NH$_3$

1. Glutamate dehydrogenase can use either oxidized nicotinamide adenine dinucleotide (NAD$^+$) or oxidized nicotinamide adenine dinucleotide phosphate (NADP$^+$) as a cofactor.

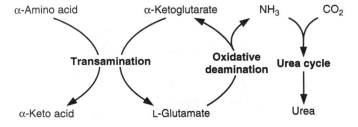

FIGURE 24-2. Metabolic flow of amino acid nitrogen.

   a. **NADPH–NADP⁺ ratio.** Under normal conditions in the liver, the ratio of reduced NADPH to oxidized NADP⁺ is high, and the ratio of reduced NADH to oxidized NAD⁺ is low. Thus, there is always a pyridine nucleotide coenzyme available in its oxidized or reduced state to participate in the above reaction in either direction.

   b. The reaction above is controlled, therefore, by the relative levels of glutamate, α-ketoglutarate, and ammonia (NH_3).

2. **Allosteric regulators**

   a. **Activators** include adenosine diphosphate (ADP) and guanosine diphosphate (GDP).

   b. **Inhibitors** include ATP, guanosine triphosphate (GTP), and NADH.

C. **Alternative mechanisms for deaminating amino acids**

1. **Direct deamination by serine and threonine dehydratase**

   a. Because of the chemistry of the hydroxyl side chain of serine and threonine (i.e., the hydroxyl group is a good leaving group), their direct deamination is facilitated.

   b. The reactions are:

$$\text{Serine} \rightarrow \text{Pyruvate} + NH_3$$

$$\text{Threonine} \rightarrow \alpha\text{-Amino-}\beta\text{-ketobutyrate} \rightarrow \text{Pyruvate} + NH_3$$

   c. **Pyridoxal phosphate** is a required cofactor.

2. **Amino acid oxidases** catalyze the reaction:

$$\text{Amino acid} + H_2O + O_2 \rightarrow \alpha\text{-Keto acid} + NH_3 + H_2O_2$$

   a. These enzymes use tightly bound **flavins** as cofactors.

   b. Amino acid oxidases occur in the kidneys and the liver; however, their physiologic significance is not clear.

D. **The urea cycle** occurs exclusively in the **liver.** The urea that is formed contains two atoms of nitrogen, one derived from NH_3 and one derived from aspartate. The overall stoichiometry of the urea cycle is:

$$CO_2 + NH_4^+ + 3\ \text{ATP} + \text{Aspartate} + 2\ H_2O \rightarrow$$
$$\text{Urea} + 2\ \text{ADP} + 2\ P_i + \text{AMP} + PP_i + \text{Fumarate}$$

1. **Reactions of the urea cycle** (Figure 24-3)

   a. **Carbamoyl phosphate synthetase** catalyzes the formation of carbamoyl phosphate formed from ammonia and carbon dioxide.

      (1) Energy requirement. Two molecules of ATP are required for this reaction.

      (2) N-Acetylglutamate is a required **positive allosteric effector.** The activity of **acetylglutamate synthetase,** the enzyme that synthesizes N-acetylglutamate, is regulated by amino acid levels.

   b. **Ornithine transcarbamoylase** catalyzes the formation of **citrulline** from carbamoyl phosphate and ornithine.

   c. **Argininosuccinate synthetase** catalyzes the formation of **argininosuccinate** from citrulline and aspartate. One molecule of **ATP is required.** The amino group of asparate provides one of the two nitrogen atoms that appear in urea.

   d. **Argininosuccinate lyase** catalyzes the formation of **arginine and fumarate** from the cleavage of argininosuccinate. As it is a citric acid cycle intermediate, **fumarate formation links the urea cycle and the citric acid cycle.**

   e. **Arginase** catalyzes the formation of **urea and ornithine** from the cleavage of arginine.

      (1) Urea is highly soluble and nontoxic. It enters the blood and is excreted in the urine.

      (2) Ornithine continues to act as an intermediate in the urea cycle (see III D 1 b).

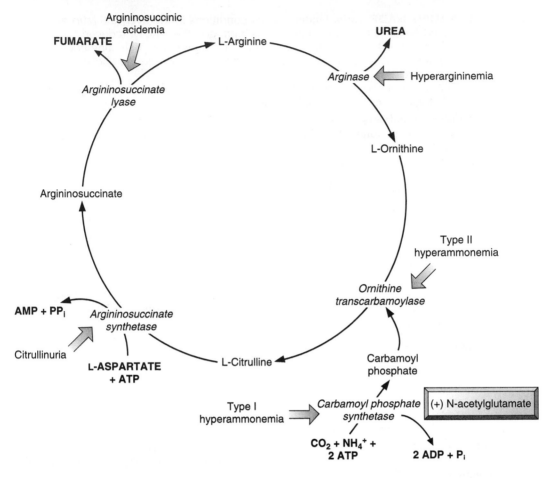

FIGURE 24-3. The urea cycle reactions. Enzyme names are in *italics.* The substrates and products of the urea cycle are indicated in *bold. Double arrows* indicate enzymes that are deficient in the indicated metabolic disorders. Activators are indicated by (+). *AMP* = adenosine monophosphate; *ATP* = adenosine triphosphate; *P_i* = inorganic phosphate; *PP_i* = inorganic pyrophosphate.

2. **Compartmentation of the urea cycle enzymes** requires that the urea cycle intermediates, ornithine and citrulline, be transported across the mitochondrial membrane (see Figure 24-3).
   a. The **mitochondria** contains carbamoyl phosphate synthetase and ornithine transcarbamoylase.
   b. The **cytosol** contains argininosuccinate synthetase, argininosuccinate lyase, and arginase.

3. **Genetic defects** have been documented for each of the urea cycle enzymes (see Figure 24-3).
   a. **Diseases**
      (1) **Type I hyperammonemia** is due to a defect in carbamoyl phosphate synthetase.
      (2) **Type II hyperammonemia** is due to a defect in ornithine transcarbamoylase.
      (3) **Citrullinuria** is due to a defect in argininosuccinate synthetase.
      (4) **Argininosuccinic acidemia** is due to a defect in argininosuccinate lyase.
      (5) **Hyperargininemia** is due to a defect in arginase.

    b. Symptoms

        (1) Hyperammonemia. High serum levels of ammonia are quite toxic and can cause brain damage.

        (2) Episodic encephalopathies, such as convulsions and ataxia, may occur in children with partial deficiencies of a urea cycle enzyme.

    c. Treatment. Infants who totally lack any of the urea cycle enzymes do not usually survive the neonatal period. Patients with defects that reduce, but do not eliminate, the activity of one of the urea cycle enzymes are more likely to respond to treatment.

        (1) Low-protein diets. Severe consequences of these disorders may be avoided when protein intake is restricted. However, very early diagnosis is critical in preventing mental retardation. A diet must be provided that provides adequate, but not excessive, amounts of essential amino acids. Arginine is not normally considered an essential amino acid because it may be synthesized by the action of the urea cycle. Therefore, low-protein diets should be supplemented with arginine.

        (2) Administration of sodium benzoate and sodium phenylacetate is beneficial in reducing the serum ammonia level. These compounds react with glycine and glutamine to form adducts, which are excreted in the urine. Serum ammonia must then be used to synthesize more of these nonessential amino acids, which helps to lower the overall ammonia level.

        (3) Blood transfusion and hemodialysis may be required to prevent brain damage from hyperammonemia.

IV. CLASSIFICATION OF AMINO ACIDS.

Amino acids are categorized by the final products of their degradation pathways (Figure 24-4).

A. **Ketogenic** amino acids are degraded to either acetyl coenzyme A (acetyl CoA) or acetoacetyl CoA, which can give rise to ketone bodies (see Chapter 22 IV A). Purely ketogenic amino acids are leucine and lysine.

B. **Glucogenic** amino acids are degraded to pyruvate or citric acid cycle intermediates, which can give rise to glucose (see Chapter 20 II). Purely glucogenic amino acids include alanine, arginine, asparagine, aspartate, cysteine, glutamate, glutamine, glycine, histidine, methionine, proline, serine, and valine.

C. **Ketogenic and glucogenic.** Some amino acids can be degraded into multiple intermediates, which classify them as both ketogenic and glucogenic. They are isoleucine, phenylalanine, threonine, tyrosine, and tryptophan.

V. FATE OF CARBON SKELETONS

A. **Three-carbon amino acids, threonine, and glycine are converted to pyruvate.**

    1. Alanine is converted by transamination with α-ketoglutarate.

    2. Serine is converted by direct deamination by serine dehydratase.

    3. Cysteine may be converted by three different pathways.

    4. Threonine (a four-carbon amino acid) is converted via an α-amino-β-ketobutyrate intermediate (see III C 1 b). This intermediate in pyruvate formation may alternatively be metabolized to acetyl CoA and glycine.

A. Ketogenic

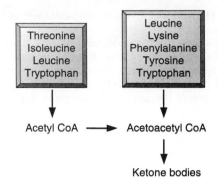

B. Glucogenic

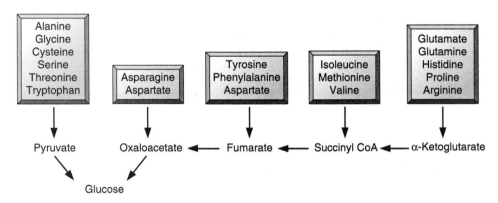

FIGURE 24-4. The metabolic fate of *(A)* ketogenic and *(B)* glucogenic amino acid carbon skeletons. *CoA* = coenzyme A.

   5. **Glycine** (a two-carbon amino acid) may be converted by serine hydroxymethyl-transferase to serine, and it is then converted to pyruvate.

B. **Four-carbon amino acids are converted to oxaloacetate.**

   1. **Aspartate** is converted by transamination with α-ketoglutarate.

   2. **Asparagine** is converted by asparaginase to aspartate and then to oxaloacetate.

C. **Some five-carbon amino acids are converted to glutamate, a precursor of α-ketoglutarate.**

   1. **Glutamine** is converted to glutamate by glutaminase.

   2. **Histidine** is converted to glutamate by a series of reactions that include the transfer of its formimino group to tetrahydrofolate (see Chapter 25 II B).

   3. **Arginine** is converted by arginase to ornithine, which may be converted to glutamate semialdehyde and oxidized to glutamate.

   4. **Proline** undergoes reactions that involve ring opening and conversion to glutamate semialdehyde and then to glutamate.

D. **Degradation of branched-chain amino acids** (Figure 24-5)

   1. **Valine, leucine, and isoleucine** all are converted to their corresponding α-keto acid by the actions of three specific aminotransferases.

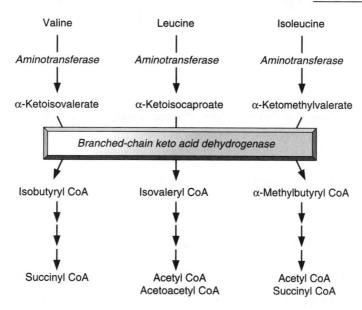

FIGURE 24-5. The catabolism of branched-chain amino acids. Enzyme names are in *italics.* CoA = coenzyme A.

2. **Branched-chain keto acid dehydrogenase is a common enzyme** that catalyzes the **oxidative decarboxylations** of each of the three α-keto acids derived from valine, leucine, and isoleucine.
   a. Branched-chain keto acid dehydrogenase is very similar to pyruvate dehydrogenase (see Chapter 18 I) and also utilizes as cofactors lipoamide, thiamine pyrophosphate (TPP), flavin adenine dinucleotide (FAD), and NAD⁺.
   b. **Maple syrup urine disease (branched-chain ketoaciduria)** is caused by a genetic defect in branched-chain keto acid dehydrogenase.
      (1) Diagnosis. Plasma and urine levels of valine, leucine, and isoleucine and their corresponding α-keto acids are abnormally high. These keto acids give the urine the characteristic odor for which the disease is named.
      (2) Treatment includes dietary restriction of valine, leucine, and isoleucine and, for acute episodes, a blood transfusion. In some cases, the defect reduces the enzyme's affinity for TPP. These patients respond to treatment with therapeutic doses of thiamine. Untreated infants do not survive long after birth.
   c. **Intermittent branched-chain ketoaciduria** is a variant of maple syrup urine disease in which the deficiency in enzyme activity is much less severe. Symptoms of this variant may not appear until later in life and may be intermittent. Treatment by dietary restriction of branched-chain amino acids is more successful than in patients with maple syrup urine disease.

3. The three CoA derivatives are then degraded by different pathways to yield different final products.
   a. **Isovaleric acidemia** is a disease caused by a **deficiency of isovaleryl CoA dehydrogenase,** an enzyme involved in the degradative pathway of leucine.
   b. **Treatment** includes dietary restriction of leucine and administration of glycine, which reacts with isovaleric acid, the toxic intermediate that accumulates in this disorder.

E. **Catabolism of amino acids to succinyl CoA** (Figure 24-6)

1. **Methionine, isoleucine, and valine** are degraded by different pathways to form succinyl CoA via L-methylmalonyl CoA.

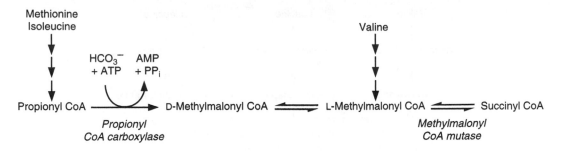

FIGURE 24-6. The catabolism of amino acids to succinyl coenzyme A *(CoA)*. *AMP* = adenosine monophosphate; *ATP* = adenosine triphosphate; *HCO₃⁻* = bicarbonate; *PPᵢ* = inorganic pyrophosphate.

2. Methionine and isoleucine are first converted to propionyl CoA, which is converted to D-methylmalonyl CoA by **propionyl CoA carboxylase, a biotin**-containing enzyme.

3. D-Methylmalonyl CoA undergoes racemization to L-methylmalonyl CoA followed by isomerization to form **succinyl CoA.**

   a. **Methylmalonyl CoA mutase** catalyzes this isomerization. It contains **5′-deoxyadenosylcobalamin** (see Chapter 14 II C 2), which is formed from vitamin B_{12} and ATP.

   b. **Methylmalonic aciduria** is caused by a defect in methylmalonyl CoA mutase. Some forms of this disorder are treatable by administration of high doses of vitamin B_{12}. Patients who do not respond to vitamin B_{12} must be placed on a diet that restricts the intake of methionine, isoleucine, and valine. This is difficult to manage because these are essential amino acids.

F. Catabolism of phenylalanine and tyrosine (Figure 24-7).

1. **Phenylalanine hydroxylase** catalyzes the **hydroxylation of phenylalanine to form tyrosine.**

   a. **Tetrahydrobiopterin** is a required cofactor. The cofactor is oxidized to dihydrobiopterin during this reaction and must be regenerated by another enzyme, **dihydrobiopteridine reductase,** which uses NADPH as a reductant.

   b. **Phenylketonuria** (PKU) is a genetic disorder associated with the inability to convert phenylalanine to tyrosine, with the subsequent accumulation of toxic derivatives of phenylalanine (e.g., phenylpyruvate).

      (1) **Classic PKU** is due to a genetic defect in phenylalanine hydroxylase. This disorder is treated with a phenylalanine-restricted diet. If not diagnosed early, mental retardation occurs in untreated infants.

      (2) **Atypical PKU** is due to a defect in dihydrobiopteridine reductase, which is needed to regenerate the reduced form of the cofactor. Tetrahydrobiopterin is also required for the synthesis of certain neurotransmitters (see Chapter 25 III A 1; IV A 2). Thus, this disorder presents neurologic problems, in addition to those seen in classic PKU, that are not abated by restricting phenylalanine.

2. **Tyrosine aminotransferase** catalyzes the reaction with α-ketoglutarate to form 4-hydroxyphenylpyruvate. **Tyrosinemia type II** is caused by a genetic defect in this enzyme.

3. **4-Hydroxyphenylpyruvate oxidase** catalyzes the conversion of 4-hydroxyphenylpyruvate to homogentisate. **Neonatal tyrosinemia** is due to a defect in this enzyme.

4. **Homogentisate oxidase** catalyzes the conversion of homogentisate to 4-maleylacetoacetate. **Alkaptonuria** is due to a genetic defect in this enzyme. Patients excrete large amounts of homogentisate in the urine, which causes it to darken after exposure to air. This disorder causes no other symptoms in children and usually is not treated. Later in life, patients may develop a form of arthritis, which is treated as such.

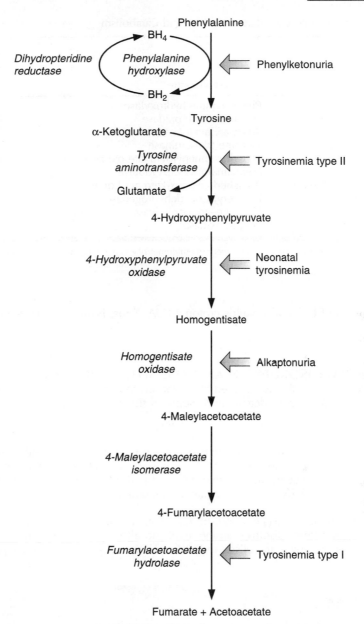

FIGURE 24-7. The catabolism of phenylalanine and tyrosine. Enzyme names are in *italics. Double arrows* indicate enzymes that are deficient in the indicated metabolic disorders. *BH$_4$* = tetrahydrobiopterin; *BH$_2$* = dihydrobiopterin.

5. **Maleylacetoacetate isomerase** converts 4-maleylacetoacetate to 4-fumarylacetoacetate.

6. Fumarylacetoacetate hydrolase cleaves 4-fumarylacetoacetate to form **fumarate,** a glucogenic product, and **acetoacetate,** a ketogenic product. **Tyrosinemia type I (tyrosinosis)** is due to a defect in this enzyme.

G. **Catabolism of tryptophan** yields crotonyl CoA, formate, and alanine. Crotonyl CoA is an intermediate in the β-oxidation of fatty acids, and thus, tryptophan is ketogenic. It is also glucogenic because alanine is also formed during its degradation.

TABLE 24-4. Some Inherited Disorders of Amino Acid Catabolism

Disorder	Defective Enzyme	Amino Acid Degradation Pathway
Phenylketonuria	Phenylalanine hydroxylase	Phe
Alkaptonuria	Homogentisate oxidase	Phe, tyr
Tyrosinemia type I	4-Fumarylacetoacetate hydrolase	Phe, tyr
Tyrosinemia type II	Tyrosine transaminase	Phe, tyr
Neonatal tyrosinemia	4-Hydroxyphenylpyruvate oxidase	Phe, tyr
Methylmalonic aciduria	Methylmalonyl CoA mutase	Met, val, ile
Maple syrup urine disease	Branched-chain α-keto acid dehydrogenase	Ile, leu, val
Isovaleric acidemia	Isovaleryl CoA dehydrogenase	Leu
Histidinemia	Histidine–ammonia lyase	His
Hyperprolinemia	Proline oxidase	Pro

His = histidine; *ile* = isoleucine; *leu* = leucine; *met* = methionine; *phe* = phenylalanine; *pro* = proline; *tyr* = tyrosine; *val* = valine.

H. **Catabolism of lysine** also yields crotonyl CoA. Thus, lysine is a ketogenic amino acid.

VI. **INHERITED DISORDERS OF AMINO ACID CATABOLISM.** Several disorders have been documented that are caused by mutations in genes that code for specific enzymes needed for amino acid degradation. Some of these disorders are summarized in Table 24-4.

A. These disorders usually lead to excessive **accumulation in the blood or urine of the intermediate** that is a substrate for that enzyme, or derivatives of that compound, and a **decrease of subsequent intermediates** in that pathway. The severity of the disorder depends on the **toxicity of the accumulated metabolites.**

B. **Treatment** often consists of a low-protein diet, which is supplemented with just enough of the unmetabolized amino acid(s) to allow normal protein synthesis but not so much as to allow catabolism and accumulation of toxic intermediates.

Case 24-1 Revisited

The low BUN levels and high levels of ammonia and glutamine (a storage form of ammonia) suggest a defect in the urea cycle. The respiratory alkalosis demonstrated by the low P_{CO_2} is due to the hyperventilation caused by the hyperammonemia. The lack of citrulline indicates a defective enzyme leading to citrulline formation. High urine levels of orotic acid, which is derived from carbamoyl phosphate, indicate a defect in an enzyme that utilizes this compound. Therefore, the defective enzyme is ornithine transcarbamoylase, which converts carbamoyl phosphate to citrulline. A defect in ornithine transcarbamoylase results in type II hyperammonemia.

The blood transfusion and hemodialysis were done to prevent brain damage from the high serum ammonia levels. Sodium benzoate and sodium phenylacetate reduce the serum ammonia level by reacting with glycine and glutamine to form adducts, which are excreted in the urine (see III D 3 c). A diet is provided that provides adequate, but not excessive, amounts of essential amino acids, to minimize the need for urea cycle function. The diet is supplemented with arginine because the normal endogenous source of this amino acid is not synthesized by the action of the urea cycle.

STUDY QUESTIONS

DIRECTIONS: Each of the numbered items or incomplete statements in this section is followed by answers or by completions of the statement. Select the **one** lettered answer or completion that is **best** in each case.

1. Which one of the following is a purely ketogenic essential amino acid?

(A) Leucine
(B) Cysteine
(C) Tyrosine
(D) Histidine
(E) Proline

2. Which one of the following statements describes the ubiquitin-mediated degradation of proteins in the cytosol?

(A) One molecule of ubiquitin binds to the protein to be degraded
(B) The process is catalyzed by a single enzyme
(C) The process depends on adenosine triphosphate (ATP)
(D) The N-terminal residue of ubiquitin becomes covalently attached to the protein to be degraded
(E) Ubiquitin becomes covalently attached to the C-terminus of the protein to be degraded

Questions 3-5

A patient with a history of urinary tract problems now suffers from kidney stones. The patient is diagnosed as having a genetic defect in an amino acid transport system, which is the cause of this problem.

3. Which one of the following amino acids is likely to be in excess in the urine of this patient?

(A) Lysine
(B) Proline
(C) Alanine
(D) Tryptophan
(E) Glutamic acid

4. Which compound crystallizes to form the kidney stones?

(A) Cysteine
(B) Lysine
(C) Arginine
(D) Cystine
(E) Indoxyl sulfate

5. Which one of the following would be a possible treatment for this patient?

(A) Administration of niacin
(B) A high-protein diet
(C) Administration of penicillamine
(D) Restriction of fluid intake
(E) A cysteine-rich diet

6. Which one of the following amino acids can undergo deamination by dehydration?

(A) Glutamine
(B) Leucine
(C) Serine
(D) Valine
(E) Lysine

7. A patient with a genetic defect in the enzyme that produces N-acetylglutamate would present with

(A) elevated levels of argininosuccinate
(B) no detectable citrulline
(C) elevated levels of arginine
(D) elevated levels of urea
(E) no detectable ornithine

DIRECTIONS: Each group of items in this section consists of lettered options followed by a set of numbered items. For each item, select the **one** lettered option that is most closely associated with it. Each lettered option may be selected once, more than once, or not at all.

Questions 8–10

Match the following statements regarding disorders of amino acid catabolism with the correct cofactor.

(A) Pyridoxal phosphate
(B) Tetrahydrobiopterin
(C) Thiamine
(D) Vitamin B_{12}
(E) Lipoamide

8. The unavailability of this cofactor causes certain symptoms consistent with a diagnosis of phenylketonuria

9. Some patients with symptoms of maple syrup urine disease respond to therapeutic doses of this compound

10. Some patients with methylmalonic aciduria respond to therapeutic doses of this compound

Questions 11–14

Match the following symptoms of disorders of amino acid catabolism with the correct treatment.

(A) A diet low in phenylalanine
(B) A leucine-restricted diet and administration of glycine
(C) Restricted intake of branched-chain amino acids
(D) A low-protein diet supplemented with arginine
(E) Therapeutic doses of vitamin B_{12}

11. High serum levels of ammonia

12. High serum levels of isovaleric acid

13. High serum levels of phenylpyruvate

14. High serum and urine levels of valine, leucine, and isoleucine and their corresponding α-keto acids

ANSWERS AND EXPLANATIONS

1. The answer is A [II A; IV A; Table 24-3]. The nine essential amino acids that cannot be synthesized by humans are leucine, isoleucine, valine, methionine, threonine, lysine, histidine, phenylalanine, and tryptophan. Although histidine is essential, it is classified as purely glucogenic because it is metabolized to α-ketoglutarate. Leucine, which is metabolized to acetyl coenzyme A (CoA) and acetoacetyl CoA, is purely ketogenic.

2. The answer is C [I B 3]. Ubiquitin plays an important role in designating the proteins to be degraded. The C-terminal residue of ubiquitin becomes covalently attached to the lysine residues of the proteins to be degraded. Multiple ubiquitin molecules may bind to a single protein. Three proteins (i.e., E1, E2, and E3) catalyze the formation of the ubiquitin-protein conjugate, which is degraded via an adenosine triphosphate (ATP)-dependent process.

3–5. The answers are: 3-A, 4-D, 5-C [I A 3 b]. Defects in amino acid transport cause increased levels of those amino acids in the urine. This patient suffers from cystinuria, a defect in the transport system for the basic amino acids (i.e., lysine and arginine), which also transports cystine, the disulfide-linked dimer of cysteine. As such, lysine is expected to accumulate in the urine. Because cystine is relatively insoluble in the urine, its accumulation leads to deposition of crystals, which may cause urinary tract infections and kidney stones. When the other amino acids accumulate, they are expected to be excreted in the soluble form. Both increasing the dietary intake of protein or cysteine or restricting fluid intake, which would decrease the volume of urine and effectively increase the concentration of cystine, would exacerbate the problem. Administration of drugs, such as penicillamine, which react with cystine in a way to render it more soluble, can be an effective treatment.

6. The answer is C [III C 1]. The amino groups of most amino acids are removed by transamination. The hydroxyl group in the side chain of serine allows the deamination of this amino acid to be coupled with the irreversible elimination of water (i.e., dehydration). The enzyme that catalyzes this reaction is serine dehydratase.

7. The answer is B [III D 1 a (2)]. N-acetylglutamate is a required positive allosteric effector of carbamoyl phosphate synthetase, the first enzyme of the urea cycle that catalyzes the formation of carbamoyl phosphate from ammonia, carbon dioxide, and adenosine triphosphate (ATP). In the urea cycle, carbamoyl phosphate next reacts with ornithine to form citrulline. In the absence of N-acetylglutamate, carbamoyl phosphate will not form. Thus, ornithine levels are high, and citrulline is undetectable. Argininosuccinate, arginine, and urea, which would be formed during subsequent reactions, would also be undetectable.

8-10. The answers are: 8-B [V F 1 b], **9-C** [V D 2], **10-D** [V E 3]. Phenylalanine is formed by the hydroxylation of tyrosine in the reaction that is catalyzed by phenylalanine hydroxylase. This enzyme requires tetrahydrobiopterin as a cofactor. Atypical phenylketonuria (PKU) is caused by a defect in dihydrobiopteridine reductase, which is needed to regenerate the cofactor after it is oxidized to dihydrobiopterin. Therefore, although phenylalanine hydroxylase is normal, the conversion of phenylalanine to tyrosine is blocked, as in classic PKU.

Branched-chain α-keto acids (which are derived from valine, leucine, and isoleucine) are all recognized by a common enzyme, branched-chain keto acid dehydrogenase, which catalyzes their oxidative decarboxylation. A defect in this enzyme is responsible for the disorder that is known as maple syrup urine disease. This enzyme utilizes as cofactors lipoamide, thiamine pyrophosphate, flavin adenine dinucleotide (FAD), and oxidized nicotinamide adenine dinucleotide (NAD+). In some cases, the defect of the enzyme reduces its affinity for the thiamine pyrophosphate cofactor. These patients may respond to treatment with therapeutic doses of thiamine.

Methylmalonyl coenzyme A (CoA) is converted to succinyl CoA by the enzyme methylmalonyl CoA mutase. A defect in this enzyme causes a disorder known as methylmalonic aciduria. The enzyme utilizes as a cofactor 5′-deoxyadenosylcobalamin, which is derived from vitamin B_{12}. Some forms of this disorder are treatable by administration of high doses of vitamin B_{12}.

11-14. The answers are: 11-D [III D 3], **12-B** [V D 3], **13-A** [V F 1], **14-C** [V D 2]. Hyperammonemia, an accumulation of ammonia in the blood, is a symptom of a defect in an enzyme of the urea cycle. Patients with partial deficiencies of a urea cycle enzyme benefit from restriction of protein intake to minimize the formation of ammonia from degradation of amino acids. Because arginine is normally synthesized by the action of the urea cycle, low-protein diets used in the treatment of urea cycle disorders should be supplemented with arginine.

Isovaleric acidemia is a disease caused by a deficiency of isovaleryl coenzyme A (CoA) dehydrogenase, an enzyme involved in the degradative pathway of leucine. Treatment includes restriction of dietary leucine and administration of glycine, which reacts with the toxic isovaleric acid to form an adduct that may be excreted in the urine.

The accumulation of toxic derivatives of phenylalanine, such as phenylpyruvate, is a symptom of phenylketonuria (PKU), which is caused by a defect in phenylalanine hydroxylase. This disorder is treated with a phenylalanine-restricted diet.

The three α-keto acids that are derived from these branched-chain amino acids are all recognized by a common enzyme, branched-chain keto acid dehydrogenase, which catalyzes their oxidative decarboxylation. A defect in this enzyme is responsible for the disorder known as maple syrup urine disease, which is characterized by high plasma and urine levels of each of these amino acids and their corresponding α-keto acids. Treatment includes restriction of dietary intake of these amino acids.

Chapter 25

Biosynthesis of Amino Acids and Amino Acid–Derived Compounds
Victor Davidson

Case 25-1

An infant appears to be normal up to 6 months of age and then begins to exhibit impaired mental development and lethargy. The condition progressively deteriorates, and the child is comatose when admitted to the hospital. Urinalysis reveals high levels of disulfide amino acids. Blood analysis reveals very high levels of homocysteine (normal = 0), no methionine (normal = 10–50 μmol/L), and no other amino acid abnormalities. Serum levels of folate are below normal. The patient is administered daily therapeutic doses of methionine, vitamin B_6, vitamin B_{12}, and folate. Dramatic improvement was observed with this treatment.

- What is the diagnosis?
- What is the rationale for the treatment?

I. BIOSYNTHESIS OF AMINO ACIDS

A. **The nine essential amino acids** must be acquired from the diet (see Chapter 24 II A).

B. **The eleven nonessential amino acids** are synthesized by mammals as follows (Figure 25-1).

1. **Alanine** is formed from pyruvate by transamination (see Chapter 24 III A).

2. **Aspartate** is formed from oxaloacetate by transamination.

3. **Asparagine** is formed by amidation of aspartate.

4. **Glutamate** is formed by reductive amination of α-ketoglutarate (see Chapter 24 III B).

5. **Glutamine** is formed by the amidation of glutamate.

6. **Arginine** is formed in the urea cycle (see Chapter 24 III D 1 d).

7. **Proline** is formed in two steps from glutamate.

8. **Serine** is synthesized from 3-phosphoglycerate, a glycolytic intermediate (see Chapter 16 III D).

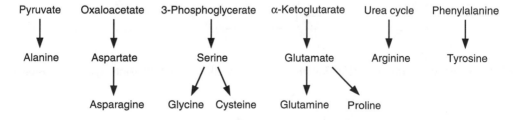

FIGURE 25-1. Precursors for the biosynthesis of nonessential amino acids.

9. **Glycine** is converted to serine by serine hydroxymethyltransferase.

10. **Cysteine** is synthesized from serine and methionine (see II C 5). Thus, it is nonessential only if methionine is provided in the diet.

11. **Tyrosine** is formed from phenylalanine (see Chapter 24 V F 1). Thus, it is nonessential only if phenylalanine is provided in the diet.

II. **AMINO ACIDS AS MAJOR INPUTS TO THE ONE-CARBON POOL.** One-carbon groups are frequently transferred during metabolism. These one-carbon fragments exist in a readily available pool. Different carriers are employed for one-carbon groups of different oxidation states.

A. **Biotin** (see Chapter 14 II B) is a carrier of carbon dioxide.

B. **Tetrahydrofolate (THF)** is derived from folic acid (see Chapter 14 II D). It carries one-carbon groups of all oxidation states (Figure 25-2) except carbon dioxide. Examples of THF-dependent enzymes include:

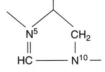

FIGURE 25-2. Tetrahydrofolate and its derivatives. Only the reactive portions of the substituted tetrahydrofolate molecules are shown.

1. **Serine hydroxymethyltransferase**

$$\text{Glycine} + N^5,N^{10}\text{-Methylene THF} \rightleftharpoons \text{Serine} + \text{THF}$$

2. **Homocysteine methyltransferase**

$$\text{Homocysteine} + N^5\text{-Methyl THF} \rightleftharpoons \text{Methionine} + \text{THF}$$

3. **Thymidylate synthase**

$$\text{2'-Deoxyuridylate} + N^5,N^{10}\text{-Methylene THF} \rightleftharpoons \text{2'-Deoxythymidylate} + \text{Dihydrofolate}$$

C. **S-Adenosylmethionine (SAM)** is the primary donor of methyl groups to a wide variety of acceptors during biosynthesis. This process occurs by a series of reactions referred to as the **activated methyl cycle** (Figure 25-3).

1. **Methionine to SAM.** In this reaction, the adenosyl group of adenosine triphosphate (ATP) is transferred to the methionine sulfur.

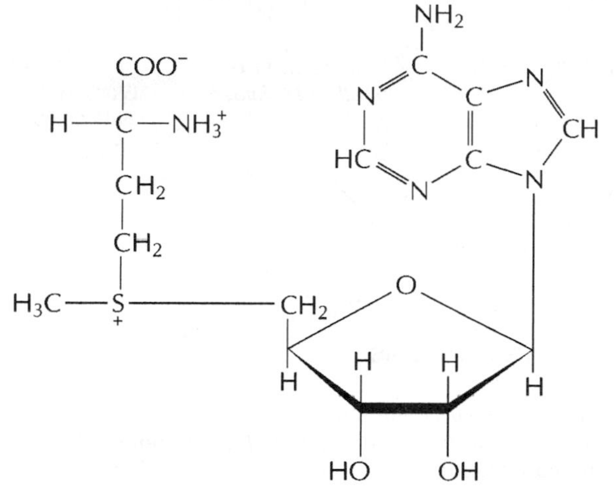

S-Adenosylmethionine

2. **Methyl transfer from SAM to an acceptor molecule.** The methyl group attached to the sulfur of SAM is transferred to an acceptor molecule to form a methylated product plus S-adenosylhomocysteine. Examples of such methylation reactions include:
   a. Norepinephrine to epinephrine
   b. Guanidinoacetate to creatine
   c. Acetylserotonin to melatonin
   d. Phosphatidylethanolamine to phosphatidylcholine
   e. Methylation of DNA

3. S-Adenosylhomocysteine is hydrolyzed to adenosine and homocysteine.

4. **Regeneration of methionine from homocysteine** is catalyzed by **homocysteine methyltransferase**, which requires two cofactors (see Figure 25-3).
   a. The **methylcobalamin** form of vitamin B_{12} (see Chapter 14 II C) provides the methyl group needed to form methionine.
   b. N^5-**methyl THF** provides a methyl group to regenerate methylcobalamin.
   c. N^5-Methyl THF must then be **regenerated.**
      (1) **Serine hydroxymethyltransferase** (see II B 1) catalyzes the conversion of THF to N^5,N^{10}-methylene THF.
      (2) N^5,N^{10}-**Methylene THF reductase** catalyzes the conversion of N^5,N^{10}-methylene THF to N^5-Methyl THF.

5. An important side reaction of the activated methyl cycle is the **synthesis of cysteine from homocysteine.**

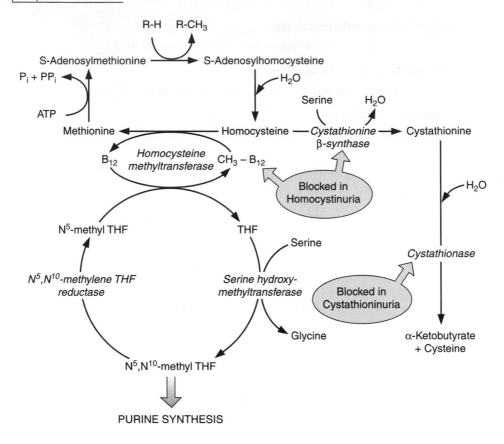

FIGURE 25-3. The activated methyl cycle and biosynthetic pathway for cysteine. Enzyme names are in *italics. ATP* = adenosine triphosphate; *B_{12}* = cobalamin; *CH_3-B_{12}* = methylcobalamin; *P_i* = inorganic phosphate; *PP_i* = inorganic pyrophosphate; *R-CH_3* = methylated product; *R-H* = substrate molecule to be methylated; *THF* = tetrahydrofolate.

    a. Cystathionine synthase catalyzes the condensation of homocysteine and serine to form cystathionine. This enzyme requires **pyridoxal phosphate (PLP)** as a cofactor.

    b. Cystathionase catalyzes the hydrolysis of cystathionine to cysteine and α-ketobutyrate. A deficiency in this enzyme causes **cystathioninuria.**

  6. Homocystinuria is the accumulation of homocystine, the disulfide-linked dimer of homocysteine, which forms when homocysteine is in excess.

    a. Causes

      (1) A defect in cystathionine synthase

      (2) A defect in homocysteine methyltransferase

      (3) The unavailability of N^5-methyl THF or methylcobalamin

    b. Treatment. Some forms of this disorder may be treated with therapeutic doses of vitamins B_6, B_{12}, or folic acid.

    c. High serum levels of homocysteine also have been implicated as a contributing factor in heart disease.

III. TYROSINE-DERIVED BIOLOGICALLY IMPORTANT COMPOUNDS (Figure 25-4; Table 25-1)

A. **Catecholamine biosynthesis** occurs in the adrenal medulla and neurons.

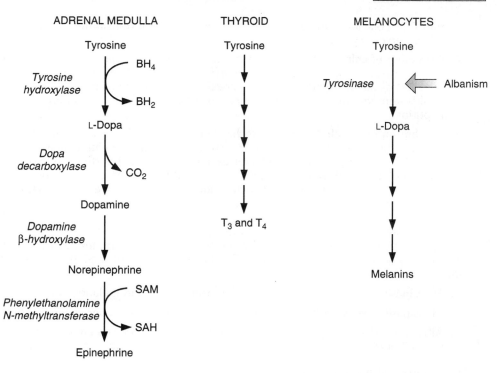

FIGURE 25-4. The biosynthesis of biologically important compounds from tyrosine. Enzyme names are in *italics*. BH_4 = tetrahydrobiopterin; BH_2 = dihydrobiopterin; *SAH* = S-adenosylhomocysteine; *SAM* = S-adenosylmethionine; T_3 = 3,3′,5-triiodothyronine; T_4 = 3,3′,5,5′-tetraiodothyronine.

TABLE 25-1. Some Amino Acid–Derived Compounds of Biologic Importance

Compound	Precursor Amino Acid	Primary Function
Carnitine	Lysine	Fatty acid transporter
Creatine phosphate	Glycine, arginine	Energy storage compound
Dopamine	Tyrosine	Neurotransmitter
Epinephrine	Tyrosine	Hormone
GABA	Glutamate	Neurotransmitter
Histamine	Histidine	Vasodilator
Melanin	Tyrosine	Pigment
Melatonin	Tryptophan	Hormone
Nitric oxide	Arginine	Vasodilator, neurotransmitter
Norepinephrine	Tyrosine	Neurotransmitter
Serotonin	Tryptophan	Vasoconstrictor
Thyroxine	Tyrosine	Hormone

GABA = γ-aminobutyric acid.

1. **Formation of dopa.** Tyrosine is hydroxylated to 3,4-dihydroxyphenylalanine (dopa) by **tyrosine hydroxylase,** which requires **tetrahydrobiopterin (BH_4)** as a cofactor. This is the **rate-limiting step** in catecholamine biosynthesis. The enzyme is allosteric, with dopamine, norepinephrine, and epinephrine acting as negative effectors.

2. **Formation of dopamine** is catalyzed by **dopa decarboxylase,** a PLP-dependent enzyme.

3. **Formation of norepinephrine. Dopamine β-hydroxylase** hydroxylates the aromatic ring of dopamine to yield norepinephrine. This enzyme requires **copper and vita-**

min C as cofactors. Norepinephrine is the **major neural transmitter** of the sympathetic nervous system.

4. **Formation of epinephrine** occurs in the adrenal medulla, where the amino group of norepinephrine is methylated by **phenylethanolamine N-methyltransferase,** using SAM as the methyl donor. The synthesis of the enzyme is induced by glucocorticoids from the surrounding adrenal cortex, and its production is inhibited by epinephrine.

5. **Catabolism of catecholamines. Catechol-O-methyl transferase** uses SAM to methylate catecholamines. This is followed by oxidation by **monoamine oxidase** and aldehyde dehydrogenase to give the major excretory product, **3-methoxy-4-hydroxymandelic acid (vanillylmandelic acid; VMA).** VMA excretion levels are used as an aid in the diagnosis of adrenal **pheochromocytomas,** which are tumors that produce huge amounts of catecholamines.

B. **Biosynthesis of melanins.** Melanins are biologic pigments. Their synthesis occurs only in pigment-producing cells called **melanocytes.** Melanins are synthesized from tyrosine by a sequence of several reactions. The first step is the conversion of tyrosine to dopa.

1. **Tyrosinase** catalyzes the conversion of tyrosine to dopa in melanocytes.

2. Tyrosinase does not require tetrahydrobiopterin, but uses **copper** as a cofactor.

3. **Albinism** is due to a genetic defect in tyrosinase, which causes afflicted individuals (i.e., **albinos**) to lack pigmentation because they cannot synthesize melanins.

C. **Biosynthesis of thyroid hormones**

1. $3,3',5,5'$-Tetraiodothyronine **(thyroxine; T_4)** and $3,3',5$-triiodothyronine **(T_3)** are hormones secreted by the thyroid gland.

2. T_4 and T_3 are formed in the follicle cells of the thyroid gland by iodination of tyrosine residues, which are in peptide linkage in chains of the protein **thyroglobulin.**

3. Iodinated thyroglobulin is stored in the lumen of the thyroid follicles until it is required. Then T_3 and T_4 are hydrolyzed off and secreted into the circulation.

IV. **TRYPTOPHAN-DERIVED BIOLOGICALLY IMPORTANT COMPOUNDS** (see Table 25-1)

A. **Serotonin** is a **potent vasoconstrictor** and stimulator of smooth muscle contraction.

1. Serotonin is synthesized by neurons in the hypothalamus and brain stem, by the pineal gland, and by chromaffin cells of the gastrointestinal tract.

2. The rate-limiting step is catalyzed by **tryptophan hydroxylase,** which requires **tetrahydrobiopterin** and forms 5-hydroxytryptophan (5-HTP) from tryptophan.

3. Decarboxylation of 5-HTP yields serotonin (5-hydroxytryptamine; 5-HT).

4. **Degradation of serotonin** is initiated by oxidative deamination by monoamine oxidase followed either by oxidation by aldehyde dehydrogenase to yield 5-hydroxyindoleacetic acid (5-HIAA) or by alcohol dehydrogenase to yield 5-hydroxytryptophol (5-HTOL). 5-HIAA and 5-HTOL are excreted in the urine.

B. **Melatonin** is a **hormone** produced by the pineal gland, which has effects on the hypothalamic–pituitary system.

1. Serotonin formed in the pineal gland is converted to 5-hydroxy-N-acetyl tryptamine by N-acetyl transferase.

2. This compound is methylated with SAM by an O-methyl transferase to melatonin.

C. The **nicotinamide ring of nicotinamide adenine dinucleotide (NAD⁺)** can be synthesized from intermediates in the catabolism of tryptophan via quinolinate.

V. **GLUTATHIONE is a tripeptide formed from glutamate, cysteine, and glycine.** Its structure is unusual in that the peptide bond to glutamate is formed with the **γ-carboxyl group** on the amino acid side chain rather than the carboxyl on the α-carbon. Glutathione has important functions in the cell.

A. It serves as a sulfhydryl buffer, **regulating the redox state of the cell** by maintaining an appropriate equilibrium between its oxidized (dimeric) and reduced (monomeric) forms.

$$\gamma\text{---Glu---Cys---Gly} \qquad \gamma\text{---Glu---Cys---Gly}$$
$$\mid \qquad\qquad\qquad\qquad\quad \mid$$
$$\text{SH} \qquad\qquad\qquad\qquad\quad \text{S}$$
$$\mid$$
$$\text{S}$$
$$\mid$$
$$\gamma\text{---Glu---Cys---Gly}$$

$$\text{(Reduced)} \qquad\qquad\qquad \text{(Oxidized)}$$

B. It plays a role in the **transport of amino acids** across the plasma membrane in certain cells.

C. It serves as a **cofactor** for certain enzymes, such as **glutathione peroxidase,** which uses reduced glutathione to detoxify peroxides.

VI. **BIOSYNTHESIS OF OTHER AMINO ACID–DERIVED COMPOUNDS** (see Table 25-1)

A. **γ-Aminobutyrate (GABA)** is formed from glutamate by **glutamate decarboxylase,** a PLP-dependent enzyme. GABA appears to be an **inhibitory transmitter** in the brain and spinal cord.

B. **Histamine is a potent vasodilator** and may be a neural transmitter. It is released during allergic reactions.

   1. Histidine decarboxylase catalyzes the formation of histamine from histidine.

   2. Antihistamine drugs are compounds that bear a structural similarity to histamine and can prevent its action.

C. **Nitric oxide (NO)** is an important biomolecule involved in vasodilation and neural transmission. It activates guanylate cyclase to produce cyclic guanidine monophosphate, an important second messenger.

   1. NO is derived from one of the guanidino nitrogens of the side chain of **arginine.** Its formation is catalyzed by **nitric oxide synthase.**

   2. NO is very short-lived and reacts with oxygen to form nitrite, which is then converted to nitrate and excreted in the urine.

D. **Carnitine** is required for transport of long-chain fatty acids across the mitochondrial membrane (see Chapter 22 II A 2).

   1. Carnitine is **derived from lysine residues** of certain proteins.

   2. The side chain amino group of lysine is trimethylated using SAM to form trimethyl-lysine.

   3. This residue is released from the protein by hydrolysis and converted in four steps to carnitine.

E. **Creatine phosphate** is a high-energy phosphate-storage compound found in muscle (see Chapter 13 IV B 3). It is formed from **glycine, arginine, and SAM.**

   1. The guanidinium group of arginine is transferred to glycine to form guanidi-noacetate.

   2. Guanidinoacetate is methylated by SAM to form creatine.

   3. ATP is used to phosphorylate creatine to creatine phosphate.

F. **Carnosine and anserine are formed from histidine and β-alanine.** Carnosine and anserine are dipeptides that occur in muscle in some species, although their function is unclear. Carnosine also is present in the olfactory pathway in the brain.

G. **Polyamines (i.e., putrescine, spermine, and spermidine) are derived from ornithine.** The polyamines are polycations at physiologic pH, and they associate with negatively charged cell components, such as membranes and nucleic acids.

H. The use of amino acids in **nucleotide metabolism** is described in Chapter 26.

VII. **HEME METABOLISM.** Heme possesses a porphyrin ring (Figure 25-5) and is the prosthetic group of several proteins and enzymes, including hemoglobin, cytochrome c, catalase, and certain peroxidases.

A. **Biosynthesis. The complex heme molecule is synthesized from two simple precursors, glycine and succinyl coenzyme A** (CoA; Figure 25-6).

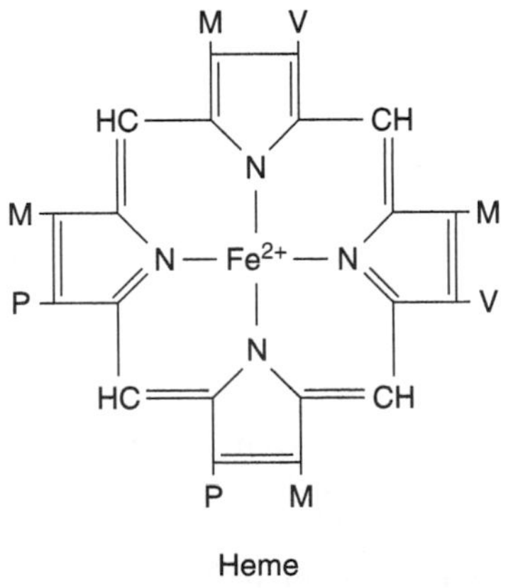

Heme

FIGURE 25-5. A heme molecule with an atom of iron *(Fe)* in the center of the porphyrin ring, and side chains abbreviated as *M* = methyl; *V* = vinyl; *P* = propionate.

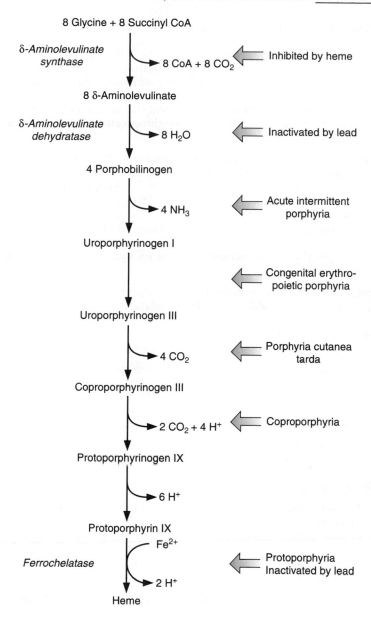

FIGURE 25-6. The biosynthesis of heme. The names of key enzymes are indicated in *italics*. Reactions that are blocked in metabolic disorders of heme synthesis are indicated by a *double arrow*. CoA = coenzyme A; CO_2 = carbon dioxide.

1. **δ-Aminolevulinate** (ALA) synthesis from glycine and succinyl CoA is catalyzed by **ALA synthase,** which utilizes **PLP** as a cofactor.
   a. **This is the rate-limiting, committed step in heme biosynthesis.**
   b. This reaction is **regulated by the level of heme.**
      (1) ALA synthase activity is inhibited by heme.
      (2) The transcription of the ALA synthase gene is repressed by heme.

2. **Porphobilinogen,** which contains a pyrrole ring, is synthesized from two molecules of ALA by ALA dehydratase (porphobilinogen synthase).

3. **Uroporphyrinogen,** a tetrapyrrole, is synthesized from four molecules of porphobilinogen.
   a. **Uroporphyrinogen synthase** catalyzes both the condensation of the four substrate molecules and the subsequent cyclization to form a tetrapyrrole ring, uroporphyrinogen I. **Acute intermittent porphyria** is due to a deficiency of this enzyme.
   b. **Uroporphyrinogen III cosynthase** catalyzes an isomerization reaction to yield uroporphyrinogen III. **Congenital erythropoietic porphyria** is due to a deficiency of this enzyme.

4. **Protoporphyrin IX** is formed from uroporphobilinogen III.
   a. **Uroporphyrinogen decarboxylase** catalyzes the decarboxylation of four of the side chains of uroporphobilinogen III to form coproporphyrinogen III. **Porphyria cutanea tarda** is due to a deficiency of this enzyme.
   b. **Coproporphyrinogen oxidase** decarboxylates two of the side chains of coproporphyrinogen III to form protoporphyrinogen IX. **Coproporphyria** is due to a deficiency of this enzyme.
   c. **Protoporphyrinogen oxidase** removes six hydrogen atoms to form **protoporphyrin IX.**

5. **Protoheme IX (heme)** is formed from protoporphyrin IX by the insertion of iron (Fe^{2+}) in a reaction catalyzed by **ferrochelatase. Protoporphyria** is due to a deficiency of this enzyme.

B. **Disorders of heme biosynthesis** (see Figure 25-6).

1. **Porphyrias** are genetic defects in enzymes of heme biosynthesis.
   a. Porphyrias result in excessive accumulation of intermediates in heme biosynthesis that cannot be further metabolized by the body.
   b. **Symptoms** of porphyrias include abdominal pain, dermatologic problems, neurologic abnormalities, and photosensitivity.

2. **Lead poisoning** affects heme biosynthesis. Two enzymes, ALA dehydratase and ferrochelatase, are inactivated by lead.

C. **Heme degradation**

1. **Red blood cell destruction** usually occurs in the spleen, although some occurs in the liver. When red cell destruction occurs elsewhere (e.g., in hemolytic anemias), two carrier proteins prevent the loss of iron via the kidney that could otherwise occur.
   a. **Haptoglobin** binds methemoglobin dimers.
   b. **Hemopexin** binds free heme.

2. **Conversion of heme to biliverdin** is catalyzed by **heme oxygenase.** The porphyrin ring is cleaved, and iron is released.

3. **Biliverdin is reduced by nicotinamide adenine dinucleotide phosphate (NADPH) to bilirubin.** Bilirubin, which is poorly soluble, is transported to the liver bound to serum albumin.

4. **In the liver, bilirubin is conjugated to glucuronic acid.** The bilirubin diglucuronide that is formed is soluble and is secreted into the bile.
   a. **Uridine diphosphate (UDP)-glucuronyl transferase** catalyzes this reaction.
   b. **Deficiencies**
      (1) **Crigler-Najjar syndrome** is due to a deficiency in this enzyme and results in severe jaundice.
      (2) **Neonatal jaundice** is a temporary condition caused by production of insufficient levels of UDP-glucuronyl transferase by the infant. This is typically treated by **phototherapy.** The products from the irradiation of bilirubin are more soluble than bilirubin and can be excreted by the liver into the bile without conjugation with glucuronic acid.

    c. Classification of bilirubin
       (1) Direct bilirubin refers to conjugated bilirubin.
       (2) Indirect bilirubin refers to free, unconjugated bilirubin.

5. Bilirubin diglucuronide is hydrolyzed to free bilirubin in the bowel, where it is converted to **urobilinogens** and **stercobilinogens,** which are excreted in the urine and feces.

6. Jaundice is a condition in which the blood contains excessive amounts of bilirubin and related compounds. Bilirubin and related compounds are deposited in the skin and mucous membranes, which gives affected patients a yellowish hue.
    a. Prehepatic jaundice is caused by diseases or intoxications that cause abnormally high levels of red blood cell destruction and excessive release of hemoglobin, which overwhelms the body's capacity to degrade heme.
    b. Hepatic jaundice is caused by disorders of the liver (e.g., hepatitis, cirrhosis) that prevent uptake of bilirubin or the conjugation of bilirubin to glucuronate.
    c. Posthepatic jaundice is caused by conditions or physical obstructions that prevent the bile from reaching the intestinal tract.

Transport and storage of iron (Fe^{3+})

1. Transport. Fe^{3+} is transported in the blood bound to a protein synthesized in the liver, **transferrin.**

2. Storage. Fe^{3+} is stored in the cells in combination with the protein **ferritin.**

Case 25-1 Revisited

The patient was suffering from homocystinuria due to the inability to convert homocysteine to methionine. The excess homocysteine reacts with itself to dimerize to homocystine, which is not normally present in significant amounts in the serum or urine. Homocystinuria may become apparent at different stages of life and may present with a variety of symptoms, depending on the severity of the condition. Common symptoms include mental retardation, thromboses, osteoporosis, and dislocated lenses in the eye. When the condition presents early in life, as in this case, immediate treatment is critical.

    The rationale for the treatment is as follows. Methionine supplementation ensures that adequate levels are present for growth. Vitamin B_6 (i.e., PLP) may increase cystathione-β-synthase activity, which decreases homocysteine levels. Vitamin B_{12} may enhance methionine formation by homocysteine methyltransferase. It is possible that these symptoms could be due to a deficiency of N^5,N^{10}-methylene THF reductase. Further tests would be required to confirm this possibility. Therapeutic doses of folate hopefully allow formation of some N^5-methyl THF by an enzyme with diminished activity. Although all four of these treatments may not have been necessary to correct the condition in this case, the emergency of the situation and rapid and dramatic response dictated this therapy.

STUDY QUESTIONS

DIRECTIONS: Each of the numbered items or incomplete statements in this section is followed by answers or by completions of the statement. Select the **one** lettered answer or completion that is **best** in each case.

1. The rate-limiting step in catecholamine biosynthesis is

(A) the hydroxylation of tyrosine
(B) the hydroxylation of phenylalanine
(C) the formation of dopamine
(D) the reduction of dihydrobiopterin
(E) the hydroxylation of dopamine

2. Epinephrine is formed from norepinephrine by which one of the following actions?

(A) Hydroxylation
(B) Decarboxylation
(C) Oxidative deamination
(D) O-Methylation
(E) N-Methylation

3. Which one of the following nutrients is a precursor for a cofactor that carries one-carbon groups of different oxidation states?

(A) Methionine
(B) Thiamine
(C) Folic acid
(D) Biotin
(E) Pryidoxine

4. During the degradation of heme, which one of the following actions occurs?

(A) Heme is initially converted to bilirubin
(B) Reduction of bilirubin yields biliverdin
(C) Bilirubin is conjugated to glucuronic acid in the liver
(D) Failure to conjugate bilirubin to glucuronic acid causes porphyria
(E) Free (unconjugated) bilirubin may be reduced to urobilinogen in the liver

DIRECTIONS: Each group of items in this section consists of lettered options followed by a set of numbered items. For each item, select the **one** lettered option that is most closely associated with it. Each lettered option may be selected once, more than once, or not at all.

Questions 5–7

Match the following descriptions with the correct medical problem.

(A) Albinism
(B) Jaundice
(C) Adrenal tumor
(D) Homocystinuria
(E) Protoporphyria

5. May be characterized by high urinary levels of vanillylmandelic acid

6. May be caused by a defect in tyrosinase

7. Is one consequence of a vitamin B_{12} deficiency

Questions 8–11

Match the following descriptions to the correct amino acid.

(A) Arginine
(B) Tyrosine
(C) Tryptophan
(D) Glycine
(E) Glutamate

8. The precursor of thyroid hormones

9. The precursor of the potent vasoconstrictor serotonin

10. The precursor of nitric oxide

11. A precursor of heme

ANSWERS AND EXPLANATIONS

1. The answer is A [III A 1]. Tyrosine hydroxylation to form dopa is the rate-limiting step in catecholamine biosynthesis. The enzyme, tyrosine hydroxylase, requires tetrahydrobiopterin as a cofactor, but the reduction of dihydrobiopterin (the oxidized form of the cofactor) is not the slow step in catecholamine biosynthesis.

2. The answer is E [III A 4]. Epinephrine is formed in the adrenal medulla from norepinephrine by N-methylation by the methyl donor S-adenosylmethionine in a reaction catalyzed by phenylethanolamine N-methyltransferase. O-Methylation and oxidative deamination are steps in the degradation of catecholamines, and hydroxylation and decarboxylation are steps in the synthesis of norepinephrine.

3. The answer is C [II B]. Folic acid is a vitamin precursor of tetrahydrofolate, which carries one-carbon groups at all levels of oxidation except carbon dioxide (CO_2). Biotin is a carrier specific for CO_2. Thiamine is the precursor of thiamine pyrophosphate, a carrier of the two-carbon acetate group. Methionine is an amino acid that is the precursor of S-adenosylmethionine, a carrier specific for the methyl group. Pyridoxine is the vitamin precursor of pyridoxal phosphate, a cofactor involved in many reactions using amino acids as substrates.

4. The answer is C [VII C 4]. The first step in heme catabolism is the cleavage of the porphyrin ring to form biliverdin, which is then reduced to form bilirubin. Normally, the insoluble bilirubin is rendered soluble by conjugation to glucuronic acid in the liver. Failure to conjugate bilirubin to glucuronic acid leads to jaundice. Bilirubin diglucuronide is excreted in the bile; in the gut, bacterial enzymes reduce the bilirubin to urobilinogen and stercobilinogen.

5-7. The answers are: 5-C [III A 5], **6-A,** [III B 3], **7-D** [II C 6]. Vanillylmandelic acid (VMA) is the end product of the catabolism of catecholamines. Pheochromocytomas are adrenal tumors that produce huge amounts of catecholamines. High VMA excretion levels are diagnostic of this condition.

Albinism is due to a genetic defect in tyrosinase or one of the enzymes that synthesizes melanins from tyrosine. In melanocytes, tyrosinase catalyzes the conversion of tyrosine to dopa, the initial step in this process.

Homocystinuria is the accumulation of homocystine, the disulfide-linked dimer of homocysteine, which forms when homocysteine is in excess. This may be caused by defects in the enzymes that utilize homocysteine, or by unavailability of an essential cofactor for the enzyme. Methylcobalamin, which is derived from vitamin B_{12}, is required by homocysteine methyltransferase.

8-11. The answers are: 8-B [III C], **9-C** [IV A], **10-A** [VI C], **11-D** [VII A 1]. Tyrosine is the precursor of thyroid hormones. It is iodinated while it is in peptide linkage in the protein thyroglobulin. Mono- and diiodotyrosines are formed, which react further to form thyroxine (T_4) and triiodothyronine (T_3).

Tryptophan is the precursor of serotonin. Tryptophan is hydroxylated by tryptophan hydroxylase and then decarboxylated to yield 5-hydroxytryptamine, which is serotonin.

Nitric oxide (NO) is an important biomolecule involved in vasodilation and neural transmission. It is derived from one of the guanidino nitrogens of the side chain of arginine. Its formation is catalyzed by nitric oxide synthase.

The complex heme molecule is synthesized from glycine and succinyl coenzyme A (CoA). The first step in this process is the reaction catalyzed by δ-aminolevulinate synthase.

Chapter 26

Nucleotide Metabolism
Susan Wellman
Donald Sittman

Case 26-1.

A 50-year-old man presents with severe pain of his left great toe (metatarsophalangeal joint). The patient reports feeling fine when he went to bed but awakening in the middle of the night because of severe toe pain. He has no memory of previously injuring his foot. The patient's history also reveals that he ate a very rich meal and consumed a good deal of wine the previous evening at a celebration. A physical examination of the foot reveals a warm, swollen, red, and extremely tender joint.

- What is the most likely diagnosis of this patient's problem?
- How would this diagnosis be confirmed?
- Do diet or any other factors affect this condition?
- What is the best course of treatment for this patient?

I. **SYNTHESIS OF PURINE AND PYRIMIDINE NUCLEOTIDES.** Most cellular nucleic acids arise from cellular synthesis because only small amounts of dietary nucleic acids are incorporated into cellular DNA. A review of the nomenclature of nucleotides and nucleosides as described in Chapter 6, Table 6-1 would be helpful for this chapter.

A. **5′-Phosphoribosyl-1-pyrophosphate (PRPP) is an intermediate of major significance in nucleotide metabolism.**

1. **Formation.** PRPP is formed from ribose-5-phosphate and adenosine triphosphate (ATP).

$$\text{Ribose-5-phosphate} + \text{ATP} \rightarrow \text{PRPP} + \text{AMP}$$

2. There are several **sources of ribose-5-phosphate.**
   a. **Glucose metabolism** (see Chapter 17 I A 2)
   b. **Nucleoside degradation** (see III B) generates ribose-1-phosphate, which can be converted to ribose-5-phosphate.

3. **PRPP** is required in:
   a. The de novo synthesis of pyrimidine and purine nucleotides
   b. The salvage pathways for purine nucleotides
   c. The biosynthesis of nucleotide coenzymes

4. **The cellular concentrations of PRPP are closely regulated and usually are low.** The formation of PRPP is catalyzed by **PRPP synthetase. Adenosine diphosphate (ADP) and 2,3-bisphosphoglycerate** (see Chapter 3 II B 3 c) inhibit PRPP synthetase as well as adenosine 5′-monophosphate (AMP), guanosine 5′-monophosphate (GMP), and inosine 5′-monophosphate (IMP) [see I B 4 a].

B. **De novo synthesis of purine nucleotides**

1. **Origin of the carbons and nitrogens of the purine ring**
   a. **Base.** The purine ring is built on a **molecule of PRPP.**

b. The **precursors** of the ring are **PRPP, glutamine, glycine, carbon dioxide** (CO_2), **aspartate,** and two one-carbon fragments from the one-carbon **folate** pool (see Chapter 25 II B).

2. **Synthesis of IMP.** The formation of IMP is a 10-step, energetically expensive process that uses 6 high-energy phosphate bonds (Figure 26-1).

3. **Synthesis of AMP and GMP from IMP** (Figure 26-2)
   a. **Adenylosuccinate** is formed by the addition of aspartate to IMP. **Fumarate** is then cleaved to yield AMP (adenylate; see Chapter 6, Table 6-1).
   b. **Xanthosine 5′-monophosphate** (xanthylate; XMP) is formed by the oxidation of IMP. An amino group from glutamine is then added to yield GMP (guanylate; see Chapter 6, Table 6-1).
   c. **Guanosine triphosphate** (GTP) is cleaved in the synthesis of AMP, and ATP is cleaved in the synthesis of GMP. This reciprocity helps to balance the levels of adenine and guanine nucleotides.

4. **De novo synthesis of purine nucleotides is regulated by feedback inhibition** (Figure 26-3).
   a. Both of the **enzymes** that catalyze the first two steps of IMP synthesis—**PRPP synthetase** and **PRPP amidotransferase** (see Figure 26-1, step 1)—are inhibited by IMP, GMP, and AMP.
   b. **PRPP amidotransferase has two allosteric sites:** one for IMP or GMP, and one for AMP. If both sites are occupied, then inhibition is synergistic.
   c. **Inhibition.** The synthesis of adenylosuccinate from IMP is inhibited by AMP, and the synthesis of XMP is inhibited by GMP.

C. **Salvage pathways for purine nucleotides.** There are two specific enzymes that catalyze the transfer of the ribose phosphate from PRPP to free purine bases, which are formed by the degradation of nucleotides (see III).

1. **Hypoxanthine–guanine phosphoribosyltransferase (HGPRT)** catalyzes the formation of nucleotides from either hypoxanthine or guanine (Figure 26-4). The enzyme is inhibited by high concentrations of its products, IMP and GMP.

$$\text{Hypoxanthine} + \text{PRPP} \rightarrow \text{IMP} + \text{PP}_i$$

$$\text{Guanine} + \text{PRPP} \rightarrow \text{GMP} + \text{PP}_i$$

2. **Adenine phosphoribosyltransferase (APRT)** catalyzes the formation of AMP from adenine (see Figure 26-4). The enzyme is inhibited by high concentrations of its product, AMP.

D. **De novo synthesis of pyrimidine nucleotides**

1. **Origin of the carbons and nitrogens of the pyrimidine ring**

FIGURE 26-1. Steps in the de novo biosynthesis of inosine 5′-monophosphate *(IMP)*. *(1)* The committed step is the formation of 5′-phosphoribosyl-1-amine from 5′-phosphoribosyl-1-pyrophosphate *(PRPP)* and an amino group from glutamine. The reaction is catalyzed by PRPP-amidotransferase. *(2)* A molecule of glycine is added to form N-glycinamide ribonucleotide. *(3)* A formyl group is transferred from N^{10}-formyltetrahydrofolate to form N-formylglycinamide ribonucleotide. *(4)* An amino group is transferred from another glutamine to form N-formylglycinamidine ribonucleotide. *(5)* With closure of the imidazole ring, 5-aminoimidazole ribonucleotide is formed. The bond that is formed is marked with an *asterisk*. *(6)* The addition of carbon dioxide *(CO_2)* forms 5-aminoimidazole-4-carboxylate ribonucleotide. *(7)* Aspartate is added, forming 5-aminoimidazole-4-N-succinocarboxamide ribonucleotide. *(8)* Fumarate is cleaved, leaving only the amine from the aspartate and forming 5-aminoimidazole-4-carboxamide ribonucleotide. *(9)* A formyl group is transferred from N^{10}-formyltetrahydrofolate to form 5-formamidoimidazole-4-carboxamide ribonucleotide. *(10)* IMP is formed by ring closure. The bond that is formed is marked with an *asterisk*. ADP = adenosine diphosphate; *ATP* = adenosine triphosphate; P_i = inorganic phosphate; PP_i = inorganic pyrophosphate. Groups that are added at each step are outlined with *dashed lines*.

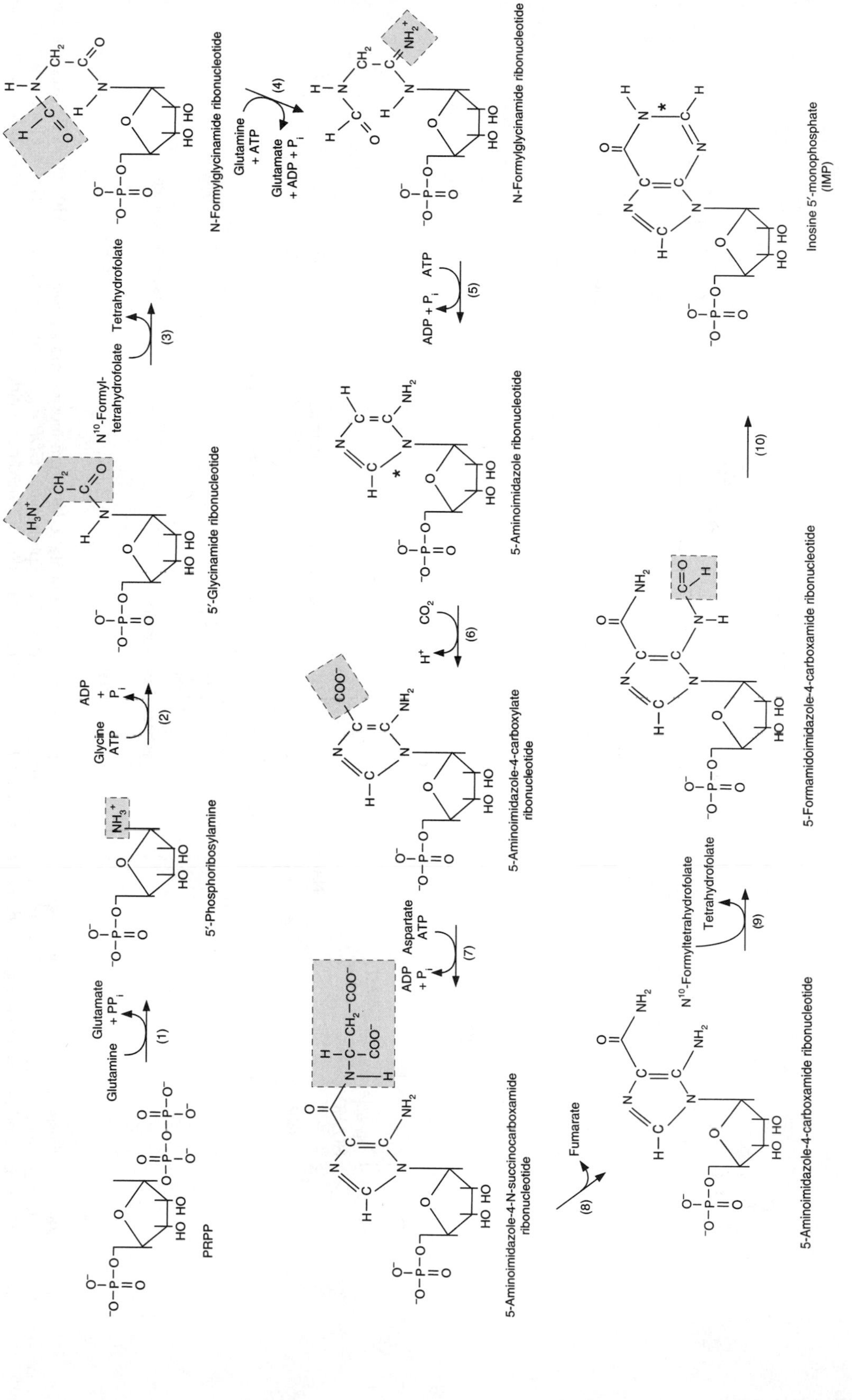

PRPP

(1) Glutamine → Glutamate + PP$_i$

5'-Phosphoribosylamine

(2) Glycine + ATP → ADP + P$_i$

5'-Glycinamide ribonucleotide

(3) N^{10}-Formyl-tetrahydrofolate → Tetrahydrofolate

N-Formylglycinamide ribonucleotide

(4) Glutamine + ATP → Glutamate + ADP + P$_i$

N-Formylglycinamidine ribonucleotide

(5) ATP → ADP + P$_i$

5-Aminoimidazole ribonucleotide

(6) CO$_2$ → H$^+$

5-Aminoimidazole-4-carboxylate ribonucleotide

(7) Aspartate + ATP → ADP + P$_i$

5-Aminoimidazole-4-N-succinocarboxamide ribonucleotide

(8) → Fumarate

5-Aminoimidazole-4-carboxamide ribonucleotide

(9) N^{10}-Formyltetrahydrofolate → Tetrahydrofolate

5-Formamidoimidazole-4-carboxamide ribonucleotide

(10)

Inosine 5'-monophosphate (IMP)

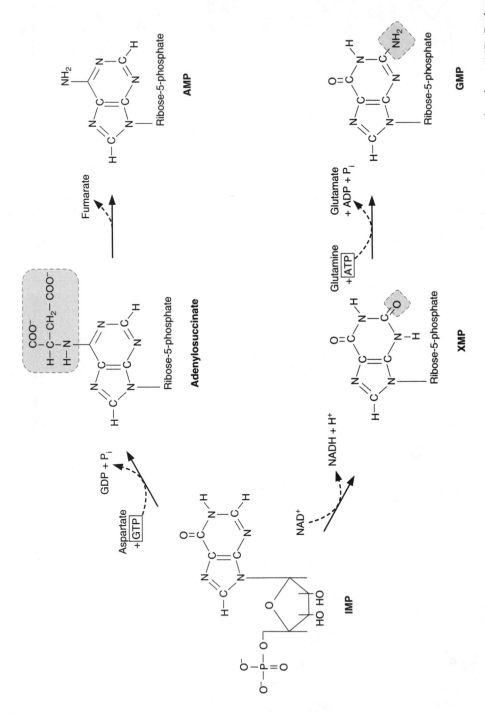

FIGURE 26-2. Synthesis of adenosine monophosphate (*AMP*) and guanosine monophosphate (*GMP*) from inosine monophosphate (*IMP*). *Dashed boxes* enclose the groups that are added at each step. *ADP* = adenosine diphosphate; *ATP* = adenosine triphosphate; *GDP* = guanosine diphosphate; *GTP* = guanosine triphosphate; *P_i* = inorganic phosphate; *NAD⁺* = oxidized nicotinamide adenine dinucleotide; *NADH* = reduced nicotinamide adenine dinucleotide; *XMP* = xanthosine 5'-monophosphate.

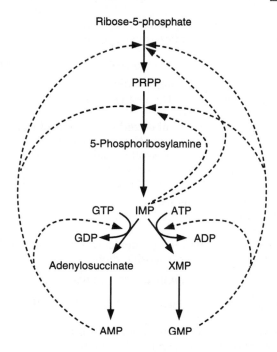

FIGURE 26-3. Regulation of synthesis of purine nucleotides. The *dashed lines* indicate where adenosine monophosphate *(AMP)*, guanosine monophosphate *(GMP)*, and inosine monophosphate *(IMP)* inhibit the steps of the pathway. *ADP* = adenosine diphosphate; *ATP* = adenosine triphosphate; *GDP* = guanosine diphosphate; *GTP* = guanosine triphosphate; *PRPP* = 5'-phosphoribosyl-1-pyrophosphate; *XMP* = xanthosine 5'-monophosphate.

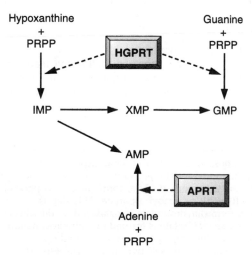

FIGURE 26-4. Salvage pathways for purine nucleotides. *AMP* = adenosine monophosphate; *APRT* = adenine phosphoribosyltransferase; *GMP* = guanosine monophosphate; *HGPRT* = hypoxanthine–guanine phosphoribosyltransferase; *IMP* = inosine monophosphate; *PRPP* = 5'-phosphoribosyl-1-pyrophosphate; *XMP* = xanthosine 5'-monophosphate.

    a. Base. The pyrimidine ring, unlike the purine ring, is not built on a molecule of PRPP. Instead, the pyrimidine ring is formed, and then it reacts with PRPP to form the nucleotide.

    b. The **precursors** of the ring are **glutamine, aspartate,** and **CO_2.**

2. **The formation of uridine 5′-monophosphate** (uridylate; UMP; see Chapter 6, Table 6-1) is shown in Figure 26-5. The first compound in the pathway is **carbamoyl phosphate.**

    a. Carbamoyl phosphate is synthesized in the **cytosol** from glutamine and CO_2 by the enzyme **carbamoyl phosphate synthetase II.**

    b. Carbamoyl phosphate also is synthesized in the **liver** as an intermediate in urea synthesis, but this synthesis takes place in the mitochondria and is catalyzed by a different enzyme, carbamoyl phosphate synthetase I (see Chapter 24 III D).

3. **UMP is converted to uridine triphosphate (UTP) in two steps.**

    a. The **first step** is catalyzed by a specific nucleoside monophosphate kinase, **UMP kinase.**

    b. The **second step** is catalyzed by **nucleoside diphosphate kinase,** an enzyme that has broad specificity for nucleoside diphosphates.

$$UMP + ATP \rightarrow UDP + ADP$$

$$UDP + ATP \rightarrow UTP + ADP$$

4. **An amino group from glutamine is donated to UTP to form cytidine triphosphate (CTP).** This reaction is catalyzed by CTP synthetase.

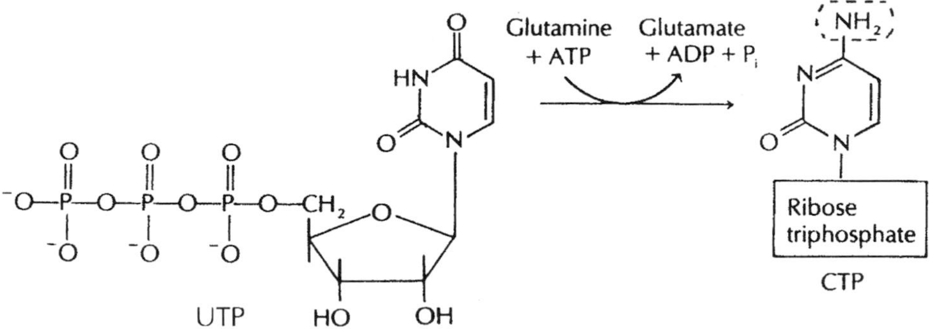

5. **Regulation of pyrimidine synthesis**

    a. In bacteria, the enzyme **aspartate carbamoyl transferase,** which catalyzes the committed step in pyrimidine synthesis (i.e., the formation of N-carbamoyl aspartate; see Figure 26-5, step 2) **is inhibited by UTP.**

FIGURE 26-5. Steps in the synthesis of uridine 5′-monophosphate (UMP). *(1)* Carbamoyl phosphate synthetase II catalyzes the combination of an NH_2 group from glutamine and a phosphate group from adenosine triphosphate *(ATP)* with carbon dioxide *(CO_2)* to form carbamoyl phosphate. *(2)* The committed step is the addition of aspartate to form N-carbamoyl aspartate. This step is catalyzed by aspartate carbamoyl transferase. *(3)* Ring closure to form dihydroorotate is catalyzed by dihydroorotase. The bond that is formed is marked with an *asterisk*. *(4)* Orotate is formed by dehydrogenation. The double bond that is formed is marked with an *asterisk*. This step is catalyzed by dihydroorotate dehydrogenase, which is a mitochondrial enzyme. All of the other enzymes of pyrimidine synthesis are cytosolic. *(5)* A ribose phosphate group from PRPP is added to form orotidine 5′-monophosphate. This reaction is catalyzed by orotate phosphoribosyltransferase. *(5)* Orotidine 5′-monophosphate (OMP) is decarboxylated to form UMP. This reaction is catalyzed by OMP-decarboxylase. *ADP* = adenosine diphosphate; *NAD^+* = oxidized nicotinamide adenine dinucleotide; *NADH* = reduced NAD; *P_i* = inorganic phosphate; *PP_i* = inorganic pyrophosphate; *PRPP* = 5′-phosphoribosyl-1-pyrophosphate.

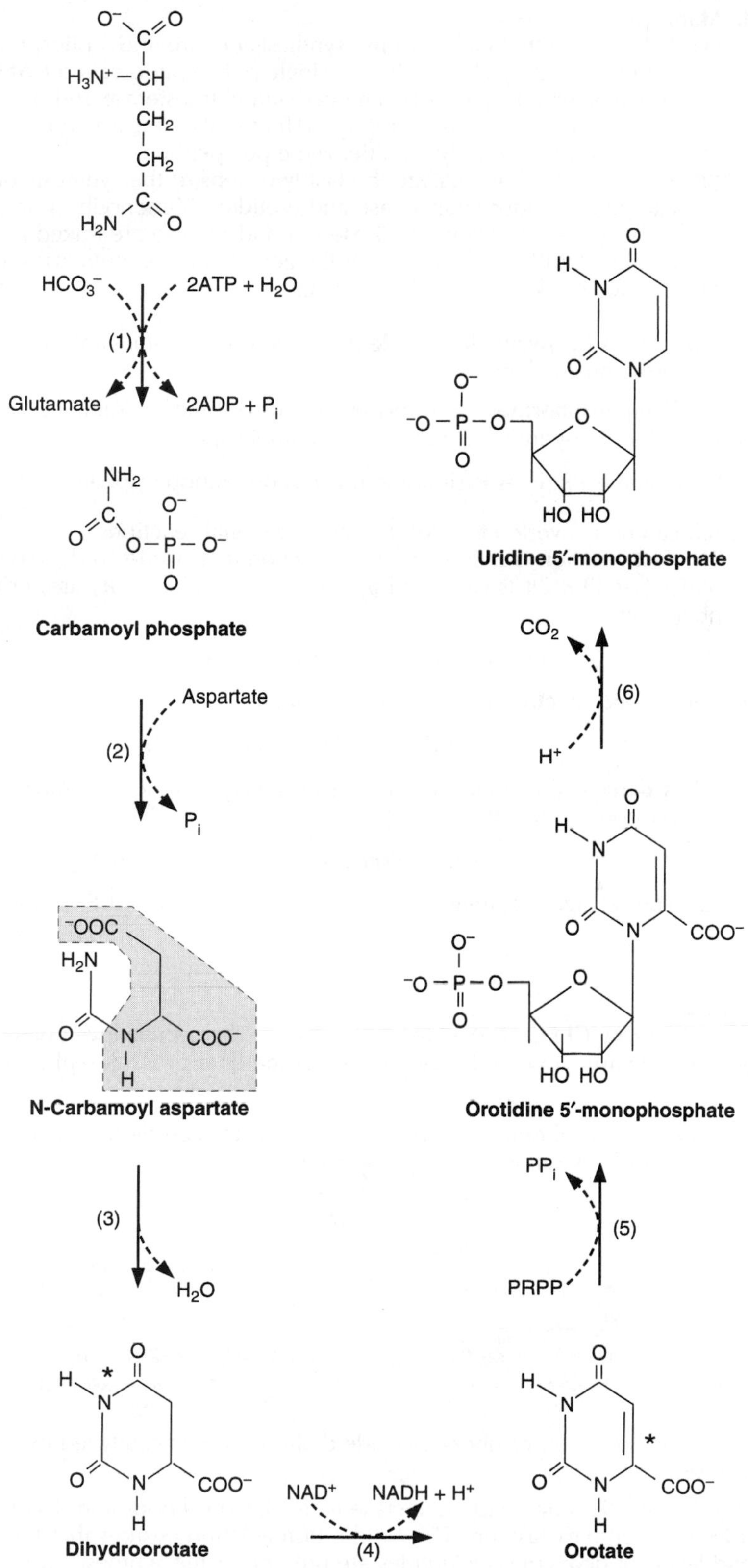

HCO_3^-
2ATP + H_2O
(1)
Glutamate
2ADP + P_i
Carbamoyl phosphate
Aspartate
(2)
P_i
N-Carbamoyl aspartate
(3)
H_2O
Dihydroorotate
NAD^+
NADH + H^+
(4)
Orotate
PRPP
(5)
PP_i
Orotidine 5′-monophosphate
H^+
(6)
CO_2
Uridine 5′-monophosphate

b. Mammals

   (1) The enzyme that catalyzes the synthesis of carbamoyl phosphate (**carbam-oyl phosphate synthetase II**) is a single polypeptide called **CAD,** which also contains the enzymes **a**spartate carbamoyl transferase and **d**ihydroorotase (see Figure 26-5, steps 2 and 3). UTP inhibits the carbamoyl phosphate synthetase II activity of this multienzyme polypeptide.

   (2) The enzymes that catalyze the last two steps of the synthesis of UMP–orotate phosphoribosyltransferase and orotidine 5′-monophosphate (OMP) decarboxylase (see Figure 26-5, steps 4 and 5), also are linked in a single polypeptide. UMP and CMP inhibit the activity of this multienzyme.

   (3) CTP feedback inhibits CTP synthetase.

E. **Salvage pathways for pyrimidine nucleotides** are not as significant in mammals as are those for purine nucleotides.

   1. Pyrimidine phosphoribosyltransferase can convert the pyrimidines, orotate, uracil, and thymine, to pyrimidine nucleoside monophosphates.

   Pyrimidine + PRPP → Pyrimidine nucleoside monophosphate + PP_i

   2. Uracil can be converted to UMP by two sequential reactions.

   a. The **first reaction** is the reverse of a reaction that occurs in degradation of nucleotides (see III B). It is catalyzed by a nucleoside phosphorylase, uridine phosphorylase.

   Uracil + Ribose-1-phosphate → Uridine + P_i

   b. The **second reaction** is catalyzed by uridine kinase.

   Uridine + ATP → UMP + ADP

   (1) **A deoxycytidine kinase** can convert deoxycytidine to deoxycytidine monophosphate (dCMP).

   Deoxycytidine + ATP → dCMP + ADP

   (2) **The salvage reactions** for thymine are described in II E.

II. **DEOXYRIBONUCLEOTIDES** are found in DNA. The cellular levels of deoxyribonucleotides are ordinarily low, and they increase at the time of DNA replication.

A. **Formation of deoxyribonucleotides.** Deoxyribonucleoside diphosphates are formed by the **reduction of ribonucleoside diphosphates.**

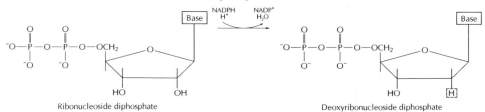

Ribonucleoside diphosphate   Deoxyribonucleoside diphosphate

B. **Enzyme.** The reduction of ribonucleoside diphosphates is catalyzed by **ribonucleotide reductase.**

   1. Regulation. Ribonucleotide reductase is regulated by ribo- and deoxyribonucleotides in a complex fashion. The pattern of regulation ensures that the proper ratios and levels of deoxyribonucleotides are present for the synthesis of DNA.

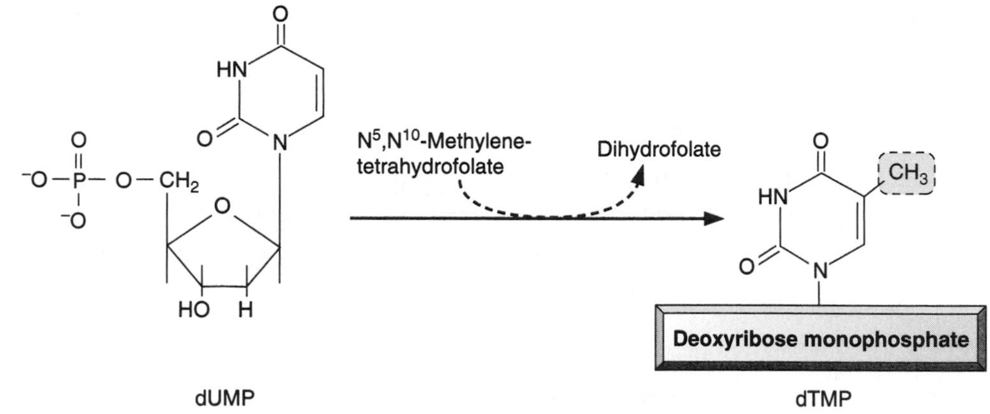

FIGURE 26-6. Synthesis of deoxythymidine 5′-monophosphate *(dTMP)* from deoxyuridine 5′-monophosphate *(dUMP)*. A *dashed box* encloses the methyl group that is added.

2. **Oxidized thioredoxin.** During the reduction of ribonucleoside diphosphates, thioredoxin, the electron donor, is oxidized. Oxidized thioredoxin is reduced by thioredoxin reductase and reduced nicotinamide adenine dinucleotide phosphate (NADPH).

C. **Deoxyribonucleotides** that are formed directly by **ribonucleotide reductase** are deoxyadenosine diphosphate (dADP), deoxycytidine diphosphate (dCDP), deoxyguanosine diphosphate (dGDP), and deoxyuridine diphosphate (dUDP).

D. For **deoxythymidine 5′-monophosphate (dTMP)** to be formed, dUDP must first be converted to deoxyuridine 5′-monophosphate (dUMP). **Thymidylate synthase** then converts dUMP to dTMP.

1. In this reaction, a methylene group from N^5,N^{10}-methylenetetrahydrofolate is transferred and reduced to a methyl group (Figure 26-6). N^5,N^{10}-Methylenetetrahydrofolate is then oxidized to dihydrofolate.

2. Tetrahydrofolate is regenerated by dihydrofolate reductase in a reaction that requires NADPH.

E. **Salvage pathway for the synthesis of thymine deoxyribonucleotides**

1. **Thymine phosphorylase** converts thymine to thymidine.

$$\text{Thymine} + \text{Deoxyribose-1-phosphate} \rightarrow \text{Thymidine} + P_i$$

2. **Thymidine kinase** converts thymidine to dTMP.

$$\text{Thymidine} + \text{ATP} \rightarrow \text{dTMP} + \text{ADP}$$

III. **DEGRADATION OF PURINE AND PYRIMIDINE NUCLEOTIDES.** A summary of the interconversions including the degradation of the bases, nucleosides, and nucleoside mono-, di- and triphosphates (i.e., nucleotides) is diagrammed in Figure 26-7. The nucleotides that result from the degradation of RNA and DNA are broken down within the cell.

A. **Nucleotidases** remove the 5′-phosphates from purine and pyrimidine ribo- and deoxyribonucleotides, converting them to ribo- and deoxyribonucleosides.

A. Purines

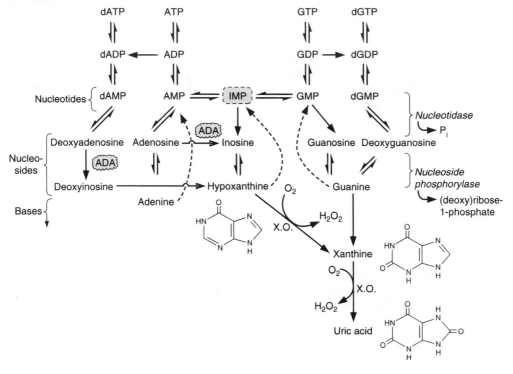

B. Pyrimidines

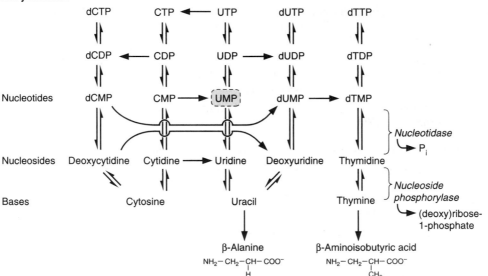

FIGURE 26-7. Interconversions and degradation of bases, nucleosides, and nucleoside mono-, di-, and triphosphates. *(A)* Purines. *(B)* Pyrimidines. In the center of each, circled with a *dashed line,* is the product of de novo synthesis, inosine 5'-monophosphate (IMP) or uridine 5'-monophosphate (UMP). Not all steps are shown for each conversion. In the degradation of purine and pyrimidine nucleotides, the first reaction is catalyzed by nucleotidases, and the second reaction is catalyzed by nucleoside phosphorylases. P_i = inorganic phosphate; *ADA* = adenosine deaminase; *X.O.* = xanthine oxidase; O_2 = oxygen; H_2O_2 = hydrogen peroxide.

1. **AMP is degraded by two pathways:** It may first be deaminated to IMP, with IMP then hydrolyzed to inosine; or it may be hydrolyzed to adenosine first, with the adenosine then deaminated to inosine by **adenosine deaminase.**

2. **Deoxy AMP (dAMP)** is hydrolyzed to deoxyadenosine, which is then deaminated to deoxyinosine by **adenosine deaminase.**

3. **GMP** and **deoxyguanosine 5'-monophosphate (dGMP)** are hydrolyzed to guanosine and deoxyguanosine respectively.

4. **Cytidine monophosphate (CMP)** may be deaminated to UMP and then hydrolyzed to uridine, or it may be hydrolyzed to cytidine and then deaminated to uridine.

5. **dCMP** may be deaminated to dUMP and then hydrolyzed to deoxyuridine, or it may be hydrolyzed to deoxycytidine and then deaminated to deoxyuridine.

6. **UMP** is hydrolyzed to uridine.

7. **dTMP** is hydrolyzed to thymidine.

B. **Nucleoside phosphorylases** catalyze the phosphorolysis of nucleosides to **free bases** and **ribose-1-phosphate** or **deoxyribose-1-phosphate.**

1. In **phosphorolysis,** a bond is cleaved by the addition of inorganic phosphate (P_i) across it:

Inosine + P_i ↔ Hypoxanthine + Ribose-1-phosphate

Deoxyinosine + P_i ↔ Hypoxanthine + Deoxyribose-1-phosphate

Guanosine + P_i ↔ Guanine + Ribose-1-phosphate

Deoxyguanosine + P_i ↔ Guanine + Deoxyribose-1-phosphate

Uridine + P_i ↔ Uracil + Ribose-1-phosphate

Deoxyuridine + P_i ↔ Uracil + Deoxyribose-1-phosphate

Thymidine + P_i ↔ Thymine + Deoxyribose-1-phosphate

2. Nucleoside phosphorylases readily catalyze the **reverse reaction,** the conversion of a free base to a nucleoside. The reverse reaction is important in salvage pathways, especially of uracil and thymine (see I E 2 and II E).

C. **The final product of purine degradation is uric acid** (see Figure 26-7), which is produced via the following pathway.

1. **Hypoxanthine,** from the breakdown of AMP, is oxidized to xanthine by the enzyme **xanthine oxidase.**

2. **Guanine,** from the breakdown of GMP, is deaminated to xanthine.

3. **Xanthine** is oxidized to uric acid by **xanthine oxidase.**
   a. **Oxygen (O_2)** is required, and **hydrogen peroxide (H_2O_2)** is generated in the oxidations by xanthine oxidase.
   b. Xanthine oxidase contains **molybdenum,** which is why this element is required in trace amounts in humans. This enzyme also contains **iron** and **sulfur.**

D. **The final products of pyrimidine degradation are β-alanine (from uracil) and β-aminoisobutyrate (from thymine)** [see Figure 26-7].

IV. BIOSYNTHESIS OF NUCLEOTIDE COENZYMES

A. **Nicotinamide adenine dinucleotide (NAD+),** a major electron acceptor in oxidative phosphorylation, is synthesized through several routes. Tryptophan, nicotinate (niacin), or nicotinamide may serve as precursors (Figure 26-8).

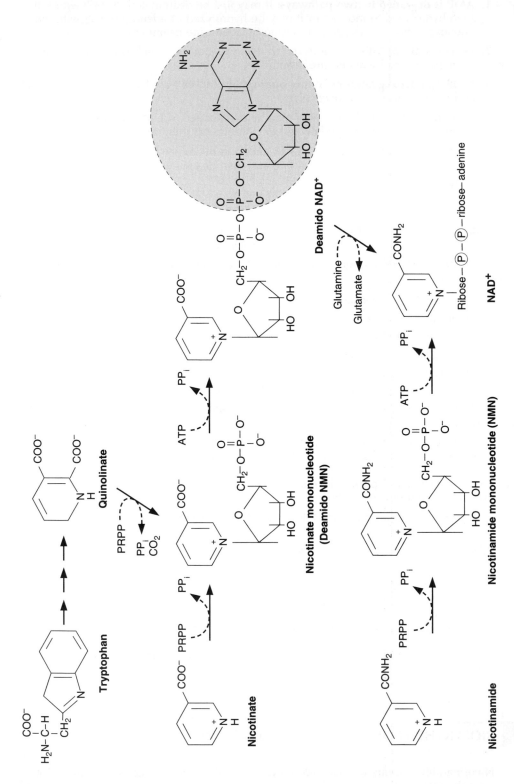

FIGURE 26-8. Synthesis of oxidized nicotinamide adenine dinucleotide *(NAD⁺)* from tryptophan, nicotinate, or nicotinamide. *ATP* = adenosine triphosphate; *PPᵢ* = inorganic pyrophosphate; *PRPP* = 5′-phosphoribosyl-1-pyrophosphate.

B. **Oxidized nicotinamide adenine dinucleotide phosphate (NADP+) is synthesized from NAD+.** NADPH, the reduced form of NADP+, is the major electron donor in biosyntheses. The 2'-hydroxyl of the adenosine ribose is phosphorylated.

$$NAD^+ + ATP \rightarrow NADP^+ + ADP$$

C. **Flavin adenine dinucleotide (FAD),** also a major electron acceptor in oxidative phosphorylation, is synthesized from riboflavin (Figure 26-9).

D. Coenzyme A (CoA), the major carrier of acyl groups in metabolism, is synthesized from pantothenate (Figure 26-10).

V. **INHIBITORS OF PURINE AND PYRIMIDINE METABOLISM.** The turnover of nucleotides in neoplastic tissues is often high. Several compounds that inhibit nucleotide synthesis are useful therapeutically in treating neoplasms. (For other nucleotide analogs, see Chapter 8 IV B.)

A. **5-Fluorouracil** is an analog of uracil. It is often used clinically to treat many cancers including those of the gastrointestinal tract and breast.

1. **5-Fluorouridine 5′-monophosphate (F-UMP).** 5-Fluorouracil undergoes conversion to the nucleoside 5′-monophosphate F-UMP in cells.
   a. **Formation.** Fluorouracil may react directly with PRPP to form F-UMP, or it may first be converted to fluorouridine and then phosphorylated to F-UMP.
   b. **Phosphorylation.** F-UMP may be phosphorylated to the nucleoside triphosphate and be incorporated into RNA, where it may have some inhibitory effect on transcription.

2. **F-UMP can be phosphorylated to the nucleoside diphosphate.** In this form, it is reduced to the deoxyribonucleotide.
   a. **F-dUMP.** The reduced nucleoside diphosphate is dephosphorylated to 5-fluoro-deoxyuridine 5′-monophosphate (F-dUMP), which is the **critical form for antineoplastic activity.**
   b. **Interaction.** F-dUMP interacts with **thymidylate synthase** and **N⁵,N¹⁰-methylene-tetrahydrofolate.** This complex resembles the transition state formed during the conversion of dUMP to dTMP (see II D).
   c. **Inhibition.** The transfer of a methylene group to the pyrimidine ring is blocked by the fluorine atom. Therefore, thymidylate synthase is trapped in a complex with F-dUMP, and synthesis of dTMP is inhibited (Figure 26-11).

B. **Methotrexate** is an analog of folic acid that **inhibits dihydrofolate reductase.** Therefore, the regeneration of tetrahydrofolate is blocked, and synthesis of dTMP is inhibited (see Figure 26-11). It is clinically used to treat many cancers including leukemias, lymphomas, and breast cancer.

C. **6-Mercaptopurine and thioguanine** are purine analogs that are used clinically in the treatment of some leukemias.

1. Both mercaptopurine and thioguanine are converted to ribonucleotides by HGPRT.
   a. The mercaptopurine ribonucleotide **6-thioIMP** inhibits the conversion of IMP to AMP and GMP.
   b. The thioguanine ribonucleotide **6-thioGMP** inhibits the conversion of IMP to GMP.

2. **Feedback inhibition.** Both 6-thioIMP and 6-thioGMP cause feedback inhibition of the controlling step of purine synthesis, the reaction of PRPP with glutamine.

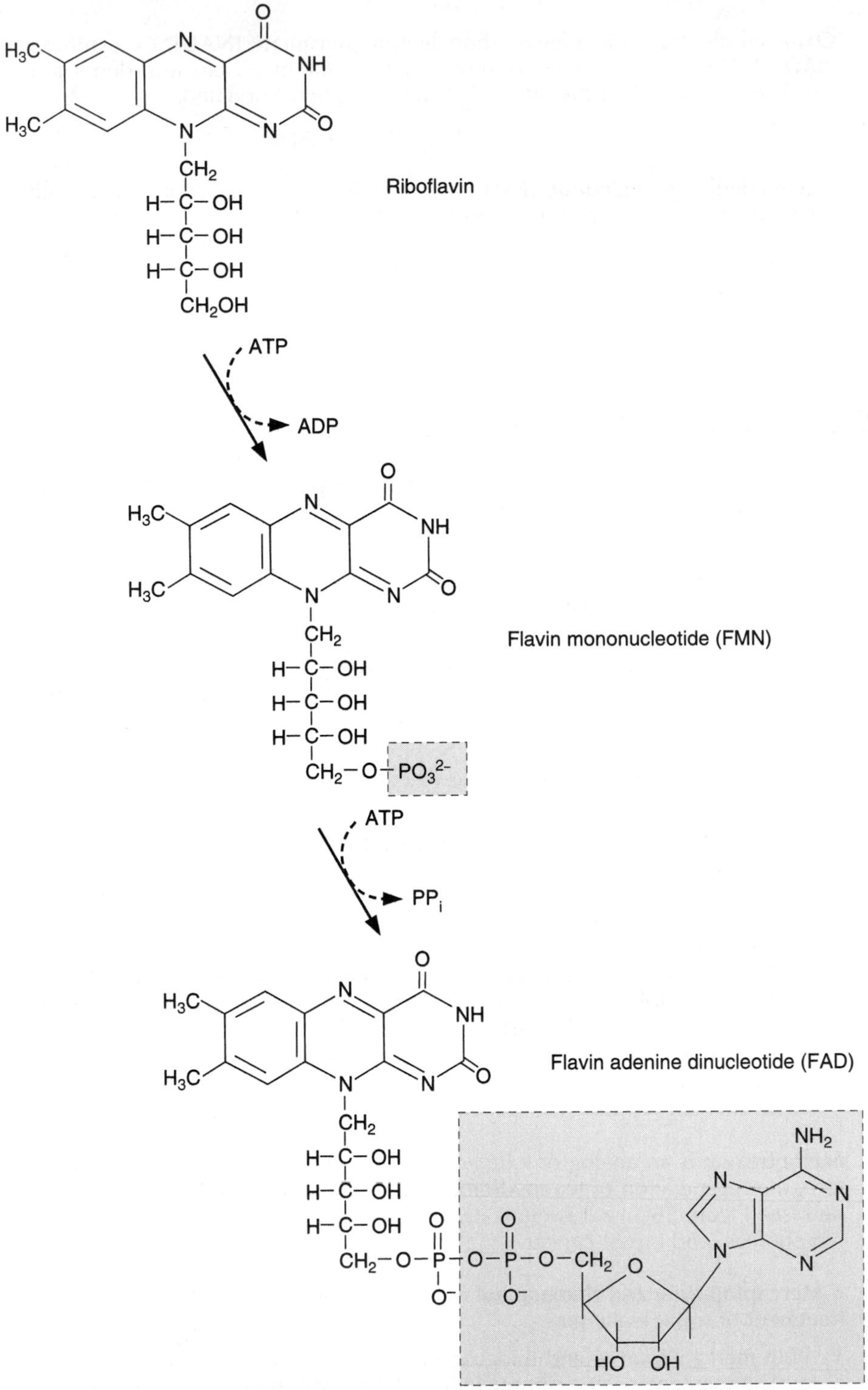

FIGURE 26-9. Synthesis of flavin adenine dinucleotide *(FAD).* A *dashed box* indicates all added groups. *ADP* = adenosine diphosphate; *ATP* = adenosine triphosphate; *PP$_i$* = inorganic pyrophosphate. (Adapted with permission from Zubay G: *Biochemistry,* 2nd ed. Macmillan, 1988, p 839.)

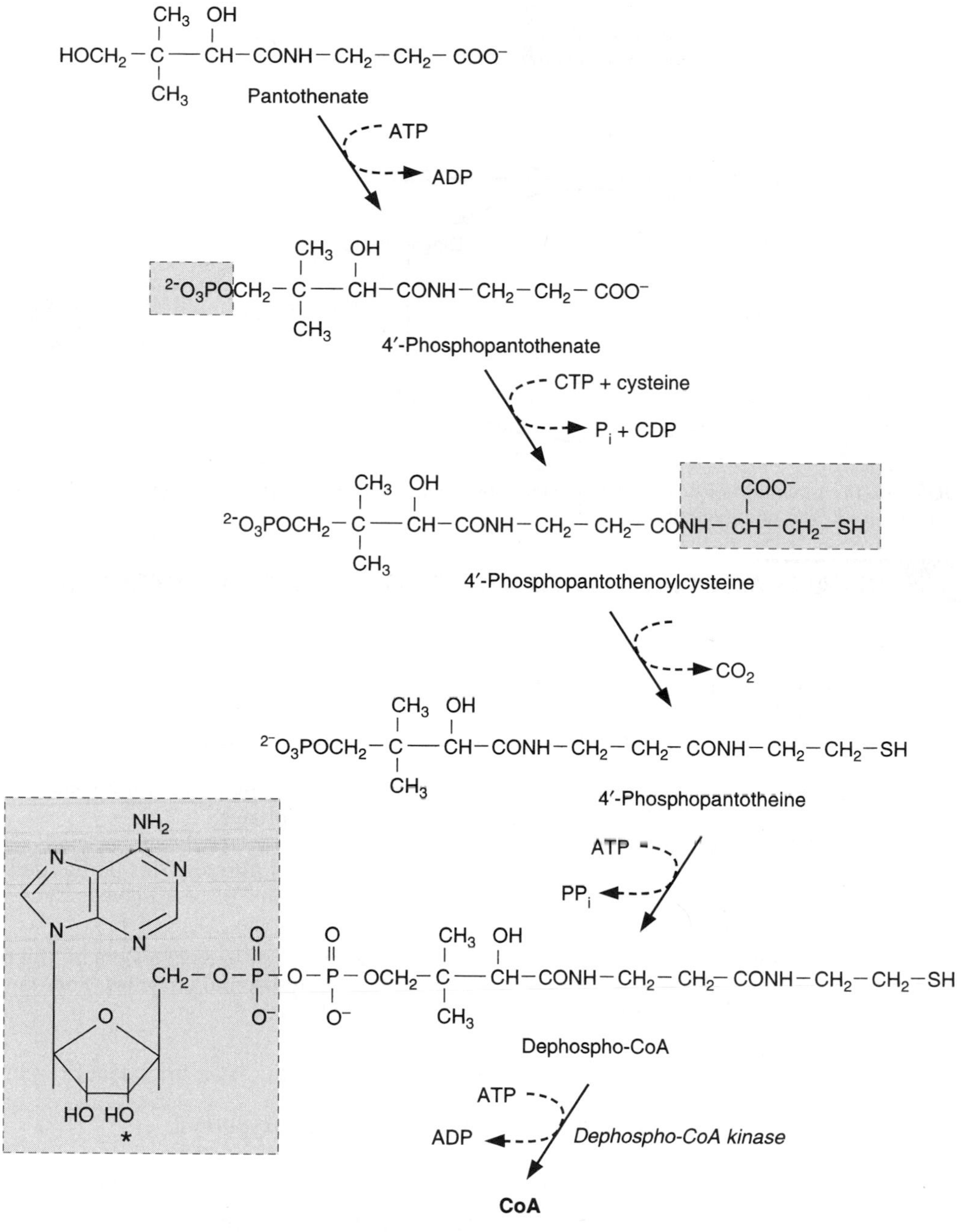

FIGURE 26-10. Synthesis of coenzyme A *(CoA)*. The second to last step shows the synthesis of dephospho-CoA. In the final step, a phosphate group is added at the position marked with an *asterisk* to form CoA. *Dashed box* indicates all other added groups. *ADP* = adenosine diphosphate; *ATP* = adenosine triphosphate; *CDP* = cytidine diphosphate; *CTP* = cytidine triphosphate; P_i = inorganic phosphate; PP_i = inorganic pyrophosphate.

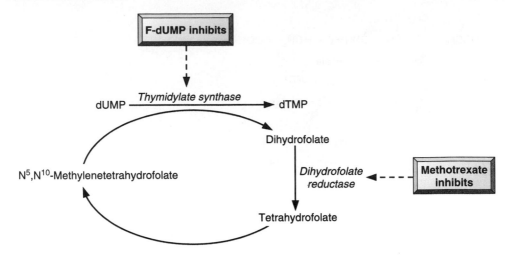

FIGURE 26-11. Inhibition of deoxythymidine monophosphate *(dTMP)* by 5-fluorodeoxyuridine 5'-monophosphate *(F-dUMP)* and methotrexate.

VI. DISEASES ASSOCIATED WITH DEFECTS OF NUCLEOTIDE METABOLISM

A. Gout

1. **Cause.** Gout is caused by the precipitation of sodium urate crystals in the joints and kidneys. Sodium urate crystals precipitate because the serum levels of urate exceed its solubility limit. Elevated uric acid levels may be due to one of several disorders.
   a. In some patients, **PRPP synthetase** (see I A 4) **is abnormal** and is not responsive to feedback inhibition by purine nucleoside diphosphates.
   b. A **partial deficiency of HGPRT** (see I C 1) leads to increased cellular levels of PRPP, which leads to increased de novo synthesis of purines. This partial deficiency does not cause any of the neurologic symptoms of Lesch-Nyhan syndrome (see VI C).

2. **Effect.** Inflammation and erosion of the joints occur when leukocytes engulf the deposited crystals and consequently rupture, releasing lysosomal enzymes. Sodium urate crystals in the urinary tract impair renal function.

3. **Treatment**
   a. **Allopurinol,** which blocks the production of uric acid, is an important drug in the treatment of gout.
      (1) Allopurinol is oxidized by xanthine oxidase to **oxypurinol.**

      Allopurinol $\xrightarrow{\ O_2\quad H_2O_2\ }$ Oxypurinol

      (2) Oxypurinol binds tightly to xanthine oxidase, inhibiting its ability to oxidize xanthine or hypoxanthine (see III C 1). This is an example of **suicide inhibition.**

(3) HGPRT (see I C 1) salvages the hypoxanthine whose levels increase upon inhibition of uric acid formation. This leads to a decrease in PRPP levels and thus to a decrease in de novo purine synthesis.

b. **Colchicine** is an anti-inflammatory drug that may be used to treat an acute gout attack. It inhibits leukocyte movement by affecting microtubule formation.

B. In **glycogen storage disease type I (von Gierke's disease),** a deficiency in glucose-6-phosphatase activity (see Chapter 21, Table 21-1) leads to an increase in cellular levels of ribose phosphates, which increases the levels of PRPP. The elevated levels of PRPP result in increased de novo synthesis of purines.

C. Lesch-Nyhan syndrome

1. **Cause.** Lesch-Nyhan syndrome is a hereditary X-linked recessive condition that is due to a severe or complete **deficiency of HGPRT activity.**
   a. **Increased synthesis of purines.** Because there is little or no HGPRT activity in people affected with Lesch-Nyhan syndrome, hypoxanthine and guanine are not salvaged. Also, the intracellular levels of PRPP increase, whereas those of IMP and GMP decrease. This leads to increased de novo synthesis of purines.
   b. **Several forms of HGPRT deficiency** have been identified in Lesch-Nyhan syndrome.
      (1) In one form, patients have normal levels of HGPRT protein, but the enzyme is inactive.
      (2) Some patients have an enzyme that is apparently unstable; its activity is higher in young red blood cells than in old.

2. The **symptoms** include hyperuricemia, gout, urinary tract stones, and the neurologic symptoms of mental retardation, spasticity, and self-mutilation. The basis for the neurologic symptoms is unknown. However, brain cells normally have much higher levels of purine salvage enzymes than other cells and may normally use salvage pathways to a greater extent.

3. **Treatment** with **allopurinol** reduces the uric acid formation but does not alleviate the neurologic symptoms. Also, because there is little or no HGPRT activity, PRPP levels and de novo purine synthesis do not decrease with allopurinol treatment. No single therapy has been found to be universally effective in treating all forms of Lesch-Nyhan syndrome.

D. Immunodeficiency disorders

1. **Adenosine deaminase (ADA) deficiency**
   a. **Cause. Deoxyadenosine and adenosine levels are high** in people with an ADA deficiency because these nucleosides are not degraded to deoxyinosine and inosine (see III A 1, 2). Lymphocytes are particularly sensitive to high levels of deoxyadenosine and adenosine. One suggested mechanism is that the increased levels of deoxyadenosine and adenosine lead to an accumulation of deoxy ATP (dATP). **High levels of dATP inhibit ribonucleotide reductase, which inhibits DNA synthesis** and accordingly the proliferation of lymphocytes.
   b. **Effect.** T-cell and B-cell functions are defective. ADA deficiency is associated with **severe combined immunodeficiency (SCID).**
      (1) **Symptoms** of SCID appear before 6 months of age and include recurrent or chronic infections and failure to thrive (growth retardation). SCID is usually fatal, often by 18 months of age.
      (2) **Treatment.** Bone marrow transplantation and enzyme replacement have been used to treat SCID. Gene therapy is an experimental treatment (see Chapter 11, Case 11-1).

2. **Purine nucleoside phosphorylase** (see III B) **deficiency**
   a. **Cause.** In the cells of people with this deficiency, deoxy GTP (dGTP) accumulates. Like dATP, dGTP inhibits ribonucleotide reductase, but not to the same degree.

    b. Effect. Purine nucleoside phosphorylase deficiency is associated with **impaired T-cell function;** B-cell function may be unaffected. The reason why primarily the function of T cells is affected is unclear.

        (1) Symptoms of T-cell deficiency include recurrent or chronic infections.

        (2) Treatment. No effective treatment exists. Affected people should not be exposed to infectious diseases.

Case 26-1 Revisited

This patient's symptoms are characteristic of acute gouty arthritis. The diagnosis of gout depends heavily on the clinical presentation. It occurs most frequently in middle-aged and older men. Usually only one joint is affected, and most commonly it is the metatarsophalangeal joint of the great toe. The inflammation of the affected joint extends to the adjacent tissue and surrounding skin. The swelling and tenderness may extend well beyond the affected joint. An untreated attack may last for several weeks.

Acute gouty arthritis is caused by the precipitation of sodium urate crystals in the joints. Sodium urate crystals precipitate because the serum levels of urate exceed its solubility limit. The patient's serum levels of urate should be checked, although it is possible that they are within a normal range and that the patient could have previously formed urate crystals within the joint. Definitive diagnosis of gout would be to aspirate, with a needle, synovial fluid from the joint and microscopically identify urate crystals.

Urate or uric acid is the final breakdown product of purine metabolism. These crystals activate an inflammatory process that results in an acute gouty arthritis attack. If the urate levels exceed the solubility of urate, then it may form insoluble crystals. Urate levels may be high in people with either abnormal PRPP synthetase or HGPRT, although other factors may predispose people to high urate levels. Various factors, often for poorly defined reasons, also may play a role in increasing normally high levels of urate in individuals to the point that urate crystals form. Some of these factors include diets high in purines (e.g., meats), heavy alcohol consumption, physical or mental stress, particular medications, and chemicals such as lead.

The first treatment for someone suffering from an acute gouty arthritis attack is to try to reduce the inflammation. Colchicine (see VI A 3 b) may be given early after onset, although nonsteroidal anti-inflammatory drugs would be safer. The patient should be encouraged to reduce the factors that may induce an attack, such as excessive alcohol consumption. If attacks continue, then treatment with allopurinol (see VI A 3 a) may be considered.

STUDY QUESTIONS

DIRECTIONS: Each of the numbered items or incomplete statements in this section is followed by answers or by completions of the statement. Select the **one** lettered answer or completion that is **best** in each case.

1. The end product of guanine catabolism in humans is

(A) xanthine
(B) uric acid
(C) β-aminoisobutyric acid
(D) urea
(E) β-alanine

2. The hereditary X-linked recessive condition known as Lesch-Nyhan syndrome is due to a severe, or complete, deficiency of

(A) 5′-phosphoribosyl-1-pyrophosphate (PRPP) synthetase activity
(B) ribonucleotide reductase activity
(C) adenine phosphoribosyltransferase activity
(D) hypoxanthine–guanine phosphoribosyltransferase (HGPRT) activity
(E) purine nucleoside phosphorylase activity

3. Deoxyribonucleotides are formed by reduction of

(A) ribonucleosides
(B) ribonucleoside monophosphates
(C) ribonucleoside diphosphates
(D) ribonucleoside triphosphates
(E) uridine triphosphates

4. The first nucleotide made by de novo purine biosynthesis is

(A) adenosine 5′-monophosphate (AMP)
(B) guanosine 5′-monophosphate (GMP)
(C) inosine 5′-monophosphate (IMP)
(D) deoxyuridine 5′-monophosphate (dUMP)
(E) cytidine 5′-monophosphate (CMP)

5. The action of allopurinol is best described as

(A) leading to the inhibition of xanthine oxidase
(B) inhibiting 5′-phosphoribosyl-1-pyrophosphate (PRPP) amidotransferase
(C) increasing the solubility of uric acid in plasma
(D) inhibiting the formation of PRPP
(E) inhibiting leukocyte movement by affecting microtubule formation

6. Which one of the following is a unique precursor of de novo pyrimidine nucleotide biosynthesis?

(A) Aspartate
(B) Carbamoyl phosphate
(C) Carbon dioxide
(D) 5′-Phosphoribosyl-1-pyrophosphate (PRPP)
(E) Glutamine

DIRECTIONS: Each group of items in this section consists of lettered options followed by a set of numbered items. For each item, select the **one** lettered option that is most closely associated with it. Each lettered option may be selected once, more than once, or not at all.

Question 7–10

For the following partial pathways showing the interconversions of purine and pyrimidine bases, nucleosides and nucleotides, match the appropriate action for the lettered step.

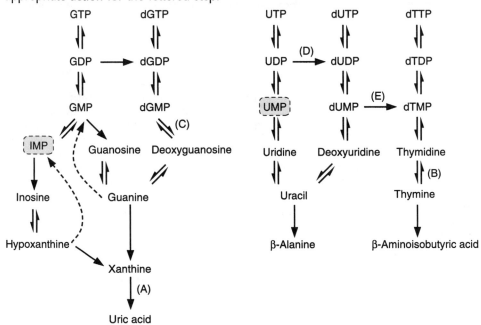

7. Inhibited by allopurinol

8. Catalyzed by ribonucleotide reductase

9. Inhibited by methotrexate

10. Catalyzed by a nucleoside phosphorylase

ANSWERS AND EXPLANATIONS

1. The answer is B [III C]. The purine nucleosides are converted to hypoxanthine (adenosine and inosine) or xanthine (guanine). The enzyme xanthine oxidase oxidizes hypoxanthine to xanthine and xanthine to uric acid, which, as the final product of purine catabolism, is excreted in the urine. The final product of pyrimidine metabolism is either β-alanine from uracil or β-aminoisobutyric acid from thymine.

2. The answer is D [VI C 1]. Lesch-Nyhan syndrome is due to severe, or complete, deficiency of hypoxanthine–guanine phosphoribosyltransferase (HGPRT) activity. Adenine phosphoribosyltransferase activity is not affected. Symptoms include hyperuricemia, gout, and neurologic problems of spasticity, mental retardation, and self-mutilation. Deficiencies of 5'-phosphoribosyl-1-pyrophosphate (PRPP) synthetase or ribonucleotide reductase would probably be lethal even if there were only a partial deficiency. A deficiency of purine nucleoside phosphorylase is associated with impaired T-cell function (with normal B-cell function) in the immune system.

3. The answer is C [II A]. Deoxyribonucleotides are formed by reduction of the corresponding ribonucleotides, which must be in the diphosphate form. The reduction of the 2'-hydroxyl group of ribose is catalyzed by ribonucleotide reductase and requires thioredoxin. Oxidized thioredoxin is reduced by thioredoxin reductase and reduced nicotinamide adenine dinucleotide phosphate (NADPH). Cytidine triphosphate is formed by the addition of an amino group from glutamine to uridine triphosphate.

4. The answer is C [I B 2, 3]. Inosine 5'-monophosphate (IMP) is the first purine nucleotide made by a 10-reaction de novo biosynthetic process. Adenosine and guanosine 5'-monophosphates (AMP and GMP) are made from IMP. The first nucleotide made by de novo pyrimidine biosynthesis is uridine 5'-monophosphate (UMP). UMP is phosphorylated to uridine triphosphate (UTP), which is converted to cytidine triphosphate (CTP) by the addition of an amino group from glutamine.

Deoxy UMP (dUMP) is the precursor to the formation of deoxythymidine 5'-monophosphate (dTMP).

5. The answer is A [VI A 3]. Allopurinol is used to reduce the formation of uric acid in patients with gout. In this condition, crystals of sodium urate accumulate in the joints. Allopurinol inhibits uric acid formation by inhibiting xanthine oxidase, which oxidizes both hypoxanthine to xanthine and xanthine to uric acid. Allopurinol does not inhibit 5'-phosphoribosyl-1-pyrophosphate (PRPP) formation. However, PRPP levels are reduced by allopurinol when the hypoxanthine, whose levels are increased, is salvaged. The decrease in PRPP levels results in a decrease in de novo purine synthesis. Colchicine is an anti-inflammatory drug that may be used to treat an acute gout attack. It inhibits leukocyte movement by affecting microtubule formation.

6. The answer is B [I A 3, B 1 b, D 1, 2 a]. The first compound to be made in the de novo biosynthesis of pyrimidines is carbamoyl phosphate. It is synthesized in the cytosol from glutamine and carbon dioxide by the enzyme carbamoyl phosphate synthetase II. Glutamine and carbon dioxide are also precursors of de novo purine biosynthesis. PRPP is required in the de novo synthesis of both purine and pyrimidine nucleotides. Purines are synthesized on a molecule of PRPP, whereas pyrimidine rings are synthesized first and in the form of orotate are added to a molecule of PRPP. Aspartate is a common precursor to both de novo purine and pyrimidine nucleotide synthesis.

7–10. The answers are: 7-A [VI A 3], **8-D** [II C], **9-E** [V B], **10-B** [III B]. Allopurinol may be used in the treatment of gout because it blocks the production of uric acid. It is oxidized by xanthine oxidase to oxypurinol, which inhibits xanthine oxidase's ability to oxidize xanthine or hypoxanthine.

Deoxyribonucleoside diphosphates are formed by the reduction of ribonucleoside diphosphates, which is catalyzed by ribonucleotide reductase. The deoxyribonucleotides that are formed directly by ribonucleotide reductase are deoxyadenosine diphosphate (dADP), deoxycytidine diphosphate (dCDP), deoxyguanosine diphosphate (dGDP), and deoxyuridine diphosphate (dUDP).

Methotrexate is an analog of folic acid that inhibits dihydrofolate reductase. Therefore, the regeneration of tetrahydrofolate is blocked, and synthesis of deoxythymidine 5′-monophosphate (dTMP) from deoxyuridine 5′-monophosphate (dUMP) is inhibited.

Nucleoside phosphorylases catalyze the phosphorolysis of nucleosides to free bases and ribose-1-phosphate or deoxyribose-1-phosphate. In phosphorolysis, a bond is cleaved by the addition of inorganic phosphate (P_i) across it. Therefore, in the degradation of thymidine, a nucleoside phosphorylase catalyzes the following reaction:

$$\text{Thymidine} + P_i \leftrightarrow \text{Thymine} + \text{Deoxyribose-1-phosphate}$$

Chapter 27

Integration of Metabolism
Victor Davidson

Case 27-1

A 20-year-old man is brought to the hospital emergency department in an unconscious state. He exhibits rapid, deep breathing, and the smell of acetone (i.e., somewhat like nail polish remover) is evident on his breath. Analysis of his blood reveals a pH of 7.1 (normal = 7.4), a bicarbonate concentration of 5 mm (normal = 24), and a blood glucose level of 350 mg/dl (normal = 30–110 mg/dl). The treatment consists of administration of insulin, intravenous fluids, electrolytes to replace lost body water, sodium, potassium, and chloride.

- What is the diagnosis?
- What is the basis for the symptoms?
- What is the rationale for the treatment?

I. **METABOLIC FUELS** are substances used by the body as **sources of carbon** or **sources of free energy,** which are used for anabolic processes and cellular functions.

A. **Caloric value of metabolic fuels** is expressed in terms of **kilocalories (kcal) per gram.** The approximate caloric values of the major types of metabolic fuels are:

1. **Carbohydrates** (e.g., glucose) = 4 kcal/g

2. **Amino acids** = 4 kcal/g

3. **Ketone bodies** = 4 kcal/g

4. **Fatty acids** = 9 kcal/g

B. **Body stores of metabolic fuels**

1. **Glucose** circulating in the blood is a major metabolic fuel.

2. **Carbohydrate** is stored primarily as glycogen in the liver and skeletal muscle.

3. **Triacylglycerols** are stored primarily in the adipose tissue. They are a source of fatty acids and glycerol, the latter of which is a substrate for gluconeogenesis.

4. **Body protein** also may be considered a source of fuel because amino acids may be converted to either glucose or ketone bodies.

II. **USE OF METABOLIC FUELS**

A. **Feeding–fasting cycle.** Any consideration of metabolism and the use of metabolic fuels must take into account the fact that humans are intermittent feeders.

1. The **fed (postprandial) state** occurs during and just after a meal. Plasma substrate levels are elevated above fasting levels, and the metabolic fuels used by tissues may be derived directly from the ingested, digested, and absorbed food molecules.

2. The **fasting (postabsorptive) state** occurs several hours after eating. Metabolic fuels used by tissues are derived from mobilized stores of fuel molecules.

3. **Starvation** occurs after extended fasting (i.e., 2 or 3 days without food).

B. **Nonhormonal regulation of metabolic pathways.** Different strategies have evolved for regulating the flow of metabolites through the different major metabolic pathways (Table 27-1).

1. **Allosteric control.** In certain pathways, the activity of a key enzyme that catalyzes the rate-limiting, committed step in the pathway is modulated by the levels of metabolites that act as activators or inhibitors.
   a. **Glycolysis**
      (1) **Phosphofructokinase** is the site of regulation (see Chapter 16 III C).
      (2) **Activators** are fructose-2,6-bisphosphate (F2,6BP)and adenosine monophosphate (AMP).
      (3) **Inhibitors** are citrate and adenosine triphosphate (ATP).
   b. **Gluconeogenesis**
      (1) **Fructose-1,6-bisphosphatase** (F1,6BPase) is the site of regulation (see Chapter 20 III E).
      (2) **Activators** are citrate and ATP.
      (3) **Inhibitors** are F2,6BP and AMP.
   c. **Fatty acid synthesis**
      (1) **Acetyl coenzyme A (CoA) carboxylase** is the site of regulation (see Chapter 22 I C 1).
      (2) The **activator** is citrate.
      (3) The **inhibitor** is palmitoyl CoA.

TABLE 27-1. Nonhormonal Regulation of Major Metabolic Pathways

Pathway	Mode of Regulation	Key Enzyme	Stimulate	Depress
Citric acid cycle	Respiratory control	—	—	—
Fatty acid oxidation	Respiratory control	—	—	—
Fatty acid synthesis	Allosteric	Acetyl CoA carboxylase	Citrate	Palmitoyl CoA
Glycogenolysis	Reaction cascade	Glycogen phosphorylase	—	—
Glycogenesis	Reaction cascade	Glycogen synthase	—	—
Glycolysis	Allosteric	Phosphofructokinase	F2,6BP, AMP	Citrate, ATP
Gluconeogenesis	Allosteric	Fructose-1,6-bis-phosphatase	Citrate	F2,6BP, AMP
Pentose phosphate pathway	Substrate availability	Glucose-6-phosphate dehydrogenase	—	—
Oxidative phosphorylation	Respiratory control	—	—	—
Urea cycle	Substrate availability	Carbamoyl phosphate synthetase	—	—

AMP = adenosine monophosphate; ATP = adenosine triphosphate; CoA = coenzyme A; F2,6BP = fructose 2,6-bisphosphate.

2. Respiratory control (see Chapter 19 III). Under respiratory control, the flux through a pathway matches the need of the cell for ATP. Pathways regulated in this manner are:
   a. Citric acid cycle (see Chapter 18 II E; III)
   b. Fatty acid synthesis (see Chapter 23 I C)
   c. Oxidative phosphorylation (see Chapter 19 III)

3. Covalent modification. Hormone-triggered reaction cascades, which result in the covalent modification of a key enzyme of a pathway, are used to regulate the following pathways.
   a. Glycogenesis. Glycogen synthase is inactive when phosphorylated and active when dephosphorylated (see Chapter 21 II B; IV A).
   b. Glycogenolysis. Glycogen phosphorylase is active when phosphorylated and inactive when dephosphorylated (see Chapter 21 III A; IV B).

4. Substrate availability primarily determines the flux of metabolites through the following:
   a. Pentose phosphate pathway (see Chapter 17 I)
   b. Urea cycle (see Chapter 24 III D)

C. **Hormonal regulation of metabolic pathways.** Certain hormones exert direct and indirect effects that regulate the flow of metabolites through certain pathways (Table 27-2).

1. Insulin signals the fed state (see II A 1) through the following actions.
   a. Insulin stimulates the synthesis of glycogen, fat, and proteins.
   b. Insulin inhibits the degradation of glycogen, fat, and proteins.

2. Glucagon and epinephrine signal the fasting state (see II A 2) through the following actions.
   a. Glucagon and epinephrine inhibit the synthesis of glycogen, fat, and proteins.
   b. Glucagon and epinephrine stimulate the degradation of glycogen, fat, and proteins.

3. Epinephrine also signals stressful states when mobilization of fuel is required.

TABLE 27-2. Hormonal Regulation of Major Metabolic Pathways

| Pathway | Effect of: | |
	Insulin	**Glucagon/Epinephrine**
Cholesterol synthesis	Stimulates	. . .
Fatty acid oxidation	Inhibits	. . .
Fatty acid synthesis	Stimulates	. . .
Gluconeogenesis	Inhibits	Stimulates
Glycogenesis	Stimulates	Inhibits
Glycogenolysis	Inhibits	Stimulates
Glycolysis	Stimulates	Inhibits
Lipogenesis	Stimulates	Inhibits
Lipolysis	Inhibits	Stimulates
Pentose phosphate pathway	Stimulates	. . .
Protein synthesis	Stimulates	. . .
Proteolysis	Inhibits	. . .

III. **THE FLOW OF KEY METABOLIC INTERMEDIATES BETWEEN DIFFERENT PATHWAYS.** Key metabolites may be used as intermediates in different processes (Figure 27-1). Control of the direction of flux of these intermediates is a major factor in integration of metabolism at the cellular level.

A. **Glucose-6-phosphate** may be converted to:

1. **Glucose** in gluconeogenic tissues (see Chapter 20 III G)

2. **Glucose-1-phosphate** and used in glycogen synthesis (see Chapter 21 II A)

3. **Pyruvate** via glycolysis (see Chapter 16 III)

4. **Ribose-5-phosphate,** a substrate for nucleotide synthesis, via the pentose phosphate pathway (see Chapter 17 I A, C)

B. **Pyruvate** may be converted to:

1. **Oxaloacetate** and metabolized via the citric acid cycle (see Chapter 18 III A)

2. **Acetyl CoA** by pyruvate dehydrogenase (see Chapter 18 I)

3. **Alanine** via transamination (see Chapter 25 I B)

4. **Lactate** in muscle tissue and red blood cells by lactate dehydrogenase (see Chapter 16 IV A)

C. **Acetyl CoA** may undergo any of the following:

1. **Oxidization to carbon dioxide (CO_2)** via the citric acid cycle (see Chapter 18 III A)

2. **Usage in fatty acid synthesis** (see Chapter 22 I B)

3. **Conversion to 3-hydroxy-3-methylglutaryl CoA (HMG CoA),** which is a precursor of:
   a. **Cholesterol** (see Chapter 23 IV A)
   b. **Ketone bodies** (see Chapter 22 IV A)

IV. **METABOLISM OF SPECIALIZED TISSUES.** All metabolic pathways are not present in all cells and tissues, and their distribution varies among the major tissues. The types of fuels that are imported, exported, and stored also vary with tissue type (Figure 27-2). Furthermore, the metabolic profiles of the major tissues vary depending on the metabolic state of the body (Table 27-3).

A. **The liver** plays a central role in metabolism in regulating the serum levels of glucose and other metabolic fuels. Most low molecular weight metabolites that appear in the blood after digestion are first carried to the liver from the intestine through the portal vein.

1. The liver is responsible for the **maintenance of blood glucose levels.**
   a. During the **fed state,** it takes up excess glucose for storage as glycogen or conversion to fatty acids.
   b. During the **fasting state,** glycogenolysis and gluconeogenesis by the liver are major sources of glucose for the rest of the body.

2. The liver serves as **the major site of fatty acid synthesis.**

3. The liver **synthesizes ketone bodies** during starvation.

4. The liver **synthesizes plasma lipoproteins.**

B. **Skeletal muscle** is the greatest consumer of metabolic fuel and oxygen, owing to its great mass compared with other tissues.

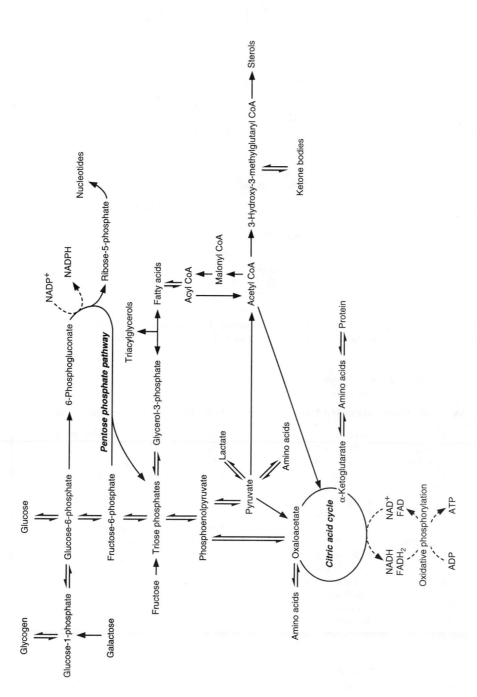

FIGURE 27-1. Integration of metabolism at the cellular level. The flow of key metabolites within and between different metabolic pathways is indicated. In some cases, the *arrows* linking metabolites represent more than a single-step conversion. *ADP* = adenosine diphosphate; *ATP* = adenosine triphosphate; *CoA* = coenzyme A; *FAD* = flavin adenine dinucleotide; $FADH_2$ = reduced FAD; NAD^+ = oxidized nicotinamide adenine dinucleotide; *NADH* = reduced nicotinamide adenine dinucleotide; *NADP*⁺ = oxidized nicotinamide adenine dinucleotide phosphate; *NADPH* = reduced nicotinamide adenine dinucleotide phosphate.

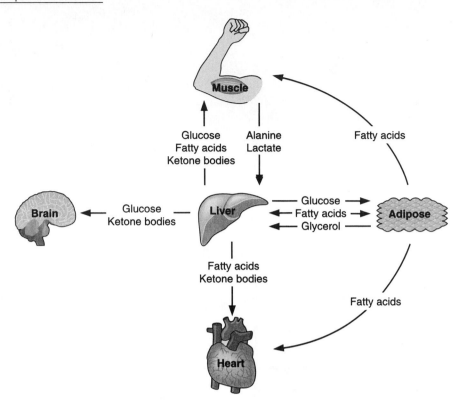

FIGURE 27-2. Integration of metabolism among major tissues of the body. The flow of key metabolites through the blood to and from the major tissues that relate to fuel metabolism is indicated by the *arrows*.

TABLE 27-3. Metabolic Profiles of Major Tissues

Tissue	Metabolic State	Imported Fuel	Exported Fuel	Stored Fuel
Liver	Fed	Glucose	Fatty acids	Glycogen
	Fasting	Fatty acids	Glucose	. . .
	Starvation	Amino acids	Ketone bodies	. . .
Muscle	Fed	Glucose	Lactate	Glycogen
	Fasting	Fatty acids	. . .	. . .
	Starvation	Fatty acids, ketone bodies	Amino acids	. . .
Adipose	Fed	Fatty acids	. . .	Triacylglycerols
	Fasting	. . .	Fatty acids, glycerol	. . .
	Starvation	. . .	Fatty acids, glycerol	. . .
Heart	Fed	Fatty acids	. . .	. . .
	Fasting	Fatty acids	. . .	. . .
	Starvation	Ketone bodies	. . .	. . .
Brain	Fed	Glucose	. . .	. . .
	Fasting	Glucose	. . .	. . .
	Starvation	Ketone bodies	. . .	. . .

1. Skeletal muscle maintains large stores of **glycogen,** which provide a source of glucose for energy during exertion.

2. In resting muscle, the preferred fuel is **fatty acids.**

3. **Muscle protein** may be mobilized as a fuel source, if no other fuel is available.

4. **Pyruvate,** the product of glycolysis, in the skeletal muscle may be converted to either lactate or alanine and exported to the liver, where it is used to regenerate glucose via gluconeogenesis (see Chapter 20 II A, B).

C. **Heart muscle** differs from skeletal muscle in the following ways.

1. Its **work load of heart muscle is much less variable** than that of skeletal muscle.

2. It is a **completely aerobic** tissue, whereas skeletal muscle has a limited capacity to function anaerobically.

3. It contains **no fuel reserves** and must be continuously supplied with fuel.

D. **Adipose tissue** stores metabolic fuel in the form of **triacylglycerols.**

1. During the **fed state,** the adipose tissue synthesizes triacylglycerols from glucose and fatty acids, which are synthesized in the liver and exported as very low-density lipoproteins.

2. During the **fasting state,** triacylglycerols are converted to glycerol and fatty acids, which are exported to the liver and other tissues.

E. **Brain tissue** uses glucose as an exclusive fuel, except during starvation, when it adapts to use ketone bodies. The brain contains no fuel reserves and must be continuously supplied with fuel.

V. ADAPTATIONS DURING STARVATION

A. **Protein.** After an overnight fast, gluconeogenesis is already providing glucose from amino acids. Gluconeogenesis from amino acids increases during the first 3 days of starvation and then declines as the body adjusts its metabolism to use ketone bodies as a primary fuel source. The decline in the use of protein as a metabolic fuel is essential for prolonged survival, because the protein represents the "fabric" and "enzymatic machinery" of the body and can be depleted only to a certain extent.

B. **Fatty acids.** Gluconeogenesis from amino acids declines as starvation continues because free fatty acids mobilized under conditions of low plasma insulin levels are oxidized preferentially. The mobilization of free fatty acids is unchecked and lasts as long as the reserves of triacylglycerols allow.

C. **Ketone bodies.** The high levels of acetyl CoA in the liver drive the formation of ketone bodies, which are produced at the maximum rate as early as the third day of starvation. Ketone bodies are readily used by cardiac and skeletal muscle as fuel and by the brain when the plasma levels of ketone bodies are high enough.

VI. DIABETES MELLITUS

A. There are **two types** of diabetes.

1. **Insulin-dependent diabetes mellitus (IDDM; type I)** is caused by an inability of the body to produce insulin.
   a. This is brought about by the destruction of the insulin-producing beta cells of the pancreatic islets.
   b. The onset of this disease is often abrupt and occurs before the age of 40. It is sometimes referred to as **juvenile-onset diabetes.**

2. Non–insulin-dependent diabetes mellitus (NIDDM; type II) is caused by a deficiency or defect in insulin receptors, or by defects in insulin-responsive cells.

    a. The body is still able to produce insulin when affected by this disorder.

    b. The onset of this disease often occurs after the age of 40. Patients are usually overweight and have a family history of diabetes. It is sometimes referred to as **adult-onset diabetes.**

B. **Metabolic abnormalities in IDDM.** Because insulin production is impaired, the level of insulin is always very low, relative to that of glucagon, regardless of the level of glucose in the blood. As such, **the metabolic profile of the body is very similar to that of starvation,** despite the presence of an abundance of metabolic fuel.

    1. Glucose uptake by tissues is impaired, despite the fact that glucose is being released by the liver.

    2. Glycolysis is depressed.

    3. Gluconeogenesis is stimulated.

    4. Lipolysis of triacylglycerols is stimulated.

    5. Synthesis of fatty acids and triacylglycerols is depressed.

    6. Fatty acid oxidation is increased.

    7. Glycogen stores are depleted.

    8. Ketone bodies are synthesized in the liver and used as fuel by other tissues.

    9. Proteins are degraded, and the amino acids are used as fuel.

    10. Levels of glucose, fatty acids, and **ketone bodies** in the blood **become very high.**

    11. Excess glucose leads to **glycosylation of hemoglobin** and other proteins.

C. **Clinical manifestations of untreated diabetes** include:

    1. Hyperglycemia (i.e., high levels of glucose in the blood)

    2. Increased urinary output

    3. Dehydration and electrolyte imbalance from increased output of urine

    4. Acidosis from high levels of ketone bodies in the blood. Acetoacetate and β-hydroxybutyrate are acids that cannot be excreted by the lungs, and this disrupts the acid–base balance by lowering pH. This can lead to coma and death if not corrected.

    5. Neuropathy due to sorbitol accumulation in Schwann cells and subsequent cell damage (see Chapter 17 IV)

    6. Renal failure

    7. Retinopathy and blindness

D. **Treatment**

    1. Administration of insulin in appropriate doses is critical for IDDM.

    2. Administration of fluids and electrolytes corrects osmotic and electrolyte imbalances.

    3. Diet therapy is extremely important for patients with NIDDM.

    4. The use of **oral hypoglycemic agents,** such as sulfonylurea, may be used in patients with NIDDM who have not responded to diet therapy.

Case 27-1 Revisited

The patient is suffering from a severe metabolic acidosis (see Chapter 1 III B). The diagnosis is diabetic ketoacidosis.

Insulin deficiency has caused an abnormal metabolic pattern in which serum glucose is not utilized, and excessive amounts of ketoacids (i.e., ketone bodies) are produced and accumulate in the blood. This lowers serum bicarbonate levels and decreases pH. The hyperventilation is an attempt by the lungs to correct the acidosis (see Chapter 1 III B).

Insulin treatment promotes glucose uptake and restoration of normal metabolism. When the hyperglycemia is corrected, the loss of water and electrolytes ceases. Although the patient's pH is low, bicarbonate therapy is not necessary. Inhibition of ketone body formation and metabolism of glucose to carbon dioxide via glycolysis and the citric acid cycle should allow the acid–base balance to return to normal. In fact, the change in bicarbonate levels on treatment serves as a guide to monitor the success of the treatment.

STUDY QUESTIONS

DIRECTIONS: Each of the numbered items or incomplete statements in this section is followed by answers or by completions of the statement. Select the **one** lettered answer or completion that is **best** in each case.

1. The postprandial state is characterized by

(A) high blood levels of glucose and low levels of insulin
(B) high blood levels of glucose and high levels of insulin
(C) high blood levels of free fatty acids and low levels of glucagon
(D) high blood levels of free fatty acids and high levels of glucagon
(E) high blood levels of insulin and glucagon

2. Which one of the following metabolic pathways is correctly matched with the key enzyme that regulates that pathway?

(A) Pentose phosphate pathway—glucokinase
(B) Glycolysis—fructose-1,6-bisphosphatase
(C) Gluconeogenesis—phosphofructokinase
(D) Fatty acid synthesis—acetyl coenzyme A (CoA) carboxylase
(E) Citric acid cycle—glucose-6-phosphate dehydrogenase

Questions 3–5

A patient is suffering from untreated insulin-dependent diabetes.

3. Which one of the following metabolic actions is occurring in this patient?

(A) Glucose is used by skeletal muscle for fuel
(B) Ketone bodies are released by the liver into the blood
(C) Glucose is used by the liver for fuel
(D) Fatty acids are transported from the liver to the adipose tissue
(E) Insulin is secreted by the pancreas into the blood

4. Which one of the following metabolic pathways is stimulated in this patient?

(A) Gluconeogenesis
(B) Glycolysis
(C) Fatty acid synthesis
(D) Protein synthesis
(E) Glycogenesis

5. Another patient with very similar symptoms is suffering from non-insulin–dependent diabetes. Serum levels of which one of the following will most likely be different in this patient?

(A) Glucose
(B) Ketone bodies
(C) Insulin
(D) Fatty acids
(E) Electrolytes

DIRECTIONS: The group of items in this section consists of lettered options followed by a set of numbered items. For each item, select the **one** lettered option that is most closely associated with it. Each lettered option may be selected once, more than once, or not at all.

Questions 6–10

(A)   Ketone bodies
(B)   Glucose
(C)   Fatty acids
(D)   Glycerol
(E)   Lactate

Match the following descriptions with the correct metabolite.

6. The preferred source of metabolic fuel for the brain

7. The primary source of metabolic fuel used by most tissues in the late stages of untreated diabetes

8. Released by the adipose tissue and converted to pyruvate by the liver

9. The preferred source of metabolic fuel for the liver in the postabsorptive state

10. Exported by skeletal muscle in the postprandial state

■ ANSWERS AND EXPLANATIONS

1. The answer is B [II A 1, C]. The postprandial state is characterized by high blood levels of glucose arising from the ingested meal. High blood glucose levels promote insulin release and inhibit the release of glucagon. The level of free fatty acids in the blood is low, and most of the circulating fat is as triacylglycerols in the form of chylomicrons or very low-density lipoproteins.

2. The answer is D [II B; Table 27-1]. Acetyl coenzyme A (CoA) carboxylase catalyzes the committed step in fatty acid synthesis. Glycolysis and gluconeogenesis also are controlled by the allosteric regulation of a key enzyme. However, in glycolysis that enzyme is phosphofructokinase, and in gluconeogenesis it is fructose-1,6-bisphosphatase. The citric acid cycle is regulated by respiratory control, and the pentose phosphate pathway is regulated by the availability of substrates.

3–5. The answers are: 3-B, 4-A, 5-C [VI; Table 27-3]. The metabolic profile of untreated diabetes is essentially identical to that of starvation except that high blood levels of glucose are present because glucose uptake by tissues is impaired in the absence of insulin. The body adapts to using ketone bodies as a major fuel source. Ketone bodies are produced primarily from amino acids in the liver and are released into the blood. Glucose uptake by the liver and muscle is impaired. The adipose tissue exhausts its supply of fatty acids after several days of starvation. Insulin, which signals high levels of blood glucose, is not secreted in insulin-dependent diabetes mellitus (IDDM).

In the absence of insulin, the body behaves as though blood glucose levels are low. Glucose-utilizing pathways such as glycolysis are depressed, as are energy-requiring biosynthetic pathways, such as fatty acid synthesis, protein synthesis, and glycogenesis. The formation of glucose by gluconeogenic tissues is stimulated.

The metabolic profile and symptoms of non–insulin-dependent diabetes mellitus (NIDDM) is essentially the same as for IDDM. The major difference is that in patients with NIDDM, insulin is being produced by the pancreas. The clinical problems are caused by a deficiency or defect in insulin receptors, or by defects in insulin-responsive cells.

6–10. The answers are: 6-B, 7-A, 8-D, 9-C, 10-E [IV; VI B; Table 27-3]. The brain normally uses glucose as an exclusive fuel. However, during starvation, when glucose is scarce, the brain can adapt to use ketone bodies as an energy source.

In patients with untreated diabetes, most tissues adopt a metabolic profile similar to that seen in starvation and use ketone bodies, which are produced by the liver, as a fuel.

During the fasting state, triacylglycerols in the adipose tissue are converted to glycerol and fatty acids, which are released into the blood. Glycerol is taken up by the liver and converted to 3-phosphoglycerate, an intermediate in both glycolysis and gluconeogenesis.

During the postabsorptive state, the liver provides glucose for the rest of the body from glycogenolysis and gluconeogenesis. However, the liver itself favors fatty acids as a fuel source.

In the fed state, muscle uses glucose as a fuel and converts it to pyruvate via glycolysis. Pyruvate is then converted to lactate or alanine and exported to the liver, where it may be used to regenerate glucose via gluconeogenesis.

Comprehensive Examination

QUESTIONS

DIRECTIONS: Each of the numbered items or incomplete statements in this section is followed by answers or by completions of the statement. Select the **one** lettered answer or completion that is **best** in each case.

Questions 1–5

A patient is suffering from untreated diabetes. His symptoms include thirst, frequent urination, weight loss, hyperventilation, and fatigue. Blood analysis reveals above normal glucose levels and below normal bicarbonate levels, pH, and partial pressure of carbon dioxide (P_{CO_2}).

1. Which one of the following conditions does this patient exhibit?

(A) Respiratory acidosis with compensatory metabolic alkalosis
(B) Respiratory alkalosis with compensatory metabolic acidosis
(C) Metabolic acidosis with compensatory respiratory alkalosis
(D) Metabolic alkalosis with compensatory respiratory acidosis
(E) Metabolic acidosis with compensatory respiratory acidosis

2. What is the primary cause of the below normal pH in this patient?

(A) Hyperventilation
(B) Water loss due to frequent urination
(C) Lactic acidosis
(D) Renal failure
(E) Ketoacidosis

3. Which one of the following metabolic pathways is most active in the liver of this patient?

(A) Gluconeogenesis
(B) Glycolysis
(C) Glycogenesis
(D) Fatty acid synthesis
(E) Lipolysis

4. Which one of the following processes is most active in the muscle of this patient?

(A) Glycolysis
(B) Proteolysis
(C) Gluconeogenesis
(D) Urea cycle
(E) Ketone body synthesis

5. Most of the glucose-6-phosphate (G6P) formed in this patient's liver is converted to

(A) ribose-5-phosphate
(B) glucose-1-phosphate
(C) glucose
(D) pyruvate
(E) fructose-6-phosphate

Questions 6–10

A 2-day-old patient exhibits extreme lethargy and hyperventilation. Blood analysis reveals a pH of 7.5, normal bicarbonate levels, below normal blood urea nitrogen (BUN), very high levels of ammonia, and below normal partial pressure of carbon dioxide (P_{CO_2}). Urinalysis reveals very high levels of orotic acid and no detectable citrulline.

6. This patient suffers from a defect in

(A) glycolysis
(B) the urea cycle
(C) heme degradation
(D) nucleotide synthesis
(E) tyrosine metabolism

7. Which one of the following enzymes is most likely deficient in this patient?

(A) Carbamoyl phosphate synthetase
(B) Ornithine transcarbamoylase
(C) Argininosuccinate synthetase
(D) Argininosuccinate lyase
(E) Arginase

8. Which one of the following best describes this patient's acid–base balance?

(A) Respiratory alkalosis
(B) Respiratory acidosis
(C) Metabolic acidosis
(D) Metabolic alkalosis
(E) Normal

9. This patient's blood will have above normal levels of

(A) pyruvate
(B) oxaloacetate
(C) α-ketoglutarate
(D) α-ketoisovalerate
(E) glutamine

10. Which one of the following is an essential amino acid for this patient?

(A) Tyrosine
(B) Glycine
(C) Arginine
(D) Glutamate
(E) Aspartate

Questions 11–13

A patient presents with an enlarged spleen and liver. Extracts of leukocytes, which were isolated from the patient's blood, exhibited β-glucosidase activity that was less than 10% of normal.

11. From what disorder is this patient suffering?

(A) von Gierke's disease
(B) Pompe's disease
(C) Gaucher's disease
(D) Niemann-Pick disease
(E) Crigler-Najjar syndrome

12. Enlargement of the organs is due to the accumulation of

(A) glycogen
(B) a sphingolipid
(C) fatty acids
(D) triacylglycerols
(E) cholesterol

13. In what subcellular location does the activity of the deficient enzyme normally occur?

(A) Cytosol
(B) Mitochondria
(C) Golgi complex
(D) Lysosomes
(E) Peroxisomes

Questions 14–16

A patient is brought to the emergency room suffering from carbon monoxide poisoning. He is ventilated with oxygen and soon recovers.

14. What metabolic process is inhibited by carbon monoxide?

(A) Citric acid cycle
(B) Mitochondrial electron transport
(C) Fatty acid oxidation
(D) Glycolysis
(E) Pentose phosphate pathway

15. Carbon monoxide inhibits respiration by binding to

(A) the oxygen-binding site of hemoglobin
(B) the oxygen-binding site of cytochrome oxidase
(C) succinate dehydrogenase
(D) coenzyme Q
(E) reduced nicotinamide adenine dinucleotide (NADH) dehydrogenase

16. The effects of carbon monoxide poisoning are very similar to those of

(A) arsenic
(B) lead
(C) ethylene glycol
(D) nerve gas
(E) cyanide

Questions 17–19

A newborn infant is placed in the intensive care unit because of very high serum levels of indirect bilirubin. After a few days of phototherapy, the levels return to near normal.

17. Inefficiency of which one of the following metabolic processes has caused this problem?

(A) Urea cycle
(B) Degradation of branched-chain amino acids
(C) Degradation of phenylalanine
(D) Degradation of heme
(E) Degradation of sphingolipids

18. Why is phototherapy effective?

(A) It activates the enzyme that degrades bilirubin
(B) It converts bilirubin to a more soluble compound
(C) It converts bilirubin to biliverdin
(D) It converts indirect bilirubin to direct bilirubin
(E) It causes bilirubin to dimerize

19. In which one of the following conditions is there an increase in the serum level of direct bilirubin?

(A) Prehepatic jaundice
(B) Decreased hepatic uptake of bilirubin
(C) Crigler-Najjar syndrome
(D) Neonatal jaundice
(E) Obstruction of the bile duct

20. The most important source of reducing equivalents for fatty acid synthesis in the liver is

(A) oxidation of glucuronic acid
(B) oxidation of acetyl coenzyme A
(C) glycolysis
(D) the citric acid cycle
(E) the pentose phosphate pathway

21. Low levels of 3-hydroxy-3-methylglutaryl coenzyme A (HMG CoA) reductase activity are most likely to result from

(A) a vegetarian diet
(B) the administration of a bile acid-sequestering resin
(C) a low-cholesterol diet
(D) familial hypercholesterolemia
(E) a long-term high-cholesterol diet

22. During long-term fasting, the major control of the rate of gluconeogenesis is the

(A) cyclic adenosine monophosphate level in the liver
(B) adenosine triphosphate level in the liver
(C) availability of free fatty acids to the liver
(D) availability of alanine in the blood
(E) insulin:glucagon ratio

23. The release of ammonia from amino acids is catalyzed by

(A) transaminases and dehydratases
(B) transaminases and glutamate dehydrogenase
(C) transaminases and amino acid oxidases
(D) dehydratases and glutamate dehydrogenase
(E) dehydratases and amino acid oxidases

24. The enzyme-catalyzed conversion of serine to glycine requires

(A) niacin and vitamin B_{12}
(B) thiamine and vitamin B_{12}
(C) thiamine and folic acid
(D) niacin and folic acid
(E) folic acid and vitamin B_{12}

25. A reaction exhibits a $\Delta G^{\circ\prime}$ of 2.8 kcal/mol. At equilibrium, what is the ratio of products to reactants?

(A) 100:1
(B) 10:1
(C) 1:1
(D) 0.1:1
(E) 0.01:1

26. Which one of the following terms best describes an enzyme that catalyzes this reaction?

$$\text{Glucose} + \text{ATP} \rightleftharpoons$$
$$\text{Glucose-6-phosphate} + \text{ADP}$$

(A) Phosphatase
(B) Kinase
(C) Phosphodiesterase
(D) Hydrolase
(E) Phosphorylase

27. The only component of the electron transport chain that is NOT firmly embedded in the inner mitochondrial membrane is

(A) cytochrome c
(B) coenzyme Q
(C) cytochrome oxidase
(D) reduced nicotinamide adenine dinucleotide (NADH) dehydrogenase
(E) succinate dehydrogenase

28. Glycogenolysis in muscle does not contribute directly to blood glucose concentration because muscle lacks the enzyme

(A) phosphorylase
(B) phosphoglucomutase
(C) glucose-6-phosphatase
(D) glucokinase
(E) phosphoglucoisomerase

29. Which one of the following metabolic pathways possesses a key enzyme that is allosterically regulated by citrate?

(A) Citric acid cycle
(B) Urea cycle
(C) Fatty acid synthesis
(D) Pentose phosphate pathway
(E) Fatty acid degradation

30. Enzymes increase the rates of reactions by

(A) increasing the free energy of activation
(B) increasing the free-energy change of the reaction
(C) changing the equilibrium constant of the reaction
(D) decreasing the energy of activation
(E) decreasing the free-energy change of the reaction

31. An enzyme involved in the catabolism of fructose to pyruvate is

(A) hexokinase
(B) phosphofructokinase
(C) 6-phosphogluconate dehydrogenase
(D) glyceraldehyde-3-phosphate (G3P) dehydrogenase
(E) phosphoglucomutase

32. The biosynthesis of triacylglycerols in adipose tissue requires

(A) elevated levels of plasma epinephrine
(B) elevated intracellular levels of cyclic adenosine monophosphate
(C) increased glucose entry into the cells
(D) increased rate of glycerol release from the cells
(E) decreased levels of plasma insulin

33. A product of the series of reactions that converts carbamoyl phosphate to urea is

(A) arginine
(B) aspartate
(C) adenosine triphosphate
(D) citrulline
(E) fumarate

34. The rate-controlling step in the biosynthesis of porphyrins is

(A) δ-aminolevulinate synthesis
(B) porphobilinogen synthesis
(C) uroporphyrinogen synthesis
(D) decarboxylation of uroporphyrinogen III
(E) conversion of protoporphyrin IX to protoheme IX

35. If the substrate concentration in an enzyme-catalyzed reaction is equal to 1/2 K_m, the initial reaction velocity is

(A) $0.25\ V_{max}$
(B) $0.33\ V_{max}$
(C) $0.50\ V_{max}$
(D) $0.67\ V_{max}$
(E) $0.75\ V_{max}$

36. Which one of the enzymes listed provides a link between glycolysis and the citric acid cycle?

(A) Acetyl coenzyme A (CoA) synthetase
(B) Lactate dehydrogenase
(C) Pyruvate kinase
(D) Citrate synthase
(E) Pyruvate dehydrogenase

37. Which one of the following amino acids is purely ketogenic?

(A) Proline
(B) Phenylalanine
(C) Isoleucine
(D) Leucine
(E) Arginine

38. Which one of the following enzymes is activated by phosphorylation?

(A) Glycogen synthase
(B) Glycogen phosphorylase
(C) Pepsin
(D) Trypsin
(E) Protein kinase

Questions 39–41

The following metabolic events are occurring in an individual. Fatty acids and glycerol are being released from the adipose tissue. Glucose is being released from the liver. Fatty acids are being taken up by the heart and skeletal muscle. Ketone body levels are very low.

39. Which one of the following best describes the metabolic state of this individual?

(A) Postprandial
(B) Postabsorptive
(C) Starvation
(D) Diabetic

40. Which one of the following is being released by the skeletal muscle in this person?

(A) Glucose
(B) Glycerol
(C) Lactate
(D) β-Hydroxybutyrate
(E) Acetoacetate

41. In this metabolic state, which tissue will preferentially use glucose as a fuel?

(A) Liver
(B) Heart
(C) Skeletal muscle
(D) Adipose
(E) Brain

42. Which one of the following would be seen in a patient with a severe thiamine deficiency?

(A) Decreased serum levels of pyruvate and lactate
(B) Increased clotting time of blood
(C) Low red cell transaminase activity
(D) Increased urinary excretion of xanthurenic acid following a tryptophan load
(E) Decreased transketolase activity in red blood cells

43. An enzyme that catalyzes an anaplerotic reaction is

(A) succinate dehydrogenase
(B) citrate lyase
(C) citrate synthetase
(D) pyruvate dehydrogenase (PDH)
(E) pyruvate carboxylase

44. High levels of citrate reduce the activity of

(A) the pentose phosphate pathway
(B) glycolysis
(C) gluconeogenesis
(D) fatty acid synthesis
(E) glycogenesis

45. Under conditions of repeated episodes of hyperglycemia, hemoglobin A_1 (Hb A_1) may be modified chemically. What is the effect of this chemical modification?

(A) Hemoglobin loses its ability to show cooperativity in the binding of oxygen
(B) Hb A_1 becomes less soluble, forming long rod-like structures that deform the erythrocyte
(C) A stable glucose derivative of Hb A_1 appears in the blood and may amount to more than 10% of the total hemoglobin
(D) The synthesis of Hb A_1 is depressed in favor of the synthesis of hemoglobin F
(E) The affinity of hemoglobin for oxygen is increased, inhibiting the release of oxygen

46. Thermal denaturation of DNA results in which one of the following?

(A) A hypochromic effect
(B) Cleavage of glycosidic bonds resulting in a hyperchromic effect
(C) A broad melting point transition
(D) A melting temperature that depends on the base content
(E) Cleavage of the phosphodiester bonds resulting in a hyperchromic effect

47. DNA polymerase I is best described by which one of the following statements? It

(A) functions as a DNA repair enzyme but is not involved in the DNA replication process
(B) requires a template and a primer to polymerize deoxyribonucleotide triphosphates
(C) joins together Okazaki fragments to complete the lagging strand during DNA replication
(D) produces Okazaki fragments linked to RNA primer chains
(E) has 5′ to 3′ exonuclease activity but lacks 3′ to 5′ exonuclease activity

48. Which one of the following is an effective antibiotic that works by inhibiting the initiation of RNA synthesis in prokaryotes through binding to the β subunit of the RNA polymerase holoenzyme?

(A) Actinomycin D
(B) Rifampin
(C) α-Amanitin
(D) Quinolones
(E) Puromycin

49. An investigator has isolated a bacterium that, in the absence of glucose, constitutively produces the proteins coded for by the *lac* operon. Which one of the following statements best explains this observation?

(A) The promoter has a mutation that prevents RNA polymerase from binding
(B) There is a missense mutation in the gene for β-galactosidase
(C) The gene for the catabolite activator protein is mutated and is inactive
(D) There is a mutation in the attenuator sequence
(E) The gene for the repressor protein is mutated and is inactive

50. Which one of the following hemoglobins cannot bind oxygen because the heme iron is in the ferric (Fe^{3+}) form?

(A) Hemoglobin A_{1c}
(B) Hemoglobin C
(C) Hemoglobin S
(D) Hemoglobin F
(E) Hemoglobin M

51. Collagen occurs in different types, which are usually classified on the basis of the

(A) type of carbohydrate present
(B) cysteine content
(C) hydroxyproline and hydroxylysine content
(D) types of peptide chains present
(E) glycine content

52. Where is the cut site (as indicated by a slash) in the restriction enzyme recognition sequence GACGTC?

(A) G/ACGTC
(B) GAC/GTC
(C) GACG/TC
(D) GACGTC/
(E) Without knowing the restriction enzyme that recognizes this sequence, the cut site cannot be predicted

53. Which one of the following restriction enzyme sequences will generate the longest 5′ sticky ends upon cleavage by the appropriate restriction enzyme (the cleavage site is indicated with a slash)?

(A) ATGCA/T
(B) TGG/CCA
(C) C/CCGGG
(D) CCTGCA/GG
(E) AT/TAAT

54. Adenosine triphosphatase (ATPase) activity needed for muscle contraction is a component of

(A) the amino-terminal globular head of myosin
(B) the carboxy-terminal tail region of myosin
(C) tropomyosin
(D) actin
(E) troponin C

55. Vitamin K is directly involved with which one of the following enzymatic actions?

(A) Activation of Factor X
(B) Regulation of blood calcium levels
(C) Conversion of fibrinogen to fibrin
(D) Synthesis of prothrombin
(E) Transcriptional control of fibrinogen synthesis

56. The substitution of valine (Val) for glutamic acid (Glu) in the sixth position on the β chain of hemoglobin produces sickle cell anemia in the homozygote because

(A) the cooperative binding of oxygen is lost because of the missing Glu-6 residue
(B) the apoprotein can no longer protect the heme iron from becoming oxidized owing to the presence of the hydrophobic Val-6
(C) the Val-6 variant loses solubility upon deoxygenation
(D) the Val-6 variant tends to retain oxygen when the oxygen tension is low
(E) the red cell is unable to sequester high enough concentrations of the Val-6 variant hemoglobin

57. In which type of nucleic acid would one expect to find the highest level of rare or modified base residues?

(A)   Heterogeneous nuclear RNA (hnRNA)
(B)   Transfer RNA (tRNA)
(C)   Small nuclear RNA (snRNA)
(D)   Messenger RNA (mRNA)
(E)   Ribosomal RNA (rRNA)

58. The portion of an operon to which a repressor binds is

(A)   the catabolite activator protein (CAP) site
(B)   a regulatory gene
(C)   a promoter
(D)   an initiation site
(E)   an operator

59. Which one of the following statements regarding eukaryotic gene expression is correct?

(A)   All regions of eukaryotic DNA are transcribed, and regulation of transcription occurs upon processing to form messenger RNA (mRNA)
(B)   Because transcription takes place near nuclear pores, eukaryotes can regulate gene expression by coupling transcription to translation
(C)   Eukaryotic promoters are analogous to prokaryotic promoters, and all are on the 5′ end of each gene, upstream of the transcriptional initiation site
(D)   mRNA that contains a poly A tail obtains it from transcription of a poly T sequence at the 3′ terminus of the gene
(E)   In eukaryotes, gene expression can be regulated by alteration of mRNA stability

60. A patient was initially treated for a particular cancer with daunorubicin and later was switched to treatment with etoposide. The cancer type was known to respond well to both of these drugs, yet this patient's cancer did not respond to the second treatment with etoposide. Which one of the following is the best explanation for why the patient did not respond to treatment by etoposide?

(A)   Etoposide and daunorubicin both inhibit cell growth by the same mechanism, and the initial treatment likely resulted from selection of cancer cells that are resistant to all drugs of this inhibitory class
(B)   The initial treatment with daunorubicin may have led to amplification of the multidrug resistance gene, which resulted in resistance to etoposide
(C)   Inhibition of eukaryotic cell replication by daunorubicin may have led to selection and amplification of a plasmid that coded for a gene that confers resistance to etoposide
(D)   An immune response may have been elicited to daunorubicin, and, because etoposide shares similar structural features to daunorubicin, the patient may have been effectively immunized to the presence of etoposide

61. Fetal hemoglobin (Hb F) is able to bind oxygen well because

(A)   fetal red blood cells have high levels of 2,3-bisphosphoglycerate (2,3-BPG)
(B)   fetal red blood cells have low levels of 2,3-BPG
(C)   Hb F binds 2,3-BPG tightly
(D)   Hb F does not bind 2,3-BPG well
(E)   the oxygen partial pressure (PO_2) levels of the placenta are high

62. Specific radioactive labeling of the RNA (not the DNA) of a cell can be done by feeding the cell radioactive

(A)   adenosine
(B)   guanosine
(C)   cytidine
(D)   thymidine
(E)   uridine

63. If a patient with adenosine deaminase deficiency-severe combined immunodeficiency (ADA-SCID) were to be treated by somatic cell gene therapy, which type of cells should be used as host cells?

(A) *Escherichia coli*
(B) Embryonic stem cells
(C) Peripheral blood lymphocytes
(D) Liver cells
(E) Red blood cells

64. Which one of the following statements regarding the supercoiling of duplex DNA is correct?

(A) DNA replication promotes positive supercoiling in advance of the replication fork
(B) DNA polymerase III can replicate positively supercoiled duplex DNA
(C) DNA topoisomerases relieve DNA supercoils by unwinding duplex DNA into single-stranded DNA chains
(D) DNA supercoils rarely exist naturally
(E) Supercoils have a lower free energy than nonsupercoiled DNA

65. A family physician suspects that a diabetic patient is not following his diet and carefully controlling his blood glucose level, although the blood glucose level is always normal when he visits the clinic. What should the physician do to determine if the suspicion is correct?

(A) Determine the percentage of the patient's hemoglobin A_2 (Hb A_2) relative to his total amount of hemoglobin
(B) Determine the percentage of the patient's Hb A_{1c} relative to his total amount of hemoglobin
(C) Determine the level of 2,3-bisphosphoglycerate (2,3-BPG) in the patient's red blood cells
(D) Determine the ratio of the patient's Hb A_2 to his 2,3-BPG
(E) Determine the ratio of the patient's Hb A_{1c} to his 2,3-BPG

66. Which one of the following compounds is responsible for the degradation of clots?

(A) Antithrombin III
(B) Thromboplastin
(C) Plasmin
(D) Thrombin
(E) Thrombomodulin

67. The peptide bond is best described by which one of the following statements? It

(A) shows rotation around the $-CN-$ bond only in α-helices
(B) exhibits conformational flexibility that allows for the different secondary structure of proteins
(C) is always planar
(D) shows rotation around the $-CN-$ bond only in β-turns

68. Where is the effector domain of an antibody located?

(A) Within the heavy chains
(B) Within the carboxy terminal domains of the heavy and light chains
(C) Within the light chains
(D) Within the variable region of the heavy and light chains
(E) Within the hinge region of the heavy chains

69. Which modification is associated with Barr bodies?

(A) Methylation
(B) Acetylation
(C) Phenylation
(D) Ubiquination
(E) Adenylation

70. Ingestion of the "death-cap" mushroom, *Amanita phalloides,* can lead to liver and kidney failure and often to death. What is the subcellular site of synthesis of the class of RNA least sensitive to the toxic effects of the death-cap mushroom?

(A) Nucleoplasm
(B) Cytoplasm
(C) Nucleolus
(D) Endoplasmic reticulum

DIRECTIONS: Each group of items in this section consists of lettered options followed by a set of numbered items. For each item, select the **one** lettered option that is most closely associated with it. Each lettered option may be selected once, more than once, or not at all.

Questions 71–74

The following drugs can be classified by their specific mechanisms of action. Match each classification with the correct drug.

(A) Rifampin
(B) Methotrexate
(C) Zidovudine
(D) Etoposide
(E) Bleomycin
(F) Doxorubicin

71. Substrate analog

72. DNA breakage

73. Antimetabolite

74. Intercalator

Questions 75–79

Match the causes of diseases listed below with the appropriate disease.

(A) Burkitt's lymphoma
(B) Xeroderma pigmentosum
(C) Lesch-Nyhan syndrome
(D) Severe combined immunodeficiency (SCID)
(E) Type IX Ehlers-Danlos syndrome

75. Deficiency in DNA repair

76. Deficiency in lysyl oxidase

77. Translocation that activates a proto-oncogene

78. Deficiency in or inactivity of hypoxanthine–guanine phosphoribosyltransferase (HGPRT)

79. Deficiency in adenosine deaminase

Questions 80–84

Match the following functions with the associated factor or protein.

(A) Sigma (σ) factor
(B) dnaA protein
(C) Catabolite activator protein (CAP)
(D) Rho (ρ) factor
(E) Transcription factor IId (TFIID)

80. Prokaryotic positive transcription regulatory factor

81. Required for proper initiation of replication in *Escherichia coli*

82. Required for termination of transcription in prokaryotes at particular termination sequences

83. Required for initiation of transcription from TATA box-containing promoters

84. Required for proper initiation of transcription in prokaryotes

Questions 85–91

Match the following mechanisms of action with the appropriate chemotherapeutic drug.

(A) Cisplatin
(B) 5-Fluorouracil
(C) 6-Mercaptopurine
(D) Bleomycin
(E) Actinomycin D
(F) Cytaribine
(G) Methotrexate

85. Causes cross-links between adjacent guanines in DNA

86. Inhibits dihydrofolate reductase

87. Inhibits conversion of inosine monophosphate (IMP) to adenosine monophosphate (AMP) and guanosine monophosphate (GMP)

88. Intercalates

89. Causes DNA breakage

90. Inhibits thymidylate synthase

91. Slows the rate of replication

Questions 92–96

Match each of the following actions with the correct hormone.

(A) Atrial natriuretic peptide
(B) Thyroxine
(C) Insulin
(D) Inositol 1,4,5-triphosphate (IP$_3$)
(E) Diacylglycerol (DAG)

92. It binds to a transmembrane tyrosine kinase and activates it

93. It diffuses into the cytosol, where it causes the release of calcium from intracellular stores

94. Its mechanism of action is the same as that of the phorbol esters

95. It forms a complex with its receptor, which acts in the nucleus to modulate gene expression

96. Its receptor is a transmembrane guanylate cyclase

Questions 97–101

Match the disease with the protein most closely linked to the disease.

(A) G$_s$
(B) *ErbB*
(C) G$_i$
(D) Adenosine deaminase
(E) eEF-2

97. Whooping cough

98. Severe combined immunodeficiency

99. Cholera

100. Diphtheria

101. Cancer

Questions 102–106

Match the following symptoms with the associated disorder.

(A) Tay-Sachs disease
(B) Niemann-Pick disease
(C) Congenital adrenal hyperplasia
(D) Maple syrup urine disease
(E) von Gierke's disease

102. Enlarged liver, lactic acidemia, fasting hypoglycemia, and hyperlipidemia

103. Mental retardation and high levels of gangliosides in brain tissue

104. Enlarged liver and spleen due to excessive accumulation of sphingomyelin

105. Elevated serum and urine levels of leucine, valine, isoleucine, and their corresponding α-keto acids

106. High serum levels of 17α-hydroxy-progesterone and very low levels of serum cortisol

Questions 107–109

Match the following functions with the correct metabolic intermediate.

(A) Fumarate
(B) Glucose-6-phosphate
(C) Pyruvate
(D) Acetyl coenzyme A
(E) Glucose-1-phosphate

107. May be converted to precursors for glycogen synthesis or nucleotide synthesis

108. Couples the actions of the urea cycle and the citric acid cycle

109. May serve as a substrate for the citric acid cycle or as a precursor for cholesterol synthesis

Questions 110–113

Match each disease characteristic with the associated disorder.

(A) Albinism
(B) Crigler-Najjar syndrome
(C) Pheochromocytomas
(D) Protoporphyria
(E) Homocystinuria

110. A defect in tyrosine metabolism

111. A deficiency in ferrochelatase

112. A deficiency in uridine diphosphate (UDP)-glucuronyl transferase

113. High urine levels of 3-methoxy-4-hydroxymandelic acid

Questions 114–118

Match each symptom of a vitamin deficiency with the appropriate vitamin.

(A) Cobalamin (vitamin B_{12})
(B) Biotin
(C) Thiamine (vitamin B_1)
(D) Ascorbic acid (vitamin C)
(E) Vitamin K

114. High serum and urine levels of leucine, valine, isoleucine, and their corresponding α-keto acids

115. High serum and urine levels of lactate, β-methylcrotonate, β-hydroxyisovalerate, and β-hydroxypropionate

116. High serum levels of methylmalonic acid

117. Defective blood clotting

118. Defective collagen synthesis

Questions 119–123

Match the symptoms below with the associated disorder.

(A) Glucose-6-phosphate dehydrogenase (G6PD) deficiency
(B) Jaundice
(C) Chronic granulomatous disease
(D) Lipoprotein lipase deficiency
(E) Tangier disease

119. Low levels of plasma cholesterol and high-density lipoproteins (HDLs)

120. High levels of serum triacylglycerols and chylomicrons

121. Elevated levels of serum bilirubin

122. Hemolytic anemia after ingestion of an oxidizing drug such as aspirin

123. The phagocytotic cells of affected individuals exhibit a reduced capacity to produce superoxide

Questions 124–128

A laboratory is designing drugs that inhibit specific enzymes. Match the desired effect of a drug with the enzyme that it must inhibit.

(A) Cyclooxygenase
(B) Xanthine oxidase
(C) 3-Hydroxy-3-methylglutaryl coenzyme A (HMG CoA) reductase
(D) Monoamine oxidase (MAO)
(E) Thymidylate synthase

124. Reduction of serum cholesterol

125. Anti-inflammatory agent

126. Treatment for gout

127. Antihypertensive agent

128. Antineoplastic agent

Questions 129–133

Match the correct physiologic function with the high-energy compound listed below.

(A) Reduced nicotinamide adenine dinucleotide (NADH)
(B) Reduced nicotinamide adenine dinucleotide phosphate (NADPH)
(C) Reduced flavin adenine dinucleotide (FADH$_2$)
(D) Uridine triphosphate (UTP)
(E) Adenosine triphosphate (ATP)

129. A major product of the reactions of the pentose phosphate pathway

130. Three moles are generated during one turn of the citric acid cycle

131. Normally tightly bound to enzymes

132. Two moles per mole of glucose are produced during anaerobic glycolysis

133. Required to synthesize the nucleotide precursor of glycogen

Questions 134–138

Match the following characteristics with the hormones listed below.

(A) Leukotrienes
(B) Thyroxine
(C) Testosterone
(D) Epinephrine
(E) Insulin

134. Is derived from cholesterol

135. May be inactivated by a protease

136. Contains covalently bound iodine

137. Tetrahydrobiopterin is required for its biosynthesis

138. Is derived from a hydroxyeicosatetra-enoic acid (5-HPETE)

DIRECTIONS: Each set of matching questions in this section consists of a list of four to twenty-six lettered options followed by several numbered items. For each numbered item, select the appropriate lettered option(s). Each lettered option may be selected once, more than once, or not at all. EACH ITEM WILL STATE THE NUMBER OF OPTIONS TO SELECT; CHOOSE EXACTLY THIS NUMBER.

Items 139–141

(A) Transformylase
(B) Transferrin
(C) Streptokinase
(D) Cyclic adenosine monophosphate (cAMP)-dependent protein kinase
(E) Protein disulfide isomerase
(F) Protein kinase C
(G) Chaperone
(H) Tissue plasminogen activator
(I) Peptidyl transferase
(J) Tyrosine kinase

For each action, select the appropriate enzyme or protein.

139. Formation of tertiary structure
(Select 2 enzymes or proteins)

140. Fibrinolysis
(Select 2 enzymes or proteins)

141. Mediation of hormone action
(Select 3 enzymes or proteins)

Items 142–144

(A) Factor XIII
(B) Kininogen
(C) Factor VIII
(D) Activated protein C
(E) Factor XII
(F) Factor XI
(G) Antithrombin III
(H) Thrombomodulin
(I) Prekallikrein
(J) Factor V

For each action, select the appropriate blood proteins.

142. Activated by thrombin
(Select 4 proteins)

143. Make contact with an abnormal surface to initiate the intrinsic pathway of clotting
(Select 3 proteins)

144. Natural inhibition of clotting
(Select 3 proteins)

Items 145–147

(A) Ribonucleoside triphosphates
(B) Primer
(C) DNA polymerase
(D) RNA polymerase
(E) Deoxynucleoside triphosphates
(F) Restriction enzyme
(G) Reverse transcriptase
(H) Plasmid vector
(I) Dideoxynucleoside triphosphates

For each procedure, select the appropriate components.

145. Formation of double-stranded complementary DNA (cDNA)
(Select 4 components)

146. Sanger method of DNA sequencing
(Select 4 components)

147. Polymerase chain reaction
(Select 3 components)

ANSWERS AND EXPLANATIONS

1–5. The answers are: 1-C [Chapter 1 III B], **2-E** [Chapter 27 VI C 4], **3-A** [Chapter 27 IV A; VI B], **4-B** [Chapter 27 IV B; VI B 9], **5-C** [Chapter 27 III A]. Metabolic acidosis is defined as a below normal level of serum bicarbonate. Respiratory alkalosis is defined as a below normal partial pressure of carbon dioxide (P_{CO_2}). The respiratory alkalosis represents an attempt by the lungs to compensate for the metabolic acidosis. If the lungs do not compensate, the blood pH is even lower.

The primary cause of low blood pH in an untreated diabetic is ketoacidosis due to high levels of ketone bodies in the blood. The ketone bodies, acetoacetate and β-hydroxybutyrate, are acids that cannot be excreted by the lungs. Hyperventilation is a response by the lungs to compensate for the metabolic acidosis. Lactate, a product of glycolysis in muscle, is not expected to be present in a diabetic state because glucose is not taken up by tissues. Although the patient may eventually experience renal failure if the condition is not treated, this is not the primary cause of the acidosis.

The metabolic profile of the liver in people with untreated diabetes is very similar to what is observed during starvation. Glucose-utilizing pathways, such as glycolysis and glycogenesis, and biosynthetic pathways, such as fatty acid synthesis, are depressed. Gluconeogenesis is stimulated in the liver so that it may continue to provide glucose for tissues. In the diabetic state, the liver has not received a signal that adequate glucose is already present in the blood. Lipolysis also occurs until triacylglycerol stores are depleted, but this occurs in adipose tissue, not the liver.

The metabolic profile of skeletal muscle in the untreated diabetic is very similar to what is observed during starvation. Glucose is not taken from the blood, and the glycogen stores are quickly depleted. Proteolysis occurs to provide amino acids as a source of energy for the body. Gluconeogenesis, ketone body synthesis, and the urea cycle are active, but these pathways are located in the liver, not the muscle.

In the diabetic state, as in the postabsorptive and starved states, the liver exports glucose generated from glycogenolysis and gluconeogenesis. The final step in gluconeogenesis is the dephosphorylation of glucose-6-phosphate (G6P). G6P also is an intermediate in glycolysis, the pentose phosphate pathway, and glycogenesis. These pathways are not active under these conditions. Fructose-6-phosphate is an intermediate in glycolysis, and pyruvate is the end product of glycolysis. Ribose-5-phosphate is a product of the pentose phosphate pathway. Glucose-1-phosphate is formed from G6P in glycogenesis.

6–10. The answers are: 6-B [Chapter 4 III D 3], **7-B** [Chapter 24 III D 1 b], **8-A** [Chapter 1 III B], **9-E** [Chapter 24 III A, B; Chapter 25 I B 5], **10-C** [Chapter 24 III D 3 c (1); Chapter 25 I B]. The low blood urea nitrogen (BUN) levels and high levels of ammonia reflect a disorder of the urea cycle, which converts ammonia that is derived from amino acid degradation to urea.

The lack of citrulline indicates a defect leading to citrulline formation. High levels of orotic acid, which is derived from carbamoyl phosphate, indicate a defect in utilization of this compound. The defective enzyme is ornithine transcarbamoylase, which converts carbamoyl phosphate to citrulline.

An above normal pH (normal = 7.4), normal bicarbonate, and below normal partial pressure of carbon dioxide is defined as respiratory alkalosis, which is due to hyperventilation caused by the hyperammonemia.

Glutamine (a storage form of ammonia) is high due to the excess ammonia driving the formation of glutamate from ammonia and α-ketoglutarate by glutamate dehydrogenase and subsequent formation of glutamine by the amidation of glutamate. Pyruvate, oxaloacetate, α-ketoglutarate, and α-ketoisovalerate are α-keto acids that may be formed from amino acids by transamination reactions. Their concentrations should be low because high glutamate and low α-ketoglutarate shift the equilibrium of the transamination reaction in favor of amino acid formation from their corresponding keto acids.

Arginine is not normally considered an essential amino acid because it is formed as an intermediate of the urea cycle. In the case of a defect in this pathway, arginine cannot be synthesized and, therefore, must be considered essential.

11–13. The answers are: 11-C [Chapter 23 II D 1; Figure 23-3], **12-B** [Chapter 7 IV B 1; Table 7-3], **13-D** [Chapter 23 II D 1]. Patients with Gaucher's disease are deficient in β-glucosidase, which is needed to degrade the sphingolipid glucocerebroside. Niemann-Pick disease is also a defect in sphingolipid metabolism, but it is due to a deficiency of sphingomyelinase. Pompe's disease and von Gierke's disease are glycogen storage diseases, and Crigler-Najjar syndrome is a disorder of heme metabolism.

Most glucocerebroside is stored in the liver and spleen, and the enlargement of these organs is a consequence of the inability to degrade it.

The degradation of glucocerebroside occurs in the lysosomes, which are the primary site of the intracellular degradation of macromolecules.

14–16. The answers are: 14-B [Chapter 19 I D 6 e], **15-B** [Chapter 19 I D 6, Figure 19-1; Chapter 3 II A 2 c (3)], **16-E** [Chapter 4 IV C 1; Chapter 16 III F 3; Chapter 17 VII B; Chapter 19 I D 6; Chapter 25 VII B 2]. Carbon monoxide inhibits mitochondrial electron transport by combining with the oxygen-binding site of cytochrome oxidase, preventing the electrons passed down the electron transport chain from interacting with oxygen.

Carbon monoxide also binds to the oxygen-binding site of hemoglobin, reducing the capacity of the blood to carry oxygen, but this function does not inhibit electron transport or cause the life-threatening symptoms that result from blocking the electron transport chain. The other choices are components of the electron transport chain but bind neither oxygen nor carbon monoxide.

Cyanide also binds to the oxygen-binding site of cytochrome oxidase, blocking respiration. Lead is an inhibitor of heme biosynthesis. Arsenate is a phosphate analog that uncouples substrate-level phosphorylation during glycolysis. Nerve gas (e.g., sarin) inhibits acetylcholine esterase. Ethylene glycol is metabolized by alcohol dehydrogenase to a toxic product.

17–19. The answers are: 17-D [Chapter 25 VII C 5], **18-B** [Chapter 25 VII C 4 b (2)], **19-E** [Chapter 25 VII C 5 c]. Jaundice is a condition in which the blood contains excessive amounts of bilirubin, an intermediate in the degradation of heme, and related compounds. Direct bilirubin refers to conjugated bilirubin. Indirect bilirubin refers to free, unconjugated bilirubin. Bilirubin and related compounds are deposited in the skin and mucous membranes, which gives affected patients a yellowish hue.

Neonatal jaundice is a temporary condition due to production of insufficient levels of uridine diphosphate (UDP)-glucuronyl transferase by the infant. This is typically treated by phototherapy. The products from the irradiation of bilirubin are more soluble than bilirubin and can be excreted by the liver into the bile without conjugation with glucuronic acid.

In an obstruction of the bile duct, there is an accumulation of the conjugated bilirubin diglucuronide, which cannot be transported by the bile from the liver to the bowel. Prehepatic jaundice occurs when the rate of bilirubin formation is greater than the capacity of the bilirubin conjugation system. In decreased hepatic uptake of bilirubin, Crigler-Najjar syndrome, and neonatal jaundice, there is an increase in free bilirubin due to the inability to form the conjugate in the liver.

20. The answer is E [Chapter 17 I A 1; Chapter 22 I A 6, B 1 b]. Reducing equivalents are required during fatty acid synthesis to convert the β-ketoacyl–acyl carrier protein (ACP) intermediate to the saturated acyl–ACP thioester. Reduced nicotinamide adenine dinucleotide phosphate (NADPH) is used as the electron donor. In the liver, it arises mainly from the oxidation of glucose-6-phosphate (G6P) via the pentose phosphate pathway. The reducing equivalents that are generated by the other pathways are primarily in the form of reduced nicotinamide adenine dinucleotide (NADH).

21. The answer is E [Chapter 23 IV A 2]. The rate-limiting and regulated step of cholesterol biosynthesis is the formation of mevalonate from 3-hydroxy-3-methylglutaryl coenzyme A (HMG CoA) catalyzed by HMG CoA reductase. This enzyme is inhibited by dietary cholesterol and endogenously synthesized cholesterol. A vegetarian diet, a diet low in cholesterol, and the administration of bile acid-sequestering resin all result in a reduced intake of cholesterol, which will not reduce

HMG CoA reductase activity. Familial hypercholesterolemia is a result of a deficiency of low-density lipoprotein receptors.

22. The answer is D [Chapter 20 II B; Chapter 27 V A]. During long-term fasting, the insulin:glucagon ratio is low, and mobilization of metabolic fuels predominates. The cyclic adenosine monophosphate levels in the liver are high due to glucagon dominance, and the adenosine triphosphate levels in the liver are always adequate. Free fatty acids from mobilized triacylglycerol stores in adipose tissue are available to the liver and other tissues. The main controlling factor for the rate of gluconeogenesis is substrate availability. The substrates for gluconeogenesis in prolonged fasting are amino acids, although after 3-4 days of fasting, the rate of supply of amino acids to the liver from peripheral tissues declines. Alanine is a major form by which amino acids arrive at the liver from muscle and other tissues.

23. The answer is B [Chapter 24 III A, B]. The first step in the degradation of most amino acids is a transamination reaction with α-ketoglutarate to form its corresponding keto acid and glutamate. Glutamate dehydrogenase then catalyzes the oxidative deamination of glutamate to regenerate α-ketoglutarate and release the amino group as ammonia.

24. The answer is E [Chapter 25 II B 1 c 4; Figure 25-3]. Serine hydroxymethyltransferase catalyzes the interconversion of serine and glycine. It requires tetrahydrofolate (THF), a derivative of folic acid, as a cofactor. With inadequate vitamin B_{12} uptake from the gut, the metabolism of folate is impaired, and there is an accumulation of the N^5-methyl THF form. This is because the only way in which N^5-methyl THF can be converted to THF is in the reaction converting homocysteine to methionine, which requires methylcobalamin, a derivative of vitamin B_{12}.

25. The answer is E [Chapter 13 III B 5]. The equilibrium ratio of products to reactants is related to $\Delta G^{\circ\prime}$ by the equation:

$$\Delta G^{\circ\prime} = -RT \ln[\text{products}]/[\text{reactants}]$$

Under standard conditions, this becomes:

$$2.8 = -1.418 \log_{10}[\text{products}]/[\text{reactants}]$$
$$[\text{products}]/[\text{reactants}] = \text{antilog}(-2.0) = 0.01$$

26. The answer is B [Chapter 4 I C; Table 4-1]. A kinase is a transferase that catalyzes the transfer of phosphate from adenosine triphosphate (ATP) to another substrate, which in this case is glucose. The participation of ATP in the reactions distinguishes a kinase from phosphatases and phosphorylases, which also transfer phosphate groups. A phosphodiesterase cleaves phosphodiester bonds such as those in nucleic acids. Hydrolases transfer water.

27. The answer is A [Chapter 19 I D 5 a]. Unlike the other components of the respiratory chain, cytochrome c is a soluble protein that binds to the membrane to perform its electron transfer role. The enzymes cytochrome oxidase (complex IV), reduced nicotinamide adenine dinucleotide (NADH) dehydrogenase (complex I), and succinate dehydrogenase (complex II) are each firmly embedded in the membrane. The electron carrier coenzyme Q is a highly lipid-soluble molecule that is also embedded in the membrane.

28. The answer is C [Chapter 20 G; Chapter 21 III]. The gluconeogenic enzyme glucose-6-phosphatase occurs in the liver and kidney. Without it, muscle cannot synthesize glucose, and glycogenolysis in exercising muscle leads to an elevation of blood lactate, which is formed via glycolysis. Lactate is an important gluconeogenic substance, so muscle contributes significantly to the level of blood glucose indirectly by providing lactate to the liver. Phosphorylase is necessary for the depolymerization of glucose to form glucose-1-phosphate. Glucokinase phosphorylates glucose in the liver. The other enzymes participate in glycolysis in both tissues.

29. The answer is C [Chapter 22 I C 1 b; Chapter 27, Table 27-1]. Citrate regulates fatty acid synthesis by allosterically affecting the acetyl coenzyme A carboxylase. The rates of the urea cycle and pentose phosphate pathway are controlled by substrate availability, and the citric acid cycle and fatty acid degradation are under respiratory control.

30. The answer is D [Chapter 4 II A 2]. A chemical reaction occurs when a substrate molecule becomes sufficiently energized to reach a transition state, where there is a high probability that a chemical bond will be formed or broken. This is the energy of activation, and the effect of a catalyst (i.e., an enzyme) is to decrease the energy of activation. Enzymes do not alter the equilibrium or the overall free-energy change of a reaction.

31. The answer is D [Chapter 16 III F, Figure 16-2; Chapter 17 III B]. Fructose is phosphorylated by fructokinase to fructose-1-phosphate. Hexokinase does not phosphorylate fructose. Fructose-1-phosphate is cleaved by phosphofructoaldolase (aldolase B) to form dihydroxyacetone phosphate (DHAP) and glyceraldehyde. DHAP is converted to glyceraldehyde-3-phosphate (G3P) by triose phosphate isomerase. G3P is converted to 1,3-bisphosphoglycerate (1,3-BPG) by G3P dehydrogenase. 1,3-BPG is further metabolized to pyruvate by glycolytic enzymes. 6-Phosphogluconate is an intermediate in the pentose phosphate pathway, which arises from glucose-6-phosphate (G6P) and not from fructose-1-phosphate. Fructose-1-phosphate derived from fructose does not give rise to G6P and, therefore, does not involve the activity of phosphoglucomutase.

32. The answer is C [Chapter 22 III B]. The biosynthesis of triacylglycerols involves the esterification of glycerol by fatty acyl coenzyme A (CoA). Adipose tissue cells cannot phosphorylate glycerol arising from lipolysis because they lack a glycerol kinase. Instead, they use dihydroxyacetone phosphate or glycerol-3-phosphate formed during glycolysis. The biosynthesis of triacylglycerols is thus stimulated by increased glucose entry into the cells. The higher the plasma insulin, the greater the rate of glycolysis, and the more glycerol-3-phosphate available for esterification of fatty acyl CoAs. Elevated plasma levels of epinephrine and of intracellular levels of cyclic adenosine monophosphate stimulate lipolysis.

33. The answer is E [Chapter 24 III D; Figure 24-3]. In liver mitochondria, carbamoyl phosphate is formed from ammonia, carbon dioxide, and adenosine triphosphate. The carbamoyl group is then transferred to ornithine by ornithine transcarbamoylase. The product is citrulline, which combines with aspartate to form argininosuccinate. This is cleaved by argininosuccinate lyase to arginine and fumarate. Arginine is then cleaved by arginase to yield urea and ornithine.

34. The answer is A [Chapter 25 VII A 1]. The synthesis of δ-aminolevulinate is the first and the rate-controlling step of porphyrin biosynthesis; the synthase that catalyzes the condensation of succinyl coenzyme A (CoA) and glycine to form δ-aminolevulinate is allosterically inhibited by protoheme IX.

35. The answer is B [Chapter 4 III A 4]. The Michaelis-Menten equation relates the velocity (v) of an enzyme-catalyzed reaction to the maximum velocity (V_{max}), the substrate concentration, and the Michaelis-Menten constant (K_m) as:

$$v = V_{max}[S]/([S] + K_m)$$

If $[S] = 1/2\ K_m$, then

$$v = V_{max}[0.5\ K_m]/([0.5\ K_m] + K_m)$$
$$= V_{max}/3 = 0.33\ V_{max}$$

36. The answer is E [Chapter 18 I A]. Pyruvate dehydrogenase catalyzes the irreversible conversion of pyruvate, the end product of glycolysis, to acetyl coenzyme A (CoA), the substrate for the citric acid cycle. Acetyl CoA synthetase generates acetyl CoA from fatty acids. Lactate dehydrogenase catalyzes the reversible interconversion of lactate and pyruvate. Pyruvate kinase is the final enzyme in glycolysis that forms pyruvate. Citrate synthase is the first enzyme of the citric acid cycle that utilizes acetyl CoA.

37. The answer is D [Chapter 24 IV 4]. Proline and arginine are catabolized to glutamate, which may be converted to α-ketoglutarate. Three carbons of α-ketoglutarate can provide a net synthesis of glucose and are, therefore, glucogenic. Isoleucine is metabolized to succinyl coenzyme A (CoA), which is glucogenic, and acetyl CoA, which is ketogenic. Phenylalanine is metabolized to fumarate (glucogenic) and acetoacetate (ketogenic). None of the carbon from leucine is glucogenic.

38. The answer is B [Chapter 21 IV; Chapter 24 I A 2]. The regulation of glycogen metabolism involves covalent modification of two key enzymes. Glycogen phosphorylase, which converts glycogen to glucose-6-phosphate, is active only when it is phosphorylated. Glycogen synthase, which forms glycogen from UDP-glucose, is inactive when phosphorylated and must be dephosphorylated by a phosphatase to regain activity. Protein kinase is the enzyme that catalyzes the phosphorylation of these enzymes. Pepsin and trypsin are each activated by a proteolytic cleavage of an inactive precursor.

39–41. The answers are: 39-B [Chapter 27 II A; Table 27-3], **40-C** [Chapter 27 IV B 4], **41-E** [Chapter 27 IV E]. This metabolic profile occurs during the postabsorptive state, several hours after a meal. The adipose tissue releases fatty acids, which are utilized by the heart, skeletal muscle, and liver for fuel. Glycerol, which is taken up by the liver and converted to glucose, also is released by adipose tissue. The liver releases glucose into the blood.

Some of the glucose, which is derived from glycogenolysis and gluconeogenesis, is taken up and used for fuel by the skeletal muscle. It releases lactate, formed from glucose via pyruvate, which is taken up by the liver and used as a substrate for gluconeogenesis. β-Hydroxybutyrate and acetoacetate are ketone bodies that would be released by the liver if the metabolic state were starvation or untreated diabetes.

Under all metabolic conditions, glucose is the preferred fuel for the brain. During starvation and in untreated diabetes, it will adapt to use ketone bodies. In the postabsorptive state, the liver, heart, and muscle preferentially use fatty acids, which are released by adipose tissue for fuel.

42. The answer is E [Chapter 14 II I 4; Chapter 17 I C 5]. Transketolase activity in erythrocytes is a sensitive indicator of body thiamine levels. In severe thiamine deficiency, transketolase activity, which requires the thiamine pyrophosphate (TPP) cofactor, is depressed. Blood levels of pyruvate and lactate would not be expected to be low; rather, pyruvate levels are increased in thiamine deficiency due to a reduced use of pyruvate by the TPP-dependent pyruvate dehydrogenase complex. Thiamine deficiency should not significantly influence the clotting time of blood, catabolism of tryptophan, or transaminase activity in red blood cells.

43. The answer is E [Chapter 18 IV B 2; Chapter 20 III A]. Reactions that increase the concentration of citric acid cycle intermediates without using other citric acid cycle intermediates are called anaplerotic. One such reaction is the carboxylation of pyruvate to oxaloacetate, which is catalyzed by pyruvate carboxylase. Succinate dehydrogenase and citrate synthetase are enzymes of the citric acid cycle and cannot provide a net synthesis of any citric acid cycle intermediates solely from acetyl coenzyme A (acetyl CoA). Citrate lyase is a cytosolic enzyme that cleaves citrate to oxaloacetate and acetyl CoA. Pyruvate dehydrogenase provides the citric acid cycle with acetyl CoA but does not increase the concentration of cycle intermediates.

44. The answer is B [Chapter 16 III C]. Citrate is an inhibitor of phosphofructokinase, the enzyme that catalyzes the committed step in glycolysis. High levels of citrate signal a high-energy state, and continued activity of an energy-generating pathway, such as glycolysis, would be wasteful. Citrate also acts as an allosteric regulator of the key enzymes involved in gluconeogenesis and fatty acid synthesis but in those pathways, citrate activates the enzymes.

45. The answer is C [Chapter 3 II B 4 a]. Hemoglobin A_1 (Hb A_1), the major circulating form in adult humans, reacts spontaneously with glucose to form a derivative known as Hb A_{1c}. Normally the level of Hb A_{1c} is very low, but in patients with diabetes mellitus, in whom blood sugar levels may be periodically high, the concentration of Hb A_{1c} may reach 12% or more of the total hemoglobin. Vigorous control of blood sugar levels in diabetic patients may reduce blood levels of Hb A_{1c} to more normal values.

46. The answer is D [Chapter 6 II D 1, 2; Figure 6-4]. The base composition affects the melting temperature (T_m). The higher the percentage of guanine–cytosine (GC) base pairs in DNA, the higher is its T_m. No damage or breaking of any covalent bonds occurs upon denaturation. In fact, duplex DNA can reform by a process called renaturation. When DNA is denatured, its absorption of light at 260 nm increases. This is the hyperchromic effect. A decrease in absorption occurs upon renaturation, which is the hypochromic effect. The melting transition that occurs upon DNA denaturation is sudden for a homogeneous piece of DNA.

47. The answer is B [Chapter 8 II A, B 1, D 2 a; VI 1 a]. DNA polymerase I (DNA pol I) requires both a template and a primer to function as a polymerizing enzyme. Both 3' and 5' exonuclease activities are also integral parts of this single-peptide protein. It functions in normal DNA replication, hydrolyzing the stretches of primer chain RNA (5' to 3' exonuclease activity) and replacing them with template-directed deoxyribonucleotides (polymerizing function). DNA pol I also is involved in the repair of DNA. For example, it participates in the excision of thymine dimers, which is a 5' to 3' exonuclease activity. During normal DNA replication, DNA pol I exhibits 3' exonuclease activity, excising incorrectly introduced deoxyribonucleotide residues. Okazaki fragments are produced by DNA pol III complex, not DNA pol I, and after the removal of the RNA primer chains, the fragments are linked by DNA ligase.

48. The answer is B [Chapter 8 IV C 1 c, D 2 a; Chapter 9 II A 4 b (2), B 2 a (3); Chapter 10 VIII B 2]. The antibiotic rifampin inhibits initiation of transcription in prokaryotes by binding to the β subunit of RNA polymerase when it is in the holoenzyme form. Because it binds only to the β subunit when the RNA polymerase is in the holoenzyme form (i.e., with the σ factor), it affects only initiation and not elongation of transcription. Actinomycin is an intercalator and as such inhibits both replication and transcription. The quinolones inhibit DNA replication by inhibiting the bacterial topoisomerase, DNA gyrase. Puromycin acts as an analog of aminoacyl transfer RNA (tRNA) and inhibits protein synthesis.

49. The answer is E [Chapter 12 I A 2, C 1–2]. A gene that is expressed at a constant, unregulated, and often low rate is said to be constitutively expressed. A mutation in either the operator sequence or the *lac I* gene, so that it produces an inactive repressor, results in an operon that cannot be regulated by the presence or absence of lactose and is thus inactive. With an inactive repressor, the *lac* operon can still be regulated by catabolite repression. With a mutated repressor and no glucose, the expression of the *lac* operon would be high because there would be no catabolite repression by glucose. In the presence of glucose, it would be expressed but at a low level. A mutated promoter that prevents RNA polymerase from binding leads to a complete inhibition of expression under all growth conditions. A missense mutation (see Chapter 8 V B 1 b) in the β-galactosidase gene is likely to reduce the activity of the enzyme but is not likely to affect its cellular levels. A mutated β-galactosidase has no effect on either of the other two enzyme products of the operon. A mutation in the catabolite activator protein (CAP) affects the ability of the *lac* operon to be regulated by catabolite repression. The *lac* operon is not regulated by attenuation (see Chapter 12 III).

50. The answer is E [Chapter 3 II B 2 b, 4 a, b (3), c]. Hemoglobin M (Hb M) refers to methemoglobin, which is found in hemoglobinopathies in which the iron is in the ferric (Fe^{3+}) form. These hemoglobinopathies arise because of mutations in either the proximal or

distal histidine residues. Normally, these histidines bond with iron in the heme group or with oxygen. Without these histidines, the ferrous form of iron (Fe^{2+}) oxidizes to the ferric form, which cannot bind iron. Hemoglobin A_{1c} (Hb A_{1c}) is a normally occurring glycosylated derivative of Hb A_1. Hemoglobin F (Hb F) is the predominant fetal hemoglobin. Both hemoglobin C (Hb C) and hemoglobin S (Hb S) are found in different hemoglobinopathies. In Hb A_{1c}, Hb C, Hb S, and Hb F, there is normal ferrous iron.

51. The answer is D [Chapter 3 V B]. Collagen types are classified by the nature of the peptide chains, which form the triple helix of procollagen. For instance, six different α1 chains are recognized, which vary in primary structure; these are labeled α1(I), α1(II), α1(III), α1(IV), α1(V), and α1(VI). The collagen of bone, skin, tendons, and scar tissue contains triple helices made up of two α1(I) chains and one α2(I) chain. Collagen of cartilage and vitreous contains three α(II) chains. Other collagens are made up of different combinations of α1, α2, and α3 chains.

52. The answer is E [Chapter 11 II A 2]. Restriction enzymes cut both strands of duplex DNA. The cuts are symmetrical and usually within the recognition sequence, but not necessarily along the axis of symmetry. A particular enzyme always makes cuts at the same position. Without experimental determination, there is no way to predict where a particular enzyme will cut DNA.

53. The answer is C [Chapter 11 II A 2; Figure 11-1]. Restriction enzymes recognize specific sequences in double-stranded DNA and make two unique sequence-specific cuts, one in each strand. These cuts generate 3′-hydroxyl and 5′-phosphate ends. Restriction enzyme cuts are symmetrical but not necessarily along the axis of symmetry. If the cuts are not along the axis of symmetry, they are said to produce sticky ends. By convention, the sequence of only one strand of double-stranded DNA sequences is written in the 5′ to 3′ direction. The products of only two of the above examples leave 5′ sticky ends, C/CCGGG and AT/TAAT. A cut in C/CCGGG would leave a four-base 5′-sticky end, whereas a cut in AT/TAAT would leave only a two-base 5′-sticky end. A cut in TGG/CCA would be right along the axis of symmetry and would generate blunt ends not sticky ends. Cuts in ATGCA/T and CCTGCA/GG would each generate 3'-sticky ends four bases in length.

54. The answer is A [Chapter 3 VI B 1 b, 2 a (1) (c), b, c; Figure 3-11]. Myosin contains the adenosine triphosphatase (ATPase) activity, which is needed to drive the contraction reactions. If myosin is cleaved with trypsin and papain, the amino-terminal globular head (which contains the light chains) can be purified and shown to contain the ATPase activity. The ATPase activity of actin serves to increase the rate of production of F actin from G actin. Troponin C is a subunit of the troponin complex that participates in the regulation of contraction by binding calcium. It exhibits no ATPase activity. The carboxy-terminal tail region contains the self-assembly activity needed to form myosin. Tropomyosin plays an integral role in contraction by regulating the interaction of actin and myosin.

55. The answer is D [Chapter 4 VII B 2 a]. Prothrombin has a high affinity for platelets, which is due to the presence of γ-carboxylated glutamate (Gla) residues. These Gla residues allow prothrombin to bind to platelets in the presence of calcium. Vitamin K is required for the completion of synthesis of prothrombin via the post-translational γ-carboxylation of prothrombin. Factors VII, IX, and X also have a high affinity for platelets because of the presence of vitamin K-dependent Gla residues. However, the vitamin K-dependent carboxylation of these factors, although crucial to clot formation, only indirectly affects the activation of Factor X. The two factors that can activate Factor X (i.e., VIIa and IXa) are enzymatically active without being γ-carboxylated; they are not in a high concentration near activated platelets. Likewise, thrombin is brought to activated platelets by the γ-carboxylation of prothrombin. In fact, thrombin loses its affinity for activated platelets upon activation. Vitamin K has no known direct effect on blood calcium levels or on the regulation of transcription.

56. The answer is C [Chapter 3 II B 4 b (1)]. Hemoglobin S (Hb S), the form of hemoglobin found in sickle cell anemia, is a mutant molecule with valine substituted for glutamic acid in the sixth position on the β chains. In the homozygote form, deoxyhemoglobin S polymerizes within the red cells. The long insoluble polymer fibers distort the erythrocyte, leading to the characteristic sickle-shaped cells. These misshapen cells are destroyed by the spleen, leading to anemia. In other respects, Hb S appears normal; the cooperative binding of oxygen and the protection of the ferrous iron by the apoprotein heme pocket are not affected.

57. The answer is B [Chapter 6 IV C 2; Chapter 9 III A 3 d]. The most heavily modified RNA is transfer RNA (tRNA). These modifications are required for structural reasons. Other RNAs, in particular heterogeneous nuclear RNA (hnRNA) and messenger RNA (mRNA), may have 5' cap structures. Ribosomal RNAs (rRNAs) are methylated. Methylation is probably involved in directing the proper processing of rRNA.

58. The answer is E [Chapter 9 II B 1; Chapter 12 I C 1 b, 2 c; II A 2]. An operator is a controlling element of an operon. A repressor inhibits transcription of an operon by binding to the operator and blocking the initiation of transcription. In the case of the *lac* operon, and many other operons, the operator spans the initiation site. The repressor specifically binds to the operator sequences, not to the single base initiation site. An operator can be positioned in an operon at other than a promoter/initiation area. This is exemplified in the *ara* operon. A catabolite activator protein (CAP) site is where a CAP binds when complexed with cyclic adenosine monophosphate (cAMP) to turn on transcription in the absence of glucose and in the presence of another sugar. A regulatory gene produces, usually constitutively, a regulatory protein that controls the expression of an operon. A promoter is responsible for directing RNA polymerase to initiate transcription at the initiation site.

59. The answer is E [Chapter 6 II E; Chapter 9 II B 1 c; III B 2 b; Chapter 12 VI B; VII D]. Alterations in RNA stability may make a considerable contribution to gene regulation in eukaryotes. Fewer than 10% of a typical eukaryotic genome codes for a product and, within any one cell, only a small percentage of the genes are expressed. Regulation of gene expression during the processing events that lead to the formation of messenger RNA (mRNA) is common in eukaryotes, but by no means is it the only mechanism of regulation. The nuclear membrane forms too great of a physical barrier to allow the coupling of transcription and translation. Therefore, eukaryotes cannot regulate gene expression by attenuation. Many, but not all, of the eukaryotic gene promoters are upstream of their transcriptional initiation sites. Genes transcribed by RNA polymerase III have promoters within the transcribed portion of the gene, downstream of the transcriptional initiation site. The addition of a poly A tail to mRNA is a post-transcriptional processing event.

60. The answer is B [Chapter 8 IV C 1 b, D 2 b; Chapter 12 VIII A 3 c; Case 12-1]. Daunorubicin and etoposide are both antineoplastic drugs. However, they inhibit cell proliferation by completely different mechanisms. Daunorubicin is a DNA intercalator, and etoposide inhibits topoisomerase II. Therefore, they are not likely to be structurally similar. The multidrug resistance gene produces a large membrane-bound glycoprotein called P glycoprotein that confers resistance to many anticancer drugs by pumping them out of the cell in an adenosine triphosphate (ATP)-dependent manner. Cells become resistant to many anticancer drugs by amplifying this gene. Because this gene confers resistance to multiple drugs, a particular chemotherapeutic treatment may lead to resistance to another drug that has never been used on a patient. Plasmids are extrachromosomal pieces of DNA that are present in many bacteria but not in eukaryotic cells. Therefore, in the unlikely event that a plasmid coded for resistance to etoposide, it would not affect a eukaryotic cancer cell.

61. The answer is D [Chapter 3 II B 3 c–d]. Fetal hemoglobin (Hb F) needs an increased affinity for oxygen because the partial pressure of oxygen (Po_2) in the placenta is, like that of most other tissues, low. Decreased levels of 2,3-bisphosphoglycerate (2,3-BPG) cause the oxygen binding affinity of hemoglobin A_1 (Hb A_1) to increase. This does not happen in fetal red blood cells because, in the absence of 2,3-BPG, Hb F has a lower affinity for oxygen than Hb A_1. The 2,3-BPG levels of fetal red blood cells are similar to those of adult red blood cells. Hb F differs from Hb A_1 by having two γ subunits instead of two β subunits. The γ subunits do not bind 2,3-BPG well, and this gives Hb F a higher oxygen binding affinity than Hb A_1.

62. The answer is E [Chapter 6 I B 2 b]. Experimentally, DNA synthesis is distinguished from RNA synthesis by whether radioactive thymidine or uridine is incorporated. DNA and RNA differ in the pyrimidines thymine and uracil. Thymines are found only in DNA, and uracils are found only in RNA. Cells can take up radioactive nucleosides, convert them to nucleoside triphosphates, and incorporate them into DNA or RNA during replication or transcription. To label the RNA of a cell, radioactive uridine should be fed to the cell.

63. The answer is C [Chapter 11 III E 2; Case 11-1; Chapter 26 VI D 1]. A deficiency in adenosine deaminase (ADA) leads to dysfunctional T cells and B cells of the peripheral blood lymphocytes. The levels of deoxyadenosine triphosphate (dATP) increase because dATP is not degraded by ADA. The high levels of dATP inhibit DNA synthesis by inhibiting ribonucleotide reductase. Therefore, T cells and B cells cannot proliferate, which leads to severe combined immunodeficiency (SCID). ADA-SCID has been successfully treated by somatic cell gene therapy by transfecting cultured T cells from the patients with a recombinant DNA vector that expresses normal ADA. *Escherichia coli,* embryonic stem cells, or liver cells could not replace the patient's deficient T cells. Red blood cells have no nuclei, so they are not amenable to gene therapy.

64. The answer is A [Chapter 6 III A; Chapter 8 II E 2; IV D 2]. DNA replication promotes positive supercoiling in advance of the replication fork. Topoisomerases are required in replication to relieve the torsional stress that results from the formation of supercoils, which are at a higher free energy than nonsupercoiled DNA. In bacteria, if the topoisomerase DNA gyrase is inhibited by antibiotics such as nalidixic acid or the fluoroquinolones, then replication is inhibited. This indicates that DNA polymerase III cannot replicate positively supercoiled DNA. Helicases, not topoisomerases, unwind duplex DNA into single-stranded DNA chains. The unwinding of DNA would induce, not relieve, supercoil formation. Supercoiled DNA exists naturally. Most naturally occurring supercoils are negative.

65. The answer is B [Chapter 3 II B 4 a]. There is no evidence that a patient's 2,3-bisphosphoglycerate (2,3-BPG) levels change depending on blood glucose levels. Hb A_2 is a minor hemoglobin tetramer in adults (2%). Instead of two β chains, Hb A_2 has two δ chains. The β subunits of Hb A_1 react spontaneously with glucose to form Hb A_{1c}. If patients have a high blood glucose level for a prolonged period of time, their percentage of Hb A_{1c} relative to the total level of hemoglobin increases significantly. Because red blood cells have a long half-life (120 days), this increase can be detected even if a patient's blood glucose level is low at the time of determination. The percentage of Hb A_{1c} relative to the total level of hemoglobin, therefore, becomes a good assay of long-term maintenance of blood glucose levels.

66. The answer is C [Chapter 4 VII B 2, C 1; VIII A 2, 4, B 1]. Plasmin, the active form of the zymogen plasminogen, is the protease that specifically degrades clots. Thrombin causes the formation of loose clots by converting fibrinogen to fibrin as well as by activating a number of other clotting factors. Thromboplastin or tissue factor is responsible for triggering the extrinsic pathway of clotting. Thrombomodulin converts thrombin from an enzyme that is crucial to clot formation to one that inhibits clot formation. Antithrombin III is a slow inhibitor of thrombin and Factors IXa, Xa, and XIa.

67. The answer is C [Chapter 2 III A 3]. The peptide bond is a planar structure with the two adjacent α-carbons, a carbonyl oxygen, an α-amino nitrogen and its associated hydrogen atom, and the carbonyl carbon all lying in the same plane. The —CN— bond has a partial double-bond character that prevents rotation around the bond axis. The peptide bond remains the same in all of the secondary structures of proteins.

68. The answer is B [Chapter 3 IV B; Figure 3-7]. The effector domain is the region of the antibody that is responsible for initiating the processes that rid the body of the antibody-bound antigens and that designates the class and distribution of an antibody. The COOH-terminal domains of the heavy (H) and light (L) chains have a constant structure that is similar between different antibodies of the same class. The amino acid sequence in this region shows very little difference between different antibodies. The effector domain lies within the constant region. The NH_2-terminal portion of both the L and H chains has a variable structure that differs in sequence considerably between different antibodies. The variable regions of paired L and H chains are adjacent to each other and form the antibody-binding

site, which binds antigen. The amino acid sequence of the variable region is the sole determinant of the specificity of binding of an antibody with an antigen. The heavy chains contain a hinge region between the first two structural domains of the constant region. As the name implies, this region is flexible and allows movement between the two antibody-binding sites.

69. The answer is A [Chapter 12 V A 2, 4]. In the cells of human females, one of the X chromosomes is made transcriptionally inactive through heterochromatinization. Methylation likely plays a role in the maintenance of inactive heterochromatin. Part of the experimental evidence for this is that inhibiting the maintenance methylase during replication can reactivate genes on Barr bodies.

70. The answer is C. [Chapter 9 II A 4 b; Table 9-1]. *Amanita phalloides* contains the toxin α-amanitin, which is primarily responsible for death from ingestion of these mushrooms. α-Amanitin acts through a differential inhibition of the eukaryotic nuclear RNA polymerases. In fact, it played a crucial role in identification of the class of RNA produced by (and the subnuclear location of) each of the three nuclear RNA polymerases. Messenger RNA (mRNA) and some of the small nuclear RNAs (snRNA) are produced by RNA polymerase II, which is located in the nucleoplasm. RNA polymerase II is most sensitive to α-amanitin. RNA polymerase III produces many of the small RNAs (e.g., tRNA, 5S rRNA) in the nucleoplasm. RNA polymerase III exhibits an intermediate sensitivity to α-amanitin. The large precursor 45S rRNA is produced by RNA polymerase I in the nucleolus. RNA polymerase I is completely resistant to inhibition by α-amanitin.

71–74. The answers are: 71-C [Chapter 8 IV B 1], **72-E** [Chapter 8 IV C 2 c], **73-B** [Chapter 8 IV A; Chapter 26 V B], **74-F** [Chapter 8 IV C 1 b]. Zidovudine (azidothymidine, AZT) is a substrate analog that is an effective inhibitor of viral DNA synthesis. It preferentially inhibits reverse transcriptase over cellular DNA polymerase. The bleomycins bind to DNA and cause DNA breakage when they interact with oxygen and ferrous iron (Fe^{2+}). Methotrexate is an antimetabolite that ultimately inhibits replication by preventing the conversion of deoxyuridine monophosphate (dUMP) to deoxythymidine monophosphate (dTMP). It does this by inhibiting dihydrofolate reductase

(DHFR), which is needed to produce the methylenetetrahydrofolate required in the conversion of dUMP to dTMP. Doxorubicin is an intercalator and, as such, blocks DNA synthesis.

75–79. The answers are: 75-B [Chapter 8 VI A 1 b], **76-E** [Chapter 3 V D 3; Table 3-2], **77-A** [Chapter 12 VIII D], **78-C** [Chapter 26 VI C], **79-D** [Chapter 26 VI D 1]. Xeroderma pigmentosum is an autosomal recessive disease that results in hypersensitivity of the skin to ultraviolet light damage and a concomitant high incidence of skin cancer. It is due to a deficiency in the repair of thymine–thymine dimers.

Type IX Ehlers-Danlos syndrome is caused by an X-linked recessive deficiency in lysyl oxidase. This results in decreased cross-linking of collagen because lysyl oxidase causes formation of intramolecular and intermolecular cross-links between lysines and hydroxylysines of tropocollagen molecules. Patients with this syndrome have hyperextensible skin and skeletal deformities.

Burkitt's lymphoma is caused by a translocation of immunoglobulin genes that leads to an activation of the *myc* proto-oncogene.

Lesch-Nyhan syndrome is a severe neurologic disorder that is due to inactive or deficient hypoxanthine–guanine phosphoribosyltransferase (HGPRT). An absence of HGPRT results in an increase in phosphoribosylpyrophosphate and a decrease in inosine monophosphate (IMP) and guanosine monophosphate (GMP).

Severe combined immunodeficiency (SCID) is due to a deficiency in adenosine deaminase. Adenosine deaminase activity is needed to degrade adenosine and deoxyadenosine. The resulting accumulation of high levels of deoxyadenosine triphosphate (dATP) inhibits DNA replication. This inhibition of proliferation strongly affects B and T cells, which are needed in the immune response.

80–84. The answers are: 80-C [Chapter 12 II A 2], **81-B** [Chapter 8 II C 2], **82-D** [Chapter 9 II C 1 b], **83-E** [Chapter 9 II B 2 b], **84-A** [Chapter 9 II A 4 a (2), B 2 a]. Catabolite activator protein (CAP), also called cyclic adenosine monophosphate (cAMP) receptor protein (CRP), is a positive transcription regulatory factor in prokaryotes. In the presence of cAMP (due to low levels of glucose), CAP greatly enhances the initiation of transcription at CAP-responsive promoters.

The dnaA protein is required for proper initiation of replication in *Escherichia coli*. It binds to specific sequences within the origin of replication, and, in the presence of adenosine triphosphate (ATP) and other components of replication, dnaA protein facilitates initiation of replication.

Although the exact mechanism is unknown, rho (ρ) protein binds as a hexamer to rho-dependent termination sequences and, upon cleavage of ATP by rho, termination of transcription takes place.

The eukaryotic transcription factor II D (TFIID) is needed to initiate transcription from TATA box promoters by RNA polymerase II. TFIID recognizes and binds to the TATA box sequences independently of RNA polymerase II.

Sigma (σ) factor is required for proper initiation of transcription in prokaryotes. It enables the RNA polymerase holoenzyme to recognize and bind to the promoter sequences and accurately initiate transcription.

85–91. The answers are: 85-A [Chapter 8 IV C 2 b], **86-G** [Chapter 26 V B], **87-C** [Chapter 26 V C], **88-E** [Chapter 8 IV C 1 c], **89-D** [Chapter 8 IV C 2 c], **90-B** [Chapter 26 V A], **91-F** [Chapter 8 IV B 2]. Cisplatin is a platinum-containing compound that reacts with nucleophiles such as the seventh nitrogen on the purine ring of guanine. This leads to the formation of cross-links between adjacent guanines in DNA.

Methotrexate is a folic acid analog that inhibits dihydrofolate reductase (DHFR). The inhibition of DHFR stops production of deoxythymidine 5'-monophosphate (dTMP), which is needed for continued DNA synthesis.

6-Mercaptopurine is converted to the mercaptopurine ribonucleotide 6-thioIMP by hypoxanthine–guanine phosphoribosyltransferase (HGPRT). 6-thioIMP inhibits the conversion of inosine monophosphate (IMP) to adenosine monophosphate (AMP) and guanosine monophosphate (GMP) and causes feedback inhibition of the controlling step of purine synthesis, the reaction of 5'-phosphoribosyl-1-pyrophosphate (PRPP) with glutamine.

Actinomycin D has a planar phenoxazone ring that intercalates between the bases of DNA. The physical insertion of intercalators into DNA causes a physical block of replication and transcription as well as a distortion of the structure of DNA.

Bleomycin binds to DNA and interacts with oxygen and ferrous iron (Fe^{2+}) to cause DNA breakage.

5-Fluorouracil is a uracil analog that is converted to 5-fluorodeoxyuridine 5′-monophosphate (F-dUMP) in the cell. F-dUMP inhibits thymidylate synthase and prevents the formation of deoxythymidine monophosphate (dTMP), which is needed as a substrate for DNA replication.

Cytaribine or cytosine arabinoside (araC) is a substrate analog that probably exerts its effect through slowing the rate of replication.

92–96. The answers are: 92-C [Chapter 15 II G 1 d], **93-D** [Chapter 15 II F 2 a], **94-E** [Chapter 15 II F 2 b, c], **95-B** [Chapter 15 III B 3, C], **96-A** [Chapter 15 II G 3]. Insulin is a protein hormone. Its receptor is a transmembrane tyrosine kinase. Insulin binds to the extracellular domain of its receptor, which stimulates the tyrosine kinase activity of the intracellular domain. The activated receptor phosphorylates itself and then phosphorylates other, unidentified proteins.

Inositol 1,4,5-triphosphate (IP_3) is produced from hydrolysis of phosphatidylinositol 4,5-bisphosphate (PIP_2), a membrane phospholipid. A water-soluble molecule, IP_3 diffuses into the cytoplasm and triggers the release of calcium from intracellular stores.

Along with IP_3, diacylglycerol (DAG) is produced from hydrolysis of PIP_2. DAG is lipid soluble; it diffuses laterally in the membrane and activates protein kinase C. Phorbol esters mimic the effects of DAG. However, they are not rapidly hydrolyzed and, therefore, have a prolonged effect relative to that of DAG.

Thyroxine is a lipophilic thyroid hormone that enters the cell and binds to an intracellular receptor. The hormone-receptor complex binds to its hormone response element, which is a specific sequence of DNA, and stimulates the transcription of specific genes.

The receptor for atrial natriuretic peptide is a transmembrane guanylate cyclase. When this receptor is activated, it catalyzes the formation of cyclic guanosine monophosphate (cGMP) from guanosine triphosphate (GTP). cGMP activates cGMP-dependent protein kinase.

97–101. The answers are: 97-C [Chapter 15 II E 2 a (2); Case 15-1], **98-D** [Chapter 11 Case 11-1; Chapter 26 VI D 1], **99-A** [Chapter 15 II D 2], **100-E** [Chapter 10 VIII C 1; Chapter 11 Case 11-1], **101-B** [Chapter 15 G 1 e]. The bacterium that causes whooping cough produces the pertussis toxin. Pertussis toxin is an enzyme that modifies the α subunit of G_i. The modification prevents G_i from exchanging guanosine diphosphate (GDP) for guanosine triphosphate (GTP). Therefore, the modified G_i protein is unable to block the activation of adenylate cyclase. When administered to animals, pertussis toxin alone produces most of the symptoms of whooping cough.

Deoxyadenosine and adenosine levels are high in people with an adenosine deaminase (ADA) deficiency because these nucleosides are not degraded to deoxyinosine and inosine. Lymphocytes are particularly sensitive to high levels of deoxyadenosine and adenosine, and ADA deficiency is associated with severe combined immunodeficiency.

Cholera toxin is an enzyme produced by the bacterium *Vibrio cholerae*. Cholera toxin modifies the α subunit of G_s, which blocks the hydrolysis of GTP to GDP. This prevents the inactivation of G_s. The result is a persistently high level of cyclic adenosine monophosphate (cAMP), which causes the epithelial cells of the intestine to transport sodium ions and water into the intestinal lumen. This results in severe diarrhea.

Diphtheria is caused by diphtheria toxin, which is produced by a lysogenic bacteriophage that infects *Corynebacterium diphtheriae*, which can infect the nasopharynx region of the respiratory tract. Diphtheria toxin catalyzes the transfer of adenosine diphosphate ribose (ADP-ribose) from oxidized nicotinamide adenine dinucleotide (NAD^+) to an already post-translationally modified histidine in eEF-2. This ADP ribosylation inactivates eEF-2 and inhibits the translocation step of elongation. Because diphtheria toxin is catalytic, only small amounts are needed to be toxic to the cell.

The oncogene *erb*B codes for an altered form of the epidermal growth factor (EGF) receptor. The *erb*B protein lacks the hormone-binding domain of the EGF receptor and is always activated. Its unregulated activity leads to unregulated growth and oncogenesis.

102–106. The answers are: 102-E [Chapter 20 IV B; Chapter 21 VI A], **103-A** [Chapter 23 II F 2 b], **104-B** [Chapter 7 IV C; Chapter 23 II C 2], **105-D** [Chapter 24 V D 2 b], **106-C** [Chapter 23 IV D 3]. Von Gierke's disease (glycogen storage disease type I) is due to a genetic defect in glucose-6-phosphatase, which prevents the liver from releasing glucose into the blood. This causes hypoglycemia (low blood glucose levels), an enlarged liver (due to glycogen accumulation), lactic acidemia (because gluconeogenesis via lactate is blocked), and hyperlipidemia (because reduced glucose production increases the mobilization of fat).

Tay-Sachs disease (G_{M2} gangliosidosis) is due to a deficiency of the lysosomal hexosaminidase, which cleaves (by hydrolysis) the terminal N-acetylgalactosamine residue from G_{M2} gangliosides. This leads to the accumulation of gangliosides in brain tissue.

Niemann-Pick disease is due to a genetic defect in sphingomyelinase, which degrades sphingomyelin to ceramide and phosphatidylcholine. This leads to excessive accumulation of sphingomyelin in tissues.

Accumulation of the branched-chain amino acids leucine, valine, and isoleucine, and the α-keto acids formed from them by transamination is diagnostic of maple syrup urine disease, which is caused by a defect in the enzyme branched-chain keto acid dehydrogenase.

Congenital adrenal hyperplasia refers to several disorders of steroid hormone metabolism caused by genetic defects in enzymes involved in the synthetic pathways. The most common form is due to a defect in the enzyme that converts 17α-hydroxyprogesterone to cortisol.

107–109. The answers are: 107-B [Chapter 16 III A 2], **108-A** [Chapter 18 III G; Chapter 24 III D 1 d], **109-D** [Chapter 18 III A; Chapter 23 IV A]. Glucose-6-phosphate may be converted to glucose-1-phosphate and used in glycogen synthesis or metabolized to ribose-5-phosphate, a substrate for nucleotide synthesis, via the pentose phosphate pathway.

Fumarate is a product of the urea cycle and an intermediate in the citric acid cycle.

Acetyl coenzyme A (CoA) is the substrate for the citric acid cycle. It also may be converted to 3-hydroxy-3-methylglutaryl CoA (HMG CoA), a precursor for cholesterol synthesis.

110–113. The answers are: 110-A [Chapter 25 III B 3], **111-D** [Chapter 25 VII A 5], **112-B** [Chapter 25 VII C 4 a], **113-C** [Chapter 25 VII A 5]. Individuals suffering from albinism cannot synthesize melanins, the major body pigment, from tyrosine. This can be caused by a deficiency of tyrosinase in the pigment-producing cells (melanocytes). Tyrosinase catalyzes the conversion of tyrosine to dopaquinone, the first step in melanin synthesis.

Ferrochelatase catalyzes the insertion of ferrous iron formation into protoporphyrin IX to form heme. A deficiency of this enzyme causes protoporphyria, an accumulation of protoporphyrin IX.

Uridine diphosphate (UDP)-glucuronyl transferase conjugates glucuronic acid to bilirubin in the liver. The bilirubin diglucuronide is much more soluble than free bilirubin and is secreted into the bile. Crigler-Najjar syndrome, a deficiency in this enzyme, causes severe jaundice.

3-Methoxy-4-hydroxymandelic acid (vanillylmandelic acid; VMA) occurs in the urine in large amounts when a medullary pheochromocytoma is present. These tumors produce huge amounts of catecholamines, which are metabolized to VMA.

114–118. The answers are: 114-C [Chapter 24 IV D 2], **115-B** [Chapter 14 II B; Chapter 20 IV A], **116-A** [Chapter 14 II C 3; Chapter 24 V E 3], **117-E** [Chapter 4 VIII; Chapter 14 III D 3], **118-D** [Chapter 3 V C; Chapter 14 II A 3]. Accumulation of these branched-chain amino acids and their corresponding α-keto acids is diagnostic of maple syrup urine disease, which is due to a defect in branched-chain keto acid dehydrogenase. Similar symptoms are observed if this enzyme is inactive because it lacks an essential cofactor. Thiamine pyrophosphate, a derivative of thiamine, is one of the cofactors required by this enzyme.

Lactate, β-methylcrotonate, β-hydroxyisovalerate, and β-hydroxypropionate are all substrates, or metabolites of substrates, for the biotin-dependent carboxylases pyruvate carboxylase, acetyl coenzyme A (CoA) carboxylase, propionyl CoA carboxylase, and β-methylcrotonyl CoA carboxylase. The activities of all of these enzymes are consequently deficient in the absence of biotin.

Methylmalonyl CoA mutase is one of only two enzymes in the body that require a cofactor derived from vitamin B_{12}. Without this vitamin, the enzyme does not function, and methylmalonic acid, a derivative of the substrate for the enzyme, accumulates.

A requirement for proper blood clotting is that certain glutamic acid residues on prothrombin are carboxylated. This process is catalyzed by a vitamin K–dependent enzyme.

During collagen biosynthesis, proline and

lysine residues on procollagen are hydroxylated by three enzymes, each of which requires ascorbic acid as a cofactor.

119–123. The answers are: 119-E [Chapter 23 V C 2 b], **120-D** [Chapter 23 V C; Table 23-1], **121-B** [Chapter 25 VII C 5], **122-A** [Chapter 17 I C 1 b], **123-C** [Chapter 19 V E]. Tangier disease is due to a deficiency of high-density lipoproteins (HDLs). The primary role of HDLs is to transport excess cholesterol from other tissues to the liver for reprocessing and conversion to bile acids. Without sufficient levels of HDLs, excess cholesterol accumulates in the plasma.

Type I hyperlipidemia is due to a deficiency in lipoprotein lipase, which removes most of the lipid from chylomicrons to form chylomicron remnants. This deficiency causes accumulation of chylomicrons in plasma as well as elevated levels of triacylglycerols.

Jaundice is a condition in which the blood contains excessive amounts of bilirubin and related compounds. It may be caused by a disease or an intoxication that causes abnormally high levels of red cell destruction and excessive release of hemoglobin, disorders of the liver that prevent the uptake of bilirubin from the plasma or the conjugation of bilirubin with glucuronic acid, and physical obstructions that prevent the bile from reaching the intestinal tract.

Erythrocytes depend on the pentose phosphate pathway for reduced nicotinamide adenine dinucleotide phosphate (NADPH), which the cells require to maintain the reduced glutathione needed to sustain the integrity of the cell membrane. Hemolytic anemia results if, because of defective glucose-6-phosphate dehydrogenase (G6PD), flux through the pentose phosphate pathway is not sufficiently high to maintain reduced glutathione levels. Certain oxidizing drugs, including aspirin, can cause hemolytic anemia in individuals deficient in G6PD, because these compounds reoxidize reduced glutathione faster than it can be regenerated by the pentose phosphate pathway.

Neutrophils and other phagocytotic cells of the immune system appear to produce superoxide intentionally as a defense mechanism. Chronic granulomatous disease is due to a genetic defect that reduces the capacity of these cells to produce superoxide. Patients with this disorder exhibit increased susceptibility to infection.

124–128. The answers are: 124-C [Chapter 23 IV A 2], **125-A** [Chapter 23 III B 1], **126-B** [Chapter 26 VI A], **127-D** [Chapter 25 III A 5; IV A 4], **128-E** [Chapter 26 II D; V A 2]. 3-Hydroxy-3-methylglutaryl coenzyme A (HMG CoA) reductase is the site of regulation of cholesterol biosynthesis. Although it has no effect on cholesterol obtained from the diet, inhibition of this enzyme prevents the synthesis of additional cholesterol by the body.

Aspirin inhibits cyclooxygenase, which is required for the synthesis of prostaglandin precursors. These compounds modulate a wide range of activities, including the inflammatory response.

Gout is caused by high serum levels of uric acid, the final product of purine degradation. Uric acid is formed in this process by the oxidation of xanthine by xanthine oxidase.

Monoamine oxidase (MAO) is involved in the degradation of catecholamine neurotransmitters, histamine and serotonin. MAO inhibitors have been used as antihypertensive agents.

Because nucleotide turnover is high in neoplastic cells, inhibitors of nucelotide synthesis are useful in treating cancer. Thymidylate synthase catalyzes the formation of deoxythymidine 5′-monophosphate (a component of DNA) and is a target for antineoplastic drugs.

129–133. The answers are: 129-B [Chapter 17 I A 1], **130-A** [Chapter 18 II D], **131-C** [Chapter 13 V C 2], **132-E** [Chapter 16 IV A], **133-D** [Chapter 21 II A]. The reduction of oxidized nicotinamide adenine dinucleotide phosphate (NADP⁺) to reduced nicotinamide adenine dinucleotide phosphate (NADPH) occurs primarily as a result of the reactions of the pentose phosphate pathway, which also generates substrates for nucleotide metabolism. Unlike reduced nicotinamide adenine dinucleotide (NADH), which is used primarily to drive oxidative phosphorylation, NADPH is used in reductive biosyntheses such as fatty acid synthesis.

A primary source of NADH is the citric acid cycle, which generates three moles per turn of the cycle.

Of the compounds listed, only reduced flavin adenine dinucleotide (FADH$_2$) is normally found tightly bound to enzymes, such as in succinate dehydrogenase.

A primary source of adenosine triphosphate (ATP) is the glycolytic pathway. During anaerobic glycolysis, two moles of ATP are produced per mole of glucose.

The nucleotide precursor of glycogen is uridine diphosphate (UDP)-glucose, which is formed from uridine triphosphate (UTP) and glucose-1-phosphate by UDP-glucose pyrophosphorylase.

134–138. The answers are: 134-C [Chapter 23 IV D 2, Figure 23-6], **135-E** [Chapter 15 I B 1], **136-B** [Chapter 25 III C], **137-D** [Chapter 25 III A], **138-A** [Chapter 23 III B 2].
Testosterone is a gonadal steroid hormone that is derived from cholesterol and synthesized in the Leydig cells of the testis.

Insulin is a peptide hormone and as such is susceptible to degradation by proteases.

Thyroxine is a thyroid hormone that is derived from tyrosine and contains three iodine atoms.

Epinephrine is a catecholamine hormone that is derived from dopa. Dopa is formed from tyrosine by tyrosine hydroxylase, which requires tetrahydrobiopterin as a cofactor.

5-Hydroxyeicosatetraenoic acid (5-HPETE), a derivative of arachidonic acid, is the precursor of the leukotrienes.

139–141. The answers are: 139-E,G [Chapter 2 IV C 3], **140-C,H** [Chapter 4 VII IX C], **141-D,F,J** [Chapter 15 II D 1 a (2), F 2 b, G 1, 2].
A peptide chain free in solution will not achieve its biologically active tertiary structure as rapidly or properly as within the cell. Within the cell, some of the proteins that facilitate proper folding include protein disulfide isomerase, which catalyzes the formation of proper disulfide bond formation between cysteine residues. Chaperones catalyze the proper folding of proteins in part by inhibiting improper folding and interactions with other peptides.

Fibrinolytics are agents that employ enzymatic reactions to dissolve clots. Two fibrinolytics commonly used to dissolve clots that cause heart attacks include streptokinase and tissue plasminogen activator (t-PA).

The second messenger, cyclic adenosine monophosphate (cAMP), relays information from particular hormone-receptor complexes to activate cAMP-dependent protein kinase. This protein upon activation activates other cellular proteins through phosphorylation. The second messenger, diacylglycerol (DAG), activates protein kinase C, which is calcium dependent. Tyrosine kinases may be transmembrane receptors that are activated upon hormone binding and then activate through phosphorylation a large number of other proteins.

142–144. The answers are: 142-A,C,F,J [Chapter 4 VII B 2 c], **143-B,E,I** [Chapter 4 VII D a], **144-D,G,H** [Chapter 4 VIII A].
Thrombin is a very specific protease that is responsible for activating a number of factors in the clotting cascade. Besides converting fibrinogen to form insoluble fibrin, which aggregates into a loose clot, thrombin activates the fibrin-stabilizing factor (Factor XIII). Thrombin also activates Factors V, VIII, and XI.

All of the factors needed for initiation of the intrinsic pathway are in the bloodstream before initiation of clotting. When a complex of Factor XII, prekallikrein, and high molecular weight kininogen makes contact with an abnormal surface, such as collagen in an open wound, the prekallikrein is converted to kallikrein, which converts Factor XII to Factor XIIa, which then initiates the activation cascade.

Antithrombin is a slow inhibitor of thrombin and Factors IXa, Xa, and XIa. Activated protein C is a vitamin K-dependent protease that inactivates the modifying proteins, Factors Va and VIIIa. Thrombomodulin converts thrombin from an enzyme that is crucial to clot formation to one that inhibits clot formation.

145-147. The answers are: 145-B,C,E,G [Chapter 11 III C 2], **146-B,C,E,I** [Chapter 11 IV E 2], **147-B,C,E** [Chapter 11 IV F].
Before the formation of a complementary DNA (cDNA) clone, a double-stranded DNA copy of an RNA must be formed. The first step in the formation of a double-stranded cDNA copy of an RNA is to make a single-strand cDNA copy of the RNA with reverse transcriptase. Reverse transcriptase is an RNA-dependent DNA polymerase and, as with all DNA polymerases, it requires a primer with a 3'-hydroxyl group. Because most cDNA are made of messenger RNA (mRNA) that usually have a 3' polyadenylate tail, a short chain oligodeoxythymidine is typically used as a primer. The second step of cDNA cloning is to make a double-stranded DNA copy so that it can be inserted into the DNA vector. A primer is needed for the formation of the second strand of a cDNA, which is usually catalyzed by a DNA-dependent DNA polymerase. The synthesis of both strands of DNA in the formation of a double-stranded cDNA requires deoxynucleoside triphosphates as substrate (see Chapter 8 II A 1).

Fundamentally, the Sanger method of DNA sequencing is the replication of a strand of

DNA from a precise start point with the replication being interrupted by base-specific termination. It requires a strand of DNA, a specific primer, a DNA polymerase, deoxynucleoside triphosphates as substrate, and base-specific chain terminators in the form of dideoxynucleoside triphosphates for each of the four bases.

The polymerase chain reaction (PCR) is a technique in which repetitive rounds of DNA synthesis between two primers are used to amplify DNA. Two opposing primers define the region of DNA to be amplified. One primer is complementary to one strand of DNA, and the other primer is complementary to the opposite strand of DNA. Because DNA synthesis requires a single-stranded template, the DNA must be heat denatured between each round of synthesis. After the DNA is heat denatured, the temperature is lowered to one that is optimal for the annealing of the primers and synthesis of DNA. Because the temperature required for heat denaturing DNA inactivates the *Escherichia coli* DNA polymerases, a thermostable DNA polymerase is used. As with all DNA polymerases, it requires deoxynucleoside triphosphates as substrate.

Index

In this index, *italic* page numbers refer to figures; the letter "t" refers to tables; *see also* refers to related topics.

A

AAUAAA sequence, 157
A bands, 48
AB blood type, 84
Abetalipoproteinemia, 366
A blood type, 83
ABO blood group, 83
Absorption
  of amino acids, 374
Acetoacetate, 352, 355
Acetone, 352
Acetylcholine, 370
Acetyl CoA, 238, 281, 294, 304, 355, 428, 460
  in fatty acid metabolism, 343–346, *344*
Acetyl CoA carboxylase, 344, 355, 426
N-Acetylglutamate, 379, 387
Acetyl transacylase, 345
Acid(s)
  amino. (*See* Amino acids; Amino acid[s]; Protein[s])
  arachidonic, 111, 360–361, *361*
  ascorbic (vitamin C), 46, 47, 248–249, *249*, 289, 317, 393–394
  bile, 38, 113–114, 363–364
  cholic, 113, *113*
  citric, 303–306, 321–322. (*See also* Citric acid cycle)
  defined, 2–3
  fatty, 105–107, 106t, 343–355. (*See also* Fatty acid metabolism)
  folic (folate), 250–251, 389, 401, 424, 451
  free fatty, 38
  D-glucuronic, 81, *81*
  hydrochloric, 373
  imino, 12, 15t
  lipoic, 303
  nucleic, 89–103. (*See also* DNA; Nucleic acids; RNA)
  pH scale and, 3
  phytanic, 349
  sialic, 109
  tricarboxylic, 303–306, 321–332
  uric, *412*, 413. (*See also* Uric acid cycle)
  uronic, 289, *290*
  vanillylmandelic (VMA), 394, 460
  weak
    behavior in presence of salts, 3–5
    dissociation of, 2–3
    physiologically relevant, 3t
Acid–base equilibrium, 2–5
  abnormalities of, 6t
  blood pH regulation, 5–6
Acidemia
  argininosuccinic, 378
  isovaleric, 381, 384t, 388
Acidic side chain amino acids, 14t–15t
Acidosis, 6, 6t
  diabetic ketoacidosis, 432, 436

lactic, 281, 303, 327
  metabolic, 449
Aciduria
  methylmalonic, 384t, 388
Aconitase, 304
Acridines, 133, 142
Actin, 51, 52, 455
Actinomycin, 454
Actinomycin D, 131, 458
Activated protein C, 71, 462
Active transport
  of carbohydrates, 274–275
Actomyosin, 375
Acute intermittent porphyria, 397
Acyl carrier protein, 355
Acyl CoA, 346–347, 452
Adaptor molecules, 166–167
Adenine phosphoribosyltransferase (APRT), 404
Adenosine deaminase (ADA), 419, 456, 459
Adenosine diphosphate (ADP), 290, 315, 321, 361, 461
Adenosine monophosphate (AMP), 275, 331, 404, *405*, 423
  cyclic. (*See* cAMP)
  deoxy (dAMP), 413
Adenosine triphosphatase (ATPase)
  muscle contractions and, 51
Adenosine triphosphate (ATP). (*See* ATP [adenosine triphosphate])
Adenosylmethionine (SAM), 391, 396
Adenylate cyclase, 261, *262*, 336
Adenylosuccinate, 404
Adipocytes, 106, 350–351
Adipose tissue, 431
ADP, 290, 315, 321, 461
Adrenal hyperplasia
  congenital, 365, 460
Adrenocortical hormones, 112–113, 364. (*See also* Steroids)
Adult-onset diabetes, 432. (*See also* Diabetes mellitus)
Affinity (absorption) chromatography, 23
Affinity labeling, 64
A-form DNA, 93
Agammaglobulinemia
  infantile X-linked (Bruton's), 42
Agarose gel electrophoresis, 195
Alanine, 14t, 281, 332, 379, 389
  in gluconeogenesis, 324, *324*
β-Alanine, 413
Albinism, 394, 401, 460
Albumin, 29, 38–39
Alcohol dehydrogenase, 293
Alcoholic cirrhosis, 243
Alcoholic hepatitis, 243
Alcoholism, 248, 252, 288–289
Alcohols
  sugar, 81
Aldehyde dehydrogenase, 293
Aldolase, 277
Aldose reductase, 291
Aldoses, 77, 81

Aldosterone, 113, *113*, 364
Aliphatic nonpolar side chain amino acids, 14t
Alkalosis, 6, 6t
  respiratory, 449
Alkaptonuria, 382, 384t
Alkylating agents, 131. (*See also* Cancer chemotherapy)
Allergy, 395
Allolactose, 208
Allopurinol, 64t, 419, 423–424
Allosteric control
  of metabolic pathways, 426
Allosteric enzymes, 275
Alpers syndrome, 317t
α-helix, 17, *17*
α-sarcin, 179
α-thalassemia trait, 37t, 38
Alternative splicing, 219
α-Amanitine toxicity, 457
Ames test, 142
Amidic amino acids, 15t
Amino acid oxidases, 377
Amino acid pool, *375*, 375–376
Amino acids. (*See also* Protein(s); *specific amino acids and related compounds*)
  amphoteric properties of, 15
  biosynthesis of, *237*, 246, *389*, 389–390
  branched-chain, 387, 460–461
  catabolism of, 379–384
    of branched-chain amino acids, 380–381
    inherited disorders of, 384, 384t
    as α-ketoglutarate precursor, 380
    as oxaloacetate, 380
    phenylalanine and tyrosine, 382–383, *383*
    as pyruvate, 379–380
    as succinyl CoA, 381–382, *382*
    tryptophan, 383–384
  classification of, 379, *379*
  composition of, 12
  compounds related to. (*See also* Nucleotides)
    τ-aminobutyrate (GABA), 395
    anserine, 396
    carnitine, 396
    carnosine, 396
    creatine phosphate, 396
    glutathione, 395
    heme, *396*, 396–399, 401
    histamine, 395
    nitric oxide (NO), 395
    polyamines, 396
    tryptophan-derived, 394–395
    tyrosine-derived, 392–394, 393t
  C-terminal, 17
  degradation of, 451
  essential, 375, 376t
  glucogenic, 325, 379
  ketogenic, 379
  ketogenic/glucogenic, 379

465

Look for These Future NMS⚕ Titles:

NMS immunology, 4th edition
NMS physiology, 4th edition
NMS surgery, 4th edition